Quick
Orthopedics
Review

Concise Summary and MCQs

Quick
Orthopedics
Review

Concise Summary and MCQs

Mukul Mohindra
MS (Ortho), DNB, MNAMS, Dip. SICOT (Belgium)
FNB (Arthroscopy and Sports Medicine)
Central Institute of Orthopaedics
Safdarjung Hospital and VMM College
New Delhi

Anish Agarwalla MBBS MS
Central Institute of Orthopaedics
Safdarjung Hospital and VMM College
New Delhi

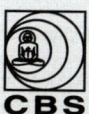

CBS

CBS Publishers & Distributors Pvt Ltd

New Delhi • Bengaluru • Chennai • Kochi • Kolkata • Mumbai
Hyderabad • Jharkhand • Nagpur • Patna • Pune • Uttarakhand

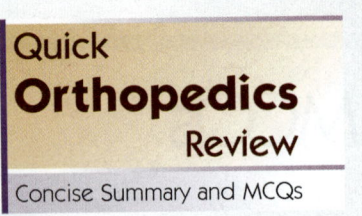

Quick
Orthopedics
Review

Concise Summary and MCQs

ISBN: 978-93-87742-87-1

Copyright © Authors and Publisher

First Edition: 2018

Published by Satish Kumar Jain and produced by Varun Jain for

CBS Publishers & Distributors Pvt Ltd

4819/XI Prahlad Street, 24 Ansari Road, Daryaganj, New Delhi 110 002, India.
Ph: 23289259, 23266861, 23266867 Website: www.cbspd.com
Fax: 011-23243014   e-mail: delhi@cbspd.com; cbspubs@airtelmail.in.
Corporate Office: 204 FIE, Industrial Area, Patparganj, Delhi 110 092

Ph: 4934 4934   Fax: 4934 4935   e-mail: publishing@cbspd.com; publicity@cbspd.com

Branches

- **Bengaluru:** Seema House 2975, 17th Cross, K.R. Road,
  Banasankari 2nd Stage, Bengaluru 560 070, Karnataka
  Ph: +91-80-26771678/79   Fax: +91-80-26771680   e-mail: bangalore@cbspd.com
- **Chennai:** 7, Subbaraya Street, Shenoy Nagar, Chennai 600 030, Tamil Nadu
  Ph: +91-44-26680620, 26681266   Fax: +91-44-42032115   e-mail: chennai@cbspd.com
- **Kochi:** Ashana House, No. 39/1904, AM Thomas Road, Valanjambalam,
  Ernakulam 682 016, Kochi, Kerala
  Ph: +91-484-4059061-65   Fax: +91-484-4059065   e-mail: kochi@cbspd.com
- **Kolkata:** 6/B, Ground Floor, Rameswar Shaw Road, Kolkata-700 014, West Bengal
  Ph: +91-33-22891126, 22891127, 22891128   e-mail: kolkata@cbspd.com
- **Mumbai:** 83-C, Dr E Moses Road, Worli, Mumbai-400018, Maharashtra
  Ph: +91-22-24902340/41   Fax: +91-22-24902342   e-mail: mumbai@cbspd.com

Representatives

- **Hyderabad** 0-9885175004 • **Jharkhand** 0-9811541605 • **Nagpur** 0-9021734563
- **Patna** 0-9334159340 • **Pune** 0-9623451994 • **Uttarakhand** 0-9716462459

Printed at Rashtriya Printers, Dilshad Garden, Delhi, India

to
my parents for their blessings,
my wife Bhumika for her unconditional love and
my family for always being there

MUKUL MOHINDRA

---

to
my parents Mr Banwarilal Agarwalla and
Smt. Sarita Agarwalla,
whose nurturing gave me courage to dream,
my bhaiya and bhabi Aman and Chandni who
has always been there whenever I needed support and
my sister Nikita who strengthened me to realize
my dreams

ANISH AGARWALLA

Contributors

Dr Anurag Gupta MS (Ortho)

Spinal injury and pediatric spine disorders
Consultant, Sanjeevani Hospital
Baran, Rajasthan

Dr Tarun Verma MS (Ortho)

Sports injury
SR (Ortho), MAMC, Delhi

Dr Kavish Singh MS (Ortho), DNB (Ortho)

Joint disorders

Dr Urmi Khanna
MD (Dermatology and Venerology)
DNB (Dermatology), MNAMS

Autoimmune disorders

Foreword

Words of Wisdom

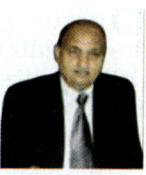

The master key to success is dedication and determination, to do that extra bit and to go that extra mile. But effort should always be well disciplined. Discipline means patience and perseverance—the ability to continue through bad times, obstacles and problems in a competent manner. This book targeted towards budding doctors who strive to pursue career in postgraduation, is an effort by a team of people to share the knowledge and experience they gained over the sleepless nights of hard work to give you the best. So get set to reach your goals with a mentor to guide and steer you through till you reach what you deserve.

Always remember the *6Ds* that demarcate the bridge between mediocrity and excellence:

Desire, Direction, Decisiveness, Dedication, Determination, Discipline.

Dr (Prof) Rajendra Sharma MD (Pmr)

Medical Superintendent
VMMC and Safdarjung Hospital
New Delhi

Foreword

Pursuing in postgraduation is any MBBS student's dream and the entrance examination for the same is getting difficult day by day. Orthopedics is a vast subject and is an indispensable part of any entrance examination. Book on orthopedics should be concise and easy to revise for competitive examinations.

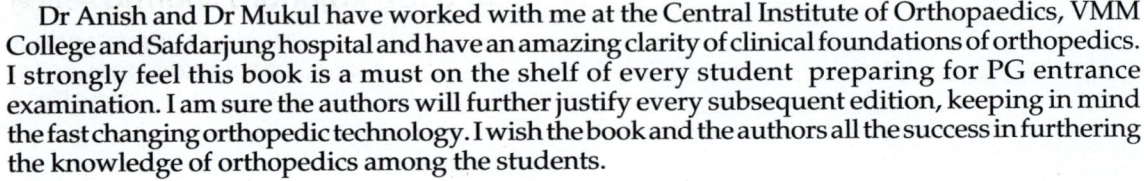

This book by Dr Anish and Dr Mukul has narratively and comprehensively explained the basic concepts of orthopedics, which students must know. The inclusion of excellent colored diagrams, 3D pictures and table depictions are highly informative, with an eye on daily orthopedic practice dealing. Having gone through a few chapters, I am fully convinced that this book with its clarity yet in-depth elaboration of orthopedic topics will be an asset to every student preparing for PG entrance examination.

Dr Anish and Dr Mukul have worked with me at the Central Institute of Orthopaedics, VMM College and Safdarjung hospital and have an amazing clarity of clinical foundations of orthopedics. I strongly feel this book is a must on the shelf of every student preparing for PG entrance examination. I am sure the authors will further justify every subsequent edition, keeping in mind the fast changing orthopedic technology. I wish the book and the authors all the success in furthering the knowledge of orthopedics among the students.

Dr Ramesh Kumar

Director Professor
Director, Central Institute of Orthopaedics
VMMC and Safdarjung Hospital
New Delhi

Foreword

Competitive examinations for PG entrance examination are getting difficult every year, with addition of new questions and topics each year, and orthopedics is of no exception. It is immensely important for MBBS students to have a thorough idea of the subject and at the same time the book should be concise for quicker revision.

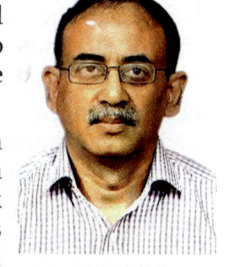

It gives me immense pleasure to write the Foreword for Dr Anish Agarwalla and Dr Mukul Mohindra. I believe that this book will fill the lacunae in undergraduate and postgraduate entrance examination teaching. The book appears to cover all the relevant topics with questions. All colored diagrams and X-rays included in this book will have a direct impact in student's learning. Important tables and figures in color make reading easy, matter easy to remember and has high recall value.

Both Anish and Mukul have a flair for teaching and it is appropriate that they have come up with this excellent book. I hope that all the undergraduates and students preparing for PG entrance examination will find it useful. I wish the authors and book success in enlightening all of us.

Dr LG Krishna
Director Professor
Central Institute of Orthopaedics
VMMC and Safdarjung Hospital
New Delhi

Preface

Today when the medical education curve is steep and long, it is our duty to guide the ones who are traversing the path we walked in the past. It is not possible for us to guide each one individually, hence this book is an attempt to do the same.

The book is our vision to prepare the PG aspirants in the best manner for the tough competition of PG entrance examination. Briefing the matter and then solving the questions by the application of what you acquire and reinforcing it again and again, so that it has an everlasting impression to carry with you for the 'D day' is what the book is aimed at.

This book is the outcome of the constant effort to provide you with the latest information in the field of orthopedics and latest trends of questions featuring in all current formats of PG entrance examination.

We wish you best of the efforts and results. In case of any doubts or queries about the material, feel free to contact the authors.

Best wishes.

Mukul Mohindra
Anish Agarwalla

Acknowledgments

This book was a dream project for both of us but efforts of a number of people stand behind the stage. Without them the dream would have never come true. It is our pleasure to acknowledge their efforts as their support formed that pillar of strength that helped us finish this herculean task with such an ease.

The seeds of this book were sown in Central Institute of Orthopaedics, VMMC and Safdarjung Hospital. It was the vision of our Director, Dr Ramesh Kumar, to motivate us to begin this journey. His visionary leadership is an encouragement to every young budding orthopod. Problems unfolded as we travelled the path but the guidance and blessings by our teachers Dr LG Krishna and Dr RK Chopra helped us pave our way through. Their vast experience and sea of knowledge helped us at every single step. Dr Naval Bhatia, Dr Vikas Gupta, Dr BP Sharma and Dr Davinder were all a source of motivation whenever we got into any dilemma. The friendly nature of Dr Narendra Kumar, Dr Hitesh Lal, Dr Jatin Talwar, Dr Tankeswar Baruah, Dr RK Beniwal, Dr Ashish Rustagi and Dr Sandeep Shaina helped us to clear many doubts and we could ring them at any time for any assistance.

I, Dr Anish, would be grateful to goddess Saraswati and Shiva for catering me good mental and physical health that made timely completion of this book possible. I would take this pleasure to thank my teachers whom I owe what I am today. My alma mater Gauhati Medical college, Guwahati and its Orthopedics department under Dr Tulsi Bhattacharjee are the reason I took orthopedics. The Central Institute of Orthopaedics, VMMC and Safdarjang Hospital carved a stone into a structure which had a meaning. I am short of words to thank Prof (Dr) LG Krishna (Director Professor) who was not just my guide but my mentor and guardian both academically and personally. I would like to remember my seniors Dr Akshat Sharma, Dr Ketan Pandey, Dr Kavish, Dr Balu, Dr Dheer Singh, Dr Abhimanyu, Dr Sathyamurthy, Dr Narendran P, Dr Vikash Moond who have always been source of inspiration. I would also like to thank my colleagues Dr Lokesh, Dr Rajesh, Dr Saumya, Dr Aditya, Dr Apoorva, Dr Nikhil and my juniors for helping me find out time to write the book. I would be failing in my duty if I do not thank my friend Dr Anurag Gupta and Dr Tarun Verma for helping me in the book and Dr Sahil, Dr Saloni Gupta, Dr Ankit Jain, Manish Agrawal, Dr Anamika Thakral, Dr Akhil Taneja for igniting that spark in me for writing the book. I would also extend my thanks to my motivator Dr Mukul Mohindra for encouraging the idea of this book and being an equal and indispensable part of this journey.

I, Dr Mukul, would like to first thank my teachers whom I owe a lot. Dr M Yamin (Director Professor, Dayanand Medical College and Hospital, Ludhiana) has been a mentor to whom I have always looked up. Dr Daljeet Singh, Dr Sandeep Puri and Dr Rajoo Singh have been the role models I aspire to be. The support and encouragement I received from Dr Hemlata Badyal, Dr Lily Walia, Dr Hitant Vohra, Dr Jagjiv Sharma, Dr Deepinder Chinna, Dr Sarit, Dr Sunil Juneja, Dr Rajneesh Garg, Dr Alka Dogra and Dr Bajwa sculpted in me the confidence to face the challenges of life. I find myself short of words when it comes to thank my guide in postgraduation, Prof (Dr) SS Sangwan (Former Vice Chancellor, University of Health Sciences, Rohtak). The skills I have today to a great extent belong to Dr RC Siwach, Dr NK Magu, Dr RK Gupta, Dr Roop Singh, Dr ZS Kundu, Dr A Devgun, Dr R Rohilla, my teachers during my postgraduation. I would be failing in my duty if I do not thank my teachers at Maulana Azad Medical College, Dr A Dhal, Dr AK Gupta, Dr VK Gautam, Dr Lalit Maini, Dr Vinod Kumar, Dr Manoj, Dr Sumit Sural and Dr Dhananjay Sabat who made me the person I am today. My job would be incomplete without extending my thanks to Dr Deepak Chaudhary, a great motivator, whose blessings infused in me the confidence to begin this journey. Problems unfolded as I travelled the path but the guidance by my teachers Dr Himanshu Kataria, Dr Deepak Joshi and Dr Vineet Jain helped me pave through. Dr Ankit Goyal, Dr Nitin Mehta, Dr Pallav Mishra, Dr Himanshu

Gupta, Dr Ajay Lal, Dr Vivek Shankar and Dr Ashutosh Jha were all a source of motivation. Never can I miss Dr George Maceras who made my training in Greece during my fellowship a memorable one. A special thanks to Dr SP Singh and Dr Shyama Gupta, Dr Anurag Jain and Dr SK Pandey for giving me the space to grow. And last but no way the least, support by my seniors, colleagues, juniors and friends was indispensable. Dr Jitesh Jain, Dr Navdeep, Dr Naveen MG, Dr Lalait Bafna, Dr Mohd. Shafi Bhat, Dr Darsh Goyal, Dr Milind Tanwar, Dr Rahul, Dr Manoj Arya, Dr Shiv Chouksey, Dr Rakesh Daripa, Dr Himanshu Bhargava, Dr Brahma Prakash, Dr Pawan Sharma, Dr Utkarsh, Dr Atul Mahajan, Dr Pankaj, Dr Sunny, Dr Dickey, Dr Chandan Jasrotia, Dr Rohit, Dr Sanjay Arora, Dr Gaurav Saini, Dr Ankit Ruhella and Dr Jitender Mishra, thank you all for being there. I would also extend my thanks to motivators cum-teachers Dr Sumer Sethi, Dr Tushar Mehta, Dr Pritish Singh and Dr Kamal Bali.

The contributors of this book deserve special thanks for the valuable time they devoted and the immense hard work and energy they had put in. Despite their busy schedules, even at a single call they stood by us to write the chapters comprehensively. Guys this project never would have been an accomplishment without your efforts.

Finally, we would like to thank CBS Publishers and Distributors and the team of Mr YN Arjuna, the real men behind the stage. Their efforts turned this dream of ours into a reality. We would be looking forward to work more with the wonderful team in the coming future.

Mukul Mohindra
Anish Agarwalla

Contents

General Orthopedics

ORTHOPEDICS—WHO'S WHO

Orthopedics was born as a specialty for correcting bony deformities in children and later Nicolas Andry (Fig. 1.1) used the word "Orthopedics", which was derived from Greek words for "correct" or "straight" (*orthos*) and "child" (*paidion*). Orthopedics evolved a lot during World War I and II. In fact many great orthopedic surgeons were military surgeons.

* Development of principles of antisepsis by Sir Joseph Lister (Fig. 1.2).
* The invention of X-rays by Wilhelm Konrad Roentgen.
* *Galen*: **Father of sports medicine**. He is also credited with describing for the first time the use of longitudinal traction for reduction of overlapping bone fragments.

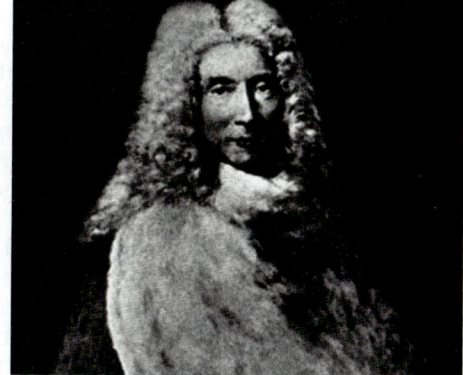

Fig. 1.1: Nicolas Andry

* *Nicolas Andry* (Fig. 1.1): He published the first book in orthopedics "L'Orthopedie" in 1741, which conferred him the title of "**father of orthopedics**". His famous engraving (Fig. 1.3) of the "crooked tree" published by him in his book soon became the symbol of orthopedics worldwide.
* *Percival Pott*: **Pott's fracture. Pott's paraplegia.** In 1756, this great English surgeon sustained a broken leg after fall from his horse. It was assumed that he had sustained a bimalleolar fracture so it began to be called Pott's fracture but in reality he had sustained a much serious open fracture of tibia.
* *Hugh Owen Thomas*: He devised the popular Thomas splint and Thomas test for flexion deformity of the hip. He is also known as "**father of British orthopedics**".

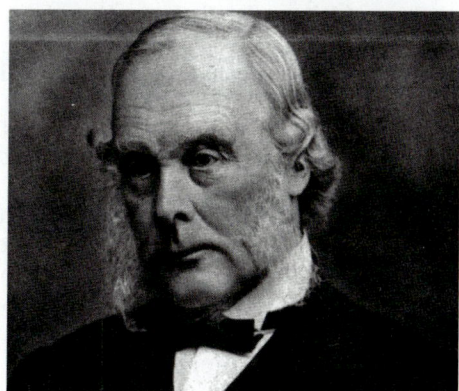

Fig. 1.2: Sir Joseph Lister

He first used TK splint for his wife's TB of knee and thus the device is known as Thomas' knee splint, while it is rarely used for knee these days.
* *James Paget*: He popularized the term 'fracture disease' to refer to stiffness that occurs following conservative treatment of fractures. He was also the first to describe 'carpal tunnel syndrome'.
* *Robert Jones*: He was the nephew of great Hugh Owen Thomas. He is known as "**father of modern orthopedics**". He described the Jones fracture and the Robert Jones bandage. He published the first report of use of X-rays in orthopedics.
* *Albin Lambotte*: Belgian surgeon, coined the term 'osteosynthesis' meaning internal fixation and is regarded as the "**father of modern internal fixation**". He also devised the first modern external fixator and was the first to describe use of biodegradable implants.

- *Martin Kirschner*: He contributed the very simple but the very useful "K wire" to orthopedics.
- *Lorenz Bohler*: **Father of trauma surgery**.
- *Austin Moore*: He performed the first metallic hip replacement. He designed the Austin Moore prosthesis, which is still in use even today.
- *Gerhard Kuntscher*: His biggest contribution to orthopedics was the intramedullary nail which revolutionized the treatment of diaphyseal fractures of long bones.
- *Raginald Watson Jones*: He devised the Watson Jones approach (anterolateral approach) to the hip joint.
- *Maurice E Muller:* He was a Swedish surgeon who was instrumental in development of internal fixation techniques (fixation of fractures with metal implants placed inside the skin). In 1958, he co-founded 'Arbeitsgemeinschaft fur Osteosynthesefragen' (German for "Association for the Study of Internal Fixation", or 'AO', a popular organization that works for improving the standard of patient care in orthopedics.

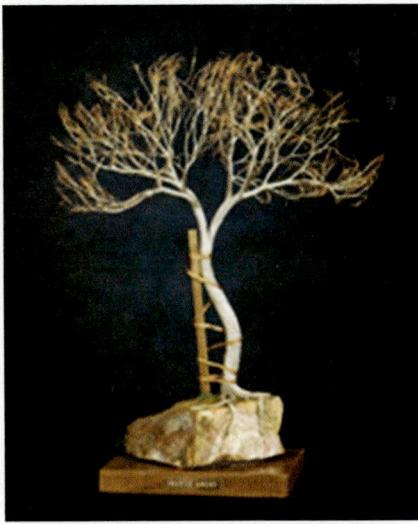

Fig. 1.3: Famous engraving of "crooked tree" from the book of Nicolas Andry

- *Paul Randall Harrington*: Harrington invented the Harrington Rod, a device that is used during corrective surgery for scoliosis.
- *John Charnley* (Fig. 1.4): **Father of total hip arthroplasty**. He was the great innovator of the modern total hip replacement and popularized the use of bone cement in total hip replacement.
- *Gavriil Abramovich Ilizarov*: He gave the famous Ilizarov theory that bone would grow if gradually distracted. His work pioneered a new way of treating some of the most difficult cases in orthopedics, viz. infected non-union, deformity correction and limb lengthening.
- *Kenji Takagi*: **Father of arthroscopy**. Takaji, a Japanese surgeon, carried out the first successful arthroscopy of a joint (knee).
- *Masaki Watanabe*: **Father of modern arthroscopy**. He performed the first arthroscopic partial meniscectomy.
- *William Enneking*: **Father of orthopedic oncology**. He gave a classification system for bone tumors.

Some Common Terms used in Orthopedics

- *Ankylosis*: Fusion of a joint due to a disease that causes abnormal adhesions between two joint surfaces.
- *Arthrocentesis*: Joint aspiration (withdrawing synovial fluid/blood from the joint).
- *Arthrodesis*: Surgically induced fusion of two joint surfaces.
- *Arthroeresis*: It refers to an operation carried on a joint to restrict an undue mobility.
- *Calcaneus*: Deformity of ankle joint with the foot fixed in dorsiflexion.
- *Calcification*: Deposition of amorphous (powdered/non-crystalline) calcium phosphate.
- *Cavus*: Exaggeration of medial longitudinal arch of the foot.
- *Planus:* Flattened medial longitudinal arch.
- *Plantaris*: Equinus that occurs at the forefoot is called plantaris (forefoot fixed in plantar flexion).
- *Chemonucleolysis*: Injection of chymopapain (a proteolytic enzyme) into disc space to dissolve the disc (as a treatment of prolapsed disc).
- *Coxa*: Pertaining to the hip.
- *Epiphyseal plate/growth plate or physis*: Hyaline cartilage present above the proximal metaphysis and below the distal metaphysis separating metaphysis from epiphysis.
- *Laminectomy*: Removal of spinal lamina (usually to decompress the spinal cord or nerves).

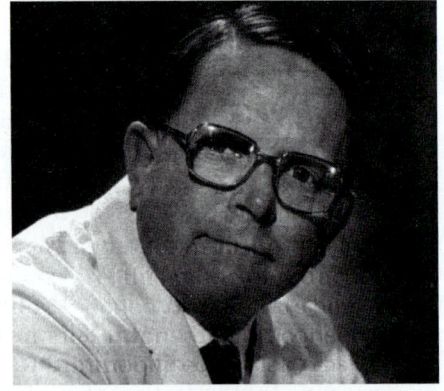

Fig. 1.4: Sir John Charnley (1911–1982)

- *Laminotomy*: Removal of a part of lamina.
- *Manus*: Pertaining to the wrist.
- *Orthotic*: Orthotic is a device that aids/supports a body part and enhances the structural and functional characteristics of the skeletal system.
- *Prosthesis*: An artificial device that replaces a body part.
- *Ossification*: Deposition of crystalline calcium phosphate to form new bone.
- *Osteoclasis*: Surgically induced fracture of the bone (to correct a bone deformity).
- *Osteogenesis*: Bone formation
- *Spondylitis*: Inflammation of vertebrae.
- *Spondylosis:* An umbrella term that refers to degenerative changes in the spine, viz. bone spurs, degenerated intervertebral discs, etc.
- *Spondylolisthesis*: Anterior or posterior translation of one segment of spine in relation to the vertebrae below.
- *Spondylolysis*: A defect in pars-interarticularis of vertebral arch. It may progress to spondylolisthesis.

BONE STRUCTURE AND COMPOSITION

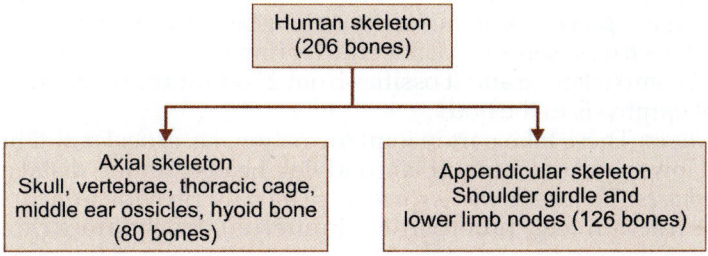

Bones are made up of (Table 1.1):
  i. Bone cells (osteoblast, osteoclast and osteocytes)
  ii. Intercellular matrix

Bone cells: There are three types of bone cells—(1) osteoblast, (2) osteoclast and (3) osteocytes.

Osteoblasts
- Mononuclear bone forming cells derived from mesenchymal precursors in the bone marrow.
- Rich in alkaline phosphatase and produce type I collagen and other non-collagenous bone proteins.
- Osteoblasts have receptors for vitamin D_3 and parathyroid hormone and they control osteoclastic activity.

Osteoclasts
- Derived from mononuclear precursors of macrophage lineage (specifically monocytes) in the marrow and are bone reabsorbing multinucleated giant cells.
- Their main function is to resorb bone and are thus involved in bone remodeling. Active osteoclasts are present in excavations in bone formed by them after erosion of the matrix, the excavations being called "Howship's lacunae" (lacunae means 'pit').

Osteocytes
- Terminally differentiated stage of osteoblasts.
- They are linked to each other via long cytoplasmic extensions called canaliculi, which are used for exchange of nutrients through gap junctions.

Table 1.1: Chemical composition of bone (based on dry weight)
• Bone cells: Make up approximately 5%
• Intercellular matrix (95%)
– *Inorganic matrix*: 65% (mainly calcium and phosphorus)
– *Organic matrix*: 30% (80% of which is type I collagen with rest being non-collagenous proteins (osteocalcin/bone Gla protein, osteopontin, osteonectin and alkaline phosphatase)

- Although they are not capable of mitotic division, they are actively involved in the routine turnover of bony matrix, through various mechanisms.
- They can also destroy bone through a rapid, transient mechanism (different from osteoclasts) called osteocytic osteolysis.

Intercellular matrix: Matrix consists of organic (biological) and inorganic (mineral) components. Organic component includes collagen fibers (mostly type I collagen). Inorganic matter is composed mainly of calcium and phosphorus in a crystalline form called "hydroxyapatite". Bone also contains other minerals in small amount, i.e. magnesium, potassium, strontium and ferrous salts, etc. Organic matter gives the bone its flexibility and elasticity while inorganic matter gives strength and hardness to the bone. Bones are densest tissue in the body due to deposition of minerals in the intercellular matrix.

Parts of a Growing Long Bone

Long bone in a growing child can be divided into epiphysis, physis (growth plate/epiphyseal plate), metaphysis and diaphysis. In mature bone epiphysis fuses with metaphysis and growth plate gets replaced by bone (visible on X-ray as epiphyseal line).

A few important facts about each of these parts:

- *Epiphysis*: Epiphysis is present on either ends of a long bone except the metacarpals, metatarsals and phalanges where it is present only at one end. It primarily consists of cancellous bone covered by a thin layer of compact bone and it ossifies from 2° ossification center.
  Various types of epiphysis in the body:
  - *Pressure epiphyses*: These take part in joint formation, i.e. *articular* and hence, weight transmission, e.g. lower end of femur, tibial condyles, head of femur, distal end of radius.
  - *Traction epiphyses*: These are *non-articular*, primarily provide attachments to ≥1 tendon which exert traction, e.g. tuberosities (humerus), trochanters (femur) and mastoid process.
  - *Atavistic epiphyses*: These are phylogenetically independent but become fused in man, e.g. coracoid process of scapula, posterior tubercle of talus, os-trigonum.
  - *Aberrant epiphyses*: These are epiphyses that are not always present, e.g. epiphysis at head of 1st metacarpal and base of other metacarpal.

  A thin layer of articular cartilage that covers up ends of pressure epiphysis (epiphysis of long bones taking part in joint formation) possesses the following features:
  - Is mostly hyaline cartilage by nature.
  - Is devoid of nerves (least pain sensitive structure in joint), blood vessels, perichondrium and ossification.
  - Cells of articular cartilage divide by mitosis.
  - Nutrition—hypochondrial vessels (of medullary cavity), vessels of synovial membrane and synovial fluid.

- *Physis*: Physis (growth plate/epiphyseal plate) is the zone of maximum growth and is responsible for the longitudinal growth of the bones (interstitial growth).
  1. Germinal zone/resting zone
  2. Proliferative zone
  3. Hypertrophic zone (maturation zone)
  4. Zone of provisional calcification (endochondral ossification)

  Since the hypertrophic zone has large-sized cells lying loosely in scanty intercellular tissue, it is the weakest zone of physis. Hence, most physeal injuries occur through this plane. In rickets, due to lack of calcification, cells accumulate in hypertrophic zone, resulting in weakened growth plates that eventually deform under body weight.
  Physis is connected to the epiphysis and metaphysis by the zone of Ranvier and the perichondral ring of LaCroix.
  - The zone of Ranvier contains germinal cells, which are responsible for the circumferential growth of the physis (appositional growth).
  - Ring of LaCroix is a fibrous structure that connects the zone of Ranvier with the periosteum of the metaphysis, thereby strengthening the metaphyseal–physeal interphase.

- *Metaphysis*: It is full of cancellous bone and hence fractures have good union rate owing to massive surface area and abundant vascularity of the cancellous bone.
  - Most common site of osteomyelitis
  - Zone of active growth
  - Highly vascularised zone
  - Hair pin arrangement of blood vessels.
  - More prone to injury.
- *Diaphysis*: It is the narrow region between the two metaphyses.
  - It ossifies from 1 primary center of ossification.
  - It is the strongest portion of bone.
  - Cortex is lined on outside by a layer of dense connective tissue called periosteum which is anchored to cortex by special fibers called **Sharpey's fibers**.

Periosteum is composed of two layers—an outer fibrous layer having abundant blood vessels and an inner cambium layer that rich in osteogenic cells. Bone formation is more than bone resorption on the periosteal surface and bone resorption is more than bone formation on the endosteal surface, so with aging, bones normally increase in diameter and marrow spaces expand. Endosteum is metabolically the most active part of a bone.

Microscopic Structure of Human Bones

Adult human skeleton having almost 80% cortical and 20% cancellous bones.

- *Cortical bones* are the long bones of the body like the femur or humerus and the small bones of the hand and foot like metacarpals and metatarsals. Cortical bone consists of a number of columns of cells called "osteon".
  - Osteon or Haversian system is the basic structural unit of compact cortical bone.
  - Each osteon has layers of bone cells (osteoblasts, osteocytes and osteoclasts arranged in a lamellar pattern) around a central canal called "Haversian canal".
  - The Haversian canal surrounds neurovascular bundle throughout the bone and communicates with the osteocytes in the lacunae through canaliculi. "Volkmann's canals" run perpendicular to the "Haversian canals" and interconnect them with each other and the periosteum and allow for the transfer of nutrients.
- *Cancellous bone* (trabecular or spongy bone) is mainly found in small bones of the wrist, the bones of the hand and mid-foot like calcaneum and talus. The epiphyseal and metaphyseal areas of long bones, flat bones (pelvis, ribs, skull, etc.), and vertebrae are also cancellous bones.
  - Cancellous bones are more porous and thus have a much larger surface area than compact bone and they are more vascular.
  - They contain sheets (lamellae) of bone called 'trabeculae' which interconnect to form open spaces giving a honeycomb appearance.
  - Spaces between these trabeculae contain red or yellow marrow depending on person's age and which bone is it.
  - Hence, spongy bone is important for production of blood cells.
- *Lamellar bone*
  - Lamellar bone pattern is one that is present in normal adult compact as well as cancellous bones.
  - Lamellar bone is stress oriented with a parallel arrangement of collagen fibers into sheets called lamellae.
- *Woven bone*
  - Random organization of collagen fibers (as the name 'woven' suggests).
  - Relatively a weak structure in comparison to lamellar bone that is mechanically stronger.
  - It is immature bone which is not stress oriented.
  - Woven bone pattern is present in all fetal bones and in the initial stages of fracture healing (later it gets replaced by lamellar bone).
  - Woven bone is quickly produced and it has a high rate of turnover compared to lamellar bone.

Some Special Types of Bones in Body

Sesamoid bones: A small independent bone or bony nodule developed in a tendon where it passes over an angular structure, typically in the hands and feet:

1. Patella— quadriceps tendon
2. Pisiform—flexor carpi ulnaris
3. Fabella—tendon of gastrocnemius muscle.
4. Foot—2 sesamoid bones are found medial and lateral to 1st MT bone near 1st MTP joint within the tendon of flexor hallucis brevis.
5. Hand—2 sesamoid bones are found in the distal portion of 1st metacarpal bone within the tendons of flexor pollicis brevis and tendon of adductor pollicis.

Pneumatic bones: Some cranial bones are air filled to make skull light weight, air resonant and air conditioning.
1. Ethmoid
2. Sphenoid
3. Maxilla
4. Frontal
5. Mastoid

Membranous bones: These include:
1. Skull vault bones
2. Facial bones
3. Clavicle

Blood Supply of Bone
- 5–10% of the cardiac output goes to the skeleton of human body, which derives its blood supply from nutrient artery, periosteal vessels and epiphyseal–metaphyseal vessels.
- The dominant supply comes from nutrient artery which supplies the inner two-thirds of the cortices and the periosteal vessels supply blood to the outer one-third of the cortex. When nutrient artery is damaged (as in nailing a bone) or when the periosteal vessels are damaged (as in plating a bone), the other artery is sufficient enough to take over the function of other.

Growth of Bones
In the embryonic period bone formation occurs either by "intramembranous ossification" or by "endochondral ossification".
- *Endochondral ossification*: Seen in the long bones where a cartilaginous structure is first formed with subsequent replacement by calcium hydroxyapatite deposition to form bone.
  The ossification centers (Table 1.2) are of two types:
  - Primary ossification centers appear in the cartilaginous model during embryonic period. These are responsible for the formation of the diaphysis of the bones.
  - Secondary ossification centers mostly appear after birth and are responsible for the formation of the epiphysis of the long bones and the extremities of flat and irregular bones.
- *Intramembranous ossification*: It occurs in flat bones and in the clavicle. Here calcium hydroxyapatite is directly deposited into a pre-existing membrane (derived from primitive connective tissue) without any intervening cartilage model stage.
  In the intrauterine period, cartilage model grows by division of chondrocytes, **interstitial growth** leads to increase in length and **appositional growth** occurs when chondroblasts in the perichondrium produce new matrix at the periphery and increase the width of cartilage model. However, adults have mature bones and they grow only by appositional growth. Cambium layer (inner layer of periosteum) is responsible for appositional growth which contains osteoprogenitor

Table 1.2: Age of appearance of some important secondary ossification centers	
Ossification center	*Age of appearance*
• Calcaneus	3–5th months
• Talus	6–7th months
• Cuboid	9th month
• Femur lower end	9th month end (at birth)
• Upper end tibia	Immediately after birth

cells. Longitudinal growth occurs before maturity and is primarily due to cartilage proliferation at the growth plate/physis, which subsequently mineralizes to form bone (Table 1.3).

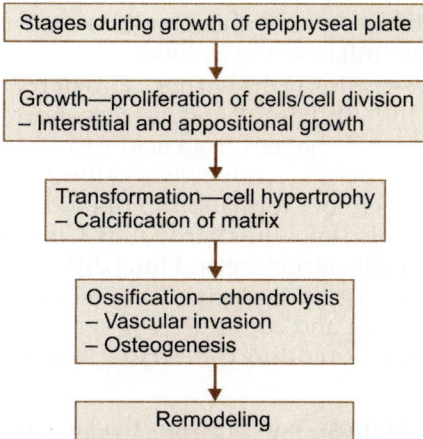

Table 1.3: Differences between ossified and calcified tissue

Ossified tissue	Calcified tissue
• Properly laid down architecture of haversian and Volkmann's canal with calcified hydroxyl-appetite crystals	• Deposition of calcium salts without bone architecture/trabeculae
• Live bone looks less white on X-rays and is strong in strength	• Dead bone looks more white on X-rays as compared to surrounding normal bone

FRACTURE

Definition

Fracture is defined as breach in the continuity of cortex (either uni or bicortical) with or without displacement.

Simple fracture/closed fracture is one where fracture does not communicate with the external environment, i.e. overlying skin and soft tissue are intact, whereas open/compound fracture communicates with external environment. In other words, fracture communication with external environment refers to hematoma draining out from the wound over or in vicinity of fracture site. Open fractures of the tibia are the commonest open long bone fractures. In open fractures, fracture hematoma is drained out and thus normal fracture healing response is disturbed.

Pain is the commonest symptom and tenderness is the most common sign of fresh fracture but the surest/diagnostic signs are abnormal mobility of bone or loss of transmitted movements. *Note*: Crepitus is not a specific sign.

Types

- Transverse—fracture line forms an angle of <30°—caused by bending force
- Oblique—fracture line forms an angle of >30°—caused by axial compression combined with bending and compression.
- Spiral—caused by twisting strain with fracture surface having wide surface area and thus more chances of union.
- Direct trauma—transverse > comminuted fracture.

Fracture Healing

There are two types and it depends upon the mode of fracture fixation:
- *Primary/direct*—here healing occurs without callus formation and is seen in cases with rigid internal fixation, e.g. compression plating and unicortical fractures (greenstick fracture).

- *Secondary/indirect*—here fracture heals with callus formation. This is the more common type, seen in conservatively managed cases (slab/cast), semirigid fixation like intramedullary nail, external fixator, Ilizarov, locked plating, etc. The process is divided into the following stages:
  - Stage of hematoma formation—forms within a few hours and fully organised within 2–3 days.
  - Stage of granulation tissue/inflammatory phase.
  - Stage of callus formation—callus is the earliest sign of fracture healing and is visible on X-ray earliest by 3 weeks. Initially it is soft and restricts shortening but not angular/rotatory movements at fracture site. pH changes from acidic to alkaline, with high oxygen tension and stability/micromovements are conducive to callus formation.
  - Stage of consolidation—woven bone formation occurs and it restricts movements in all planes as it is hard and strong, thus also known as hard callus. Clinically plaster can be discontinued after this stage. It lacks lamellar structure and thus different from mature bone.
  - Stage of remodeling—it consists of replacing woven bone by lamellar structure and thus termed modeling/remodeling and continued for years till normal structure is regained. Osteoclast removes the bone (k/a **cutting cones/Howship's lacunae**) and osteoblast deposits bone (**closing cones**).

Wolff's law: It states that in areas of stress/compression, thicker lamellar bone is laid (i.e. osteoblasts are active there) and in areas of tension/no stress unwanted bone is carved away (i.e. osteoclasts are more active) to regain normal anatomical shape.

Markers of bone formation

- Serum bone specific ALP.
- Serum osteocalcin (diagnostic/most specific).
- Serum peptide or type I procollagen.
- Type I collagen extension peptide.

Markers of bone resorption

- Urine and serum cross-linked N-telopeptide.
- Urine and serum cross-linked C-telopeptide.
- Urine hydroxyproline.
- Urine total free deoxypyridinoline.
- Urine hydroxylysine glycosides.
- Serum tartarate resistant acid phosphatase (TrAP).
- Serum bone sialoprotein.

Rate of newly formed osteoid can be estimated by **tetracycline labeling**. When tetracycline is infused it gets fixed with newly formed mineralized bone giving a specific fluorescence under UV light. Thus when 2 doses of tetracycline are infused in days apart, 2 bands of fluorescence are visible separated by a clear zone which depicts new bone that was formed during the period between the two doses.

Delayed Union, Nonunion, Union

When fracture takes more than usual time to unite depending on the type and site of fracture, but shows some progression towards union over time is known as delayed union. Delayed union often can be treated successfully by a cast that allows as much function as possible. Nonunion—according to USFDA is defined as "When union does not take place in 9 months after fracture and fracture shows no visible progressive signs of healing for at least 3 months". A fracture with long-term nonunion generally forms a structural resemblance to a fibrous joint, and is often called a "false joint" or **pseudoarthrosis**.

Types of Nonunion

- Hypertrophic type—viable fracture ends with abundant callus formation. Ends are vascular and micromotion must have existed which lead to callus formation, i.e. bone biology is adequate problem is with fixation. Bone graft is not required in these cases.
- Atrophic type—non-viable ends with no callus formation. Ends are avascular and there must be excess motion, absolutely no motion or distraction at the fracture site which leads to absent callus formation. Biology is not adequate, thus bone graft is required.

Factors favoring union: Head injury/ICU patients, alkalinity (high pH), high oxygen tension, immobilisation and micromotion at fracture site, stability, compression at fracture site, platelet products (platelet rich plasma), etc. favor callus formation and union. Younger age, closed fracture, fracture in cancellous bone and spiral fracture heal better. Pediatric patients has high union and remodeling rate.

Factors hindering union: Inadequate immobilization (commonest cause), old age, open fracture, distraction at fracture site, soft tissue interposition at fracture site, malnutrition, smoking, alcohol, comorbidities, radiation therapy, infection, pathological fracture, intra-articular fractures, all heal poorly. **However, osteoporosis per se does not lead to nonunion.**

Common Sites of Nonunion
- Fracture neck of femur
- Scaphoid
- Talus
- Lower third of tibia (overall commonest site)
- Lateral condyle of humerus

Malunion is mostly seen in metaphyseal fractures (cancellous bone), viz. supracondylar fracture of humerus, Colles' fracture, clavicle, intertrochanteric fractures, etc.

Principles of treatment in nonunion—open reduction is done with freshening of fracture margins till bleeding bone ends are found and removal of all fibrous tissue, stable internal fixation with **bone grafting (mandatory step)**. Postoperatively the limb is supported with a splint/slab. However, if the nonunion is infected, then the choice of fixation changes:
- LRS (limb reconstruction system; a special type of external fixator)
- Ilizarov—if bone gap/bone loss present and bone lengthening is desired.

Chemicals speeding up fracture union—bone marrow aspirate, platelet-rich plasma, bone morphogenetic proteins (BMP 2 and 7), etc.

Bone Grafting
Ideal bone graft should have the property of osteogenesis (supplying bone forming cells), osteoconduction (providing a scaffold for bone formation) and osteoinduction (recruiting host cells to form new bone).

Different types of bone grafts
- Cancellous —possesses all three properties. The cancellous bone graft is slowly replaced by new bone by a complex process known as "creeping substitution". Graft donor sites—iliac crest (for large amount of graft), metaphyseal area of bones (for small graft)—olecranon, tibia metaphysis, radial styloid, greater trochanter, distal femoral condyle, etc. Bone graft from iliac crest is most commonly taken from highest point of iliac crest. However, considering the percutaneous location, posterosuperior iliac spine is the best source of cancellous bone graft.
- Cortical—no osteogenic property, poor induction but better osteoconduction. Fibula is the ideal and most common site of cortical bone graft. Other sites—ribs.
- Tricortical bone graft—all three properties. Iliac crest is the most common site. Anterior iliac crest is the best source of bicortical and corticocancellous graft.
- Vascularized grafting—here along with the bone graft its vessels are also grafted to the recipient site, most commonly done using fibula. In nonunion where larger gap is present, vascularized fibular graft may be done to enhance chances of union.

Pathological Fracture
Fractures occurring in diseased bones subjected to trivial trauma are known as pathogical fractures. Here fractures occur after a trivial force in a pathologically weakened bone, not enough to cause fracture in a normal bone. Pathological cause may be systemic disease (osteoporosis, rickets, scurvy) or localized (infection, malignancy or metastasis). Vertebral bodies (DL spine) are the most common site of fracture followed by neck of femur and distal end radius. Most common cause—<60 years is metastasis and after >60 years/overall is osteoporosis. In India, most common cause is nutritional osteoporosis.

Osteoporosis or other generalized diseases causing pathological fracture per se do not lead to non-union. However, benign bony lesion may lead to delayed union and malignant lesion/ infection may lead to non-union. Fractures may be the initial/presenting symptom in a pathological fracture.

The term pathological fracture is generally used for neoplastic lesion while "fragility fractures" is reserved for osteoporotic fractures.

Stress Fracture

It is caused by abnormal amount of load applied in a rhythmic, repeated, subthreshold and non-violent manner in a relatively normal bone.

- Fatigue fracture—normal bone is subjected to abnormal stress leading to mechanical failure/ fracture over time.
- Insufficiency fracture—caused by normal physiological stress in a weaker bone.

Sites

- Most common site is distal tibia (posteromedial compression side).
- Pubic rami.
- Femoral neck—superior (tensile) side is more dangerous and require treatment while inferior/ compression side is more common.
- Runners fracture—distal fibula.
- March fracture—shaft fracture of 2nd > 3rd metatarsal bone.
- Upper limb—olecranon is the most common site in upper limb.
- Spine—pars interarticularis of 5th lumbar vertebra is the most common site and may lead to spondylolysis.

Clinical features: Pain (may be bilateral) with relatively normal X-ray. Localized tenderness with haziness in the X-ray (due to periosteal reaction) clinches the diagnosis. When X-rays are normal but clinical suspicion is high, MRI is the IOC (diagnose the fracture by bone edema). In B/L cases, bone scan is preferred.

Treatment: Mostly symptomatic with cessation of activity and cast application. Sometimes in high-risk areas with stress fracture, prophylactic fixation can be done (e.g. superior/tensile surface neck femur).

Periprosthetic Fracture

Fracture occurring in and around prosthesis (total hip, knee replacement, Austin Moore, Thompson prosthesis). Classified by Vancouver classification.

Xtra Edge

- In human skeleton, osteocytes are the most abundant (90%) and most long-lived cells.
- Osteocalcin is exclusively produced by osteoblasts and is a marker of bone. Thus its concentration in the blood is a direct measure of osteoblastic activity.
- A long bone is defined as one which has length more than width. By this definition, phalanx followed by metacarpal/metatarsal is the shortest long bone in the body.
- Porosity of cortical bones mostly falls in the range of 5 to 10%, while that of cancellous bones ranges between 75 and 95%. Hence cancellous bones are highly porous.
- Vertebrae have maximum ratio of cancellous bone compared to any other bone in the body (their cancellous to cortical bone ratio is 75:25).
- Trabecular bone is also lamellar bone, but it does not contain Haversian systems.
- Physis / growth plate is a hyaline cartilage plate conventionally taken to be a part of metaphysis. It can be considered a temporary primary cartilaginous joint.
- Hueter Volkmann law: According to this law, compression forces across the physis inhibit growth while tensile forces across the physis stimulate growth.
- Endosteum is the most metabolically active part of a bone.
- By rule, there is generally one primary center that appears before birth for every diaphysis except in clavicle that has two primary centers for its diaphysis.
- The first bone to start ossifying in the human skeleton is the clavicle. It is only long bone to ossify by intramembranous ossification. The clavicle is also the last bone to complete ossification when its medial end fuses with the shaft.

- The mandible is the second bone to ossify after clavicle by intramembranous ossification.
- *Law of ossification*: The secondary center which appears first fuses last and the bone that does not obey this law is "fibula".
- Secondary center of ossification is present in the heads of all metacarpals except the first where it is present in the base.
- *Ossification of carpals*: Carpal bones ossify by rule from one center only. Capitate is the 1st carpal bone to ossify (at 2 months) and before three years of age, only capitate and hamate ossify in a child's hand. Pisiform is the last to ossify around 12 years.

MULTIPLE CHOICE QUESTIONS

1. **Increase callus or cartilage formation is seen in:**
   A. Rigid immobilization
   B. Necrosis of bone ends
   C. Increase mobilization
   D. Compression plating

2. **Adult bone trabeculae are differentiated from fetal bone trabeculae by the presence of:**
   A. Harversian system
   B. Lamellar structure
   C. Certain special staining characteristics
   D. Different types of bone cells in each

3. **The tensile strength of a bone is due to:**
   A. Strands of collagen
   B. Hydroxyapatite crystals
   C. Periosteum
   D. Metaphysis

4. **Callus formation is seen between what duration of fracture healing:**
   A. 0–2 weeks   B. 2–4 weeks
   C. 4–12 weeks   D. 12–16 weeks

5. **Most metabolically active part in bone is:**
   A. Cortical bone   B. Cancellous bone
   C. Periosteal surface D. Endosteal surface

6. **Wolff's law states that:**
   A. If a bone is continuously subjected to a particular stress, it will adapt to become stronger to resist that loading
   B. Only diaphysis allows longitudinal growth in childhood
   C. Any infection not showing periosteal reaction within 1 week of symptoms can be ruled out to be osteomyelitis
   D. Angular deformities will progress till the closure of physis

7. **Bone resorption is inhibited by:**
   A. Parathyroid hormone
   B. Thyroid hormones
   C. Cortisol
   D. Estrogen

8. **Indicators of bone formation and resorption— which of the following is false?**
   A. Osteocalcin is marker of bone formation
   B. Hydroxyproline is marker of bone resorption
   C. N and C terminal procollagen for bone formation
   D. N and C terminal telopeptide for bone formation

9. **Marker for bone formation is:**
   A. Tartrate resistant acid phosphate
   B. Osteocalcin
   C. Urinary calcium
   D. Serum nucleotidase

10. **Rate of mineralization of newly formed osteoid can be estimated by the following:**
    A. von Kossa staining for calcium
    B. Alzarin red stain
    C. Labelled tetracycline
    D. Immunofluorescence

11. **Bone apposition is best seen in:**
    A. Endochondral ossification
    B. Osteoblastic activity in Howship's lacunae
    C. Subperiosteal cambium layer
    D. Osteoblastic activity at the area of stress

12. **Regarding bone remodeling, all are true *except*:**
    A. Osteoclastic activity at the compression site
    B. Osteoclastic activity at the tension site
    C. Osteoclastic activity and osteoblastic activity both are needed for bone remodeling in cortical and cancellous bones
    D. Osteoblasts transform into osteocytes

13. **The first center of primary ossification appears at:**
    A. At the end of 2 months in intrauterine life
    B. Beginning of 3rd month
    C. End of 3rd month
    D. End of 4th month

14. **Diagnostic sign of a fracture:**
    A. Abnormal mobility at fracture site
    B. Pain at the fracture site
    C. Tenderness
    D. Swelling

15. **The most common sign of fresh fracture is:**
    A. Crepitus   B. Bony tenderness
    C. Deformity   D. Abnormal mobility
    E. Shortening of bone

16. **A child falls from a chair. Complains of pain in the mid leg. No visible deformity. He is unable to bear his weight on standing. What is the diagnosis?**
    A. Oblique fracture
    B. Spiral fracture
    C. Comminuted fracture
    D. Fracture of epiphysis

17. **Direct impact on the bone will produce a:**
    A. Transverse fracture
    B. Oblique fracture
    C. Spiral fracture
    D. Comminuted fracture

18. **All of the following factors facilitate non-union *except*:**
    A. Hematoma formation
    B. Periosteal injuries
    C. Absence of nerve supply
    D. Chronic infection

19. **Delayed union of fracture of a bone following a surgical treatment may be due to:**
    A. Infection
    B. Inadequate circulation
    C. Inadequate mobilization
    D. All of the above

20. **Callus induction is not hampered in:**
    A. Hypoxemia
    B. Micromovements
    C. Muscle interposition
    D. Multiple bone fragments

21. **Which of the following injuries can be classified as Gustilo-Anderson Grade III injuries?**
    A. Open fracture with clean wounds less than 1 cm long
    B. Open fractures with a laceration more than 1 cm long usually up to 10 cm, with extension tissue damage, flaps or avulsions
    C. Open segmental fractures, open fracture with extensive soft tissue damage
    D. Compartment syndrome with an open fracture

22. **Open fracture in children is managed by:**
    A. Debridement
    B. External fixation
    C. Open reduction and internal fixation
    D. Intramedullary nail

23. **A patient with gunshot wound in tibia presents with comminuted fracture tibia with 2 cm wound. This belongs to what grade of Gustilo-Anderson classification of open fractures:**
    A. Grade 1   B. Grade 2
    C. Grade 3a   D. Grade 3b

24. **Vascular repair to be done in which Gustilo-Anderson type:**
    A. IIIC   B. I
    C. II   D. IIIB

25. **A patient presents with open fracture of tibia with 1.5 cm opening in skin. Which grade it belongs?**
    A. Grade I   B. Grade II
    C. Grade IIIA   D. Grade IIIB

26. **Internal fixation is primarily used in all *except*:**
    A. Compound fractures
    B. Multiple fractures
    C. Fractures in elderly patient
    D. Fracture neck of femur

27. **Hypertrophic nonunion following a fracture, most appropriate treatment would be:**
    A. Stabilisation
    B. Bone grafting
    C. Stabilisation and bone grafting
    D. None of the above

28. **Following are immediate complications of fracture:**
    A. Vascular ischemia
    B. Neuronal injury
    C. Malunion
    D. Compartment syndrome
    E. Avascular necrosis

29. **Which of the following cause malunion?**
    A. Open fracture
    B. Infection
    C. Bone grafting
    D. Soft tissue interposition
    E. Proper alignment of fracture

30. **True about fracture healing *except*:**
    A. Nutrition affects healing
    B. Stable fixation promotes healing
    C. Compression at fracture site causes non-union
    D. Hormonal status may affect healing

31. **Fracture healing is affected by all *except*:**
    A. Osteoporosis
    B. Infection
    C. Poor blood supply
    D. Soft tissue interposition

32. **Factors affecting bone healing are all *except*:**
    A. Age   B. Sex
    C. Vascularity   D. Comminution

33. **The time necessary for healing of fracture depends on the following factors:**
    A. Age of the patient
    B. Location of the fracture
    C. Type of the fracture
    D. Degree of damage to soft tissues
    E. All of the above

34. **Provisional callus is seen on X-ray earliest by:**
    A. 2 weeks   B. 3 weeks
    C. 6 weeks   D. 8 weeks

35. **Initial stage of clinical union of bone is equivalent to:**
    A. Callus formation
    B. Woven bone
    C. Hematoma formation
    D. Calcification only

36. **The most common cause of nonunion is:**
    A. Infection
    B. Inadequate immobilization
    C. Ischemia
    D. Soft tissue interposition

37. **Commonest 1st order site for bone grafting:**
    A. Iliac crest   B. Tibial metaphysic
    C. Medial malleolus   D. Femoral condyle

38. **An 8-year-old boy with a history of fall from 10 feet height complains of pain in the right ankle. X-ray taken at that time of injury was normal without any evident fracture line. But after 2 years, he developed a calcaneovalgus deformity in the foot. The missed diagnosis seem to be:**
    A. Undiagnosed malunited fracture
    B. Avascular necrosis talus
    C. Distal tibial epiphyseal injury
    D. Ligamentous injury of ankle joint

39. **Commonest site of epiphyseal injury in children:**
    A. Lower end radius
    B. Lateral condyle humerus
    C. Upper end femur
    D. Lower end femur

40. **What is the type of joint seen in the growth plate?**
    A. Plane synovial
    B. Primary cartilaginous
    C. Secondary cartilaginous
    D. Fibrous

41. **Traumatic dislocation of the epiphyseal plate of distal femur occurs (PGI type):**
    A. Medially   B. Laterally
    C. Posteriorly   D. Anteriorly
    E. Rotationally

42. **In children, best remodeling is seen in fractures with:**
    A. Angulation in diaphysis
    B. Angulation in metaphysis
    C. Rotation in diaphysis
    D. Rotation in metaphysis

43. **Commonest fracture in children:**
    A. Fracture clavicle
    B. Green stick fracture of lower end of radius
    C. Supracondylar fracture
    D. All of the above

44. **A 6-year-old child falls on to his right side and develops a crack in only the dorsal cortex of mid region of radius. The best treatment is:**
    A. Antibiotics and sedative
    B. Bone plating and external fixation
    C. Slab with wait for bone imperfect
    D. Break the cortex other side and immobilisation by POP

45. **Thomas splint was devised by Sir HO Thomas:**
    A. To splint fracture shaft of femur
    B. To stabilize cervical spine after trauma
    C. For transportation of polytrauma patients
    D. For treating tuberculosis of knee

46. **Thomas splint is not used for:**
    A. Injuries around knee joint
    B. Knee dislocation
    C. Infective arthritis of knee
    D. Fracture femur

47. **Plaster of Paris was discovered by:**
    A. Percival Potts   B. Abraham Colles
    C. John Charnley   D. Anotonius Mathysen

48. **Which side of plaster is manipulated for wedging?**
    A. Anterior   B. Posterior
    C. Concave   D. Convex

49. **Crush syndrome:**
    A. Most common in earthquakes and bombings
    B. Causes acute glomerulonephritis
    C. Release of myoglobin in blood
    D. Occurs due to massive crushing of muscles
    E. Causes acute tubular necrosis

50. **Which of the following is not a component of the crush syndrome?**
    A. Myohemoglobinuria
    B. Massive crushing of muscles
    C. Acute tubular necrosis
    D. Bleeding diathesis

51. **Crush syndrome is managed by:**
    A. 20% dextrose
    B. Hydrocortisone
    C. Maintaining high urine output
    D. Acidification of urine

52. **Pathological fracture not found in:**
    A. Bone cyst
    B. Osteoporosis
    C. Chronic osteomyelitis
    D. Osteochondroma
    E. Osteogenesis imperfect

53. **Most common cause of pathological fracture in India is:**
    A. Paget's   B. Sarcoidosis
    C. Nutritional   D. Steroids

54. **The commonest cause of pathological fracture is generalized affection is:**
    A. Carcinoma   B. Osteoporosis
    C. Cyst   D. All of the above

55. **The treatment of choice in pathological fractures is:**
    A. Internal fixation
    B. Plaster of Paris casts
    C. Skin traction
    D. External skeletal fixation

56. Investigation of choice in stress fracture:
  A. MRI   B. CT
  C. Bone scan   D. X-ray

57. Differential diagnosis of stress fracture:
  A. Infection   B. Tumor
  C. Neuropathic joints   D. Osteochondritis

58. An army recruit, smoker and 6 months into training started complaining of pain at posteromedial aspect of both legs. There was acute point tenderness and the pain was aggravated on physical activity. The most likely diagnosis is:

  A. Buerger's disease
  B. Gout
  C. Lumbar canal stenosis
  D. Stress fracture

59. What is March fracture?
  A. Fracture of 2nd metatarsal
  B. Fracture of 4th metatarsal
  C. Fracture of cuboids
  D. Fracture of tibia

60. Stress fracture is treated by:
  A. Rest   B. Cast immobilization
  C. Closed reduction   D. Internal fixation

ANSWERS

1. C. Increase mobilization
2. B. Lamellar structure
3. A. Strands of collagen
4. C. 4–12 weeks
5. D. Endosteal surface
6. A. If a bone is continuously subjected to a particular stress, it will adapt to become stronger to resist that loading
7. D. Estrogen
8. D. N and C terminal telopeptide for bone formation
9. B. Osteocalcin
10. C. Labelled tetracycline
11. C. Subperiosteal cambium layer
12. A. Osteoclastic activity at the compression site
13. A. At the end of 2 months in intrauterine life
14. A. Abnormal mobility at fracture site
15. B. Bony tenderness
16. B. Spiral fracture (because the nature of trauma is a twisting injury)
17. A > D. Transverse fracture > Comminuted fracture
18. A. Hematoma formation
19. D. All of the above
20. B. Micromovements
21. C. Open segmental fractures, open fracture extensive soft tissue damage
22. A. Debridement
23. C. Grade 3a (comminuted fracture)
24. A. IIIC
25. B. Grade II
26. A. Compound fracture
27. A. Stabilisation
28. A. Vascular ischemia and B. Neuronal injury
29. C. Bone grafting and E. Proper alignment of fracture
30. C. Compression at fracture site causes non-union
31. A. Osteoporosis
32. B. Sex
33. E. All of the above

34. B. 3 weeks
35. B. Woven bone
36. B. Inadequate immobilization
37. A. Iliac crest
38. C. Distal tibial epiphyseal injury
39. A. Lower end radius
40. B. Primary cartilaginous
41. B, D. Laterally and anteriorly
42. B. Angulation in metaphysis. (Angulation re-models better than rotation and metaphysis being cancellous active vascular bone remodels best).
43. B. Green stick fracture of lower end of radius
44. D. Break the cortex other side and immobilisation by POP (in unicortical fractures/green stick fractures, other cortex is also broken while applying cast to make it a complete fracture, otherwise growth deformity may occur).
45. D. For treating tuberculosis of knee
46. None. (Thomas splint can be used in all these conditions for a temporary stabilization).
47. D. Anotonius Mathysen
48. C. Concave
49. All are correct
50. D. Bleeding diathesis
51. C. Maintaining high urine output
52. None
49. All are correct
50. D. Bleeding diathesis
51. C. Maintaining high urine output
52. None
53. C. Nutritional
54. B. Osteoporosis
55. A. Internal fixation
56. A. MRI
57. A. Infection
58. D. Stress fracture
59. A. Fracture of 2nd metatarsal
60. B. Cast immobilization

2

Fracture Management Principles

Musculoskeletal injuries can be managed conservatively or by surgery (both have their indications and contraindications).

Surgical management: Fracture reduction either by closed reduction/open reduction followed by fracture fixation with implants internally/externally (called internal/external fixation) (discussed later).

NON-OPERATIVE MANAGEMENT

Non-operative management: Traction, immobilization with POP cast/slab, functional brace, splint, etc.

Splints, Plaster and Braces

Splint is any material which supports the fracture and immobilizes the fracture site. It may be used temporarily during transportation or when awaiting surgery to decrease swelling/pain. When used as definite mode of treatment, then fracture is first reduced and then slab/cast is applied till union. The principle of immobilization is always one joint above and below.

- **Cast/slab:** When the plaster is placed only on one surface of limb it is called "slab" but when it encircles the limb circumferentially, it is called "cast". In acute trauma, there may be swelling, so slab is preferred, but when swelling decreases it is changed to cast. Cast application in swollen limb may lead to compartment syndrome (tight cast syndrome). Slab/cast may be of plaster of Paris (POP; most common) or synthetic fibre (Scotch cast). POP bandage consists of a roll of muslin cloth stiffened by dextrose/starch and impregnated with calcium sulfate hemihydrate (gypsum). When water is added, the more soluble form of calcium sulfate returns to the relatively insoluble form, and heat is produced.

$$2 \, (CaSO_4 \cdot \tfrac{1}{2} \, H_2O) + 3 \, H_2O \longrightarrow 2 \, (CaSO_4 \cdot 2H_2O) + Heat$$

The setting of unmodified plaster starts about 10 minutes after mixing and is complete in about 45 minutes (crystalizes; setting time); however, the cast is not fully dry (drying time) for 48–72 hours.

- Spica is one where cast encircles lower trunk/spine with hip/pelvis and limbs. For example: Hip spica used in fracture shaft femur in children.
- Brace: A splint made of POP/polyethylene that can be used for supporting a part of body. When function of adjacent joints is not hampered, then it is called a functional brace (concept by Sarmiento).
- Some non-operatively managed fractures
  - Fracture clavicle, metacarpal fractures, Colles' fracture, undisplaced scaphoid, shaft fibula, metatarsal fracture and most pediatric fractures (except intra-articular fractures).

Xtra Edge
Milwaukee shoulder: Destructive shoulder arthropathy due to deposition of hydroxyapatite crystals in and around shoulder joint.

Table 2.1: Some important cast/slabs and their uses

Name	Use
U slab/hanging cast	Fracture shaft humerus
Shoulder spica	Shoulder immobilisation
Sugar tong	Fracture humerus
Distal sugar tong/reverse sugar tong	Distal forearm fracture
Colles'/handshaking cast	Colles' fracture
Glass holding cast	Fracture scaphoid
Minerva cast	Cervical/upper thoracic spine disease
Turn buckle cast	Scoliosis
Risser's cast	Scoliosis
Hip spica	Fracture femur in children
Cylindrical cast	Patella fracture
PTB cast	Fracture tibia
Platform slab	Metatarsal fracture

Table 2.2: Splints/braces/traction systems

Name	Use
Upper limb	
Figure of 8 bandage	Fracture clavicle
Velpeau sling/swathe	AC dislocation > shoulder dislocation
Triangular sling	Fracture proximal humerus
Aeroplane splint	Brachial plexus injury
Dunlop traction	Fracture supracondylar humerus
Smith's traction	Fracture supracondylar humerus
Volkmann's splint/turn buckle splint	VIC
Cock up splint	Radial nerve palsy> fracture metacarpal
Knuckle bender splint	Ulnar/median nerve palsy
Gutter splint	Metacarpal/phalangeal fracture
Thumb spica splint	Scaphoid/metacarpal fracture
	Game keeper's thumb
Buddy strapping	Phalanx fracture
Crammer wire	For emergency immobilization (U/L and L/L)
Aluminium splint	Immobilization of fingers
Lower limb	
Broom stick cast (Petrie's cast)	Perthes' disease
Pavlik harness, Von Rosen splint, Ilfeld hip abduction splint, craig splint, bachelor cast	DDH
Agnes Hunt traction	Correction of hip deformity
Well leg traction	Correction of abduction hip deformity
Russell's traction	Fracture intertrochanteric femur
Gallows traction	Fracture SOF in <2 yrs or <12 kg child
Bryant's traction	Fracture SOF in <2 yrs child
90–90 traction	Fracture proximal SOF in children>adults
Perkins traction	Fracture SOF in adults
Thomas splint	Fracture femur, knee immobilization
Bohler Braun splint	Fracture femur, knee, tibia
Dennis Brown splint	CTEV
Toe raising splint	Foot drop
Buck's traction	Skin traction

(Contd.)

Table 2.2: Splints/braces/traction systems (Contd.)	
Name	Use
Spine	
Head halter traction	Cervical spine injury
Crutchfield traction	Cervical spine injury
Four post collar, Philadelphia collar	Neck immobilisation
SOMI (sterno-occipital mandibular immobilization) brace	Cervical spine injury
Halo	Cervical spine immobilization
Minerva cast	Cervical spine
ASHE (anterior spinal hyperextension) brace	DL spine injury/TB
Taylor's brace	DL spine
Milwaukee brace, Boston brace, Risser's cast, Halo pelvic traction	Scoliosis
Goldthwaite brace	Lumbar spine (TB)
Lumbar corset	Backache

Tractions

Traction is applied in fracture to decrease over riding of bone (i.e. maintain length) and to correct deformity.

Types: Fixed traction (e.g. Thomas splint)—where countertraction is provided by a part of the splint itself and balanced/sliding traction is one where patient's body weight provides countertraction.

Modes: Skin or skeletal traction.

Skin traction—applied by adhesive/nonadhesive bandage or Buck's apparatus (Fig. 2.1). Skin traction applied when mild/moderate force is required and maximum weight permitted is 6 kg.

Skeletal traction—applied when moderate severe force is required. Maximum weight permitted is up to 20 kg (up to 25–30% body weight).

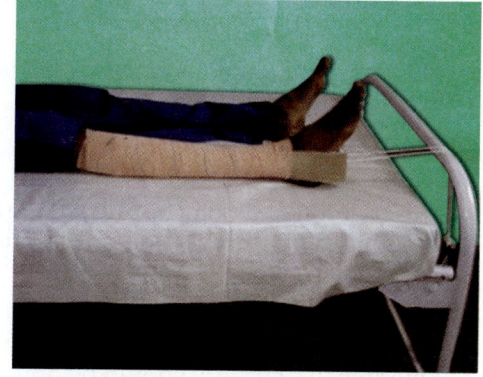

Fig 2.1: Buck's traction

Different means of skeletal traction are: Steinman's pin, Denham pin, K-wire, Ilizarov wire, crutchfield tong (Fig. 2.2), etc. Steinman's pin is pointed at one end (K-wire pointed at both ends) and nonthreaded, used in cortical/nonosteoporotic bones, whereas Denham pin is threaded in middle and used in cancellous or osteoporotic/elderly patients. K-wire/Ilizarov wires are used for traction in pediatric patients.

Thomas knee splint (Fig. 2.3)—may be used for immobilization/splintage or fixed traction. It was first used by Thomas for his wife's TB knee immobilization, since then its use has increased multifold and now it is most commonly used for hip/thigh immobilization.

Functional Cast Brace

- A concept of Sarmiento which works by hydraulic principle. When the fracture ends become sticky (i.e.

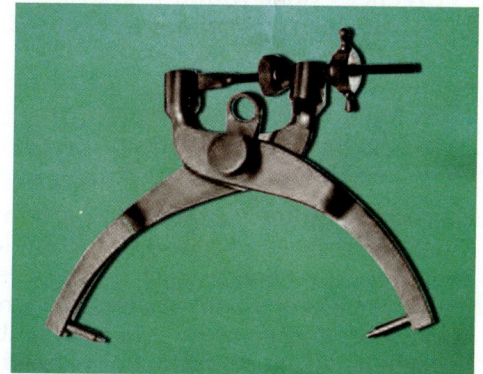

Fig. 2.2: Crutchfield tongs for cervical traction

after initial callus formation), Sarmiento cast is applied after moulding it to the fractured limb. Weight bearing is allowed (after 2 days of cast application), whereby fracture site is compressed and fastens healing. Nearby joints are not included in cast, thus their function is not compromised (therefore no joint stiffness).

- Indications—fracture humerus (commonest), tibia (PTB cast—misnomer), ulna, etc.
- It does not help primarily in reducing a fracture but the hydrostatic pressure helps in maintaining the reduction achieved while cast application.
- It is not useful in open fractures.

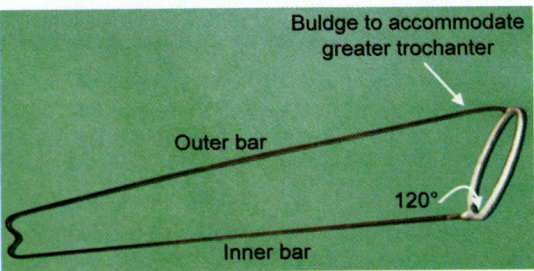

Fig. 2.3: Thomas splint [Two outer bars attached proximally by a ring suspended at 120°, outer bar is bent to accommodate the greater trochanter. Inner part of the ring is most troublesome, may cause sore in groin]

Physiotherapy

It deals with physical exercises, mechanical and electrotherapy for various indications, like pain relief, joint stiffness, range of movement, etc.

Heat Therapy

- Superficial heat penetrates only the superficial structures (skin and subcutaneous tissue).
  - For example, hot bath, paraffin wax bath, infrared lamp, moist air cabinet.
- Deep heat penetrates till muscle.
  - Short wave diathermy, microwave diathermy, ultrasonic therapy.

Electrotherapy

- TENS: Transcutaneous electrical nerve stimulation.
- Interferential therapy.

OPERATIVE MANAGEMENT

AO Principles

- Preservation of blood supply of bone during dissection
- Acceptable (preferably anatomical) reduction of fracture
- Stable internal fixation and
- Active mobilization of joints.

Timing of Surgery

- Emergency—surgery should be done as early as possible in life/limb threatening injuries
  - Vascular injury, irreducible dislocation/fracture dislocation of major joints, fracture dislocation with vascular injury (knee), compartment syndrome, compound fracture with bone exposed, any abscess, septic arthritis, spinal injuries (cauda equina, with deteriorating neurological deficit).
- Urgency—done within 1–2 days
  - Intra-articular fracture, fracture NOF, pediatric fracture (lateral condyle humerus/displaced supracondylar humerus).
- Elective—surgery can be done after proper planning in a length of time
  - Joint replacement surgery
  - Ligament surgeries (arthroscopic surgery).
  - Long bone fracture.

Closed Reduction v/s Open Reduction

The basic essence of closed reduction is that fracture site is not opened and thus the fracture hematoma is retained, which has high osteogenic potential, therefore, this mode of reduction has higher chances of union, whereas in open reduction fracture site is opened and fracture hematoma is exposed. Closed reduction is aided by C-arm guidance/image intensifier. In conservative management, reduction is done by closed reduction and fracture is immobilised by slab/cast. While in surgical management, reduction can be either done by open or closed reduction and fracture fixed with an implant which may be internal/external fixation. In closed reduction, implant is inserted percutaneously without exposing the fracture site. In pediatric patients, reduction is generally done by closed reduction accepting some malalignment because of higher union/remodelling rate. Pediatric cases are generally managed conservatively, if operative indication is present then also reduction is attempted closed, if failed then open reduction is done. However, in adults intra-articular fracture, accurate anatomical reduction is desired (to prevent arthritis), thus open reduction is done.

Internal Fixation v/s External Fixation

In internal fixation, implant is not exposed to exterior and is under the cover of skin/soft tissues. While in external fixation implant is visible outside.

Internal Fixation

For example: Tension band wiring (TBW), plates, nails, wires.

- TBW/plates—they are applied on convex/tensile surface and work on the same principle of "tensile forces are converted to compressive forces". TBW indications—fracture olecranon, patella, medial or lateral malleolus, etc.
- Plates*—they are mainly used for upper limb diaphyseal fractures (humerus, radius, ulna) and for periarticular fractures in both upper/lower limb. Rarely plating may also be done for lower limb diaphyseal fracture also. They are applied by open reduction.

  Types:
  - Dynamic compression plate (DCP): Compresses the fracture site.
  - Low contact DCP (LC-DCP): Work on same principle as above, but mechanically superior as it has low contact with bone and thus preserves bone vascularity. Both these plates provide rigid fixation.
  - Locking compression plate (LCP): Here screws are locked in plate and has very little contact with bone working as internal fixator, providing relative stability to the fracture site. Indications—pathological bone, osteoporotic bone, metaphyseal area/periarticular fracture, periprosthetic fracture.
- Nails*—intramedullary nails are mainly done for lower limb diaphyseal fractures, ideally done closed (CRIF), if failed then open reduction is done (ORIF).
  - Kuntscher nail (K-nail) was the first intramedullary nail used without any locking bolts and worked on the principle of "3-point bony fixation". It is hollow, cross section being clover leaf shaped and has a longitudinal slot facing on the tensile side. The nail is elastic and when passed intramedullary, gets deformed to take the shape of canal, allowing 3-point fixation at the two ends and at isthmus. In present day, its only indication is transverse/oblique fracture at isthmus.
  - ILN—interlocking nail is mainly used nowadays, which provides rotational stability by locking bolts which fix the nail to bolt. The length of nail can be calculated from olecranon tip to tip of little finger and diameter of nail corresponds to size of isthmus.
  - Rush nail/Enders nail/K-nail—all are less frequently used nowadays and never used in traction application.
- Wires*—Kirschner wire has varied range of uses. Used as definite management in pediatric fractures, e.g. fracture supracondylar humerus (closed reduction) and lateral condyle fracture (open reduction). It may also be used intra-operatively for provisional fixation of fractures.
- Others*
  - Herbert screw (headless screw)—scaphoid, femoral head, capitellum, radial head, etc.
  - Cannulated cancellous screw—fracture neck of femur, intra-articular fractures.
  - Dynamic hip screw (DHS)—intertrochanteric fractures.
  - Proximal femoral nail (PFN)—reverse oblique or unstable intertrochanteric fracture femur, subtrochanteric femur fracture.
  - PHILOS —proximal humerus locking plate.

---

*Images of all implants are given in fracture chapters.

External Fixation
- External fixator (AO fixator) (Fig. 2.4A) used in compound fractures, where main aim of external fixator remains to maintain length of bone and wound management, not fracture union (i.e. it is used for temporary management). It provides relative stability.
- Ilizarov (Russian) external fixator (Fig. 2.4B) may be used in compound periarticular fractures (as definite management), bone deformity correction, malunion, nonunion, CTEV, bone lengthening. It works on the principle of "distraction histiogenesis". In bone lengthening, a corticotomy (not osteotomy) is done in metaphyseal area and corticotomy site is distracted by 1 mm per day, where new bone (i.e. histiogenesis) is formed subsequently.
- JESS—by Dr BB Joshi (Mumbai) is an Indian external fixator.

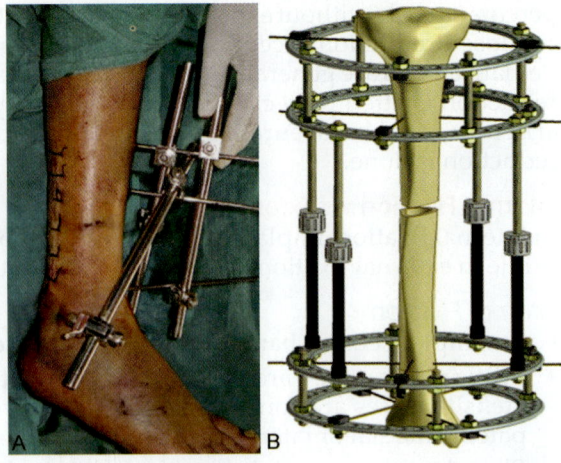

Fig. 2.4A and B: (A) AO external fixator (note longitudinal tubular rod), (B) Ilizarov external fixator (note ring system)

Implant composition: Alloy of stainless steel (316 L) or cobalt or titanium.

Mode of Healing in Different Types of Management
- 1° healing/minimal callus formation—seen in rigid fixation, e.g. compression plating (DCP, LCDCP).
- 2° healing/healing with callus formation—seen in cases with relative stability—conservative management, interlocking nail, locked plating, external fixator, Ilizarov fixator.

Surgical Excision
- Excision can be done in fractures of bone where fracture fragment is very small/extra-articular/ does not lead to instability/unreconstructible with ORIF; e.g. patella, olecranon, radial head (outer 1/3rd). Surgical excision is also a part in replacement arthroplasty, e.g. THR, where femur head and neck are excised and replaced with prosthesis.
- Surgical excision is contraindicated in:
  - Fracture olecranon where it may lead to elbow instability, e.g. fracture extending distally to coronoid, here excision of such big fragment will lead to elbow instability/triceps weakness/ loss of elbow movement.
  - In radial head fracture in children or associated ligament injury or terrible triad injury.
  - Growth plate injury, e.g. lateral condyle humerus injury.

Articular Fractures
They should always be managed with accurate reduction and stable internal fixation (TOC), else may lead to post-traumatic osteoarthritis. Surgery should be done as early as possible after swelling is decreased (wrinkles appear on skin). Articular fracture should always be mobilized (joint movement) in postoperative period else may lead to joint stiffness.

Other Modes of Management
- Aspiration of hematoma to decrease swelling and pain.
- If small intra-articular fragment acting as loose body-excision.
- Conservative on slab/cast—only if fracture is undisplaced.
- Arthrodesis—after 2° osteoarthritis sets in, to provide stable painless joint in physically active young adults (e.g. labourer). Most common cause of ankle arthrodesis is post-traumatic arthritis.
- Replacement arthroplasty—e.g. total hip replacement in femur head fracture.

MULTIPLE CHOICE QUESTIONS

1. **Identify the use of the instrument?**

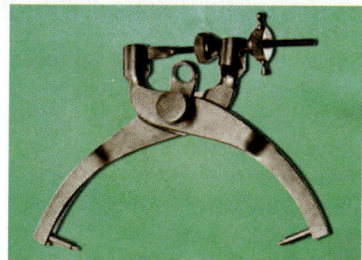

   A. Lumbar traction   B. Cervical traction
   C. Tibia traction   D. Femur traction

2. **Identify the type of fixation?**

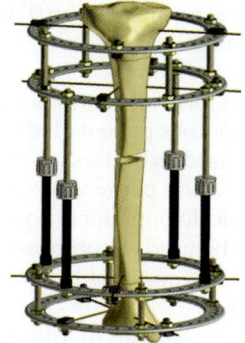

   A. Internal fixator
   B. AO external fixator
   C. Ilizarov external fixator
   D. JESS fixator.

3. **Brace used in scoliosis is:**
   A. Milwaukee brace   B. LS belt
   C. Taylor's brace   D. Four post collar

4. **Weight allowed in skeletal traction up to:**
   A. 5 kg   B. 10 kg
   C. 20 kg   D. 30 kg

5. **Cast syndrome is a complication of:**
   A. Hip spica   B. Below elbow cast
   C. Above elbow cast   D. PTB cast

6. **Treatment of choice for fracture shaft femur in a child less than 2 years of age:**
   A. Gallows traction   B. Hip spica
   C. Russell traction   D. Intramedullary nail

7. **All of the following are true regarding application of POP cast** *except*:
   A. Putting the plaster roll in water hastens setting time
   B. It is anhydrous calcium phosphate
   C. It should be carefully applied in presence of swelling
   D. Gangrene is known complication of a tight plaster cast

8. **Which of the following casts/splints is used for fracture shaft humerus?**
   A. Hanging casts
   B. Knuckle bender splint
   C. Aeroplane splint
   D. Above elbow cast

9. **Milwaukee brace is used in:**
   A. Congenital kyphosis
   B. Scheuermann's disease
   C. Adolescent idiopathic scoliosis
   D. Spondylolisthesis

10. **Identify the use of this type of fixation.**

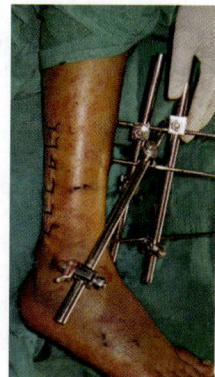

   A. Articular fracture   B. Open fracture
   C. Closed fracture   D. Spinal fracture

11. **What about Denham pin is true?**
   A. It is used to give skeletal traction
   B. It has threads in the center of pin
   C. It is used to give skeletal traction through calcaneum
   D. All of the above

12. **Gallow's traction is used in management of fracture shaft:**
   A. Femur   B. Tibia
   C. Humerus   D. Ulna

13. **Identify the splint:**

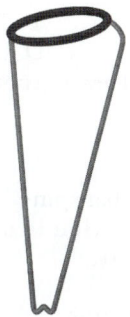

   A. Thomas knee splint   B. Thomas thigh splint
   C. BB splint   D. Krammer wire

14. **Thomas splint was not used for:**
    A. Injuries around knee joint
    B. Knee dislocation
    C. Infective arthritis of knee
    D. Fracture femur

15. **Commonest indication for ankle arthrodesis is:**
    A. Rheumatoid arthritis
    B. Post-traumatic arthritis
    C. Post-infective arthritis
    D. Failed total ankle arthroplasty

16. **Which of the following is included in management of intra-articular fracture?**
    A. Arthrodesis   B. Excision
    C. K-wire   D. All of the above

17. **Which of the following conditions should be given most priority in case of fracture?**
    A. Open fracture   B. Dislocated fracture
    C. Vascular injury   D. Malunited fracture
    E. Compartment syndrome

18. **K nail can be used for all of the following fractures *except*:**
    A. Isthmic femur shaft fractures
    B. Intertrochanteric fractures
    C. Low subtrochanteric fractures
    D. Distal femur shaft fractures

19. **Bone transport can be used in the management of:**
    A. Gap nonunion
    B. Deformity correction
    C. Comminuted shaft femur fracture
    D. Avascular necrosis of femoral head

20. **Functional bracing is now the gold standard in nonoperative management of which fractures?**
    A. Fracture shaft humerus
    B. Fracture of both bones of the forearm
    C. Fracture shaft tibia
    D. Fracture shaft femur

21. **Traction not used in lower limb:**
    A. Gallows   B. Bryant
    C. Dunlop   D. Perkin

22. **Thomas splint is used for immobilizing fractures of:**
    A. Femur   B. Tibia
    C. Radius   D. Ulna

23. **Functional cast bracing not used in fracture of:**
    A. Humerus
    B. Tibia
    C. Ulna
    D. Thoracolumbar spin

24. **Halopelvic traction is used for correcting which deformity:**
    A. Spine
    B. Pectus carinatum
    C. Spondyloptosis
    D. Coxa vara

25. **Maximum weight for skin traction:**
    A. 1–2 kg   B. 4–5 kg
    C. 10–15 kg   D. 15–20 kg

26. **All of the following are used for giving skeletal traction *except*:**
    A. Steinmann's   B. Kirschner's wire
    C. Bohler's stirrup   D. Rush pin

27. **Which is not a deep heat therapy:**
    A. Shortwave diathermy
    B. Ultrasound therapy
    C. Infrared therapy
    D. Microwave therapy

28. **Which of the following requires surgical correction:**
    A. Pathological fracture
    B. Fracture humerus shaft with radial nerve palsy
    C. Fracture humerus shaft with vascular involvement
    D. Polytrauma patient

29. **True about locking compression plate:**
    A. In osteoporotic patients, it should not be used
    B. Can be used as buttress plate
    C. Usually cause periosteal plate
    D. Mechanically superior to a conventional plate
    E. Cannot be used as compression plate

30. **Contraindication for skin traction:**
    A. Dermatitis
    B. Compromised vascularity of limb
    C. Abrasions
    D. Hypopigmentation (vitiligo)
    E. Bony deformity

31. **Most common bone for which nailing is done?**
    A. Radius
    B. Ulna
    C. Tibia
    D. Humerus

32. **In the management of long bone fracture, following can be done:**
    A. Intramedullary nailing
    B. Plating
    C. External fixation
    D. Tension band wiring
    E. Screw

33. **Action of intramedullary 'K' nail is:**
    A. Two-point fixation
    B. Three-point fixation
    C. Compression
    D. Weight concentration

34. **Skeletal traction is given by:**
    A. K-wire
    B. Pavlik harness
    C. Denham pin
    D. Steinmann's pin
    E. Rush pin

ANSWERS

1. B. Cervical traction
2. C. Ilizarov external fixator
3. A. Milwaukee brace
4. C. 20 kg
5. A. Hip spica
   Hip spica or scoliosis cast can press on superior mesenteric artery compressing 3rd part of duodenum known as cast syndrome.
6. B. Hip spica
7. B. It is anhydrous calcium phosphate
8. A. Hanging casts
9. C. Adolescent idiopathic scoliosis
10. B. Open fracture
11. D. All of the above
12. A. Femur
13. A. Thomas knee splint
14. C. Infective arthritis of knee
15. B. Post-traumatic arthritis
16. D. All of the above
17. A. Open fracture; B Dislocated fracture; C. Vascular injury; E. Compartment syndrome.
18. B. Intertrochanteric fractures
19. A. Gap nonunion
20. A. Fracture shaft humerus
21. C. Dunlop
22. A. Femur
23. D. Thoracolumbar spin
24. A. Spine
25. B. 4–5 kg
26. D. Rush pin
27. C. Infrared therapy
28. A. Pathological fracture; C. Fracture humerus shaft with vascular involvement and D. Polytrauma patient
29. B. Can be used as buttress plate and D. Mechanically superior to a conventional plate
30. A. Dermatitis; B. Compromised vascularity of limb
31. C. Tibia
32. A. Intramedullary nailing, B. Plating and C. External fixation
33. B. Three-point fixation
34. A. K-wire; C. Denham pin; D. Steinmann's pin

3

Orthopedic Radiology

Radiology plays a very important role in management of orthopedic patients. Radiological applications like X-rays, ultrasonography (USG), CT scan, magnetic resonance imaging (MRI) and nuclear imaging, all have specific roles in different orthopedic pathologies.

X-RAYS

Discovered accidentally by Wilhelm Conrad Roentgen (Fig. 3.1) in 1895, X-rays are electromagnetic waves in the wavelength 0.01–10 nm. X-rays are produced when high energy electrons strike the tungsten target in a special X-ray tube (cathode ray tube). X-rays are the first line radiographic investigation in most orthopedic cases. Uses of X-rays in orthopedics are given in Table 3.1.

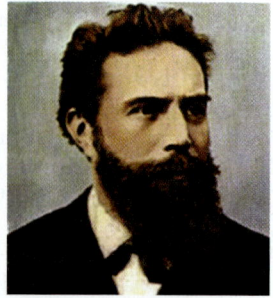

Fig. 3.1: Wilhelm Conrad Roentgen (REDRAW)

Table 3.1: Uses of X-rays in orthopedics

Use in trauma:
- Usually the first investigation in trauma
- To see location and type of fracture
- A joint above and a joint below should be covered in X-ray of a fracture bone to rule out a possible dislocation/subluxation
- At least two X-ray views are recommended to confirm a fracture
- Glass pieces can be seen on X-ray due to presence of lead within them
- Also used after fracture reduction by plaster fixation/nailing to confirm proper fixation of fracture fragments

Use in infection (osteomyelitis):
- Soft tissue planes are also visualised in X-rays and doctors often miss this part. In fact loss of soft tissue planes is the first change in pyogenic osteomyelitis (OM) (24–48 hours)
- Periosteal reaction is the first bone change (7–10 days)
- No periosteal reaction in tuberculosis (TB) osteomyelitis
- Chronic OM shows sclerosed dead bone (sequestrum) with thick onion peel type of periosteal reaction (differential diagnoses—Ewing's sarcoma)
- Air pockets may be seen in soft tissues in spread of infection to soft tissues—necrotizing fasciitis

Use in bone tumors:
- Tumor location: Epiphyseal, metaphyseal or diaphyseal
- Tumor matrix: Cartilaginous tumors have characteristic rings and arcs pattern of calcification, bone-forming tumors like osteosarcoma show osteoid tumor matrix
- Periosteal reaction, adjacent soft tissue involvement

Use in degenerative arthritis:
- Reduced joint space in involved joint (indicates cartilage damage as cartilage is not visualized on X-ray and forms the joint space)
- Osteophytes, subchondral cysts, subchondral sclerosis—seen in osteoarthritis

Taken from Fundamentals of Orthopedics by Mohindra and Jain (2nd ed., Jaypee publishers).

OSTEOPHYTE

Osteophytes (Fig. 3.2) are seen in degenerative arthritis. "Osteo" means bone and "phyte" means growth and are seen in cases of joint damage.

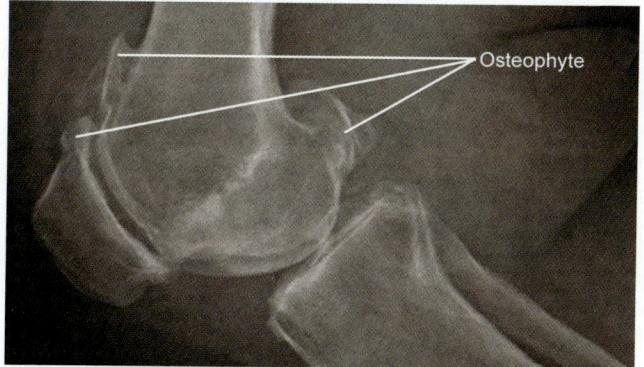

Fig. 3.2: X-ray of knee joint showing osteophytes (label as shown)

In spine pathology, new bone formations have different names according to their appearance (Fig. 3.3).

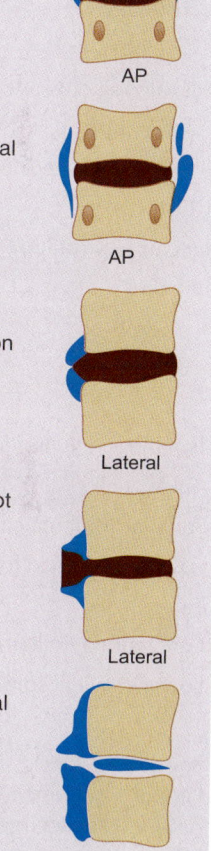

Syndesmophytes
Ossification of the annulus fibrosus. Thin, vertical and symmetrical. When extreme results in the "bamboo spine".
1. Ankylosing spondylitis
2. Alkaptonuria

AP

Paravertebral ossification
Ossification of paravertebral connective tissue which is separated from the edge of the vertebral body and disc. Large, coarse and asymmetrical.
1. Reiter's syndrome
2. Psoriatic arthropathy

AP

Claw osteophytes
Arising from the vertebral margin with no gap and having an obvious claw appearance.
1. Stress response—but in the absence of disc space narrowing does not indicate disc degeneration

Lateral

Traction spurs
Osteophytes with a gap between the end-plate and the base of the osteophyte and with tip not protruding beyond the horizontal plane of the vertebral end-plate.
1. Shear stresses across the disc—more likely to be associated with a degenerative disc.

Lateral

Undulating anterior ossification
Undulating ossification of the anterior longitudinal ligament, intervertebral disc and paravertebral connective tissue.
1. Diffuse idiopathic skeletal hyperostosis (DISH).

Fig. 3.3: New bone formation in spinal pathologies

Some Important X-ray Views (Fig. 3.4)

Bone	Name of the X-ray view
Sternoclavicular joint	Serendepity view (to diagnose dislocation)
	Hobb's view
Acromioclavicular joint	Zanca's view
Shoulder joint	Scapular Y view
	Grashey's view (True AP view)
Bony Bankart	West point view
Hills Sach's lesion	Stryker notch view
	Internal rotation view
Radiocapitellar view	Greenspan view
Evaluation of reduction in fracture supracondylar humerus	Jone's view
Scaphoid	Ulnar oblique
	Zitter view
Thumb CMC joint	Robert's view
Metacarpal head fracture	Brewerton view
Hook of hamate fracture	Carpal tunnel view
Wrist/hand	Norgaard view
	Allslate
Visualizing erosions in RA hand	Ball catchers view
Acetabulum	Judet's view (obturator oblique + iliac oblique)
Full profile of neck of femur	Internal rotation view
CDH	Von Rosen view
Lateral view of hip joint intra-op SCFE	Frog leg view
Patella	Axial
	Skyline view
	Merchant view
	Sunrise view
Trochlear notch of femur	Tunnel view
Ankle	Mortise view (15° internal rotation)
Subtalar joint (calcaneum)	Harris-Beath view
Calcaneum (used for intra-op evaluation)	Broden view
Talus (neck)	Canale view
Calcaneonavicular coalition	Sloman view
Lower cervical spine (C6, C7, T1)	Swimmer's view
	Shoulder pull down view
Spondylolisthesis	Ferguson view
Far out syndrome (5th root compression produced by a large transverse process of 5th lumbar vertebrae against the ala of the sacrum)	

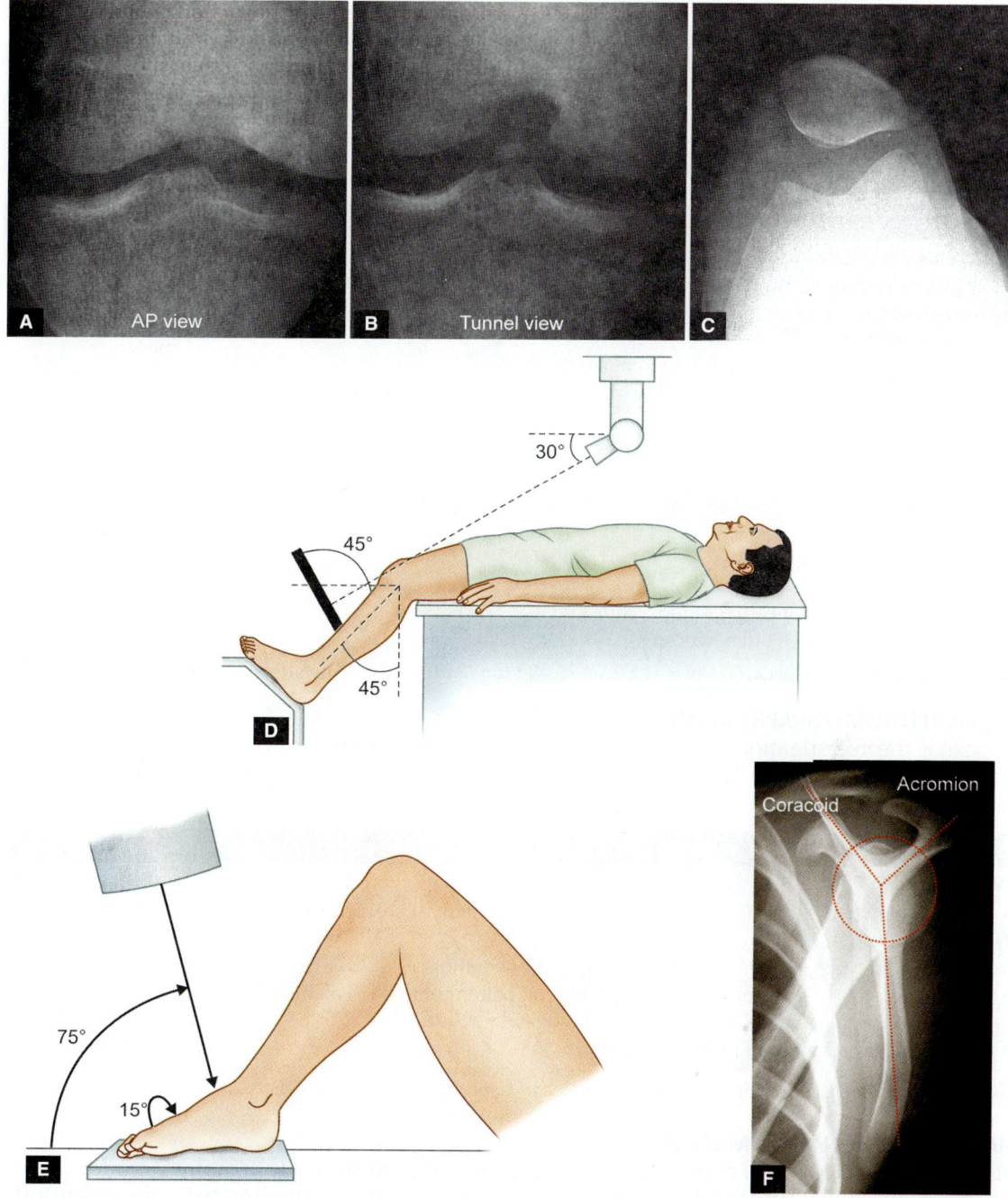

Fig. 3.4A to F: Important X-ray views. (A) AP view knee joint. (B) Tunnel view knee joint. (C) and (D) Merchant view knee joint. (E) Canale view for talar neck. (F) Scapular 'Y' view

ULTRASONOGRAPHY
USG in orthopedics has a long learning curve and has recently gained popularity in the assessment of joint and soft tissue pathologies.
- High frequency sound waves are used (2–18 MHz) and are produced by a special effect called "piezoelectric effect".
- Images are produced as hyper-/hypo-echoic.

- It provides the benefit of real-time imaging and evaluation of soft tissue near a metallic orthopedic hardware without the artifact that limits MR imaging.
- Its use in joint and soft tissue pathologies (muscle/tendon) is based on the fact that it is very sensitive to detect fluid signals (post-traumatic effusions and blood collections, pus collections) but due to subjective variation and long learning curve its use has been replaced by MRI in most of the indications.

Its main uses are listed in Table 3.2.

Table 3.2: Uses of ultrasound in orthopedics
Infection/inflammatory arthritis
• Useful for evaluation of soft tissue infections, any abscesses, muscle edema and status of draining lymph nodes
• Joint effusion can be noted best for visualization of septations or internal echoes within the joint fluid that are often seen in septic arthritis
• USG-guided aspiration of joint fluid to make diagnosis
• Thickened synovium with increased vascularity (pannus formation) is seen in rheumatoid arthritis
Trauma
• Mainly used for evaluation of vessels by using color Doppler: Vascular injury with a localized hematoma can be well appreciated in short time.
• Traumatic tendon tears: Acute or chronic tendon tears can be seen on USG, facilitated by dynamic evaluation.
Degenerative
• Tendon tears, muscle atrophy
Nerve compression
• Useful in evaluation of carpal tunnel syndrome
As a screening test in DDH in newborn.

Taken from Fundamentals of Orthopedics by Mohindra and Jain (2nd ed., Jaypee publishers)

COMPUTED TOMOGRAPHY SCAN

CT scan is the investigation for pathologies involving cortex and new bone formation (not useful for marrow involvement). It was developed by Godfrey Hounsfield. Uses of CT scan have been tabulated in Table 3.3.

Table 3.3: Uses of CT scan in orthopedics
Trauma
• Usually done after X-rays for better preoperative evaluation/3D reconstruction of joints or bones
Tumors
• MRI and X-rays are more often used to interpret bone tumors
• CT scan has role in selected cases to show extent, pattern of matrix calcification, status of adjacent bone cortex, periosteal reaction, presence of pathological fracture.
• CT angiography is a useful tool for vascular injury.

Taken from Fundamentals of Orthopedics by Mohindra and Jain (2nd ed., Jaypee publishers).

MAGNETIC RESONANCE IMAGING

MRI is the investigation of choice (IOC) for marrow, soft tissue (muscle, ligament, tendon, nerve, vessels, brain, spinal cord) and cartilage involvement. While CT scan principally shows only the bony structures, MRI shows the soft tissues very well. However, the IOC for stress fracture is MRI only as the marrow edema that is the earliest sign (even before cortical break) is best picked up by MRI.

Important MRI pulse sequences and their characteristics are as follows:

- *Proton density (PD) images:* Useful for meniscal pathology and anatomic details.
- *Gradient echo-T2 image:* Calcified areas and hemorrhage (appear hypointense/dark) are better identified, in fact, said to 'bloom' out. This characteristic can be useful in detecting loose bodies and pathologies like PVNS. Fibrocartilage, i.e. meniscus in knee and labrum in shoulder, can be visualized very nicely. 3D reconstruction of the images can be done.

Uses of MRI in orthopedics are given in Table 3.4.

Table 3.4: Uses of MRI in orthopedics
Investigation of choice in soft tissue (marrow, brain, spine, muscles, tendons, ligaments, cartilage, nerves) pathology detection
Trauma • Not routinely used • Investigation of choice (IOC) for unilateral stress fracture (bone scan can be preferred for bilateral stress fracture) and occult fracture like occult fracture neck of femur • Bone contusions can be seen, even when cortex is intact • Traumatic tendon ruptures, hematomas
Infection/inflammation • MRI is IOC in acute, subacute and chronic OM as it shows status of marrow of involved bone as well as adjacent soft tissues • Also, the preferred modality in septic arthritis and soft-tissue infections like pyo-myositis, necrotizing fasciitis
Tumors • Useful in assessing intramedullary spread, skip lesions, soft-tissue extent, status of adjacent neurovascular bundles • (The gold standard investigation for tumors is biopsy) Avascular necrosis/Perthes' disease—MRI is the investigation of choice

Taken from Fundamentals of Orthopedics by Mohindra and Jain (2nd ed., Jaypee publishers)

Role of contrast in MRI: Both CT scan and MRI employ use of contrast medium to further enhance the pathology and make its identification easier. While CT scans use iodine or barium compounds as contrast, gadolinium compounds are commonly employed as contrast material in MRI.

For visualizing joint pathologies, contrast materials can either be given by intravenous injection (indirect arthrography) or can be directly injected into the joint (direct arthrography).

BONE SCAN

Bone scan is a nuclear medicine test, i.e. it makes use of a small amount of radioactive substance (technetium 99m—labeled methylene diphosphonate) called tracer, to scan body tissues, especially bones. The tracer is injected into a vein and as it perfuses various tissues, the activity (radiations emitted by various tissues with uptake) is detected by using a gamma camera.

Activity in bone scan is recorded in three phases:

1. Early perfusion/flow phase (image taken 2–5 seconds after injection)
2. Middle blood pooling phase (image taken 5 min after injection)
3. Delayed bone phase (image taken 2–4 hours after injection): After 2–4 hours, most of isotope in blood is metabolized while the rest is taken up by bone, so bone pathologies can be elucidated. Areas with increased bone turnover/osteoblastic activity appear as areas of increased uptake (hot spots) on the scan and vice versa.

Uses of bone scan are given in Table 3.5.

Table 3.5: Uses of bone scan
Hot spots (*increased tracer uptake*): Metastasis, trauma, neoplasm, infection.
Cold spots (*decreased tracer uptake*): Multiple myeloma, histiocytosis X, metastasis from renal cell carcinoma/thyroid carcinoma (due to replacement of normal bone or marrow).
Superscan (*generalized/diffuse increased uptake*): Hyperparathyroidism, renal osteodystrophy, widespread Paget's disease, diffuse metastasis.

Taken from Fundamentals of Orthopedics by Mohindra and Jain (2nd ed., Jaypee publishers)

Some important points about bone scan to remember:
- In stress fracture, MRI is the investigation of choice but in cases with B/L stress fracture bone scan becomes the IOC.
- Lesions with lytic activity do not show activity in bone scan, e.g. multiple myeloma.
- Bone scan cannot identify the source of unknown primary but it can pick up tumors with bone to bone metastasis, e.g. (pneumonic) ONE: Osteosarcoma, neuroblastoma, Ewing's sarcoma.

PET-CT SCAN

It is combination of two modalities—positron emission tomography (PET) and CT scan. Unlike bone scan that is indicative of only osteoblastic activity, PET-CT detects any tumor cell activity. 18-FDG (fluorodeoxyglucose) is the most commonly used agent to study metabolism while 13-N ammonia is most commonly used agent to study perfusion.

In orthopedics, PET-CT is mainly used for finding occult primary in suspected patients with bone tumors, in follow-up of oncologic imaging to assess treatment response and for assessing distant/widespread metastasis.

Limitation: Osteoblastic lesions have limited uptake on PET so bone scan may be more valuable.
For metastasis IOC:
- Single lesion, soft tissue extension: MRI
- Multiple osteoblastic metastasis: Bone scan
- Multiple metastasis: PET scan.

Xtra Edge

- Gold standard for diagnosis is always tissue diagnosis. Infection and tumors can mimic each other (e.g. Ewing's sarcoma mimics osteomyelitis) clinically and radiologically as both arise from metaphysis and need tissue diagnosis for differentiation. Hence, all tissues obtained during a surgical procedure should be cultured and biopsied.
- For osteomyelitis, MRI gives the earliest diagnosis (within 24 hours) and is the IOC. Bone scan is next in preference to MRI, and can establish the diagnosis within 48–72 hours (the area of infection has increased uptake due to osteoblastic activity). Pyogenic osteomyelitis on X-rays will show loss of soft tissue planes after 24–48 hours (1st change). Day 7–10 solid periosteal reaction is identified (1st bony change). In tuberculosis, there is no periosteal reaction. The gold standard is aspiration of pus and isolation of organism (i.e. culture and sensitivity testing).
- Bone tumor: X-rays are used to localise the tumor, CT scan is for extent and cortical lesions, MRI is also the IOC for evaluating marrow extent, micrometastasis, skip lesions and soft tissue involvement in cases of bone tumors. PET scan and bone scan for multiple lesions. However, for confirming diagnoses of any tumor, biopsy is the gold standard.
- DDH: USG is considered the screening tool for DDH in neonatal age group as it allows evaluation of cartilaginous femoral head prior to appearance of ossific nucleus, subluxation, dislocation, pulvinar or inverted labrum, hypoplastic ossific nucleus, acetabular dysplasia and ossification. However, MRI allows assessment of complete disease spectrum, management and complications of DDH. T1W image displays exact position of the cartilage and T2W images are useful for complications like ischemic necrosis (AVN) and effusions which are not demonstrated with USG/X-ray.

  IOC for DDH depends on the type of que:
  - In first 6 months of life—USG is the IOC—as femoral head is primarily cartilaginous, so USG picks up well and getting MRI is unnecessary and challenging in this age group.
  - After 6 months of life—MRI is the IOC as femoral head starts ossifying, USG cannot pick up bone. X-ray can still diagnose after 6 months but MRI is the IOC to evaluate complete disease process. If question is asked simply IOC for DDH—MRI.
- *Rule of two in imaging*: Always obtain an X-ray of one joint above and one joint below the site of injury, in any suspected fracture.
- Order of investigations in inflammatory joint swelling (e.g. septic arthritis): X-ray → USG-guided aspiration of joint fluid → MRI.
- In general, fat has a high signal (bright) on T1-weighted MR images and fluid has a high signal on T2-weighted MR images. Structures with little water or fat, such as cortical bone, tendons, and ligaments, are hypointense (dark) in all types of sequences.
- In heterotopic ossification, the earliest detection can be done by a bone scan. However, the screening investigation for the purpose is alkaline phosphatase levels and prostaglandin E_2 level in 24-hour urine sample. A sudden increase in 24-hour urinary excretion of PGE_2 is an indication for bone scan.
- When patient has problems around a prosthetic joint, bone scan can be used to differentiate between infection and aseptic (non-infective) loosening of the prosthesis.

- Bone scan is highly sensitive for osteoblastic (sclerotic) lesions while FDG-PET CT is more sensitive for osteolytic lesions and marrow involvement. Hence, investigation of choice for osteoblastic/sclerotic metastasis is bone scan while for osteolytic metastasis it is FDG-PET CT.

Some commonly asked images in orthopedic radiology:

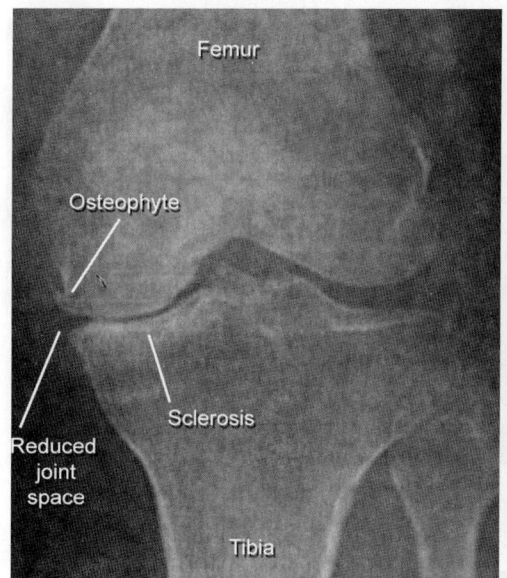
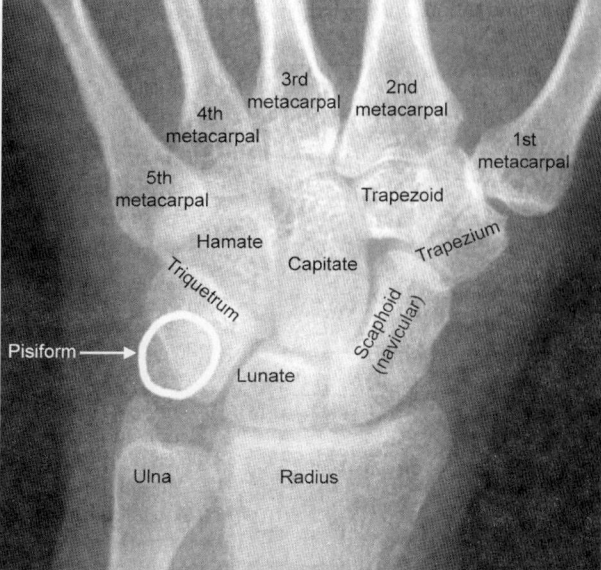

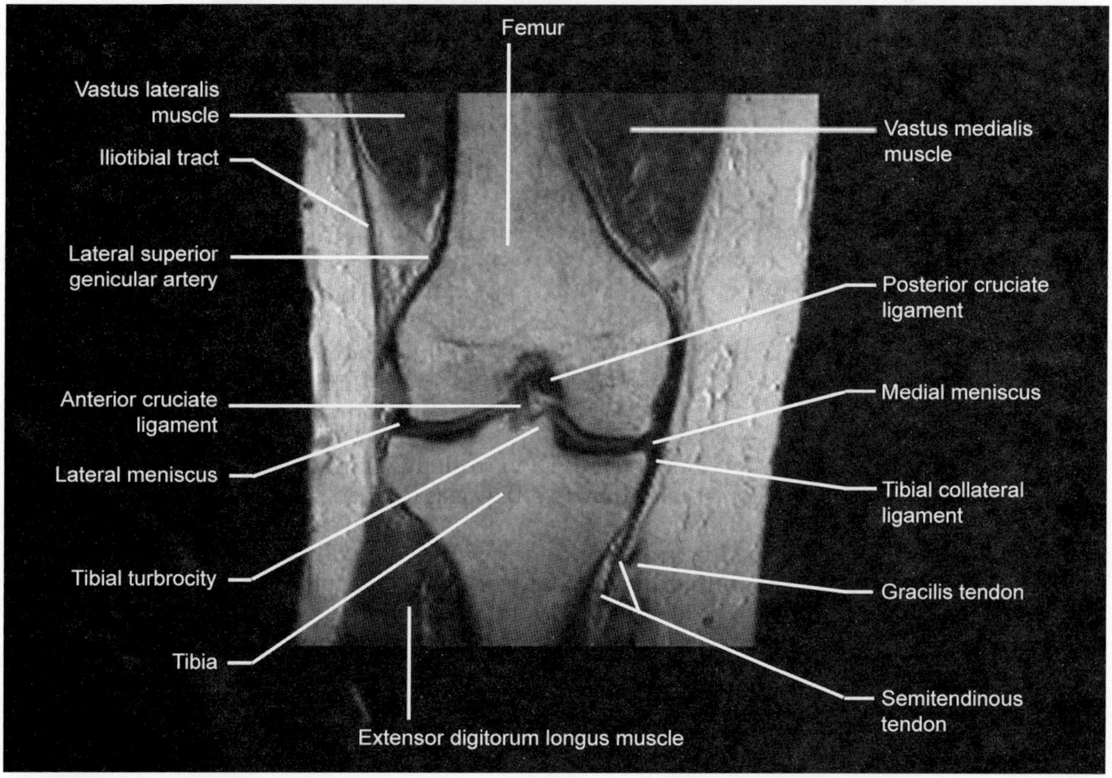

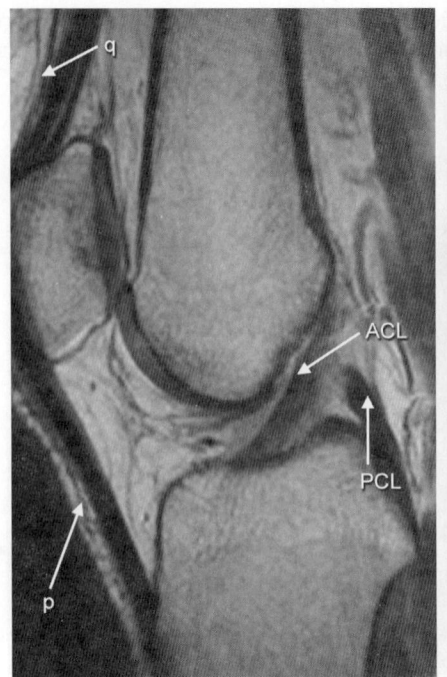

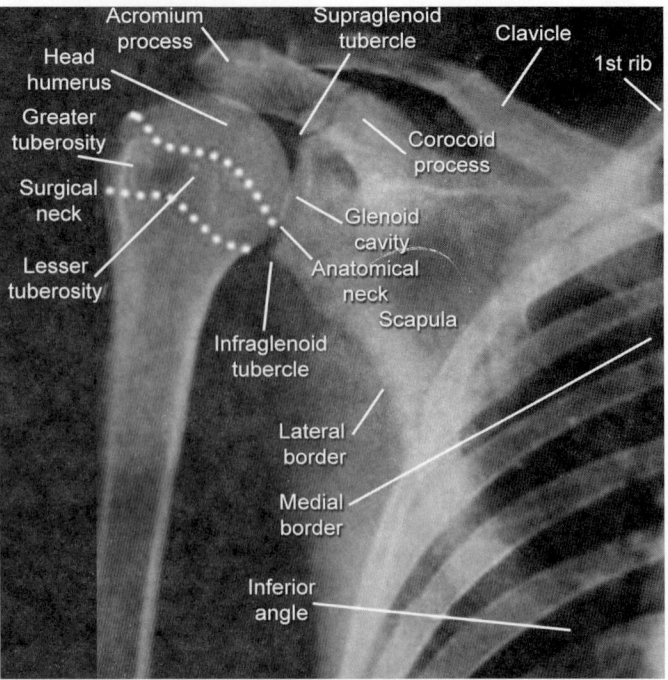

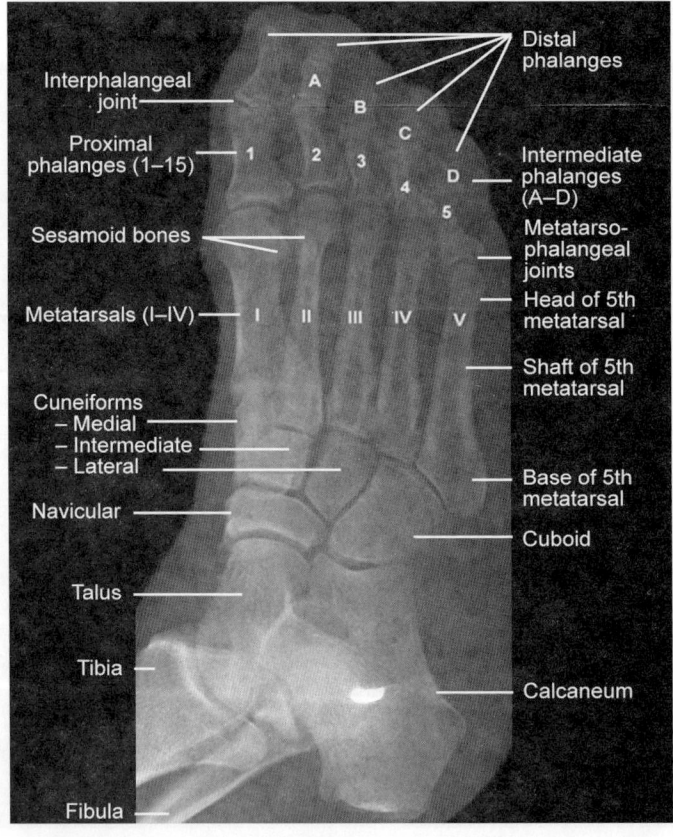

MULTIPLE CHOICE QUESTIONS

1. Acute osteomyelitis, earliest bone change can be seen by:
   - A. PET CT
   - B. MRI
   - C. Bone scan
   - D. X-ray

2. Stress fractures are diagnosed by:
   - A. X-ray
   - B. CT
   - C. MRI
   - D. Bone scan

3. Occult fracture NOF is diagnosed by:
   - A. CT
   - B. MRI
   - C. Bone scan
   - D. None

4. Which of the following is the IOC for Perthes' disease?
   - A. MRI
   - B. CT
   - C. X-ray
   - D. USG

5. Sunray appearance on X-ray is seen in:
   - A. Osteosarcoma
   - B. Osteochondroma
   - C. Osteoclastoma
   - D. Chondroblastoma

6. Sunray appearance in osteosarcoma is due to:
   - A. Blood vessel calcification
   - B. Bone resorption
   - C. Periosteal reaction
   - D. Muscle fiber calcification

7. Glass pieces in hand IOC:
   - A. X-ray
   - B. USG
   - C. MRI
   - D. CT scan

8. DDH best diagnostic modality is:
   - A. USG
   - B. MRI
   - C. X-ray
   - D. Clinical

9. Screening tool of neonatal hip instability:
   - A. USG
   - B. MRI
   - C. X-ray
   - D. CT scan

10. A 5-year-old girl child has presented with complaints of fever and mass in thigh. On X-ray, there is bony destruction and periosteal reaction. Next investigation to be done is:
    - A. CT scan
    - B. Blood culture
    - C. Bone biopsy
    - D. Bone scan

11. Periosteal reaction is seen in:
    - A. Osteomyelitis
    - B. Syphilis
    - C. Tumor
    - D. AL

12. A 4-year-old child complains of pain and swelling of left tibia. On evaluation, patient has high ESR, leucocytosis and X-ray depicts tibial lesion, best investigation is:
    - A. Blood C/S
    - B. MRI
    - C. Pus C/S
    - D. Biopsy

13. TB of spine best diagnostic modality is:
    - A. CT-guided biopsy
    - B. MRI
    - C. Clinical
    - D. X-ray

14. Best investigation for multiple bone metastasis?
    - A. PET-CT
    - B. MRI
    - C. Bone scan
    - D. CT

15. What is the earliest change of osteomyelitis on X-ray?
    - A. Loss of soft tissue planes
    - B. Sequestrum
    - C. Periosteal reaction
    - D. Lytic defects

16. What is the earliest bony change of osteomyelitis on X-rays?
    - A. Loss of soft tissue planes
    - B. Sequestrum
    - C. Periosteal reaction
    - D. Lytic defects

17. B/L stress fractures are diagnosed by:
    - A. X-ray
    - B. CT scan
    - C. Bone scan
    - D. MRI

18. A 45-year-old female has a history of fall in bathroom with C/O pain in right hip, tenderness in Scarpa's triangle and normal X-ray. Next investigation is:
    - A. MRI
    - B. CT
    - C. USG-guided aspiration
    - D. Bone scan

19. Dense regular connective tissue fibers are seen in all except:
    - A. Periosteum
    - B. Tendon
    - C. Ligament
    - D. Aponeurosis

20. A 10-year-old obese child from endocrinology department was referred to emergency department for painful limp with hip pain, which of the following is not required?
    - A. X-ray of hip
    - B. CT scan of hip
    - C. USG
    - D. MRI

ANSWERS

1. MRI > Bone scan
2. MRI (IOC for U/L is MRI and for B/L is bone scan), bone scan becomes the answer only when B/L is mentioned
3. B. MRI
4. A. MRI

5. A. Osteosarcoma
6. C. Periosteal reaction
7. A. X-ray
8. B. MRI
9. A. USG

10. C. Bone biopsy (all non-invasive investigation should be done before invasive investigation in tumors. Sequence is: X-ray > MRI > Biopsy)

11. All

12. D. Biopsy

13. A. CT-guided biopsy (tissue diagnosis is always better than any radiological diagnosis. If the question would have been best radiological modality, then the answer would have been MRI)

14. A. PET-CT

15. A. Loss of soft tissue planes

16. C. Periosteal reaction.

17. C. Bone scan

18. A. MRI (for stress fracture or occult fracture NOF marrow edema is seen in MRI)

19. A. Periosteum

20. B. CT scan

Any inflammatory joint swelling order of investigation is:

Non-invasive followed by invasive: X-ray > MRI/USG > USG-guided aspiration

D/D in this case are: Osteomyelitis, septic arthritis, Perthes, SCFE, transient synovitis of hip

4

Polytrauma

INTRODUCTION

Polytrauma patients are those patients who have sustained two or more severe injuries which endanger life (injury severity score > 18). The leading cause of polytrauma and death are road traffic accidents and mostly involved are the young and active population of society.

Three peak times of death after trauma
- 50% within the first minute of sustaining the injury caused by massive blood loss or neurologic injury.
- 30% within the first few days most commonly from neurologic injury.
- 20% within days to weeks following injury, multisystem organ failure and infection are leading causes.

Golden hour
- Period of time when life-threatening and limb-threatening injuries should be treated in order to decrease mortality.
- Estimated 60% of preventable deaths can occur during this time ranging from minutes to hours.

Use of an airbag in a head-on collision significantly decreases the rate of
- Closed head injuries
- Facial fractures
- Thoracoabdominal injuries
- Need for extraction

TRIAGE

This is a system deciding which patients should be treated first, depending on how severe are they injured. Patients are sorted into four color-coded groups of priority based on their need for evacuation and immediate treatment as outlined below.

1. **Priority 1 (red)**—immediate care needed
   - These patients cannot survive without immediate treatment, but have a chance of survival with immediate intervention.
2. **Priority 2 (yellow)**—urgent care needed
   - These patients are stable for the moment but require observation in a hospital.
   - These patients have injuries that are less severe than red categories, but may be life or limb threatening if treatment is delayed beyond several hours.
   - These patients may require a re-triage.
3. **Priority 3 (green)**—delayed care needed
   - These patients have only minor injuries and are tagged as walking wounded.
   - Treated after the red and yellow category patients have been treated.
4. **Priority 4 (black)**—dead. These are patients without obvious vitals signs.
   Priority 1 patients are those who are likely to deteriorate without medical help (requiring immediate intervention to save life) are attended first while injured, but walking in patients with stable vitals, classified into delayed (priority 3) category, are attended later as situation permits.

SEQUENCE IN MANAGEMENT OF POLYTRAUMA PATIENTS

Once triage has been done the patients who need emergency management are isolated. If a patient is found to be in cardiac arrest (absent carotid pulse and breathing for 10 seconds), immediate cardiopulmonary resuscitation is instituted using the Basic Life Support (BLS) or Advanced Cardiac Life Support (ACLS) protocols. For those patients who are not in cardiac arrest, a quick evaluation is started using the Advanced Trauma Life Support (ATLS) protocol to avoid an impending cardiac arrest in them.

ADVANCED TRAUMA LIFE SUPPORT (ATLS)

Concept behind ATLS is that save the life (i.e. prevent an impending cardiac arrest) by addressing the most dangerous threat to life first. Correct sequence for assessment and management of a polytraumatized patient (not in cardiac arrest or revived from arrest) is
- triage
- primary survey (identification of life-threatening injuries)
- adjuncts to primary survey
- patient transfer, if needed
- secondary survey (identification of non-life-threatening injuries)
- adjuncts to secondary survey
- re-evaluation and definitive care.

Prehospital Phase
- Airway maintenance
- Control of external bleeding and shock
- Immobilization of the patient
- Immediate transport to closest appropriate facility

Hospital Phase
- Triage
- Primary survey (A to F)
  A. Airway management with cervical spine management
    - Any patient with polytrauma or altered consciousness or blunt trauma above the level of clavicle is assumed to have cervical spine injury unless proved otherwise.
    - The patient should be logrolled.
    - Airway patency should be checked by chin lift or jaw thrust maneuver.
    - Causes of airway blockage may be foreign body, facial fractures, blood clots; but most common cause is the tongue that falls back and obstructs the airway in an unconscious patient.
    - *Management:* Oropharyngeal or nasopharyngeal airway
      Tracheal intubation: Indications
      - Inability to maintain adequate airway by above mentioned maneuver
      - The risk of aspiration
      - GCS score less than 8.
  B. Breathing and ventilation
    - Adequate breathing and ventilation require proper functioning of chest wall, diaphragm and lung.
    - The most serious injuries that can compromise breathing in a polytrauma patient include tension pneumothorax, massive hemothorax and flail chest.
  C. Circulation and hemorrhage control
    - External/internal bleeding should be controlled.
    - Sites of occult blood loss include chest, abdomen, retroperitoneum, pelvis and long bones.
  D. Disability and neurological status
    - Level of consciousness is conventionally assessed by GCS.
    - A practical approach of rapid assessment is simply asking the name or details of the accident and rating the patient as per the AVPU Scale: Alert, voice responsive, pain responsive or unresponsive. Patients with score below 'A' level must be carefully assessed by a formal GCS.

- Indications for neurological referral include deterioration in GCS, GCS less than 8, seizures, focal neurological signs and CSF leak.
  APVU Scale (Table 4.1)
  Glasgow Coma Scale (Table 4.2)
E. Exposure/environmental control:
  - Undress the patient and examine body parts.
  - Examination of back requires logrolling of the patient and requires at least five team members for the same.
  - Prevent hypothermia
F. Fracture splintage
  - The joints above and below must be immobilized.

Table 4.1: APVU Scale	
A	Awake and alert, spontaneous eye opening
B	Patient does not open eye spontaneously, but opens to verbal stimulation
C	Patient only respond to painful stimulation
D	Unresponsive patient

Table 4.2: Glasgow Coma Scale	
Eye-opening (E)	
• Spontaneous	4
• To speech	3
• To pain	2
• Nil	1
Best motor response (M)	
• Obeys	6
• Localises	5
• Withdraws	4
• Abnormal flexion	3
• Extensor response	2
• Nil	1
Verbal response (V)	
• Orientated	5
• Confused conversation	4
• Inappropriate words	3
• Incomprehensible sounds	2
• Nil	1
Coma score = E + M + V	
• Minimum	3
• Maximum	15

BASIC LIFE SUPPORT (BLS)

- This is a protocol for cardiopulmonary resuscitation that includes a series of steps that are instituted on emergency basis in any collapsed patient suspected to have a cardiac arrest.
- The protocol is designed to be performed not just by a doctor but a medical technician, a paramedic or even a qualified bystander who identifies such a patient.
  The steps in BLS are:
  - Chest compression— it takes priority over all other steps in patiens with cardiac arrest.
  - Airway management

- Breathing
- Defibrillation

The BLS protocol continues until:
- The patient regains a pulse
- The rescuer is relieved with another rescuer of higher training (i.e. an ALS team member)
- The rescuer is too physically tired to continue CPR
- The patient is pronounced dead by a doctor.

ADVANCED LIFE SUPPORT (ALS) AND ADVANCED CARDIOVASCULAR LIFE SUPPORT (ACLS)

- The most important point to highlight in the advanced life support system is the use of cardiac monitors to analyse the patient's heart rhythm (Table 4.3).
- In contrast to an AED in BLS, where the machine decides when and how to shock a patient, the ACLS team leader makes those decisions based on rhythms on the monitor and patient's vital signs.
- The legitimate factor in the decision to terminate resuscitation is an $ETCO_2$ (End tidal CO_2 production) of less than 10 mm Hg, measured on waveform capnography, after at least 20 minutes of resuscitation.

Table 4.3: Drugs used in ALS protocol for CPR	
Rhythm	*Drugs**
Shockable	Adrenaline 1 mg after 2nd shock and then every 2nd cycle Amiodarone 300 mg after 3rd shock
Non-shockable	Adrenaline 1 mg immediately and then every 2nd cycle

Caution: Routine atropine use is no longer recommended unless there is high risk for bradycardia

DAMAGE CONTROL ORTHOPEDICS (DCO)

Involves staging definitive management to avoid adding trauma to patient during vulnerable period. It is well known that intraoperative hypotension increases mortality rate in patients with head injury. So staging definitive management in such polytrauma patients would improve the outcome.

- Parameters that help decide who should be treated with DCO
  - Injury Severity Score* (ISS)>40 (without thoracic trauma)
  - ISS >20 with thoracic trauma
  - GCS of 8 or below
  - Multiple injuries with severe pelvic/abdominal trauma and hemorrhagic shock
  - Bilateral femoral fractures
  - Pulmonary contusion noted on radiographs
  - Hypothermia <35°C
  - Head injury with AIS of 3 or greater

Optimal Time of Surgery

The decision to operate and surgical timing on multiple injured trauma patients remains controversial. Patients are at increased risk of ARDS and multisystem failure during acute inflammatory window (period from 2 to 5 days characterized by a surge in inflammatory markers), therefore, only potentially life-threatening injuries should be treated in this period including:

- Compartment syndrome
- Fractures with vascular injuries
- Unreduced dislocations
- Long bone fractures
- Unstable spine fractures
- Open fractures

---

*Each injury is assigned an AIS (abbreviated injury score) and six body regions (head, face, chest, abdomen, extremities, including pelvis and external) are taken into consideration. Only the highest AIS score in each body region is used. The ISS score is the sum of squares of scores of three most severely injured regions. The score helps predict chances of survival.

In Pelvic Fractures
- Early temporary fracture stabilization followed by staged definitive management is the goal.
- Includes initial pelvic volume reduction via sheet, pelvic packing, skeletal traction, binder, or external fixation
- If hemodynamically stable
  - proceed with further imaging including CT chest, abdomen, pelvis
- If not hemodynamically stable
  - consider pelvic angiography and embolization
- Definitive treatment delayed for 7–10 days for pelvic fractures

In femur and tibial fractures, optimal time for surgery
- Within 3 weeks for femur fractures (conversion from external fixator to intramedullary nail)
- 7–10 days for tibia fractures (conversion from external fixation to intramedullary nail)

CRUSH SYNDROME (TRAUMATIC RHABDOMYOLYSIS)
- It is the systemic manifestation of extensive muscle injury due to severe crushing of muscles and subsequent release of cellular components of muscle cells into circulation.
- Process starts with crushing and compression opening stretch activated channels and shutting down Na/K channels at the cellular level. This leads to increased intracellular calcium, which in turn stimulates protease activity in cell leading to cellular lysis. After extrication (i.e. removal from entangled situation) restoration of blood flow to injured muscles, causes reperfusion injury. The limb may swell up rapidly leading to compartment syndrome.
- Biochemical features:
  - Influx of myoglobin, potassium, and phosphorus into the circulation
  - Hypocalcemia, hyponatremia, hypovolemic shock
- Renal injury is the most significant complication. Myoglobin released from the damaged myocytes precipitates in the PCT of kidney leading to renal failure.
- These results strongly suggest that free-radical scavengers are beneficial in attenuating or preventing reperfusion-induced injury to ischemic skeletal muscles and consequently to other organs, particularly the kidneys;
- These scavengers should be administered before crushed muscles are decompressed or as early as possible during reperfusion in order to prevent irreversible damage to ischemic cell.

Lab Investigations
- Urine myoglobin
- Serum CPK
- Chemistry panel (calcium, phosphrus, electrolytes)

Treatment
- Fluid requirements to be fulfilled
- Alkalinization of urine to be done
  - bicarbonate
  - acetazolamide
- Medical therapy involves
  - mannitol
  - allopurinol
  - benzamil
  - amiloride
  - K^+-sparing diuretic drug
- Dehydration is predisposing factor for renal failure
- Avoid IV calcium
  - unless there is danger of hyperkalemic arrhythmia, infusion of calcium is not indicated;
  - unless calcium is constantly infused, its administration will correct hypocalcemia only temporarily; most infused calcium is deposited in injured muscles, thus aggravating rhabdomyolysis and causing metastatic calcification.

- Metastatic calcification
  - danger that mild metabolic alkalosis resulting from mannitol—alkaline diuresis therapy may enhance metastatic calcification.

COMPOUND FRACTURES

Simple fracture/closed fracture—a fracture not communicating with the external environment, i.e. overlying skin and soft tissue are intact such that fracture hematoma does not drain into the external environment.

Open/compound fracture—that communicates with external environment, or in other words, where the hematoma is draining out from the wound due to disruption of soft tissues and skin in vicinity of fracture site. Open fractures of the tibia are the commonest open long bone fractures.

Gustilo-Anderson classification (Table 4.4) is the most commonly used classification system for open fractures and must be done after debridement of the wound as the grading can change after debridement.

Table 4.4: Gustilo-Anderson classification of compound fractures*	
Type/Grade	Features
I	Fracture wound <1 cm with minimal soft tissue injury and fracture comminution. Usually it is low energy trauma with clean wound.
II	Fracture wound >1 cm without extensive soft tissue damage and fracture comminution. There is mild-to-moderate soft tissue injury and mild-to-moderate wound contamination.
IIIA	Fracture wound >10 cm with extensive soft tissue injury and wound contamination, but with adequate soft tissue coverage (at least periosteum over bone is intact).
IIIB	Fracture wound >10 cm with extensive soft tissue damage and contamination. Soft tissue coverage is inadequate (periosteal stripping occurs and bone may be exposed) and require skin or flap grafting
IIIC	Any size of open wound with major vascular injury requiring repair.

*Gunshot wounds with fractures and open segmental fractures are classified as type III Gustilo-Anderson injuries.

General Management
- Open fractures are high velocity injuries and require management according to damage control orthopedics.
- 1st step is patient resuscitation and immediate shifting to OT.
- 2nd is IV antibiotics even before opening dressing.
- Thorough wound lavage and debridement.
- Assessment of muscle viability by 4 Cs (color, consistency, contraction, circulation).

Table 4.5: Open fracture management recommendations				
Type of fracture	Infection risk	Prophylactic antibiotics	Recommended saline irrigation	Wound closure
G-A type I	Increased (0–2%)	1st generation cephalosporin	With 3 liters	Usually, immediately after surgical intervention
G-A type II	Much increased (2–10%)	1st generation cephalosporin plus aminoglycoside	With 6 liters	Immediate or early (within 24 to 72 hours)
G-A type III	Maximum (10–50%)	1st generation cephalosporin plus aminoglycoside	With 9 liters	Immediate or early or delayed (after 72 hours)

Fracture Management

- Gustilo type I to IIIA can be safely managed by internal fixation and wound closure under antibiotic coverage.
- Type IIIB requires external fixation with wound coverage by plastic surgery like flaps or skin graft.
- Type IIIC requires external fixation and vascular repair.

Other Scores for Open Fractures

- Ganga score
- AO score (scoring system both open/closed fractures)
- Tscherene's score (scoring system both open/closed fractures).

MULTIPLE CHOICE QUESTIONS

1. **What is the GCS of a patient presenting after injury, confused, eye opening on painful stimuli, flexion withdrawal on left side and pointing on right side?**
   A. 8   B. 9
   C. 10   D. 11

2. **Some patients present with injury in casualty. Which of these needs to be first evaluated by the orthopedician?**
   A. Decrease capillary refill in the fingers of the patient
   B. Fracture with intra articular extension
   C. Patient with weakness of wrist extensors
   D. Patient with abrasion >10 cm over the fracture site

3. **A 30 years male suffers from road traffic accident and a car runs over his right leg. On examination, vitals are stable. The right leg is crushed with exposed muscles and bones. The debate about limb survival can be resolved to an extent by MESS score which includes all *except*:**
   A. BP   B. Nerve injury
   C. Velocity of trauma   D. Distal circulation

4. **A person falls from height of 35 feet according to an eye witness. He landed on his feet on the ground which does correlate with his statement if following fractures are present:**
   A. Foramen ring fracture with lumbar spine injury
   B. Depressed skull fracture with lumbar spine injury
   C. Gutter fracture with cervical injury
   D. Pelvic fracture with cervical spine injury

5. **Permissible ischemia time for a proximal limb amputation is:**
   A. 4 hours   B. 6 hours
   C. 8 hours   D. 12 hours

6. **Severely injured patient presents with spinal fracture and unconsciousness. First thing to be done is:**
   A. GCS scoring
   B. Spinal stabilization by cervical collar

   C. Mannitol drip to decrease ICT
   D. Airway maintenance

7. **Which of the following is not a component of the crush syndrome?**
   A. Myohemoglobinuria
   B. Massive crushing of muscles
   C. Acute tubular necrosis
   D. Bleeding diathesis

8. **Open fracture is treated by:**
   A. Tourniquet   B. Internal fixation
   C. Debridement   D. External fixation

9. **A compound fracture is initially treated by antibiotics, wound toilet and:**
   A. Skin cover   B. External splintage
   C. Prosthesis   D. Internal fixation

10. **All of the following factors evaluate the chances of amputation in a limb, *except*:**
    A. Age   B. BP
    C. Velocity of trauma   D. Presence of infection

11. **Motorcyclist's fracture is**
    A. Ring fracture of base of skull
    B. Comminuted fracture
    C. A hinged fracture where the skull separates into anterior and posterior halves
    D. Fracture base of skull

12. **A female child with abuse has fracture pelvis, multiple injuries and is bleeding per vaginum. The immediate step on presenting to the hospital is:**
    A. Inform the police
    B. Airway assessment
    C. External fixator application for pelvic fracture
    D. Blood transfusion

13. **In cardiopulmonary resuscitation, the commonly fractured ribs are:**
    A. 1st and 2nd
    B. 3rd and 4th
    C. 5th and 6th
    D. 8th and 9th

14. **Which of the following structures is fixed first during re-implantation of an amputated digit?**
   A. Bone
   B. Artery
   C. Vein
   D. Nerve
15. **In crush injuries of hand the greatest priority is given to repair of:**
   A. Tendons
   B. Skin
   C. Bone
   D. Arteries
16. **A victim of RTA with fracture shaft of femur, 1st line of management is:**
   A. IV fluids
   B. Splint
   C. Airway maintenance
   D. Breathing
17. **In cardiopulmonary resuscitation, the ribs that are fractured are:**
   A. 1st and 2nd
   B. 3rd and 4th
   C. 5th and 6th
   D. 8th and 9th
18. **Which of the following is not a component of crush syndrome?**
   A. Myohemoglobinuria
   B. Massive crushing of muscles
   C. Acute tubular necrosis
   D. Bleeding diathesis
19. **Crush syndrome is managed by:**
   A. 20% dextrose
   B. Hydrocortisone
   C. Maintaining high urine output
   D. Acidification of urine
20. **Compound fracture is:**
   A. Fracture with artery involvement
   B. Fracture with nerve involvement
   C. Fracture with skin involvement
   D. Fracture with muscle involvement
21. **Vascular repair is required in which Gustilo-Anderson type of fracture?**
   A. II
   B. I
   C. IIIB
   D. IIIC
22. **Tibial fracture with >1 cm wound, slight comminution and moderate crushing is:**
   A. Grade I
   B. Grade II
   C. Gade IIIA
   D. Grade IIIB
23. **In shotgun injuries**
   A. Each and every shot should be removed
   B. All the shots within accessible limits may be removed and thorough debridement of all the tissues are done
   C. Shots lodged in joints must be removed
   D. All the above are true
24. **Following are principles in the treatment of compound fractures _except:_**
   A. Wound debridement
   B. Immediate wound closure
   C. Tendon repair
   D. Aggressive antibiotic therapy
25. **Which of the following is the most appropriate hospital treatment of a patient with compound fracture?**
   A. Under anesthesia, thorough scrubbing and cleaning of the area getting the fracture end inside, suturing the wound and applying continuous skeletal traction with adequate antibiotic cover
   B. Cleaning and suturing the wound, applying plaster spica under traction on a Harly's table and administering antibiotics round the clock
   C. Scrubbing and cleaning the area. Resecting the protruding one inch of the bone, suturing the wound, bringing the fractured ends into alignment and applying plaster Spica with continuous antibiotic cover
   D. Thorough cleaning of the area, extending the wound bringing the fragments into alignment under vision, fixing them with intramedullary nail and giving antibiotics to the patient
26. **Internal splints are used in all _except:_**
   A. Compound fractures
   B. Multiple fractures
   C. Fractures in elderly patients
   D. Fracture neck of femur
27. **A compound fracture is initially treated by antibiotics, wound toilet and**
   A. Skin cover
   B. External splintage
   C. Prosthesis
   D. Internal fixation
28. **Immediate treatment of compound fracture of tibia is**
   A. Intravenous antibiotics
   B. Thorough irrigation of wound with saline and splintage
   C. Wound debridement
   D. Internal fixation of fracture

ANSWERS

1. D. 11
2. A. Decrease capillary refill in the fingers of the patient
3. B. Nerve injury
4. A. Foramen ring fracture with lumbar spine injury
4. B. 6 hours
   Irreversible necrotic changes begin in muscles after 6 hours of ischemia (warm

ischemia time), it is preferable to begin the replantation of parts with good muscular bulk (viz. parts proximal to palms and foot) within this time. With cooling (to 4°C), this time may be extended to 12 hours (cold ischemia time)

6. D. Airway maintenance

   Concept behind ATLS is that save the life (i.e. prevent an impending cardiac arrest) by addressing the most dangerous threat to life first.

7. D. Bleeding diathesis

8. C, D

   This is an incomplete question, as grade is not mentioned and treatment depends on type/grade of open fracture. However, debridement is done in all grades and followed by internal/external fixation. Thus the best answer here is debridement.

9. B. External splintage

10. D. Presence of infection

11. C. A hinged fracture where the skull separates into anterior and posterior

12. B. Airway assessment

13. C. 5th and 6th

   The most commonly fractured ribs are 5th, 6th and 7th

14. A. Bone

15. B. Skin

   But while the concerned digit/amputated part is addressed skin is preserved first, for adequate skin coverage for deeper structures and palmar skin is very important as its sensation is not reproducible by skin graft.

16. C. Airway maintenance

17. C. 5th and 6th

18. D. Bleeding diathesis

19. C. Maintaining high urine output

20. C. Fracture with skin involvement

21. D. IIIC

22. B. Grade II

23. B. All the shots within accessible limits may be removed and thorough debridement of all the tissues are done.
   Only accessible pellets should be attempted to remove, else more harm would be done than good in removing the pellets.

24. B. Immediate wound closure

25. A. Under anesthesia, thorough scrubbing and cleaning of the area getting the fracture end inside, suturing the wound and applying continuous skeletal traction with adequate antibiotic cover

26. A. Compound fractures
   In compound fractures external splintage is done rather than internal.

27. B. External splintage

28. B. Thorough irrigation of wound with saline and splintage

5

Amputations

INTRODUCTION

- **Amputation** is a surgical/traumatic removal of a part or all of a limb through one or more bones.
- When the disarticulation occurs through a joint, then it is called disarticulation.

Most common cause
- *India:* RTA
- *World:* Peripheral vascular disease (e.g. Buerger's disease) and diabetes.
  Approximately half of amputations for PVD is performed in patients with diabetes
- *Children:* Congenital limb deficiency followed by trauma.

Indications

Absolute Indications

In real sense, the only absolute indication for amputation is irreversible ischemia in a diseased or traumatized limb.
- **Trauma:** Leading to irreversible loss of blood supply
  - Vascular injury with warm-ischemia time > 6 hours.
  - Gustilo-Anderson Grade IIIC injury
  - Open tibial fractures that include complete disruption of tibial nerve.
- **Gas gangrene:** Clostridial infection causes severe myonecrosis that spreads rapidly within 24 hours and has a typical mousy odor. Such limbs may better be amputated to prevent a fulminant life-threatening toxemia.
- **Microvascular disease:** Buerger's gangrene.
- **Diabetic gangrene:** The cause of amputation in diabetes is both peripheral neuropathy and microvascular disease. Peripheral neuropathy causes insensate limb leading to repeated trauma and non-healing ulcers which is further aggravated by microvascular problems which delays healing and infection due to favorable local environment.
  - The most significant predictor of amputation in diabetes is peripheral neuropathy.

Relative Indications

- **Infection**
- **Frostbite:** In sharp contrast to traumatic and other amputation, amputation in frostbite should be delayed till clear demarcation of viable tissue is visible which may take as long as 2–6 months.
  - The only exception to the above rule in frostbite is removal of a circumferentially constricting eschar.
- Tumors
- Burn
- Trauma leading to nonfunctional limb
- Chronic osteomyelitis
- Congenital anomalies.

Immediate Care of a Traumatic Amputation

ATLS guidelines in traumatic amputation changes from "ABC" to "CABC", i.e. immediate control of major bleeding by ligatures/tourniquet, etc. A patient with traumatic amputation is much more likely to die with hemorrhage rather than airway problem, so control of bleeding comes first.

PREDICTOR OF AMPUTATION IN A PATIENT WITH TRAUMA
- Mangled extremity severity score (MESS)
- Ganga Score (score ≥14 will lead eventually to amputation)
- Limb salvage index.

MESS
It is a score which predicts salvagibility of limb in a patient of trauma.

	Score	
V: Velocity of trauma	1–4	
I: Ischemia	1–4	
S: Shock	0–2	VISA to death
A: Age	0–1	
Total	11	

Higher the score, higher are the chances of amputation, with a score of ≥ 7 leading to eventual amputation.

Types
1. **Closed amputation**
   - When the skin over the stump is closed, then its k/a closed amputation.
   - Bone is always kept shorter than soft tissue to facilitate closure of stump.
   - Nerves are gently retracted and cut sharply so that they are not superficial on stump and cause pain and cut sharply to avoid neuroma formation.
   - Muscles are always divided at least 5 cm distal to bone resection.
   - Thus nerves are cut most proximal; more than bone or muscles.
2. **Open (guillotine) amputation**
   - Limb is transacted at one level through skin, muscle and bone.
   - The skin is not closed over the end of the stump.
   - It always requires a second operation for closure, re-amputation, plastic repair.
   - It is indicated in infections and severe traumatic amputations with extensive tissue destruction and gross contamination.
     - Therefore purpose of guillotine is to prevent/eliminate infection and preserve length.
   - Nowadays typical guillotine amputation is not performed and only fish mouth flaps are preferred so that bone is not left exposed.

For stabilization of stump muscles, either of the two methods is used:
- **Myodesis:** Here the muscles are attached to bone end by drill holes. This is the preferred method, but contraindicated in patients with severe limb ischemia (e.g. PVD) because increased tension in muscle will further deteriorate vascularity.
- **Myoplasty:** Here muscle is sutured to periosteum, fascia or muscle of an antagonist group. Muscles should preferably be divided around 5 cm distal to the bony resection level.

Myodesis is better because it helps maximize strength and minimize atrophy and it continues counterbalancing its anatagonists and thereby preventing contractures and maximizing residual limb function.

Once muscles have been stabilized, the skin flaps can be fashioned in either of the following ways:
- *Skewed:* When there is a long posterior flap, commonly preferred method for below knee amputation.
- *Scandinavian:* Where there are equal medial and lateral flaps; mainly used in cases of PVD.

One must also know how to handle the neurovascular bundle. The blood vessels must be doubly ligated with nonabsorbable sutures to prevent any accidental bleeding postoperatively. Nerves are gently pulled and transacted with a sharp knife to ensure that end retracts proximal to the bone ends, thereby preventing the formation of a painful neuroma at the stump. Large nerves like sciatic nerve carry their vasa vasora along and hence should be ligated before transacting.

Use of Tourniquet
- The use is desirable as it lessens the blood loss and provides a clear surgical field.
- But the limb must be properly exsanguinated before inflating the tourniquet.
- However, exsanguination is contraindicated in cases where indication is an infection or malignancy for the fear of spreading the pathology proximally.

IDEAL STUMP
1. Nontender
2. Well healed
3. Nonadherent
4. Nonbulbous
5. Skin at the end of stump is mobile and sensate
6. Stump shape properly constructed for proper prosthetic fitting.

RECOMMENDED LEVELS IN VARIOUS AMPUTATIONS
Golden rule—preserve as much length as possible because shorter stumps consume more energy in walking.
- *Above knee amputation:* 18 cm below the tip of greater trochanter or 12 cm from the medial joint line.
- *Below knee amputation:* 15 cm from the medial joint line (ideally at the musculotendinous junction of gastrocnemius)
- *Above elbow amputation:* 20 cm from the acromion
- *Below elbow amputation:* 18 cm from the tip of olecranon.
  Rule of thumb for selecting the level of bone resection—allow 2.5 cm (1 inch) of bone length for each 30 cm (1 foot) of body height.

Energy expenditure with amputation at various levels is inversely proportional to length of remaining limb
  - Long below knee amputation: 10%
  - Medium below knee amputation: 25%
  - Short below knee amputation: 40%
  - Average above knee amputation: 65%
  - Hip disarticulation: 100%

Thus length should always be preserved. Conversely, a non-ambulatory patient with a knee flexion contracture should not undergo a *trans*-tibial amputation because a *trans*-femoral amputation or knee disarticulation provides better function and less risk.

NOMENCLATURE FOR SOME SPECIFIC AMPUTATIONS (Figs 5.1A and B)

Lower Limb Amputations (Fig. 5.2)
- *Hindquarter amputation:* Whole of the lower limb with half of the ilium is removed
- *Lisfranc's amputation:* Amputation at tarsometatarsal junction
- *Chopart's amputation:* Midtarsal joint amputation
- *Syme's amputation:* Talus and calcaneus are removed with rotation of heel pad to close the stump through the dome of the ankle. Distal tibia and fibula 0.6 mm proximal to the periphery of the ankle joint are also removed.
  - Modifications of Syme's amputation:
    - Sarmiento's amputation: Distal tibia and fibula are cut 1.3 mm proximal to the ankle joint with excision of medial and lateral malleoli.
    - Boyd's amputation: In Boyd's amputation, after telectomy calcaneus is shifted forward and calcaneotibial arthrodesis is done.
    - Pirogoff's amputation: Vertical section of the calcaneus is performed through the middle and calcaneus is rotated forward to fuse to the tibia. Talectomy is performed as well. Basically, both Boyd and Pirogoff's amputation involve calcaneotibial arthrodesis.

Upper Limb Amputations
- **Forequarter amputation:** Removal of scapula along with a portion of clavicle and whole of the upper limb.

- **Krukenberg amputation:** It is done in below elbow amputation to provide a pincer grasp. It is primarily indicated in blind bilateral hand amputee. This amputation separates the radius and ulna in a shape of forceps (motored by pronator teres muscle) to be used as a makeshift pincer (Fig. 5.3).
- **Ray amputation:** Removal of a finger/toe with respective metacarpal/metatarsal

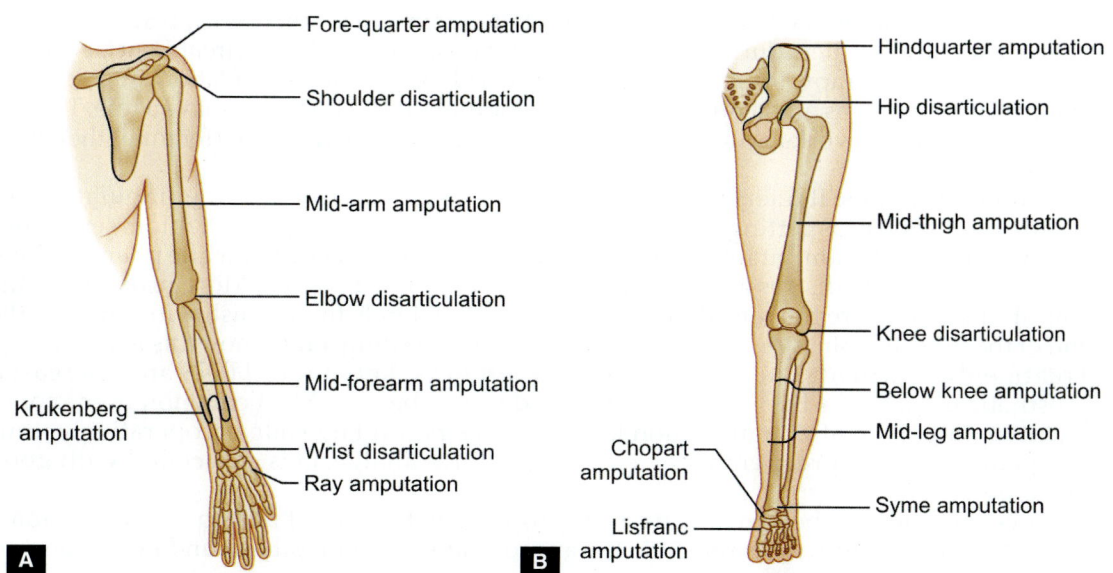

Figs. 5.1A and B: Levels of various amputations. (A) Upper limb and (B) Lower limb

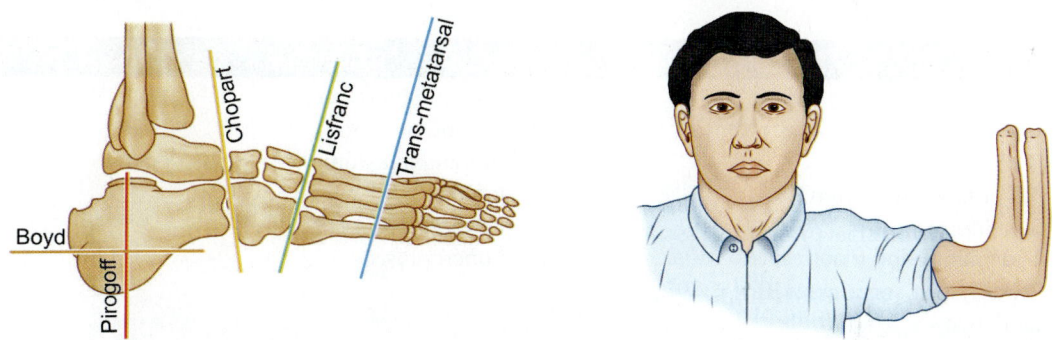

Fig. 5.2: Sites of bone resection in different types of amputation   **Fig. 5.3:** Krukenberg amputation

Special Considerations in Children
- For performing an amputation in children, Krajbich principles are often looked at.
  1. In children aim should be to preserve the growth plates
  2. Preserve all length possible.
  3. In lower limb amputations, wherever possible knee joint should be preserved.
  4. Disarticulation is preferred over transosseous amputation.
  5. Stabilize and normalize the proximal portion of the limb.
  6. The most common issue that bothers in most cases is the terminal bone growth that sometimes needs revision. One way of dealing with this problem is to use epiphyseal caps to cover medullary canals.
- Complications after surgery tends to be less severe in children
- Painful phantom sensations do not develop

- Neuromas rarely are troublesome
- Psychological problems after amputation are rare in children.

COMPLICATIONS
- Bleeding
- Skin flap necrosis
- Infection
- **Postamputation neuroma:** To prevent postamputation painful neuroma the nerves are generally pulled before cutting them during amputation and in case it forms, the best treatment is excision. While ultrasonic therapy is not much effective, pulsed radiofrequency ablation, interferential therapy (IFT) and transcutaneous electrical nerve stimulation (TENS) may have a role. TENS is most preferred and works by inhibiting pain gate pathway (TENS > Interferential therapy > USG).
- **Phantom sensations:** It refers to a situation where the patient feels that the amputated part is still present and he is getting discomforting sensations from that part. Phantom sensations are so common after amputation that they must be considered normal while phantom limb pains are extremely distressing and are present in 30–80% patients. More proximal is the amputation, more are the sensations felt. The problem tends to diminish with time. By the end of the first year phantom limb gradually shortens to stump end (known as telescoping). Treatment is difficult and antidepressants, opioids, ketamine, TENS and increased prosthetic use all have been reported to provide some benefit. Most common predictor of phantom limb pain after amputation is unbearable painful episode preoperatively, thus adequate analgesia preoperatively, e.g. via epidural analgesia is associated with good outcomes.
- **Joint contractures:** These result from improper positioning of stump and inadequate physiotherapy. Contractures preclude the appropriate use of prosthesis and hence must be prevented.
- **Sequestrum:** Excessive periosteal stripping during the procedure should be avoided as if this gets complicated further by infection, a ring sequestrum may form at the stump (Table 5.1).

Table 5.1: Different types of sequestra	
Ring sequestrum	Amputation stumps
	Around pin tracts
Conical sequestrum	Amputation stump
Pencil-like sequestrum	Infants
Coralliform	Perthes' disease
Rice grain sequestrum	Tuberculosis
Coke-shaped sequestrum	
Sand type sequestrum	
Kissing sequestrum	Paradiscal tuberculosis of spine
Feathery sequestrum	Tuberculosis > Syphilis
Ivory sequestrum	Syphilis
Tubular sequestrum	Hematogenous osteomyelitis
	Segmental fractures (middle segment)
Button sequestrum	Pheochromocytoma
Bombay sequestrum	On the exposed surface of bone due to hydrogen sulphide deposition
Colored sequestrum	Fungal
Black sequestrum	Gunshot
	Actinomycosis
Linear/flake sequestrum	Only one cortex involved
Muscle	Volkmann's ischemic contracture

EXTRA EDGE

- Interesting historical facts about amputations:
  - Amboise Pare, a French military surgeon, introduced the use of ligatures in 1529. He is called *father of amputation surgery*. He also performed the first elbow disarticulation.
  - First hip disarticulation was performed by William Kerr of England.
  - Antiseptic techniques were introduced by Joseph Lister (father of antiseptic surgery, 1867).
- Most common amputation overall: Transtibial.
- Risk of wound complications is increased when the patient has a low total lymphocyte count (TLC) level and a low serum albumin level.
- In diabetics, a below knee amputation is relatively contraindicated due to vascular issues.
- Knee disarticulation and Syme's amputation have end-bearing stumps. End-bearing stumps are those stumps where bone ends are metaphyseal and weight can be taken through the end of the stump.
- Lisfranc and Chopart amputations have a severe tendency to go into equinus.
- Amputees are advised to walk slow and take longer steps rather than taking several short steps to lower their energy consumption.
- There is no phantom limb sensation in congenital limb deficiencies and patients with brain damage.
- Syme's amputation (Edinberg; James Syme; 1843)
  - It is more energy efficient than mid-foot amputation even though it is more proximal.
  - Stable heel pad is the most important factor in Syme's amputation as migration of the heel pad is the most important complication. It has been used successfully to treat forefoot gangrene in diabetics, but the patent tibialis posterior artery is a prerequisite.

PROSTHOTICS

Prosthesis is an artificial device (metallic or non-metallic) that replaces a body part. It is a functional replacement for an amputated or congenitally malformed or missing limb. A prosthesis can replace an internal body part (e.g. hemiarthroplasty prosthesis) or replaces the part externally (e.g. artificial limb). It is easier to design a prosthesis for a lower limb but in upper limb, considering the dexterity, functional demand and cosmesis, still a lot of advancement is needed to achieve satisfactory designs.

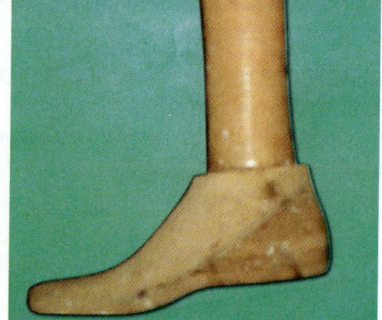

Fig. 5.4: SACH foot

Pylon prosthesis—a temporary prosthesis in immediate postoperative period wherein a metal pylon with a prosthetic foot is attached to the cast and properly aligned for ambulation.

Some commonly used prostheses are:

- *Above knee prosthesis:* Quadrilateral socket prosthesis
- *Below knee amputation:* Patellar tendon bearing prosthesis
- *Syme's amputation:* Canadian Syme's prosthesis
- *Partial foot amputations:* Shoe fillers.

Foot prosthesis for amputation stump (Table 5.2)

Solid ankle cushion heel (SACH) foot (Fig. 5.4)

Jaipur foot (designed by Dr PK Sethi) (Fig. 5.5)

ORTHOTICS

Orthosis is a device that aids or supports a body part and enhances its structural and functional characteristics.

Floor reaction orthosis: This is an AFO that is generally used with patients affected by neurological conditions such as spina bifida, cerebral palsy, and post-polio paralysis. In these cases, the floor

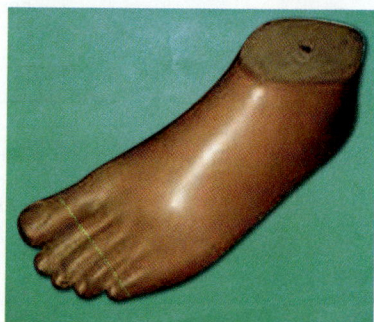

Fig. 5.5: Jaipur foot

Table 5.2: Differences between Jaipur and SACH foot

Jaipur foot	SACH foot
It looks like a normal foot so the patient does not need to wear shoe over it. However, amputee can use shoe satisfactorily over it. For the same reason barefoot walking is possible.	It requires a shoe over it for walking and also to hide it. Barefoot walking is not possible.
It has metallic keel which is confined to the ankle only and allows for dorsiflexion and plantar flexion to take place and thus allowing for squatting.	It has a rigid wooden keel which does not allow for dorsiflexion and plantar flexion and thus squatting is not possible.
Jaipur foot allows for adequate inversion and eversion of terminal piece so walking on uneven and muddy surface is comfortable.	Walking only on level ground is comfortable as it does not allow for inversion and eversion at "sub-tarsal" level.
Cross-legged sitting is possible due to adequate forefoot adduction and transverse rotation of the foot.	Cross-legged sitting is not possible.
It is very cheaper than an SACH foot. It can be made from locally available material by rural artisan.	It is very costlier than Jaipur foot. Modern technology with skilled personnel is required to manufacture it.
Shock absorbing capacity is less than a SACH foot.	The shock absorbing capacity is more than a Jaipur foot.
It meets the sociocultural needs (bare foot walking, cross-legged sitting) of Indian and many Asian populations.	It does not meet such needs and is more useful for western lifestyle.

reaction AFO functions to increase knee extension during midstance and compensate for weak or gastrosoleus muscles.

REIMPLANTATION OF AMPUTATED PARTS

The order of repair is given below (Fig. 5.6). But while the concerned digit/amputated part is addressed skin is preserved first, for adequate skin coverage for deeper structures and palmar skin is very important as its sensation is not reproducible by skin graft.

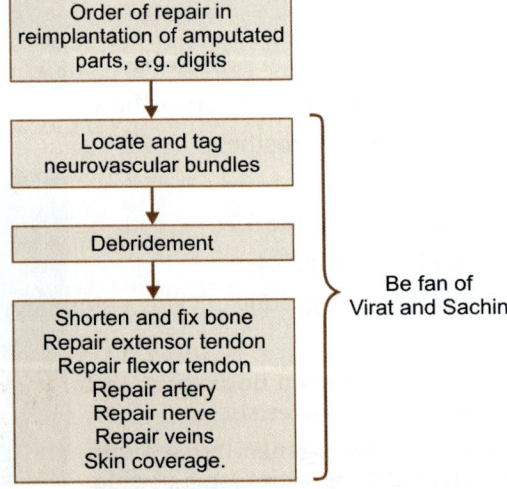

Fig. 5.6: Reimplantation of amputated parts

MULTIPLE CHOICE QUESTIONS

1. **Which of the following is the ideal length of bone for a below knee stump?**
   A. 12.5 cm to 17.5 cm
   B. Less than 5 cm long
   C. 7.5 cm to 10 cm long
   D. 20 cm long

2. **Procedure contraindicated in diabetics:**
   A. Ray amputation
   B. Forefoot amputation
   C. Syme's amputation
   D. Below knee amputation

3. **Best treatment modality for postamputation neuroma is:**
   A. Compression bandage
   B. Ultrasound
   C. Infrared
   D. Interferential therapy

4. **Pain due to postamputation neuroma is best treated by:**
   A. Infrared therapy
   B. Interference therapy
   C. Ultrasound therapy
   D. Surgical excision

5. **Pain due to postamputation neuroma can be managed by all *except*:**
   A. Infrared therapy
   B. Interference therapy
   C. Ultrasound therapy
   D. Stump bandaging

6. **An amputation through forearm where you make a fork of the two forearm bones is k/a:**
   A. Chopart's amputation
   B. Krukenberg's amputation
   C. Pirogoff amputation
   D. Syme's amputation

7. **Energy consumption in an above knee amputation is approximately:**
   A. 20%   B. 40%
   C. 55%   D. 65%

8. **Regarding SACH foot, all are true *except*:**
   A. Solid ankle cushion heel
   B. Prosthesis
   C. Squatting is easy
   D. Does not look like a normal foot

9. **In flap method of amputation which structure is kept shorter than the level of amputation**
   A. Bone
   B. Muscles
   C. Nerves
   D. Skin
   E. Vessels

10. **Myodesis is employed in amputations for all of the following indications *except*:**
    A. Trauma   B. Tumor
    C. Children   D. Ischemia

11. **Lisfranc's fracture dislocation/amputation:**
    A. Fracture dislocation through tarsometatarsal joint
    B. Fracture dislocation through ankle joint
    C. Fracture dislocation through subtalar joint
    D. Fracture dislocation through midtarsal joint

12. **Tarsometatarsal amputation is k/a:**
    A. Chopart's amputation
    B. Lisfranc's amputation
    C. Pirogoff's amputation
    D. Syme's amputation

13. **Amputation is often not required in:**
    A. Gas gangrene
    B. Buerger's disease
    C. Chronic osteomyelitis
    D. Diabetic gangrene

14. **B/K amputation:**
    A. 5 cm below tibial tuberosity
    B. 10 cm below tibial tuberosity
    C. 15 cm below tibial tuberosity
    D. 5 cm below patella
    E. 10 cm below patella

15. **In below elbow amputation the length of the stump (distance from olecranon should be):**
    A. 10–15 cm   B. 15–20 cm
    C. 20–25 cm   D. 5–10 cm

16. **Ring sequestrum is seen in:**
    A. Typhoid osteomyelitis
    B. Chronic osteomyelitis
    C. Amputation stump
    D. Tubercular osteomyelitis

17. **Which of the following is true regarding a phantom limb?**
    A. Occurs in leprosy
    B. Follows amputation
    C. Follows a psychiatric illness

18. **All of the following are true about SACH foot *except*:**
    A. SACH stands for "solid ankle cushion heel"
    B. Forms the base of a lower limb prosthesis
    C. May wear out with time
    D. Wooden keel absorbs the impact on heel strike

19. **Most common cause of amputation in India is:**
    A. Diabetic gangrene   B. RTA
    C. Gas gangrene   D. Tumors

20. **Jaipur foot was invented by?**
    A. BL Sehgal   B. PK Sethi
    C. Rajnath   D. SK Verma

21. **Principle of TENS for alleviating pain around joints and nerve:**
    A. Referred pain
    B. Gate control theory of pain
    C. Interferential therapy
    D. Compression bandage

22. **In reconstruction of limb, what is done first?**
    A. Nerve repair
    B. Bone fixation
    C. Artery repair
    D. Vein repair

ANSWERS

1. A. 12.5 cm to 17.5 cm
2. D. Below knee amputation
   Below knee amputation is avoided in Biabetics due to vascular issues
3. D. Interferential therapy
4. D. Surgical excision
5. C. Ultrasound therapy
6. B. Krukenberg's amputation
7. D. 65%
8. C. Squatting is easy
9. C. Nerves >, A. Bone
10. D. Ischemia
11. A. Fracture dislocation through tarso-metatarsal joint
12. B. Lisfranc's amputation
13. C. Chronic osteomyelitis
    Its a relative/rare indication for amputation, while all others are absolute indication.
14. C. 15 cm below tibial tuberosity
15. B. 15–20 cm from olecranon
16. C. Amputation stump
17. B. Follows amputation
18. D. Wooden keel absorbs the impact on heel strike. The heel absorbs the impact of heel strike and provides pseudoplantar flexion (flexibility), whereas the rigid wooden keel provides midstance stability.
19. B. RTA
20. B. PK Sethi
21. B. Gate control theory of pain
22. B Bone fixation

6

Upper Limb Fractures

ACUTE SHOULDER SUBLUXATION/DISLOCATION

Anatomy

Shoulder joint is a ball and socket joint with maximum range of movement because it is inherently unstable. Glenoid fossa is a flattened dish-like structure with humeral head sitting over it, like a golf ball on a tee. Only 1/4th of humeral head articulates with glenoid at any range of movement. The depth of glenoid cavity is increased by fibrocartilaginous labrum by 50%, thus increasing stability. Humeral head is rotated by 15–20° posteriorly (i.e. retroverted) in relation to the shaft.

Static stabiliser of joint
- Capsule—inferior part of the capsule is the weakest part.
- Glenohumeral ligaments , labrum , negative intra-articular pressure.

Dynamic stabiliser
- Rotator cuff—**minor SIT:** Supraspinatus, infraspinatus and teres minor (inserts on GT) and subscapularis (inserts on LT) are rotator cuff muscles.
- Deltoid and biceps.

Anterior Shoulder Dislocation

It is the most common type of shoulder dislocation and head lies subcoracoid > subglenoid > subclavicular > intrathoracic. Mechanism of injury is a hyperabduction and external rotation force (shoulder in throwing position).
- Arm lies in slight abduction
- Loss of normal rounded contour of shoulder
- Tests of dislocated shoulder—(**Bryant, DCH**)
  - Bryant's test—anterior axillary fold is at a lower level.
  - Dugas' test—patient cannot touch opposite shoulder, i.e. limited adduction and internal rotation.
  - Callaway's test—vertical circumference (distance from shoulder top till base of axilla) of shoulder is increased due to dislocated head occupying this space.
  - Hamilton ruler test—due to absent deltoid bulge, a straight ruler can touch the tip of acromian and the lateral epicondyle of humerus at the same time.

  X-ray is confirmatory (Fig. 6.1B).

Treatment: Closed reduction under sedation/general anesthesia and after reduction, the arm is immobilised in sling/chest arm bandage (Velpeau). Reduction maneuver are as follows:
- Stimpson's gravity method
- Kocher's method
- Hippocratic method

Complication
- Recurrent subluxation/dislocation—at the time of initial trauma leading to dislocation, if capsule/ligament/labrum/bone cartilage is also injured, it may lead to recurrent subluxation/dislocation. It is the most common complication in young patients/overall.

- Rotator cuff injury—most common complication in older patients.
- Nerve injury—it is the most common early complication and usually neuropraxia. Circumflex branch of axillary nerve is the most common nerve injury in anterior dislocation. Radial nerve/musculocutaneous nerve/ brachial plexus may be injured rarely.

Posterior Dislocation

Head is dislocated posteriorly, subtypes—subacromial > subglenoid > subspinous. Mechanism of injury is marked and sudden adduction and internal rotation force as seen in fits, convulsion or an electric shock. Arm is held in adduction and internal rotation, coracoids process becomes prominent anteriorly and humeral head may be palpable posteriorly. Diagnosis is often missed and thus also known as missed injury. X-ray may be normal/electric bulb sign/empty glenoid sign (Fig. 6.1C).

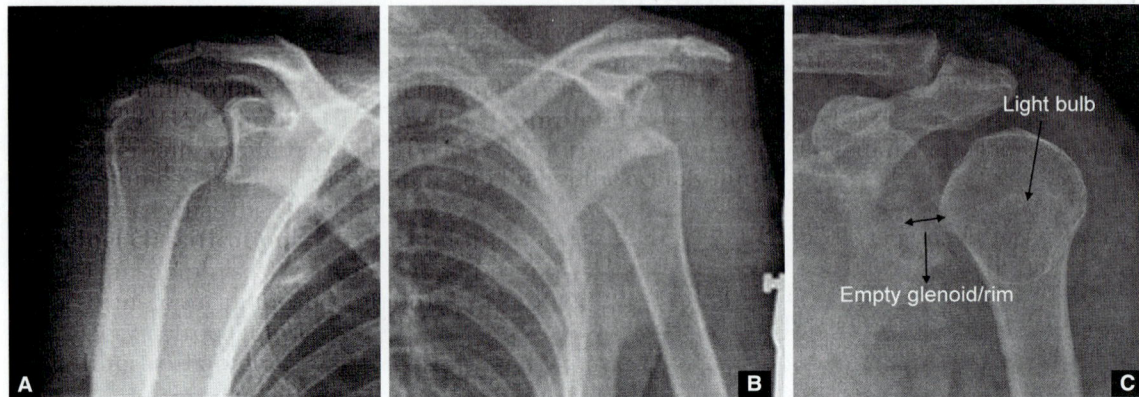

Fig. 6.1: (A) Normal shoulder X-ray, (B) anterior dislocation (subcoracoid), (C) posterior dislocation.

Inferior Dislocation/Luxatio Erecta

It is the rarest variety caused by a severe hyperabduction force. The arm is locked in full abduction, with patient's forearm resting on his head. It may lead to severe neurovascular injury, axillary nerve is the most common nerve injured. Inferior dislocation is generally seen in patients with hyperlaxity, and they usually have multidirectional instability and frequent dislocation of other joints as well.

FRACTURES AROUND SHOULDER AND ARM

Fracture Clavicle

- Peculiarities of clavicle:
  - 1st bone to start ossification and last long bone epiphysis to fuse (medial end).
  - Only long bone to lie horizontally, ossifies by intramembranous ossification, only long bone with no intramedullary cavity and has 2 primary centers of ossification for shaft.
- Fracture clavicle is the most common bone to fracture (overall) and during childbirth.
- Most common site is middle 1/3rd (esp. junction of medial–lateral 1/3rd) > lateral 1/3rd (acromial part) > medial 1/3rd (sternal part) (rare).
- Middle 1/3rd is most common because of its sudden change of curvature and is the weakest part of bone.
- X-ray—Zanca's view.
- Treatment—mid 1/3rd is managed conservatively with a figure of '8' bandage/clavicle brace with an arm sling.
- Operative indications—displaced lateral 1/3rd clavicle; middle 1/3rd with open injury, segmental fracture >2 cm shortening, floating shoulder, B/L clavicle fracture, neurovascular injury, tenting of skin by elevated fragment, symptomatic non-union. Surgical option is plating >K-wire fixation.
- Complication—most common is malunion >> non-union.

Clavicle fracture may l/t brachial plexus injury (lower trunk) and thoracic outlet syndrome.

Floating Shoulder
A glenoid neck fracture with an associated clavicle fracture is k/a floating shoulder, as glenohumeral joint is left with no intact bony contact with rest of the body. It is aka "**SSSC**"—superior suspensory shoulder complex.

Acromioclavicular Joint Dislocation
Common in sports person. AC joint stability is maintained by AC joint capsule and AC ligaments (AP stability) and coracoclavicular ligaments (superior-inferior stability). When these are torn AC joint dislocation results and is classified by Rockwood into 6 types.

X-ray: Zanca's view.

Treatment: Type I–III managed conservatively by RJ bandage/Velpeau bandage (Fig. 6.2) (other uses: Clavicle fracture and shoulder dislocation) and type IV–VI by surgery.

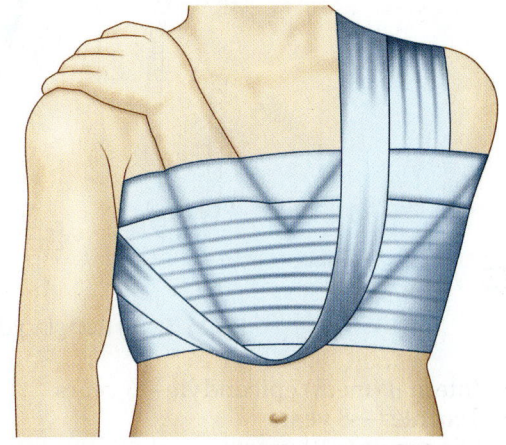

Fig. 6.2: Velpeau bandage (concept—anything which immobilises in this position is Velpeau)

Fracture Proximal Humerus
Fracture of proximal humerus is a low energy trauma, common in **elderly females**. GT, LT, head and shaft constitute the proximal humerus and Neer classified fractures based on displacement of the above fragments. A part is displaced if >1 cm of displacement or >45° angulation is seen. Axillary nerve > suprascapular is the most common nerve injured in fracture surgical neck of humerus.

Treatment: Depends on Neer type, age, functional demand, etc.
- Type I—most are undisplaced/impacted fracture, treated by sling/Velpeau/shoulder immobiliser and functional range of movement started early (TOC if specific type is not mentioned).
- Type II
  - Fracture surgical neck (most common) can be managed by closed reduction and arm sling/shoulder immobiliser application or closed reduction and fixation with K-wires. If closed reduction is not possible, then ORIF.
  - Fracture of GT is mostly associated with anterior shoulder dislocation and GT is reduced with shoulder reduction. If it is displaced >5 mm (lower threshold for GT), then CRIF or ORIF is done. Supraspinatus, infraspinatus and teres minor (SIT) are the muscle inserted in GT and if not fixed, then movements of these will be affected.
- Type III—ORIF with PHILOS (a plate).
- Type IV— high chances of AVN and hemiarthroplasty is indicated in elderly.

Fracture Shaft of Humerus
Mostly managed conservatively in a hanging cast or U-slab/cast (Fig. 6.3A). Vascular injury/high grade open injury is an indication of operative management of fracture SOH. Anatomical reduction is not necessary and some malreduction is accepted. Most common cause of delayed/non-union is distraction at fracture site due to gravity or weight of plaster. Radial nerve injury is the most common complication (neuropraxia) and recovers spontaneously, exploration of nerve is only required in open injury cases or injury of nerve during closed reduction. One such cause of injury is spiral fracture of lower third **(Holstein Lewis fragment)** (Fig. 6.3B).

ELBOW
Ossification centers around elbow appears in the following sequence **(CRITOL)**:
- Capitellum—2 years
- Radial head— 4 years

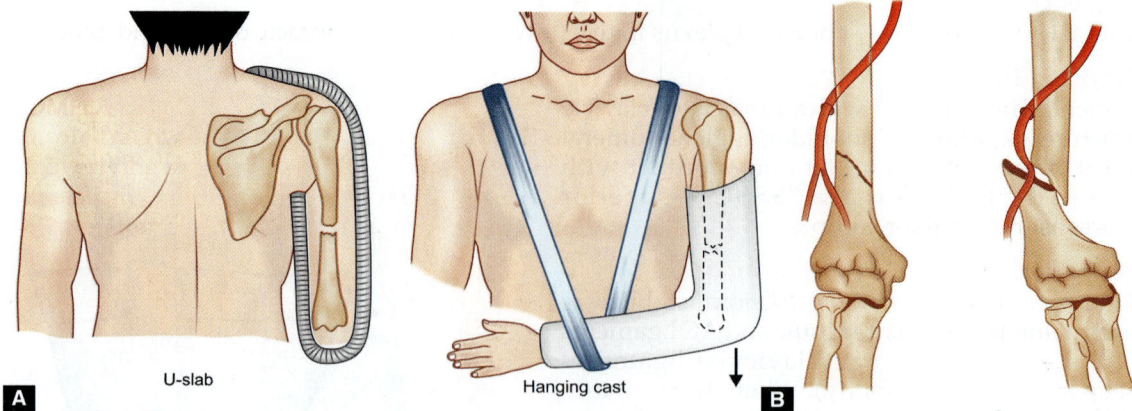

Fig. 6.3: (A) Hanging/U-cast, (B) Holstein Lewis fragment

- Internal (med.) epicondyle—6 years
- Trochlea—8 years
- Olecranon—10 years
- Lateral epicondyle—12 years

Anatomy

- Elbow movements, supination/pronation takes place at radioulnar joint and flexion/extension at ulnohumeral joint.
- MCL and LCL are ligamentous restraint to valgus and varus force.
- Carrying angle—angle between long axis of arm-forearm, in fully extended and supinated position. Angle is 14° in female and 11° in males, owing to relatively lower level of trochlea in females and larger hips, allowing arms to swing freely without hitting hips. Decreased angle is k/a cubitus varus (most common in **malunited** fracture S/C humerus) and increased is cubitus valgus (most common in non-union fracture lateral epicondyle).
- **3-point bony relationship**—two epicondyles and tip of olecranon forms a straight horizontal line in fully extended position and near isosceles triangle in 90° flexed position. This relationship is maintained in supracondylar fractures but disrupted in fractures below this level, e.g. increased intercondylar distance—medial/lateral epicondyle fracture or intra-articular fractures and maintained intercondylar distance—olecranon fracture or elbow dislocation.
- Anconeus triangle/posterolateral triangle—formed by radial head, tip of olecranon and lateral epicondyle, covered by anconeus muscle.

Supracondylar Humerus Fracture

This is the most common pediatric elbow injury, seen most common in 5–8 years age group. Extension type is the most common fracture pattern, with flexion seen in only 2% cases. **Mechanism** is: Fall on outstretched supinated hand (**FOOSH**). **Displacement** is:

DIM: Dorsal displacement and tilt (extension), impaction (proximal shift), medial tilt/shift/rotation (i.e. pronation). Extension type fracture may be posteromedially > posterolaterally displaced.

Classification: Gartland

Type	Clinically	X-ray	Treatment
Type I	Undisplaced	Fat pad sign	Slab in flexion and pronation
Type II	Posterior angulation	Intact posterior cortex	CRIF with K-wires
Type III	Completely displaced, S-shaped deformity	Both cortex broken	CRIF or ORIF with K-wires

If swelling is large, then initially managed to reduce swelling by traction—skin traction (Dunlop traction) or skeletal traction (Smith's traction).

Xtra edge
- Post-reduction on X-ray, varus tilt is judged by **Baumann's angle** (increased in cubitus varus) and posterior tilt by tear drop. Fish tail sign predicts abnormal horizontal rotation.
- **Jones view** is used to done to see elbow in flexion.
- Brachial artery injury is most common arterial injury. If pulse absent pre-reduction, fracture is reduced with lesser degree of flexion and assessed for pulse which generally reappears. If pulse absent post-reduction, then it means that artery is entrapped between fracture fragments and is an indication for open surgical exploration of artery. Management of pulseless pink hand (i.e. CRT is normal) is observation.
- Most common nerve injury is AIN > Median > radial (these three in extension type) > ulnar (in flexion type and post-surgery). AIN injury is most common seen after posterolateral displacement, radial nerve after posteromedial displacement. But posterolateral displacement is more commonly associated with nerve injury, thus injury of AIN > radial nerve. Mostly neuropraxia and recovers with time. These are early complication, a late nerve injury is seen when median nerve is entrapped in fracture callus and appears on X-ray as hole in callus known as Metev's sign.
- Compartment syndrome/myositis ossificans/VIC/elbow stiffness—most common cause is fracture S/C humerus.
- Malunion >> non-union (rare). Because of posteromedial displacement, if malunites, it leads to cubitus (elbow) varus deformity aka "gun stock deformity", since it does not involve growth plate, it is static (i.e. nonprogressive) in nature. Treated by lateral closing wedge osteotomy aka French/modified French osteotomy.

Fracture Lateral Condyle

Most common distal humeral epiphyseal fractures and 2nd most common elbow fractures in children, seen most common in 5–15 years age group, requiring surgery always, thus termed **"fracture of necessity"** by speed. 3-point bony elation is not maintained with increased intercondylar distance. **Milch** classified into two types:
- Type I—salter Harris type IV: Fracture line extends laterally to the trochlear groove, thus trochlea remains attached to shaft and elbow is stable.
- Type II—salter Harris type II: Fracture line extends medially to the trochlear groove, thus trochlea is a part of fracture fragment and elbow is stable. Type II is more coomon than type I.

X-ray: Fracture always appears smaller because of cartilageneous nature of fragment.

Treatment: Always open reduction and fixation with K-wires (as it is fracture of necessity), else will l/t nonunion.

Complications
- Lateral spur formation is the most common complication due to callus formation laterally, l/t **pseudo-cubitus varus** deformity. No treatment is required.
- Nonunion >> malunion leads to **cubitus valgus** deformity, which is progressive in nature (as it involves growth plate). Nonunion/cubitus valgus is the most common complication requiring treatment (Milch osteotomy). In valgus deformity, due to stretch on ulnar nerve "**tardy ulnar nerve palsy**" is seen, which develops years after the fracture (thus known as tardy). May be rarely seen after cubitus varus deformity. Most common symptom is tingling sensation in ulnar nerve area > claw hand. Treatment is anterior transposition of ulnar nerve in elbow to decrease stress on nerve.

Compartment Syndrome

Increased intrafascial compartment pressure (in a closed compartment) leading to loss of microcirculation/muscle hypoxia and a vicious cycle of events is known as compartment syndrome. Most common site is deep posterior compartment of leg (overall/adults) > deep flexor compartment of forearm (most common in children). In open fractures, compartment syndrome can be seen, but rare; as compartment is not closed.

Causes
- Most common cause (overall/adults) is closed fracture tibia > fracture S/C humerus (most common cause in children).
- Other causes—snakebite, crush injury, burn, exercise and tight plaster/circumferential dressing (thus also known as **tight cast syndrome**).

Clinical features
- Pain out of proportion to injury is the 1st/most common symptom and pain on passive stretch is the most common sign. Passive ankle dorsiflexion assesses superficial posterior leg compartment of leg (gastrosoleus is a superficial muscle) and toe DF is for deep posterior compartment of leg (FHL is a deep muscle).
- Others–**Ps**: Pain, puffiness (swelling), pallor, pulselessness; paresthesia and paralysis (late). Earliest and most significant is pain on passive stretch, while pulse is not a reliable indicator, may be present/absent.
- Most common muscle involved is FDP > FPL in forearm. Most common nerve involved in compartment syndrome is AIN.

Diagnosis: Is mainly clinical, but intra-compartmental pressure >30 mm Hg is diagnostic with compartment syndrome or difference between diastolic compartment pressure is <30 mm Hg. Normal calf pressure is 8–10 mm Hg (during walking is 200–300 mm Hg).

Treatment
- Prevention—immediate removal of any tight bandage/fracture reduction.
- Impending compartment syndrome—limb elevation at heart level.
- Established compartment syndrome—surgery/fasciotomy to decrease pressure followed by fracture fixation by external fixator. Compartment release (i.e. fasciotomy) should be done within 12–24 hours, after 72 hours it has no role and may lead to crush syndrome (discussed in Chapter 4).

Xtra edge
- In a hypotensive patient a lower threshold of pressure is used for diagnosis of compartment syndrome.
- In an impending compartment syndrome of leg due to fracture tibia, an unreamed intramedullary nailing should be done, reaming of medullary canal increases pressure.
- Complication of compartment syndrome: VIC in forearm.

Volkmann Ischemic Contracture (VIC)

VIC is due to irreversible tissue ischemia (muscle sequestrum) leading to muscle contracture seen after mismanaged case of compartment syndrome, seen most commonly in forearm (deep compartment) after S/C fracture humerus. Most common or earliest muscle involved is FDP > FPL and most common nerve involved is AIN and artery is brachial artery.

Deformity: Elbow flexion, forearm pronation, wrist flexion, thumb adduction, finger flexion.

Treatment: Early stage is managed by dynamic splint (turn buckle splint—Fig. 6.4) to prevent wrist contracture and in moderate cases/fibrotic muscles, muscle sliding operation is done "Max page operation". In severe cases, excision of necrotic muscle, bone shortening, neurolysis and tendon transfer is done.

Myositis Ossificans/Heterotopic Ossificans

It is a reactive lesion occurring in soft tissues and rarely near bone or periosteum but always outside the bone. It is a misnomer as there is no itis (inflammation) and rarely ossification of muscle occurs (because no true bone matrix is found, it is simply calcification, not ossification). After injury hematoma is ossified by migration of osteoblast, which are formed by metaplasia of fibroblast at the site of injury. Most

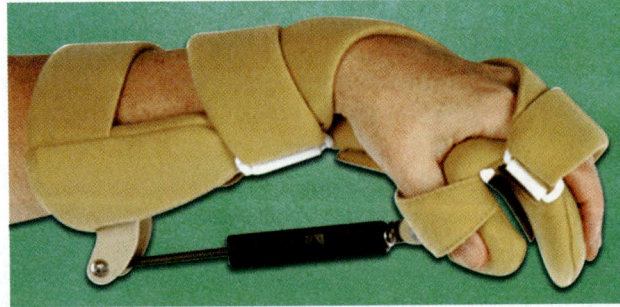

Fig. 6.4: Turn buckle splint

common site is elbow > hip joint and most common muscle involved is brachialis. Other muscles are quadriceps femoris and adductor muscles of thigh.

Risk factors
- Most common risk factor is injury/trauma f/b massage of the part and vigorous passive stretching.
- Burns/surgical trauma (elbow/hip surgery—anterior approach).
- Neurological disorder (pseudomalignant MO—not a/w trauma): Hypoxic brain injury/head injury (ICU patients), polio, GBS, AIDS, encephalopathy.

Zonal phenomena: Described by CT > USG : Periphery shows more mature ossification and central lucency (cellular area lacking bone), opposite is seen in osteosarcoma, i.e. MO matures from periphery to central.

X-ray: Peripheral opacity and central lucency, always at a distance from bone. If continuous with bone, then it might be a neoplastic bone pathology or infection. Mass appears as dotted veil/cotton wool.
- Active MO—warm, edema, painful and tender, growing in size (clinically/X-ray).
- Silent/mature MO—no local rise of temp, not painful, size is at a standstill and on X-ray margins are clear and no central lucency.

Treatment: When MO is active, immobilisation is the best treatment and any attempt at removal of the mass is hazardous. When silent and ALP/ESR levels are normal, it can safely be removed (generally after 1.5 year) if causing block in movements. Indomethacin/low dose radiation/bisphosphonates can be given prophylactically in high risk patients to prevent MO formation.

Xtra edge
- The disease is self-limiting in 30% cases and resolves spontaneously without treatment.
- Prussian disease—MO in deltoid muscle, seen in soldiers who carry heavy rifle in their shoulders.
- It is different from tumor calcinosis (metabolic disorder) which is often B/L, painless and associated hyperphosphatemia (not increased ALP level).

Myositis Ossificans Progressiva
Rare AD fatal disorder seen in children <6 years old with defective regulation of the induction of endochondral ossification.
- Abnormality/microdactyly of great toe clinches the diagnosis.
- They progress in axial-appendicular, cranial to caudal, proximal to distal. Neck, spine and shoulder regions are the most common sequence/site of involvement. Limitation of movement follows the same sequence.
- Sternocleidomastoid muscle is the most common muscle involved and most often presents initially with torticollis.
- Cardiac muscle/smooth muscle, extraocular muscle, diaphragm are always spared.
- Death is the usual outcome due to respiratory failure (restrictive lung disease > pneumonia).

Elbow Dislocation
The most common elbow dislocation is posterior or posterolateral. After fall/trauma it may result due to ligamentous injury (simple) or due to fracture (complex). Most commonly it is simple dislocation and elbow attains at flexed attitude after dislocation and olecranon becomes prominent posteriorly, disrupting 3-point bony relationship.
- Most common joint to dislocate in children.
- In complex dislocation—most common fracture is that of medial epicondyle of humerus.
- Early complication—most common arterial injury is brachial and most common nerve is ulnar > media and radial.
- Late complication—myositis ossificans, elbow stiffness, recurrent dislocation.
- Terrible triad—elbow dislocation with fracture of radial head and coronoid process.

X-ray
- In all degree of flexion and extension of elbow, if a line is drawn from head of radius proximally, it always passes through capitellum, if not, then elbow is said to be dislocated.
- Elbow perched attitude and coronoid process is posterior to humerus (Fig. 6.5).

Treatment: Urgent closed reduction in simple dislocation and ORIF for complex cases.

Pulled Elbow/Nursemaid's Elbow

In an extended and pronated forearm, when traction is given (lifting the child by arm), radial head subluxates out of annular ligament with an audible snap, and when traction is released ligament gets trapped between radial head and capitellum. It is most common in 1–4 years of age (rare after >5 years).

Clinical feature: Child starts crying immediately and elbow is held in neutral-partial pronation and 20–30° short of full extension. Tenderness over radial head, rubbery resistance to passive supination and full extension. X-rays are always normal.

Reduction is performed without anesthesia. Elbow is supinated and flexed with an audible click during reduction. Child stops crying immediately and starts using the limb within a few minutes of reduction. Many a times, before the child reports to emergency, elbow gets reduced spontaneously by

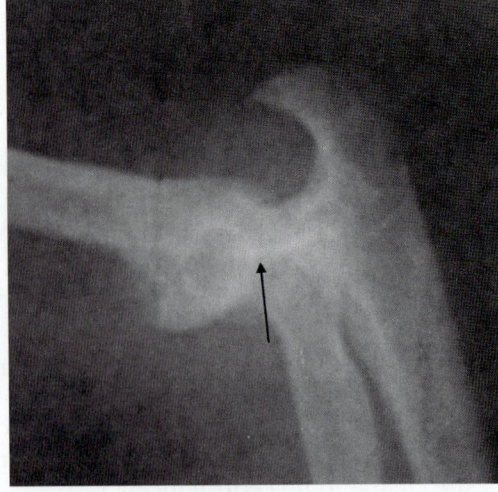

Fig. 6.5: Elbow dislocation showing coronoid process posterior to humerus, and perched attitude of olecranon with respect to humerus

gravity (as supination is a gravity dependent movement). No role of X-ray in checking reduction. No role of slab after reduction, simply a sling is advised.

Radial Head Fracture

Radial head fracture is common in adults (a type of valgus injury), while in children radial neck fractures are more common. Fracture may be associated with elbow dislocation, MCL/LCL injury or injury to interosseous membrane (known as Essex Lopresti lesion). Diagnosis of Essex Lopresti can be made by noting tenderness in forearm in addition to elbow. Fracture is classified by **Mason's** classification.

Treatment: Undisplaced fracture can be managed conservatively. If small fragment/outer 1/3rd extra-articular fragment, it can be excised easily. In displaced fractures ORIF is done. Screws (Herbert) or plate are applied in posterolateral part of head which does not take part in articulation with capitellum/sup RU joint known as safe zone. Fractures which are highly comminuted, either radial head excision or radial head replacement is done (Fig. 6.6). Radial head excision is contraindicated in fractures with associated ligament injury or Essex Lopresti injury/terrible traid injury, because after excision radius will migrate proximally (as head is now absent) and cause inferior RU joint subluxation leading to wrist/forearm pain. Excision is always contraindication in children because of growth disturbance between radius and ulna, proximal migration of radius leading to inferior RU joint subluxation > elbow instability and cubitus valgus deformity.

Xtra edge

- Essex Lopresti lesion is radial head fracture with interosseous membrane injury wth inferior RU joint dislocation.
- Most common complication of radial head fracture is joint stiffness.
- Herbert screws are used in intra-articular fractures, e.g. scaphoid, capitellum, radial head, femoral head.
- Metaizeau's technique is used for radial neck fracture in children.

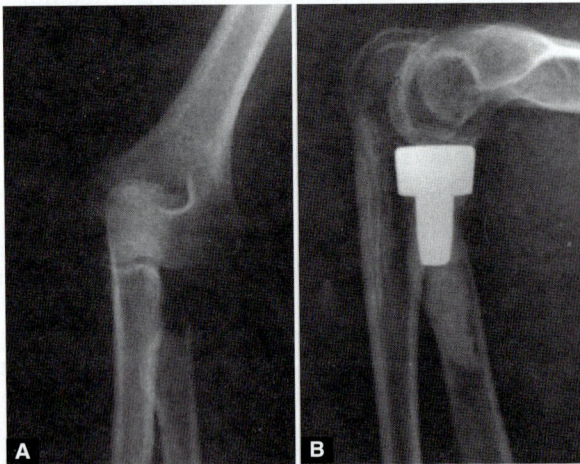

Fig. 6.6: (A) Radial head excision and (B) replacement

- Floating elbow—when there is fracture of I/L humerus and forearm leading to unsupported elbow, requiring fixation of both the fractures.

Olecranon Fracture/Javellin Throwers Fracture
Due to direct fall or avulsion by triceps pull.

Treatment
- Simple transverse fracture—tension band wiring (TBW).
- Comminuted fracture/fracture extending distally towards shaft—plate fixation.
- Small extra-articular fragment—excision. Excision is C/I where it may lead to elbow instability, e.g. fracture extending distally to coronoid, here excision of such big fragment will leading to elbow instability/triceps weakness/loss of elbow movement.

Xtra edge
- Excision can be done in fractures of bone where fracture fragment is very small/extra-articular/does not lead to instability/unreconstructible with ORIF, e.g. patella, olecranon, radial head.
- TBW indications—fracture patella, olecranon, medial malleolus, GT of humerus/femur.

INJURIES OF FOREARM
Fracture Both Bones Forearm (BBFA)
Radius and ulna functions as a unit in forearm and often fractures together. They are joined by proximal radio-ulnar joint (PRUJ), DRUJ and interosseous membrane. Movement taking place between these joints is supination and pronation, with radius moving around static ulna. Axis of rotation runs from the center of the radial head to the center of the distal ulna. Twisting force causes spiral fracture of BBFA at different levels (radius usually at higher level) and direct blow/angulating force causes transverse fracture of BBFA at same level. Forearm supinators are biceps and supinator muscle attached proximally and pronators are pronator teres and quadratus muscle attached at mid and distal forearm respectively.

Treatment
- Children—conservative with closed reduction and cast. Position of cast depends on level of fracture. In proximal fracture cast is applied in supination, because proximal fragment is supinated by attached muscles. In fractures of mid shaft, cast is applied in mid rotation, as proximal fragment is in mid rotation by attached supinator/biceps and teres muscle. In fractures of distal third, cast is applied in pronation because the proximal fragment is pronated by pronator quadrates muscle.
- Adults—always ORIF by **compression** plating (i.e. fracture site is compressed by plate).

Xtra edge
- Cross union is a complication in fractures at same level where radius unites with ulna and this is most common in head injury patients where there is hypertrophic callus response. It leads to loss of forearm rotator movements.
- *Plastic deformation*—pediatric bones are elastic, they gets deformed without concomitant fracture.
- *Green stick fracture*—unicortical undisplaced fracture.
- *Night stick fracture*—bicortical undisplaced fracture of ulna.

Monteggia Fracture
Fracture of proximal third ulna with associated radial head dislocation (PRUJ dislocation) is known as Monteggia fracture (a type of hyperpronation injury). Most commonly seen in children and missed if X-ray of elbow is not done, thinking it to be isolated fracture of ulna. Bado classified it (Fig. 6.7), based on direction of radial head dislocation.

Treatment: Principle is to reduce fracture ulna (i.e. regain length of ulna) and it automatically reduces dislocated radial head. In children, it is done by CR and cast application, whereas in adults by ORIF of ulna. If after ORIF of ulna, radial head is not automatically reduced, then open reduction of radial head should be done.

Type	Direction of radial head dislocation	Ulna fracture angulation
I (M/C in children, overall)	Anterior	Anterior
II (M/C in adults)	Posterior/posterolateral	Posterior
III(exclusive in children)	Lateral/anterolateral	Lateral
IV (exclusive in adults)	Anterior	Fracture BBFA at prox 1/3rd, at same level

Xtra edge
- Most commonly nerve injury is that of PIN. Most commonly injured in type II/III.
- Most commonly Monteggia equivalent is fracture of proximal ulna with fracture radial neck/radial epiphysis with anterior PRUJ dislocation.
- D/D— congenital radial head dislocation, where dislocation is B/L and posteriorly, radial head is enlarged due to absent growth modulation by capitellum.

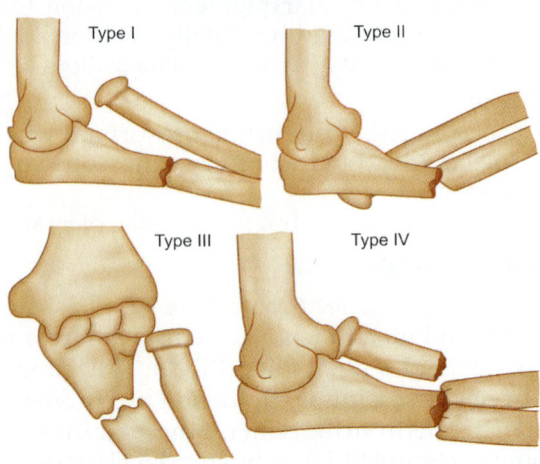

Fig. 6.7: Monteggia fractures

Galeazzi Fracture

Fracture of distal third of radius with DRUJ dislocation. Galeazzi fracture is more common than Monteggia fracture. It is more common in adults than children. In children CR and cast is done, while in adults ORIF is done. After radius is fixed, DRUJ (dislocated ulna) is automatically reduced, and if it is unstable (DRUJ), then DRUJ is fixed by transverse K-wire (from ulna to radius) and if DRUJ is not reduced automatically, then impingement by ECU tendon should be suspected and managed by open reduction of DRUJ (Fig. 6.8).

Xtra edge: Reverse Galeazzi fracture—fracture of distal third ulna with DRUJ dislocation.

FRACTURE DISTAL END RADIUS (DER)

Colles' Fracture

It is the fracture of DER at its cortico-cancellous junction (about 2–2.5 cm proximal to articular surface), occurring most commonly in elderly postmeno-pausal females, i.e. it is a fragility fracture (occurring 2° to osteoporosis). Most common mechanism is fall on pronated and dorsiflexed wrist. Therefore, displacement typically seen in Colles' fracture is:

DILS—Dorsal displacement/tilt, **I**mpaction (proximal shift), **L**ateral displacement/tilt and **S**upination **(dinner fork deformity).**

Treatment: Conservative in **below elbow** cast, forces applied opposite to the deformity: Traction >pronation–palmar flexion–ulnar deviation **(Cotton-Loder position)**. When traction is applied reduction is achieved by ligamentotaxis **(Agee's maneuver)**. Most important deformity to be corrected is restoration of radial length. Cotton-Loder position can lead to increased carpal tunnel pressure. In adults near normal function can be

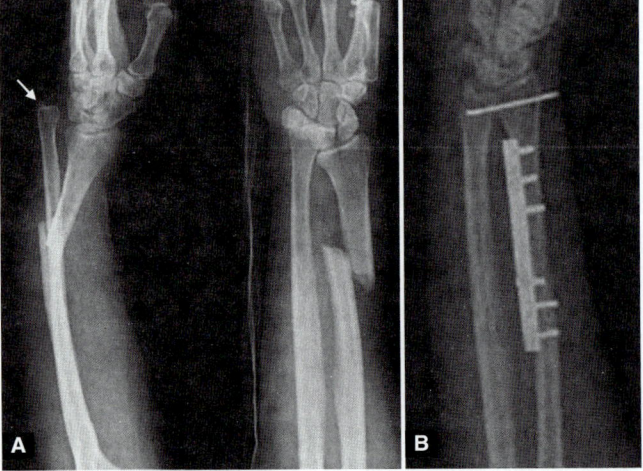

Fig. 6.8: (A) Galeazzi fracture in adult, (B) managed by ORIF of radius and a transverse K-wire fixation of unstable DRUJ

expected. In elderly/unstable fracture where reduction is lost, fixation can be done by K-wires/ radial distractor.

Complications
- Joint/finger stiffness > malunion (not nonunion).
- Rupture of EPL tendon.
- Sudeck's osteodystrophy.
- Carpal tunnel syndrome.
- Most common associated injury is ulnar styloid fracture > TFCC injury and DRUJ instability.

Smith's Fracture
Similar to Colles' fracture except displacement is opposite: Volar/anterior angulation, ulnar deviation and pronation producing garden spade deformity. Treated in **above elbow** cast in dorsal angulation, lateral deviation in supination.

Barton's Fracture
This is an intra-articular fracture of DER in which carpus and a rim of distal radius are displaced together, thus it is fracture dislocation. If displaces anteriorly known as "volar Barton" (M/C) and if posterior then dorsal Barton. They are managed by ORIF and plate is applied on volar surface (Fig. 6.9). (So if you are asked a question on fracture DER, with an image showing plate application on volar surface, diagnosis is volar Barton for MCQ purpose).

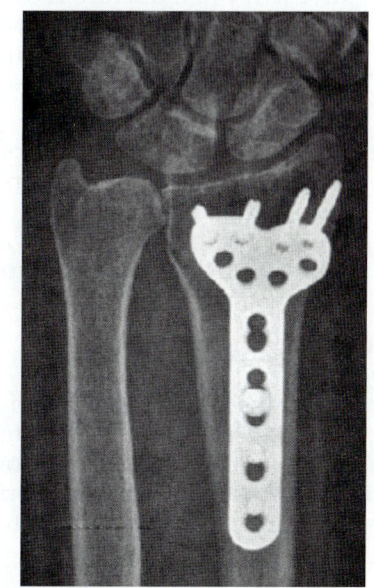

Xtra edge
- Chauffeur's fracture—fracture of radial styloid.
- Die-punch fracture—comminuted fracture DER with impacted/depressed medial articular surface (Lunate fossa) while lateral surface remains intact.

Complex Regional Pain Syndrome (CRPS)
Also known as—Causalgia/reflex sympathetic dystrophy/ Sudeck's osteodystrophy/algodystrophy.

CRPS I—chronic regional pain syndrome, burning in nature (causalgia), that develops after soft tissue / bony trauma, not confined to the distribution of a single peripheral nerve.

Fig. 6.9: Fracture volar Barton managed by volar plate application

CRPS II—it develops after injury of a single peripheral nerve/major nerve trunk. Initially pain is confined to the distribution of nerve, later whole limb is involved. Median > sciatic are the most common nerve involved.

The symptoms are unrelated (out of proportion) to the severity of initial trauma, and is said to be due to imbalance between sympathetic/parasympathetic nervous system.
- Initially—pain (most common symptom), paresthesia, edema (most common sign), vasomotor symptoms. Skin is dry, hot and pink later turns into blue, cold and sweaty.
- Later—skin is thinned out and shiny with brittle and fragile skin, nail and hairs.
- Psychological element is also involved and patients are hypersensitive.
- Stiffness in the joint is very common.

Most common cause is Colles' fracture. X-ray shows localised/patchy osteopenia due to increased blood flow.

Treatment: Multidisciplinary approach with early mobilisation and physical therapy (i.e. immobilisation of limb is avoided). Desensitisation is usually helpful. The following drugs are of proven benefits—NSAIDs, glucocorticoid, centrally acting analgesics like amitryptiline, Ca channel blocker, calcitonin, adrenergic blockers and stellate ganglion block. Recovery takes a very long time and complete relief is never a reality.

CARPAL INJURIES
Scaphoid > triquetral > trapezium are the M/C fractures of carpal bone.

Scaphoid Fracture

Parts of scaphoid are proximal pole, waist and distal pole. Blood supply of scaphoid is via a single major artery which enters distally through distal pole and travels proximally in a retrograde manner. Fracture of waist is most common scaphoid fracture in adults. In children (fracture scaphoid is rare) distal pole avulsion is the most common site of fracture. Fracture of waist most commonly leads to AVN of proximal pole.

Clinical features: Pain, tenderness and fullness in anatomical snuff box; painful thumb movements and pain with axial compression of thumb are other features. X-rays (ulnar deviated oblique view) may be negative initially in undisplaced fracture and should be repeated after10–14 days if suspicion is high. MRI is the IOC for occult fracture.

Treatment: Cast should always be applied initially in cases with positive clinical findings and negative X-ray , till fracture is ruled out.
- *Undisplaced fracture*: Scaphoid cast/glass holding cast (it is a below elbow cast, distally till MCP joints and including the proximal phalanx of thumb, in a glass holding position).
- *Displaced fracture*: Closed reduction/open reduction and internal fixation with headless screws (Herbert screw).

Complication: Nonunion (humpback deformity) > AVN.
- In cases of nonunion, vascularised muscle pedicle graft can be done, taken most common from pronator quadrates.
- *AVN*—most common due to waist fracture, but more proximal the fracture is, more is the chances of AVN. Proximal pole fracture has the highest incidence of AVN. MRI is the IOC to diagnose AVN.

Wrist Dislocations

Types
- Lunate dislocation—lunate dislocates anteriorly, while other carpal bone remains in place.
- Perilunate dislocation—lunate stays in place while other carpal bones dislocate posteriorly.
    Perilunate dislocation is the more common type, and when it is associated with fracture scaphoid, it is known as *trans*-scaphoid perilunate fracture dislocation. Median nerve is the most common nerve injury in lunate/perilunate dislocation.

X-ray
- Disruption of Gilula's line.
- Scapholunate dissociation (scapholunate ligament) produces "**Terry Thomas sign**".
- Lunate dislocation—"**spilled tea pot sign**" and "**piece of pie sign**".

Treatment: CR and fixation by K-wires. Reduction is done by "**Tavernier's maneuver**".

HAND INJURY/METACARPAL INJURY

Metacarpal has four parts—base, shaft, neck and head. Neck fractures are most common and most common metacarpal bone to fracture is 5th metacarpal at neck, known as Boxer's fracture (5th >4th). Most metacarpal fractures are stable fracture and managed by CR and cast immobilisation.

1st metacarpal base fracture: May be extra/intra-articular fracture. Intra-articular fractures are a type of carpo-metacarpal fracture dislocation.
- *Bennet's fracture*: Most common fracture of base of thumb. Oblique intra-articular fracture of base of 1st metacarpal , with distal fragment pulled laterally and proximally by unopposed pull of abductor pollicis longus. It is common in boxers and treated by closed reduction and K-wire fixation by "**Wagner technique**". In boxers, boxer's fracture is more common than Bennett's fracture (Fig. 6.10).
- *Rolando fracture*: V or Y or T shaped intra-articular fracture of base of 1st metacarpal. Distal fragment is not displaced as seen in Bennett's fracture (Fig. 6.10).
- *Complication of both*: Post-traumatic osteoarthritis of 1st CMC joint.

Kaplan injury: Irreducible dorsal dislocation of finger at MCP joint, most commonly involving 2nd finger. It almost always requires open reduction.

Bennett fracture   **Rolando fracture**

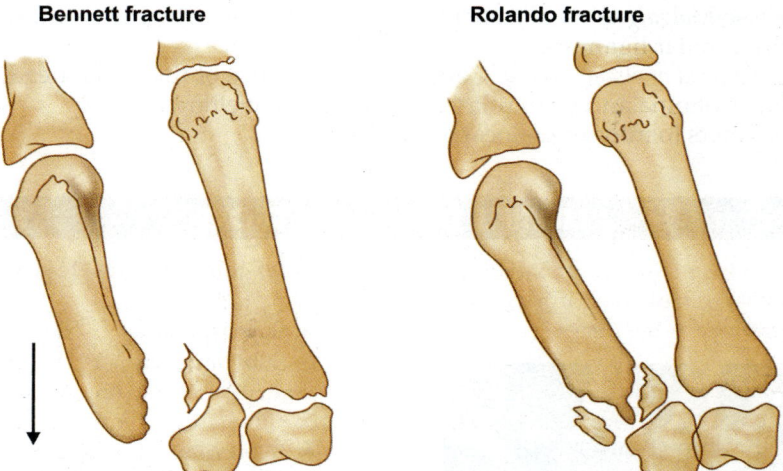

Fig. 6.10: Schematic diagram of Bennett's and Rolando fractures

Phalangeal fracture: Treated by buddy strapping, i.e. two adjacent fingers are strapped by an adhesive bandage.

UPPER LIMB FRACTURE EPONYMS

- *Mallet finger*: Avulsion or rupture of extensor tendon from the base of the distal phalanx.
- *Jersey finger*: Avulsion of flexor tendon (FDP) from base of distal phalanx.
- *Gamekeeper's/Skier's thumb*: Avulsion of the ulnar collateral ligament at MCP joint of thumb from base of proximal phalanx.
- *Bennett's fracture dislocation*: Oblique, displaced intra-articular fracture of the base of the first metacarpal with subluxation of the trapeziometacarpal joint such that the shaft of the first metacarpal is displaced laterally by abductor pollicis longus.
- *Rolando fracture*: Intra-articular Y-shaped fracture of the base of the first metacarpal with same but relatively less of diaphyseal displacements as a Bennett's fracture.
- *Boxer's fracture*: Fracture through the neck of the 5th metacarpal, usually occurs in boxers.
- *Kaplan's dislocation*: Dislocation of the MCP joint (classically of index finger).
- *Colles' fracture*: A fracture at the corticocancellous junction of the distal end of the radius with dorsal tilt of distal fragment, commonly seen in postmenopausal osteoporotic females.
- *Smith's fracture*: A fracture at the corticocancellous junction of the distal end of the radius with ventral tilt of distal fragment (also called Reverse Colles' fracture).
- *Barton's fracture*: Intra-articular fractures through the distal articular surface of the radius, taking a margin of radius with the carpals, displaced anteriorly or posteriorly.
- *Chauffeur's fracture*: A fracture of the styloid process of the radius.
- *Die-punch fracture*: A comminuted impacted fracture of distal radius.
- *Torus fracture*: Special fracture pattern seen in children where a single cortex of bone is buckled inside. It is mostly seen in distal radius.
- *Greenstick fracture*: A special fracture pattern seen classically in children (due to elastic bones and a thick periosteum) where there is break in a single cortex of bone and on X-ray one finds only bending of bones.
- *Night stick fracture*: A fracture of the shaft of ulna sustained while trying to protect from a stick blow.
- *Monteggia fracture*: Fracture of the proximal third of the ulna with dislocation of the radial head. Galeazzi fracture (Piedmont fracture): Fracture of the distal third of radius with subluxation of the distal radioulnar joint.
- *Side-swipe injury (Baby car fracture)*: It is an elbow injury sustained when one's elbow is projecting out of a car and is side swept by another vehicle. The patient sustains fractures of the distal end of humerus with fractures of proximal ends of radius and ulna.

- *Nursemaid's elbow/Malgaigne's subluxation*: Refers to pulled elbow which is subluxation of radial head out of the annular ligament
- *Hotchkiss terrible triad of elbow injury*: Comminuted fracture of the radial head, fracture of the coronoid process of ulna and posterolateral dislocation of elbow.
- *Luxatio erecta*: Refers to inferior dislocation of shoulder.

MULTIPLE CHOICE QUESTIONS

1. **A patient with history of fall on outstretched hand will most probably have injury to which of the marked area in the image?**

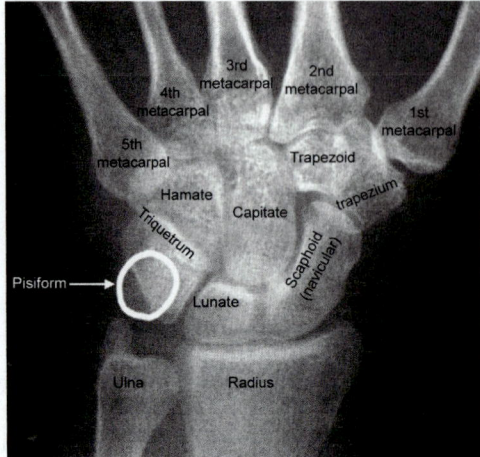

   A. Radius   B. Ulna
   C. 3rd metacarpal   D. Capitate

2. **In fasciotomy for compartment syndrome which structures are released?**
   A. Skin
   B. Skin, subcutaneous tissue
   C. Skin, subcutaneous tissue, superficial fascia
   D. Skin, subcutaneous tissue, superficial fascia and deep fascia

3. **What is the normal orientation of human head?**
   A. Retroversion of 80 degrees
   B. Retroversion of 30 degrees
   C. Anteversion of 15 degrees
   D. Anteversion of 50 degrees

4. **Dynamic stabilisers of shoulder joint:**
   A. Glenoid labrum
   B. Rotator cuff muscles
   C. Glenohumeral ligament
   D. Coracohumeral ligament

5. **For long the muscle was not given its due importance and was called forgotten muscle of rotator cuff. Which one is the muscle?**
   A. Subscapularis
   B. Supraspinatus
   C. Infraspinatus
   D. Teres minor

6. **Most common muscle damaged in rotator cuff:**
   A. Supraspinatus   B. Infraspinatus
   C. Subscapularis   D. Teres minor

7. **Painful arc syndrome is caused by impingement of:**
   A. Subacromial bursa   B. Subdeltoid bursa
   C. Rotator cuff tendon   D. Biceps tendon

8. **All are true for rotator cuff muscle *expect*:**
   A. Supraspinatus   B. Subscapularis
   C. Teres minor   D Teres major

9. **Rotator interval is between:**
   A. Supraspinatus and teres minor
   B. Teres major and teres minor
   C. Supraspinatus and subscapularis
   D. Subscapularis and infraspinatus

10. **Muscle crossing through the shoulder joint is:**
    A. Biceps short head   B. Biceps long head
    C. Triceps long head   D. Coracobrachialis

11. **Weakest portion of shoulder join capsule is:**
    A. Anterior   B. Posterior
    C. Inferior   D. Superior

12. **Which of the following is true about anterior shoulder dislocation?**
    A. It is most common type of shoulder dislocation
    B. It is most commonly subclavicular
    C. Patient keeps his arm in saluting position
    D. Injury to brachial plexus may occur

13. **Hamilton Ruler test sign is positive in which of the above mentioned conditions?**
    A. Anterior dislocation of shoulder
    B. Acromioclavicular joint dislocation
    C. Posterior dislocation of shoulder
    D. Luxatio erecta

14. **Following defect (lesion) is NOT responsible for recurrent anterior dislocation of shoulder:**
    A. Bankart's lesion
    B. Hill-Sachs lesion
    C. Bristow's lesion
    D. A defect in the anterior-inferior capsule

15. **All are seen in anterior shoulder dislocation *except*:**
    A. Elevated anterior axillary fold
    B. Duga's positive

C. Hamilton Rules positive
D. Increases vertical circumference

16. **Commonest type of shoulder dislocation:**
    A. Subcoracoid   B. Subglenoid
    C. Posterior   D. Subclavicular

17. **Uncomplicated shoulder dislocation most commonly occurs in the following direction:**
    A. Anterior   B. Posterior
    C. Superior   D. Medially

18. **An adult patient reported to emergency with limited adduction/IR with the following X-ray, diagnosis is:**

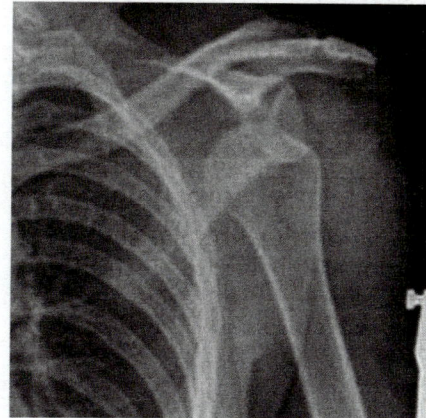

    A. Anterior dislocation of shoulder
    B. Posterior dislocation of shoulder
    C. Superior dislocation of shoulder
    D. Inferior dislocation of shoulder

19. **Nerve injured in anterior dislocation of shoulder:**
    A. Radial   B. Axillary
    C. Long thoracic   D. Median

20. **Neglected shoulder dislocation in a young labourer is?**
    A. Medically managed
    B. Surgically managed
    C. Neglected
    D. Counselled

21. **In recurrent anterior dislocation of shoulder, the movement that causes dislocation is:**
    A. Flexion and internal rotation
    B. Abduction and external rotation
    C. Abduction and internal rotation
    D. Extension

22. **Recurrent dislocations are least commonly seen in:**
    A. Ankle   B. Hip
    C. Shoulder   D. Patella

23. **All are related to recurrent shoulder dislocation *except*:**
    A. Hill-Sachs defect   B. Bankart lesion
    C. Lax capsule   D. Rotator cuff injury

24. **Traumatic Glenohumeral instability in one direction with Bankart's lesion are treated by:**
    A. Conservative methods
    B. Surgery
    C. Rehabilitation
    D. Inferior capsule shift

25. **Following anterior dislocation of the shoulder, a patient develops weakness of flexion at elbow and lack of sensation over the lateral aspect forearm: Nerve injured is:**
    A. Radial nerve
    B. Musculocutaneous nerve
    C. Axillary nerve
    D. Ulnar nerve

26. **Light bulb sign is seen in:**
    A. Anterior dislocation of shoulder
    B. Posterior dislocation of shoulder
    C. Fracture acromion
    D. Clavicular fracture

27. **40-year-old male who was unconscious and presented with bilateral adduction and internal rotation of shoulder:**
    A. Anterior dislocation
    B. Posterior dislocation
    C. Cleidocranial dislocation
    D. Brachial plexus injury

28. **In posterior dislocation of shoulder Hill-Sachs lesion is seen in:**
    A. Anterior   B. Anteromedial
    C. Posterior   D. Posteromedial

29. **Which is true about shoulder dislocation?**
    A. Anterior dislocation is more common than posterior
    B. Fixed medial rotation in posterior dislocation
    C. Kocher's maneuver is effective in anterior dislocation
    D. All of the above

30. **Which is true regarding shoulder dislocation?**
    A. Posterior dislocation is often over-looked
    B. Pain is severe in anterior dislocation
    C. Radiography may be misleading in posterior dislocation
    D. All of the above

31. **Which of the following is test of posterior glenohumeral instability?**
    A. Fulcrum
    B. Sulcus test
    C. Jerk test
    D. Crank test

32. **A 6-year-old boy a history of recurrent dislocation of the right shoulder. On examination, the orthopedician puts the patient in the supine position and abducts his arm to 90° with the bed as the fulcrum and then externally rotates it but the boy does not allow**

the test to be performed. The test done by the orthopedician:
A. Apprehension test   B. Sulcus test
C. Dugas test   D. McMurray's test

33. **Most common bone to fracture in body:**
A. Clavicle   B. Humerus
C. Tibia   D. Femur

34. **Shoulder X-ray highest bony landmark is:**

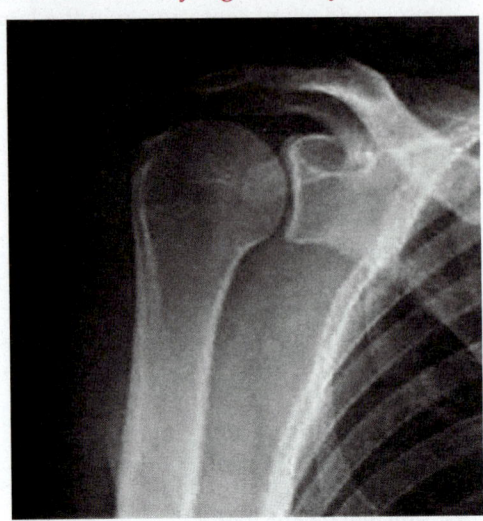

A. Greater tuberosity B. Lesser tuberosity
C. Head   D. Acromion

35. **The most common bone fractures during birth:**
A. Clavicle   B. Scapula
C. Radius   D. Humerus

36. **Clavicular fracture is usually treated by:**
A. Traction
B. Open reduction and internal fixation
C. Figure of eight bandage
D. Plate and screw fixation

37. **A patient had met with an accident and he cannot abduct his right arm and cannot lift it. On examination tenderness felt near right upper arm. X-ray showed fracture surgical neck of humerus. Muscle that that was paralysed was:**
A. Subscapularis
B. Supraspinatus
C. Infraspinatus
D. Teres major

38. **In fracture of surgical neck of humerus which nerve is involved?**
A. Axillary   B. Median
C. Ulnar   D. Radial

39. **Zanca's view is done for:**
A. AC joint dislocation
B. Shoulder dislocation
C. Cervical spine
D. Sterno-clavicular joint dislocation

40. **Most common complication of midshaft humerus fracture is:**
A. Radial nerve palsy
B. Median nerve palsy
C. Nonunion
D. Malunion

41. **Which of the following is least likely associated with vascular injury?**
A. Fracture supracondylar femur
B. Fracture supracondylar humerus
C. Fracture shaft of femur
D. Fracture shaft humerus

42. **Nerve injured in fracture of medial epicondyle of humerus:**
A. Anterior interosseous
B. Median
C. Ulnar
D. Radial

43. **Proximal humerus fracture which has maximum chances of avascular necrosis?**
A. One part   B. Two part
C. Three part   D. Four part

44. **Trauma to neck of humerus, nerve damaged:**
A. Radial   B. Ulnar
C. Median   D. Axillary

45. **Posterior elbow dislocation most common nerve involved is:**
A. Ulnar   B. Median
C. Radial   D. Musculocutaneous

46. **Name of this type of immobilisation:**

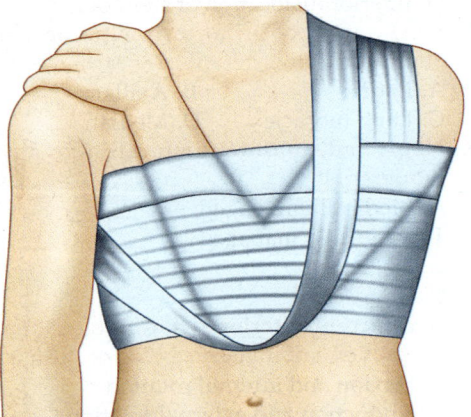

A. Velpaeu bandage
B. Cuff and collar sling
C. Arm pouch
D. Aeroplane splint

47. **Treatment of choice for fracture neck of humerus in a 70-year-old male:**
A. Analgesic with triangular sling
B. U-slab
C. Arthroplasty
D. Open reduction—internal fixation

48. Which of the following movement will be affected if the greater tubercle of the humerus is lost?
    A. Abduction and lateral rotation
    B. Adduction and flexion
    C. Adduction and medial rotation
    D. Flexion and medial rotation

49. Fracture neck humerus is common in:
    A. Elderly women   B. Young lady
    C. Children   D. All of the above

50. Hanging cast is used in?
    A. Fracture femur   B. Fracture radius
    C. Fracture tibia   D. Fracture humerus

51. The most important cause of non-union of fracture of humeral shaft is:
    A. Comminuted fracture
    B. Compound (open) fracture
    C. Overriding of fracture ends
    D. Distraction at fracture site

52. First appear amongst the ossification centers about the elbow is:
    A. Radial head   B. Olecranon
    C. Lateral epicondyle D. Capitellum

53. Three-bony point relationship is maintained in:
    A. Supracondylar fracture humerus
    B. Dislocation of elbow
    C. Fracture lateral condyle
    D. Intercondylar fracture

54. Posterolateral anconeus triangle is formed by:
    A. Head of radius, lateral epicondyle, medial epicondyle
    B. Head of radius, lateral epicondyle, olecranon
    C. Olecranon, medial epicondyle, neck of radius
    D. Neck of radius, head of redius, lateral epicondyle

55. Supracondylar fracture humerus, true is:
    A. Flexion type is the most common type
    B. Malunion causing gunstock deformity is the MC complication
    C. Definitive management requires open reduction
    D. Radial nerve injury is commonly seen

56. A child presents with the following deformity, most common etiology is:

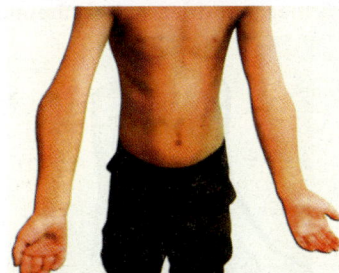

    A. Supracondylar humerus fracture
    B. Lateral condyle humerus fracture
    C. Radial head dislocation
    D. Monteggia fracture dislocation

57. Preferred treatment of cubitus varus is:
    A. Medial closing wedge osteotomy
    B. Lateral closing wedge osteotomy
    C. Medial opening wedge osteotomy
    D. Lateral opening wedge osteotomy

58. All are false regarding supracondylar humerus fracture in children *except:*
    A. Extension type is more common than flexion type
    B. Gartland classification is used for flexion type injury
    C. Gartland lll fracture shows fat pad sign
    D. Cubitus valgus is most common complication

59. In supracondylar fracture of humerus in children if the radial pulse is absent, what is the next line of management?
    A. Emergency brachial artery exploration
    B. Closed reduction of fracture and look of reappearance of pulse
    C. Closed reduction, above elbow slab plaster and observe
    D. Open reduction and internal fixation of fracture

60. Most common type of supracondylar fracture in children:
    A. Posteromedial extension
    B. Posterolateral extension
    C. Anteromedial flexion
    D. Anterolateral flexion

61. True about supracondylar fracture:
    A. Most common fracture in adults
    B. Posterior medial displacement of posterior fragment
    C. Ulnar nerve is most commonly injured
    D. Brachial artery is least commonly injured

62. The most common complication after supracondylar fracture humerus is:
    A. Cubitus varus
    B. Cubitus valgus
    C. Median nerve injury
    D. Ulnar nerve injury

63. Pointing index is a complication seen in:
    A. Lateral humeral condyle fracture
    B. Supracondylar fracture of humerus
    C. Shoulder dislocation
    D. Fracture of shaft of humerus

64. The most common type of elbow dislocation is:
    A. Posterior   B. Posteromedial
    C. Posterolateral   D. Lateral

65. Cubitus varus (gunstock) deformity is a complication of?
    A. Supracondylar fracture of humerus
    B. Fracture of lateral condyle of humerus
    C. Fracture of shaft of humerus
    D. Old unreduced elbow dislocation

66. All of the following are complications of supracondylar fracture of humerus in children, *except*:
    A. Compartment syndrome
    B. Myositis ossificans
    C. Malunion
    D. Nonunion

67. Malunited supracondylar fracture humerus causes:
    A. Static cubitus varus
    B. Progressive cubitus varus
    C. Cubitus valgus
    D. Shortening

68. Supracondylar fracture true:
    A. Distal segment displaced anterior is more common
    B. Cubitus valgus malunion more common than varus
    C. Nerve injury transitory
    D. Elbow flexion weakness

69. Late complication of elbow dislocation:
    A. Median nerve injury
    B. Brachial artery injury
    C. Myositis ossification
    D. All of the above

70. True about supracondylar fracture of humerus:
    A. Common in adults
    B. Extension type most common
    C. Flexion type is most common
    D. None

71. In extension type of supracondylar fracture, the usual displacement is:
    A. Anteromedial   B. Anterolateral
    C. Posteromedial   D. Posterolateral

72. Deformity in posterior elbow dislocation:
    A. Flexion   B. Extension
    C. Both   D. None

73. Commonest dislocation of elbow:
    A. Anterior   B. Posterior
    C. Both same   D. Medial

74. What is seen on X-ray with posterior elbow dislocation?
    A. Coronoid process posterior to humerus
    B. Coronoid process anterior to humerus
    C. Coronoid process below humerus
    D. None

75. In posterior dislocation of elbow, most prominent part:
    A. Coronoid
    B. Radial head
    C. Olecranon
    D. None

76. Supracondylar fracture humerus treatment is:
    A. Open reduction and K-wire fixation
    B. Closed reduction and K-wire fixation
    C. Excision
    D. Below elbow slab

77. Elbow dislocation going into most commonly:
    A. Posterolateral   B. Posteromedial
    C. Anterior   D. Lateral

78. Microcirculation blockade is a feature of:
    A. Sudeck's dystrophy
    B. Myositis ossifications
    C. Compartment syndrome
    D. Crush syndrome

79. The following fracture are known for non-union *except*:
    A. Fracture of lower half of tibia
    B. Fracture of neck of femur
    C. Fracture of scaphoid
    D. Supracondylar fracture of humerus

80. A 10-year-old boy presenting with a cubitus varus deformity and a history of trauma 3 months back on clinical examination, has the preserved 3 bony point relationship of the elbow. The most probable diagnosis is:
    A. Old unreduced dislocation of elbow
    B. Nonunion lateral condylar humerus
    C. Malunited intercondylar fracture of humerus
    D. Malunited supracondylar fracture of humerus

81. Supracondylar fracture is usually caused:
    A. Hyperflexion injury
    B. Axial rotation
    C. Extension injury
    D. Hyperextension injury

82. Most common elbow injury in adolescents is:
    A. Dislocation
    B. Physeal injury
    C. Supracondylar fracture
    D. Olecranon fracture

83. A six-year-old child presented with a valgus deformity at his right elbow since 3 years that is gradually progressive. He has a history of cast applied for 6 weeks after fall on outstretched hand 3 years back. The probable fracture was:
    A. Lateral condylar fracture of humerus
    B. Supracondylar fracture of humerus
    C. Posterior dislocation of elbow
    D. Fracture medial condyle of humerus

84. Identify the cause of deformity in the image below:

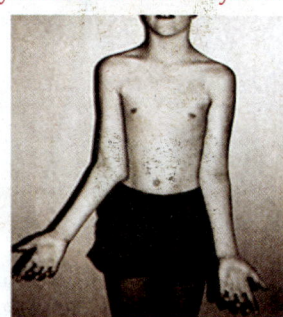

    A. Humerus lateral condylar fracture
    B. Supracondylar fracture humerus

C. Fracture shaft humerus

D. Medial condyle fracture of humerus

85. **The most common complication of lateral humeral condyle fracture in children is:**
    A. Valgus deformity   B. Varus deformity
    C. Malunion   D. Hyperextension

86. **Most common complication of lateral condyle humerus fracture:**
    A. Malunion   B. Nonunion
    C. VIC   D. Median nerve injury

87. **Which fracture requires open reduction in children?**
    A. Fracture of both bones of forearm
    B. Epiphyseal separation of tibia
    C. Intercondylar fracture of femur
    D. Lateral condyle fracture humerus

88. **A 6-year-old child has an accident and had fracture elbow, after 4 years presented with tingling and numbness in the ulnar side of finger, fracture is:**
    A. Supracondylar fracture humerus
    B. Lateral condylar fracture humerus
    C. Olecranon fracture
    D. Dislocation of elbow

89. **Tardy ulnar nerve palsy seen in:**
    A. Medial condyle fracture humerus
    B. Lateral condylar fracture humerus
    C. Supracondylar fracture humerus
    D. Fracture shaft humerus

90. **Fracture lateral condyle of humerus is a common injury in children. Which one of the following is the most ideal treatment for a displaced fracture lateral condyle of the humerus in a 7-year-old child?**
    A. Open reduction and plaster immobilization
    B. Closed reduction and plaster immobilization
    C. Open reduction and internal fixation
    D. Excision of the fracture fragment

91. **Which is the earliest reliable sign of compartment syndrome?**
    A. Stretch pain   B. Pulselessness
    C. Paraesthesia   D. Pallor

92. **The typical clinical picture of established Volkmann's ischemic contracture includes A/E:**
    A. Elbow flexion   B. Forearm pronation
    C. Wrist flexion   D. Thumb abduction

93. **Use of this splint:**

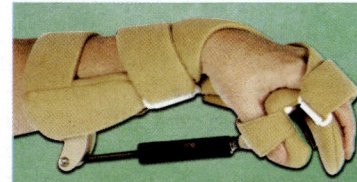

A. VIC   B. Radial nerve injury
C. Myositis ossificans D. Claw hand

94. **In supracondylar fracture of humerus in children if the radial pulse is absent, what is next line management?**
    A. Emergency brachial artery exploration
    B. Closed reduction of fracture and look for reappearance of pulse
    C. Closed reduction, about elbow slab plaster and observe
    D. Open reduction and internal fixation of fracture

95. **A cause of comminuted fracture of tibia presenting with severe pain in the calf on dorsiflexion of the foot. There is also numbers on the sole of foot. Distal pulses are present. What is the probable diagnosis?**
    A. Rupture of Achilles tendon
    B. Gastrocnemius and soleus muscle tear
    C. Compartment syndrome
    D. Tarsal tunnel syndrome

96. **Most common cause of acute compartment syndrome in children is:**
    A. Fracture supracondylar humerus
    B. Transphyseal humerus fracture
    C. Fracture radius/ulna
    D. Fracture shaft humerus

97. **Volkmann ischaemic contracture:**
    A. Due to injury of nerves
    B. Flexor digitalis superficialis usually involved
    C. Treated by releasing flexor pulleys
    D. Anterior interossei nerve is involved

98. **Which among the following is the earliest sign of compartment syndrome?**
    A. Stretch pain   B. Paresthesia
    C. Pulselessness   D. Loss of movement

99. **The earliest sign/symptom of compartment syndrome is:**
    A. Pain   B. Absence of pulse
    C. Paralysis   D. Sensory disturbance

100. **"Volkmann's ischemic contracture" mostly involves which muscle in upper limb?**
    A. Flexor digitorum superficialis
    B. Pronator teres
    C. Flexor digitorum profundus
    D. Flexor carpi radialis longus

101. **First sign of compartment syndrome is:**
    A. Pain on stretch   B. Tingling
    C. Loss of pulse   D. Loss of movement

102. **Volkmann's contracture, which artery is involved?**
    A. Radial   B. Brachial
    C. Ulnar   D. Interosseous

103. **Calf pressure during walking is:**
    A. 200–300 mm Hg
    B. 200–300 cm of H_2O
    C. 20–30 mm Hg
    D. 20–30 cm of H_2O

104. **Dye is injected in one of the extremities in a child and is followed by pain and swelling of upper limb, paresthesias of fingers, stretch pain and normal peripheral pulses, management is:**
    A. Aspiration   B. Anti-inflammatory
    C. Observation   D. Fasciotomy

105. **In posterior compartment syndrome which passive movement causes pain?**
    A. Dorsiflexion of foot
    B. Foot inversion
    C. Toe dorsiflexion
    D. Toe plantar flexion

106. **All are correct regarding compartment syndrome except:**
    A. Pulse is a reliable indicator
    B. Pain on passive stretching
    C. Interstitial pressure > capillary pressure
    D. Paresthesias are seen late

107. **The first sign of compartment is:**
    A. Paresthesia
    B. Pain on passive extension of fingers
    C. Pain on active extension of fingers
    D. Swelling of fingers

108. **The most common cause of Volkmann ischemic contracture (VIC) in a child is:**
    A. Intercondylar fracture of humerus
    B. Fracture both bone of forearm
    C. Fracture lateral condyle of humerus
    D. Supracondylar fracture of humerus

109. **The most common nerve involved in Volkmann's ischemic contracture:**
    A. Radial   B. Ulnar
    C. Median   D. Posterior interosseous

110. **Volkmann's ischemic contracture mostly involves:**
    A. Flexor digitorum superficialis
    B. Pronator teres
    C. Flexor digitorum profundus
    D. Flexor carpi radialis longus

111. **All of the following are features of myositis ossificans except:**
    A. Commonly occurs around the elbow
    B. It matures from inside out
    C. Massage is a known associated factor
    D. Can be post-traumatic

112. **Most common site of myositis ossificans:**
    A. Knee   B. Elbow
    C. Shoulder   D. Wrist

113. **False about myositis ossificans progressiva (child with heterotopic ossifications) is:**
    A. Pneumonia is common
    B. Life longevity is common
    C. Most common site involved is the spine
    D. Onset is before 6 years

114. **In myositis ossificans mature bone is seen:**
    A. At periphery
    B. In center
    C. Whole muscle mass
    D. In the joint capsule

115. **A person of 60 years age is suffering from myositis ossificans progressiva. The usual cause of death:**
    A. Nutritional deficiency
    B. Bed sore
    C. Lung disease
    D. Septicemia

116. **Myositis ossificans is most common around the joints:**
    A. Knee   B. Elbow
    C. Wrist   D. Hip

117. **Treatment of acute myositis ossificans is:**
    A. Active mobilization
    B. Passive mobilization
    C. Infra-red therapy
    D. Immobilization

118. **Myositis ossificans is due to:**
    A. Migration of osteoblasts to hematoma
    B. New bone formation
    C. Ossification of subperiosteal hematoma
    D. All of the above

119. **What is not true about pulled elbow?**
    A. Occurs due to sudden axial pull on extended elbow
    B. Forearm is held in pronation and extension
    C. Most commonly occurs between 2 and 5 years of age
    D. Treatment is quick pronation and flexion of elbow

120. **A mother catches her 3-year-old child by wrist and lifts her. The child does not move her elbow and cries, most likely cause is:**
    A. Shoulder dislocation
    B. Elbow dislocation
    C. Pulled elbow
    D. Colles' fracture

121. **Pulled elbow means?**
    A. Fracture of head of radius
    B. Subluxation of head of radius
    C. Fracture dislocation of elbow
    D. Fracture ulna

122. **A one-and-a-half-year-old child holding her father's hand slipped and fell but did not let go of her father's hand. After that she continued to cry and hold the forearm in pronated position and refused to move the affected extremity. Which of the following management at this stage is most appropriate?**
    A. Supinate the forearm
    B. Examine the child under GA

C. Elevate the limb and observe

D. Investigate for osteomyelitis

123. Name the type of surgery done in this case:

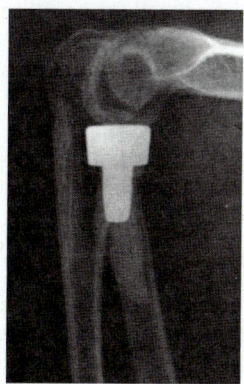

A. Radial head replacement

B. ORIF for radial head

C. Total elbow replacement

D. Fixation for radial neck

124. Essex-Lopresti lesion in upper limb:

A. Injury to interosseous membrane

B. Radial head fracture

C. Radial shaft fracture

D. Radial shaft and radio-ulnar joint fracture

125. Excision of head of radius in a child should not be done because:

A. It produces instability of elbow joint

B. It leads to secondary osteoarthritis of elbow

C. It causes subluxation of inferior radioulnar joint

D. It causes myositis ossificans

126. Open reduction is not required in which fracture?

A. Patella

B. Outer 1/3 of radius head

C. Condyle of humerus

D. Olecranon displaced fracture

127. If head of the radius is removed, it will result in:

A. Lengthening of limb

B. Valgus deformity

C. Varus deformity

D. No deformity

128. In fracture of the olecranon, excision of the proximal fragment is indicated in all of the following situation *except*?

A. Old ununited fractures

B. Non-articular fractures

C. Fracture extending to coronoid process

D. Elderly patient

129. An oblique fracture of olecranon. If displaced proximally the treatment:

A. Excision and resuturing

B. Tension band wiring

C. Elbow is immobilised by cast

D. Open reduction and external fixation

130. What is the diagnosis of this fracture?

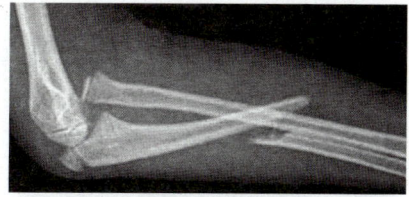

A. Monteggia fracture type

B. Side swipe fracture

C. Galeazzi fracture

131. Name of the fracture for which this surgery is done:

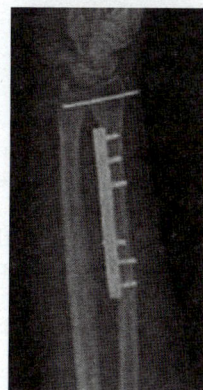

A. Galeazzi fracture   B. Monteggia fracture

C. Wrist subluxation   D. Fracture radius

132. Monteggia fracture is a:

A. Fracture of atlas

B. Fracture of radial styloid

C. Fracture of proximal 1/3 of ulna with dislocation of proximal radioulnar

D. Fracture of distal 1/3 of radius with dislocation of distal radioulnar joint

133. Monteggia fracture is the fracture of?

A. Distal radius   B. Proximal radius

C. Distal ulna   D. Proximal ulna

134. In Monteggia fracture, which is true about ulnar fracture and head of radius most commonly?

A. Both ulnar fracture and head of radius is displaced posteriorly

B. Both ulnar fracture and head of radius is displaced anteriorly

C. Ulnar fracture is posteriorly and head of radius is displaced anteriorly

D. Ulnar fracture is anteriorly and head of radius is displaced posteriorly

135. Posterior interosseous nerve is injured in:

A. Posterior dislocation of elbow

B. Monteggia fracture dislocation

C. Reversed Monteggia fracture dislocation

D. Supracondylar fracture of humerus

136. Anteroposterior and lateral view of wrist is given. What is your diagnosis?

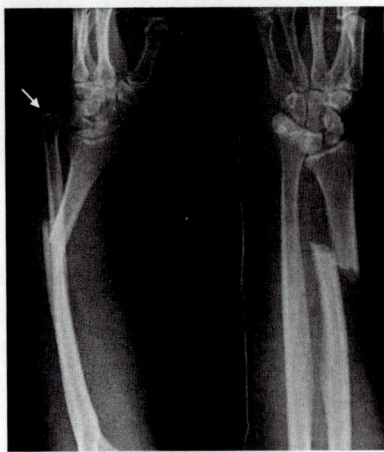

A. Galeazzi   B. Monteggia
C. Smith   D. Colles

137. Galeazzi fracture is:
A. Supracondylar fracture of the humerus
B. Fracture of the distal radius with inferior radioulnar joint dislocation
C. Fracture of radius in the proximal site and dislocation of the elbow
D. Fracture of the radial head

138. Fracture of proximal BBFA, cast position is:
A. Pronated flexion
B. Neutral position
C. Supinated position
D. Position does not matter

139. Fracture of both forearm at same level, position of the arm in plaster is:
A. Full supination   B. 10 degree supination
C. Full pronation   D. Mid-prone

140. The treatment of choice of fracture of radius and ulna in an adult is:
A. Plaster for 4 weeks
B. Closed reduction and calipers
C. Reduction and stabilization with plating
D. Küntscher nails

141. Which of the following is true about Colles fracture?
A. Volar angulation with radius deviation occurs
B. It is an intra-articular fracture
C. It may lead to gunstock deformity due to malunion
D. It is associated with dorsal angulation.

142. Colles' fracture:
A. Fracture line is at radioulnar joint
B. Fracture line extends to the carpal joint
C. 2 cm proximal to the radiocarpal joint
D. Distal fragment is ulnar deviated

143. All are true about Colles' fracture *except*:
A. In old age
B. Dorsal shift
C. At corticocancellous junction
D. Garden spade deformity

144. Colles' fracture—which of the following is not true?
A. Dorsal tilt
B. Volar tilt
C. Lateral displacement
D. Supination

145. Commonest fracture in elderly with fall on outstretched hand is:
A. Colles' fracture   B. Bennett's fracture
C. Galeazzi fracture   D. Monteggia fracture

146. Common fracture in children are all *except*:
A. Lateral condyle humerus
B. Supracondylar humerus
C. Fracture of hand
D. Radius-ulna fracture

147. Modified Allen's test is used to assess proper arterial supply at the:
A. Arm   B. Forearm
C. Wrist   D. Elbow

148. Dinner fork deformity is seen in;
A. Colles' fracture
B. March fracture
C. Lateral condyle fracture
D. Supracondylar fracture

149. Most common complication of Colles' fracture:
A. Malunion
B. Avascular necrosis
C. Finger stiffness
D. Rupture of EPL tendon

150. Position on wrist in case of Colles' fracture is:
A. Palmar deviation and pronation
B. Palmar deviation and supination
C. Dorsal deviation and pronation
D. Dorsal deviation and supination

151. Following displacement seen in Colles' fracture *except*:
A. Dorsal tilt
B. Ventral tilt
C. Dorsal displacement
D. Lateral displacement

152. Colles' fracture is:
A. Common is adolescence
B. A fracture about the ankle joint
C. Common in elderly women
D. A fracture of head of the radius

153. All of the following can be the complications of a malunited Colles' fracture *except*?
A. Rupture of flexor pollicis longus tendon
B. Reflex sympathetic dystrophy (RDS)

C. Carpal tunnel syndrome
D. Carpal instability

154. CPRS is:
A. Type 1 due to nerve injury
B. Type 2 due to fracture complication
C. Tissue necrosis and gangrene are common feature
D. Burning pain is seen

155. A lady with Colles' fracture. The fracture healed but after a few days patient develops pain and swelling over wrist and forearm, red hot and shiny skin and on X-ray patchy osteopenia is seen. Diagnosis is:
A. Sudeck's osteodystrophy
B. Causalgia
C. Non-union
D. Nerve injury

156. Sudeck's dystrophy symptoms are all except?
A. Pain
B. Increased bone density
C. Sweating
D. Stiffness

157. Regarding Sudeck's osteodystrophy all are true except?
A. Burning pain
B. Stiffness and swelling
C. Erythematous and cyanotic discoloration
D. Self liming and good prognosis

158. Sudeck's atrophy is associated with?
A. Osteopetrosis
B. Osteophyte formation
C. Osteopenia
D. Osteochondritis

159. Stellate ganglion block is useful in:
A. Sudeck's osteodystrophy
B. Compound palmar ganglion
C. Tenosynovitis
D. Osteoarthritis of first CMC joint

160. A 40-year-old female presented to the clinic after 3 months of traumatic tibial fracture with history of pain and swelling of right leg since 8–10 days. Here skin of that was shiny, cold and edematous. There was no history of hypertension and diabetes. What is the diagnosis?
A. Complex regional pain syndrome I
B. Complex regional pain syndrome II
C. Fibromyalgia neuropathy
D. Peripheral neuropathy

161. Garden spade deformity is seen in:
A. Barton's fracture   B. Colles' fracture
C. Smith's fracture   D. Bennett's fracture

162. Smith's fracture involves which bone?
A. Distal radius   B. Proximal ulna
C. Metatarsal   D. Patella

163. Management of Smith's fracture is:
A. Open reduction and fixation
B. Plaster cast with forearm in pronation
C. Closed reduction with below-elbow cast
D. Above-elbow cast with forearm in supination

164. Barton's fracture of the wrist:
A. Involved radiocarpal subluxation
B. Is a severe form of Colles' fracture
C. Is often treated by cast
D. All of the above

165. Ossification center of scaphoid appears at:
A. 1–6 months   B. 1 to 2 years
C. 2 to 6 years   D. 4 to 6 years

166. Axis of upper limb passes through:
A. Capitulum   B. Trochlea
C. Olecranon   D. Radial styloid

167. Most common complication of scaphoid fracture:
A. Malunion   B. Avascular necrosis
C. Wrist stiffness   D. Arthritis

168. All are proximal row carpal bones except:
A. Scaphoid   B. Lunate
C. Trapezium   D. Triquetral

169. Which one of the following statements is not correct regarding fracture of the scaphoid?
A. It is the most commonly fractured carpal bone
B. Persistent tenderness in the anatomical snuffbox is highly suggestive of fracture
C. Immediate X-ray of hand may not reveal fracture line
D. Malunion is a frequent complication

170. A patient reported with a history of fall on a outstretched hand, complains of pain in the anatomical snuffbox and clinically no deformities visible. The diagnosis is:
A. Colles' fracture   B. Lunate dislocation
C. Barton's fracture   D. Scaphoid fracture

171. In children fracture scaphoid is though rare but usually involves:
A. Waist   B. Proximal pole
C. Neck   D. Distal pole

172. Most common site of scaphoid fracture is:
A. Waist   B. Proximal fragment
C. Distal fragment   D. Tilting of the lunate

173. The best radiological view for fracture scaphoid is:
A. AP   B. PA
C. Lateral   D. Oblique

174. In nonunion of scaphoid vascularized muscle pedicle graft is taken from:
A. Pronator teres
B. Brachioradialis
C. Pronator quadratus
D. Extensor pollicis longus

175. Bennett's fracture is an:
A. Extra-articular fracture of the 1st metacarpal
B. Extra-articular fracture of the 2nd metacarpal

C. Intra-articular fracture of the 1st metacarpal
D. Intra-articular fracture of the 2nd metacarpal

176. One of the common fracture that occur during boxing by hitting with a closed first is:
A. Monteggia fracture dislocation
B. Galeazzi fracture dislocation
C. Bennett's fracture dislocation
D. Smith's fracture

177. Boxer's fracture is:
A. Radial styloid fracture
B. Reverse Colles' fracture
C. 5th metacarpal fracture
D. 1st metacarpal fracture

178. Rolando fracture involves base of:
A. 1st metacarpal
B. 2nd metacarpal
C. 3rd metacarpal
D. 4th metacarpal

179. Bennett's fracture is fracture dislocation of base of metacarpal:
A. 4th   B. 3rd
C. 2nd   D. 1st

180. A Bennett's fracture is difficult to maintain in a reduced position mainly because of the pull of the:
A. Flexor pollicis longus
B. Flexor pollicis brevis
C. Extensor pollicis longus
D. Abductor pollicis

181. The term Bennett's fracture is used to describe:
A. Fracture dislocation of metacarpophalangeal joint of thumb
B. Interphalangeal fracture dislocation of thumb
C. Anterior marginal fracture of distal end of radius
D. Fracture dislocation of trapeziometacarpal joint

ANSWERS

1. A. Radius
2. D. Skin, subcutaneous tissue, superficial fascia and deep fascia (complete release of fascia is important to decompress the closed compartment of increased pressure)
3. B. Retroversion of 30 degrees
4. B. Rotator cuff muscles
5. A. Subscapularis
6. A. Supraspinatus
7. C. Rotator cuff tendon
8. D. Teres major
9. C. Supraspinatus and subscapularis
10. B. Biceps long head
11. C. Inferior
12. A. It is most common type of shoulder dislocation
13. A. Anterior dislocation of shoulder
14. C. Bristow's lesion
15. A. Elevated anterior axillary fold
16. A. Subcoracoid
17. A. Anterior
18. A. Anterior dislocation of shoulder
19. B. Axillary
20. B. Surgically managed
21. B. Abduction and external rotation
22. A. Ankle
23. D. Rotator cuff injury
24. B. Surgery
25. B. Musculocutaneous nerve
26. B. Posterior dislocation of shoulder
27. B. Posterior dislocation
28. B. Anteromedial
29. D. All of the above
30. D. All of the above
31. C. Jerk test
32. A. Apprehension test
33. A. Clavicle
34. D. Acromion
    • See the normal X-ray of shoulder joint to know the bony landmarks.
35. A. Clavicle
36. C. Figure of eight bandage
37. B. Supraspinatus
38. A. Axillary
39. A. AC joint dislocation
40. A. Radial nerve palsy
41. D. Fracture shaft humerus
42. C. Ulnar
43. D. Four part
44. D. Axillary
45. A. Ulnar
46. A. Velpaeu bandage
47. A. Analgesic with triangular sling
48. A. Abduction and lateral rotation
49. A. Elderly women
50. D. Fracture humerus
51. D. Distraction at fracture site
52. D. Capitellum
53. A. Supracondylar fracture humerus
54. B. Head of radius, lateral epicondyle, olecranon
55. B. Malunion causing gunstock deformity is the MC complication
56. A. Supracondylar humerus fracture
57. B. Lateral closing wedge osteotomy
58. A. Extension type is more common than flexion type
59. B. Closed reduction of fracture and look of reappearance of pulse

60. A. Posteromedial extension
61. B. Posterior medial displacement of posterior fragment
62. A. Cubitus varus
63. B. Supracondylar fracture of humerus
  - M/C nerve injury is AIN > Median > radial (these three in extension type) > ulnar (in flexion type and post surgery). AIN/median nerve injury will lead to pointing index sign.
64. A. Posterior
65. A. Supracondylar fracture of humerus
66. D. Nonunion
67. A. Static cubitus varus
68. C. Nerve injury transitory
69. C. Myositis ossification
70. B. Extension type most common
71. C. Posteromedial
72. A. Flexion
73. B. Posterior
74. A. Coronoid process posterior to humerus
75. C. Olecranon
76. B. Closed reduction and K-wire fixation
77. A. Posterolateral
78. C. Compartment syndrome
79. D. Supracondylar fracture of humerus
80. D. Malunited supracondylar fracture of humerus
81. D. Hyperextension injury
82. B. Physeal injury
83. A. Lateral condylar fracture of humerus
84. A. Humerus lateral condylar fracture
85. A. Valgus deformity
86. B. Nonunion
87. D. Lateral condyle fracture humerus
88. B. Lateral condylar fracture humerus
89. B. Lateral condylar fracture humerus > 'C' Supracondylar fracture humerus
90. C. Open reduction and internal fixation
91. A. Stretch pain
92. D. Thumb abduction
93. A. VIC
94. B. Closed reduction of fracture and look for reappearance of pulse
95. C. Compartment syndrome
96. A. Fracture supracondylar humerus
97. D. Anterior interossei nerve is involved
98. A. Stretch pain
99. A. Pain
100. C. Flexor digitorum profundus
101. A. Pain of stretch
102. B. Brachial
103. A. 200–300 mm Hg
104. D. Fasciotomy
105. C. Toe dorsiflexion
106. A. Pulse is a reliable indicator

107. B. Pain on passive extension of fingers
108. D. Supracondylar fracture of humerus
109. C. Median
110. C. Flexor digitorum profundus
111. B. It matures from inside out
112. B. Elbow
113. B. Life longevity is common
114. A. At periphery
115. C. Lung disease
116. B. Elbow
117. D. Immobilization
118. D. All of the above
119. D. Treatment is quick pronation and flexion of elbow
120. C. Pulled elbow
121. B. Subluxation of head of radius
122. A. Supinate the forearm
123. A. Radial head replacement
124. A. Injury to interosseous membrane
125. C. It causes subluxation of inferior radioulnar joint
126. B. Outer 1/3 of radius head
127. B. Valgus deformity
128. C. Fracture extending to coronoid process
129. B. Tension band wiring
130. A. Monteggia fracture type
131. A. Galeazzi fracture
132. C. Fracture of proximal 1/3 of ulna with dislocation of proximal radioulnar
133. D. Proximal ulna
134. B. Both ulnar fracture and head of radius is displaced anteriorly
135. B. Monteggia fracture dislocation
136. A. Galleazzi
137. B. Fracture of the distal radius with inferior radioulnar joint dislocation
138. C. Supinated position
139. D. Mid-prone
140. C. Reduction and stabilization with plating
141. D. It is associated with dorsal angulation
142. C. 2 cm proximal to the radiocarpal joint
143. D. Garden spade deformity
144. B. Volar tilt
145. A. Colles' fracture
146. A. Lateral condyle humerus
147. C. Wrist
148. A. Colles' fracture
149. C. Finger stiffness
150. A. Palmar deviation and pronation
151. B. Ventral tilt
152. C. Common in elderly women
153. A. Rupture of flexor pollicis longus tendon
154. D. Burning pain is seen
155. A. Sudeck's osteodystrophy
156. B. Increased bone density

157. D. Self liming and good prognosis
158. C. Osteopenia
159. A. Sudeck's osteodystrophy
160. A. Complex regional pain syndrome I
161. C. Smith's fracture
162. A. Distal radius
163. D. Above-elbow cast with forearm in supination
164. A. Involved radiocarpal subluxation
165. D. 4 to 6 years
166. A. Capitulum
167. B. Avascular necrosis
168. C. Trapezium
169. D. Malunion is a frequent complication

170. D. Scaphoid fracture
171. D. Distal pole
172. A. Waist
173. D. Oblique
174. C. Pronator quadratus
175. C. Intra-articular fracture of the 1st metacarpal
176. C. Bennett's fracture dislocation
177. C. 5th metacarpal fracture
178. A. 1st metacarpal
179. D. 1st
180. D. Abductor pollicis
181. D. Fracture dislocation of trapeziometacarpal joint

7

Pelvis and Hip Fractures

HIP JOINT APPLIED ANATOMY

Hip joint is a ball and socket synovial joint. Neck shaft angle at birth is 140° and femoral anteversion is 40°. When the child starts walking (i.e. bearing weight), neck shaft angle decreases to adult value of 125°+/– 5° and anteversion to 15–20°, this happens till 8 years of age, after which there are no changes. Acetabulum also has 15–20° anteversion and 45° inferior inclination. Thus in hip replacement surgery, we try to reproduce 45° angulation of acetabular cup and 15–20° anteversion.

Xtra edge

- Coxa vara— neck shaft angle <120°.
- Coxa valga—neck shaft angle >130°.
- Ligament of Bigelow (iliofemoral ligament) is the strongest ligament in the body and prevents pelvis from titling backwards and limits abduction.
- Hip joint capsule is weakest posteriorly.
- Neck of femur has three sets of trabeculae, 1°/2° compressive; 1°/2° tensile and greater trochanteric group.

GAIT

Biomechanics

Biomechanics upon standing on two legs, the center of gravity is just anterior (~5 cm) to S2 vertebrae and femoral head is subjected to the following three forces:
- Body weight
- Joint reaction force (as per Newton's third law)
- Abductor muscular force.

On a single leg stance (standing), the opposite (unsupported) pelvis has a tendency to dip down due to gravity and this is prevented by abductor muscle of the supported leg. Abductor muscles (mainly gluteus medius) arise from iliac crest and insert on greater trochanter. While on single leg stance, they contract and raise the opposite/unsupported side of the pelvis by "cantilever mechanism". If abductor muscles are defective, they cannot raise the unsupported side and it dips down on single leg stance, which forms the basis of Trendelenburg test/gait (discussed later).

Gait

Normal adult pattern of gait is acquired by 5 years of age, and once motion is started, steady gait pattern is accomplished in approx 3 steps. In normal gait, each leg goes through a stance phase and a swing phase.
- *Stance phase*—when foot is on the ground (60% of the gait cycle) and is divided into (in sequence)—heel strike–foot flat–midstance–heel off–toe off (preswing).
- *Swing*—when the foot is off the ground (40% of gait cycle) and is divided into—acceleration, midswing, deacceleration.
- *Double support phase*—when both the foot is on the ground and forms 11% of gait cycle.

Different gaits

- Antalgic gait—due to painful hip, hip lurches on the same side, to decrease hip joint reactive force. Other way to decrease hip pain is to take a cane on opposite hand.
- Scissoring gait—seen in cerebral palsy.
- Crouch gait—seen in cerebral palsy.
- Hand to knee gait—seen in polio.
- Foot drop/high stepping gait—in CPN/sciatic nerve palsy.
- Short limb gait—due to one limb shortening. To compensate, patient may keep short limb in equinus or longer limb's hip/knee in flexion.
- Trendelenburg gait—when the pathological hip is in single stance phase, if abductor mechanism is weak it l/t **D**ropping of the pelvis in **O**pposite side and **L**urching on the **A**ffected side of pathology (**DOLA**).

For a normal gait, one requires intact hip abductor mechanism which acts through an intact fulcrum (head), lever (neck of femur) and power (abductors). So pathology in any of the above will lead to a positive Trendelenburg test/gait, *for example*, defective left side abductor will cause drooping of right-sided pelvis.

Causes of Trendelenburg gait/test

- Defect in fulcrum—hip dislocation, head destruction like in—advanced TB hip/AVN, Perthes, SCFE, DDH, sequelae of septic arthritis.
- Defect in lever arm—fracture of head/NOF/trochanter, coxa vara.
- Power paralysis—polio, superior gluteal nerve palsy (supply gluteus medius and minimus), disc prolapsed L4–5 compressing L5 root which supply gluteus medius and minimus; TFL, ITB and sartorius palsy can also lead to Trendelenburg gait.

Xtra edge

- In straight leg raise test (SLR) hip joint is subjected to force equal to 3 times the body weight.
- Least kinetic energy is at heel strike and maximum potential energy is at midstance.
- Preswing is the only phase of gait cycle where all muscle groups are silent.
- Trendelenburg test positive in both hip lead to waddling gait (like a duck).
- Eccentric contraction means muscle lengthens despite electrical contraction, e.g. tibialis anterior and gastro-soleus.

EXAMINATION OF HIP JOINT

Examination of hip joint starts right from the point patient enters the room by looking at his gait and attitude while lying supine.

Tests for Limb Length Discrepancy (LLD)

In diseases of hip joint shortening is more common than lengthening. Hip joint compensates for LLD by developing a deformity in the coronal plane to acquire a normal gait. Shortening is compensated by developing abduction deformity and lengthening by adduction deformity. Shortening may be due to diseases above trochanteric level k/a supratrochanteric shortening (most common) and if below trochanteric level then infratrochanteric shortening.

Qualitative assessment of **supratrochanteric shortening (Fig. 7.1)**

1. **Schoemaker's line**—a line joining tip of greater trochanter and ASIS, when extrapolated on both sides will meet at the center at/below umbilicus in normal cases. If there is supratrochanteric shortening, greater trochanter will migrate proximally and then the line will meet the opposite line below the umbilicus and on the opposite side. (Remember it looks like a shoelace and thus the name.)
2. **Chiene's parallelogram**—if both ASIS are joined and both tip of GT are joined, it forms two lines which are parallel to each other (thus the name of the test), if there is supratrochanteric shortening, then lines on that side will converge.
3. **Morris bitrochanteric test**—distance from the tip of GT to pubic symphysis are equal on both sides. If GT is externally rotated or displaced back, then distance will increase on that side or vice versa, e.g. central dislocation.
4. **Nélaton's line**—patients lies on lateral position, with the affected side up and hip flexed 90°. A line drawn from ischial tuberosity to ASIS will pass through the tip of GT. In case of supratrochanteric shortening, the line will pass below the tip of GT and vice versa.

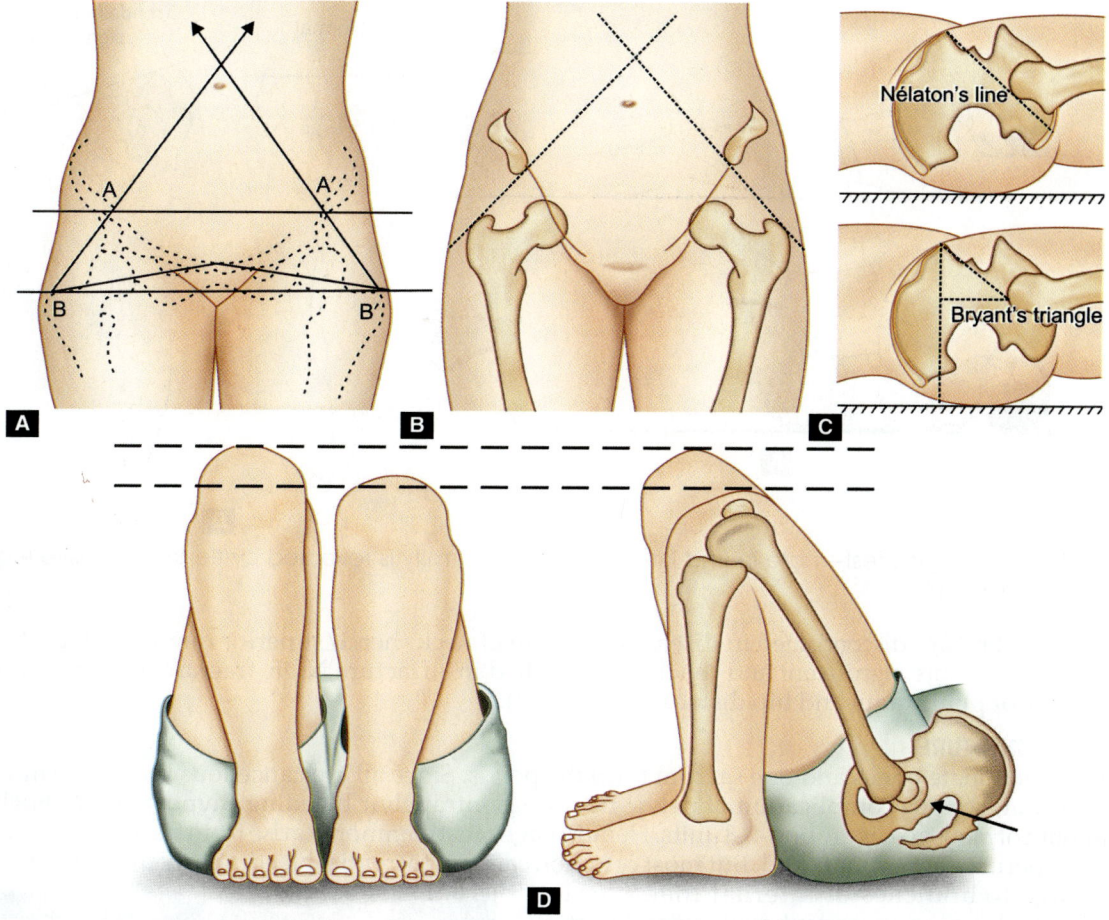

Fig. 7.1: (A) Lines of qualitative assessment, (B) schoemaker line, (C) Nélaton's line and Bryant's triangle, (D) Galeazzi test

5. **Galeazzi test**—used in DDH for visual examination of limb shortening.
   • **Quantitative** assessment—**Bryant's triangle** (Fig. 7.1C).

Test for Flexion Deformity
Hip develops flexion deformity and to conceal the same/for normal gait pattern hip biomechanics develops increased lumbar lordosis. Up to 30° flexion deformity of the hip can be compensated by lumbar lordosis. Thomas' test is done to measure/reveal fixed flexion deformity of hip by neutralising lumbar lordosis (Fig. 7.2A).

Test of Hip Instability
• Active SLRT (passive SLRT is done for disc prolapsed)
• Telescopy test
• Other test (used in DDH)—Barlow and Ortolani test.

Test for Abductor Insufficiency
Trendelenburg test—patient is asked to stand on the affected hip, normal limb off the ground. If abductor insufficiency is present, then the normal side of pelvis will deep down. Causes—as discussed earlier (Fig. 7.2B).

X-ray Signs
• **Shenton's line**—when an imaginary line is drawn from medial cortex of neck of femur till inferior border of superior pubic ramii, then a semicircular line is formed known as Shenton's line. It

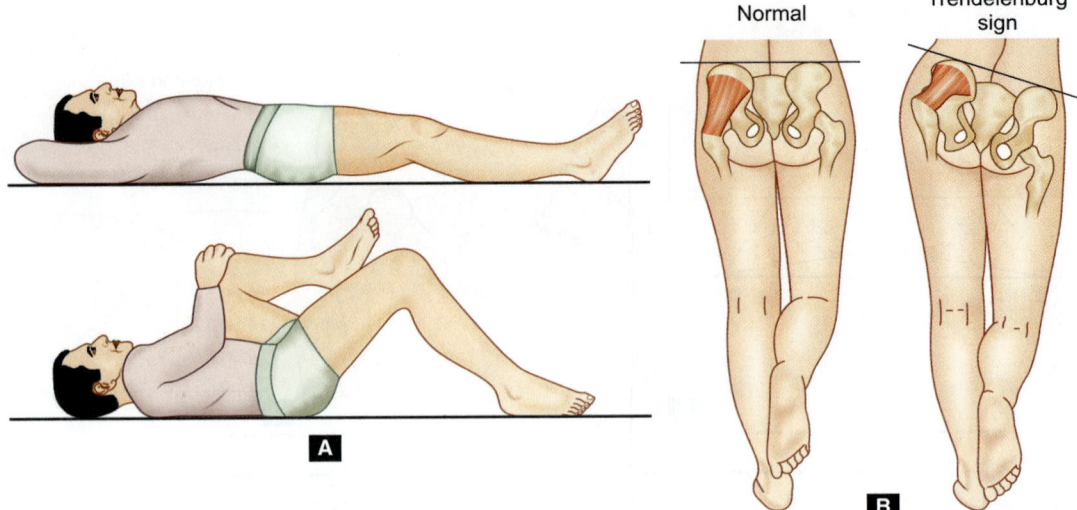

Fig. 7.2: (A) Thomas test—note in 2nd image flexion deformity is revealed by flexing opposite leg, (B) Trendelenburg test

may be broken/discontinued in diseases/fracture of neck/head/superior ramii. Neck part of the line is more significant and the line is breached in—fracture NOF, fracture head, fracture superior pubic ramii and hip dislocation (Fig. 7.3).

PELVIC FRACTURE

Two innominate bones and one sacrum form the pelvis. Since all are cancellous bones, the most important/serious complication of pelvic fracture is intrapelvic bleeding/hypovolemic shock. Amount of blood loss is around 4–8 units. Hemorrhage most commonly arise from fractured surface > retroperitoneal venous blood. But most common cause of torrential bleeding which occurs from damage to branches of internal iliac arteries; superior gluteal artery and internal pudendal artery are amongst the most common injured branches. Hypovolemic shock and head injury are the major causes of early death after pelvic fracture, while sepsis and multiorgan failure are the late causes of death. Most common pelvic fracture is ischio-pubic ramii fracture.

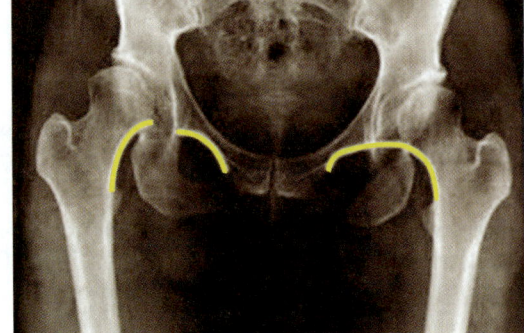

Classification
- Young and Burgess—based on direction of force (AP, lateral, vertical, combined).
- Tile
  - A—stable fracture (e.g. avulsion fracture).
  - B—rotationally unstable but vertically stable, e.g. open book injury/bucket handle injury

Fig. 7.3: Shenton's line. Note broken Shenton's line on left side due to hip dislocation

  - C—both rotationally and vertically unstable, e.g. limb length discrepancy may be present due to vertical displacement.

Radiological signs indicating unstable pelvis
- Pubic diastasis >2–2.5 cm with posterior pelvic injury or injury to anterior/posterior sacroiliac ligament or sacrospinous ligament.
- Posterior sacroiliac complex displacement >1 cm.
- Avulsion fracture of sacral/ischial end of the sacrospinous ligament.
- Presence of gap rather than impaction in the posterior pelvic ring.
- Avulsion fractures of the L5 transverse process.

Treatment

- **Emergency:** First ATLS protocol and a pelvic binder to decrease pelvic volume and create tamponade to stop/decrease intrapelvic hemorrhage. Pelvic binder may be in the form of commercially available, rolled sheet, MAST (military antishock trouser), external fixator. For anterior ring injury external fixator is applied (e.g. open book injury) but for posterior ring injury pelvic C-clamp is preferred.
- **Definitive treatment**
  - Type A—rest is sufficient.
  - Type B—external fixator is sufficient if pubic diastasis is <2.5 cm. If >2.5 cm then anterior fixation is combined with an external fixator.
  - Type C—posterior instability is addressed by posterior fixation (e.g. SI joint screw/plate) in combination with an external fixator.

Eponyms

- **Straddle fracture:** Bilateral superior and inferior pubic rami fractures.
- **Open book fracture:** A pelvic fracture due to anteroposterior compression of pelvis where the pubic symphysis is disrupted and pelvis opens up like a book.
- **Malgaigne's fracture:** A type of pelvis fracture due to side-to-side compression of pelvis where there is fracture of pubic rami anteriorly and sacroiliac joint or ilium posteriorly but on the same side.
- **Bucket handle fracture:** A type of pelvis fracture due to side-to-side compression of pelvis where there is fracture of pubic rami anteriorly and sacroiliac joint or ilium posteriorly but on the opposite side.
- **Wind swept pelvis:** It is a lateral compression injury of ipsilateral hemipelvis and open book or external rotation type injury of contralateral hemipelvis.
- **Duverney fracture:** Isolated iliac wing fracture.
- **Crescent fracture:** Iliac wing fracture in pelvis that enters into SI joint.
- **Jumper's fracture:** Transverse fracture of sacrum seen in patients who have a fall from height during a suicidal attempt. It is characterized by 'H'or 'U' shaped fracture line involving upper sacrum (S1 and S2).

Complication

Hypovolemic shock, sciatic nerve injury (neuropraxia), abdominal viscera/urethral injury, sexual dysfunction, Morel-Lavalle lesion.

- **Morel-Lavallée lesion**—it is a post-traumatic, closed, internal degloving injury resulting from a shearing force applied to the skin, in which skin and subcutaneous tissue is separated from underlying fascia, thus creating a potential space where blood, seroanguinous fluid and necrotic fat get collected. It is mostly seen in pelvic and acetabular fracture and the M/c site is around the greater trochanter in anterolateral thigh. Surgery through the lesion is C/I as it has been a/w higher incidence of infection and wound dehiscence. In such cases, fractures can be treated by ilio-inguinal approach thus, avoiding the affected area.

ACETABULUM FRACTURE

Understanding acetabulum and its anatomical landmarks in radiology: The articular socket (incomplete hemisphere/inverted horseshoe shaped) is composed of and supported by two columns of bone, described by Letournel and Judet as an inverted Y. The anterior column is composed of the anterior half of the iliac crest, the iliac spines, the anterior half of the acetabulum, and the pubis. The posterior column is the ischium, the ischial spine, the posterior half of the acetabulum, and the dense bone forming the sciatic notch. The shorter posterior column ends at its intersection with anterior column at the top of the sciatic notch. This column concept is used by Judet and Letournel in classification, treatment and prognosis (Fig. 7.4).

- The iliopectineal line is the major landmark of anterior column.
- The ilioischial line is the major landmark of posterior column.
- Posterior column fracture is the most common type of acetabular fracture.
- Bicolumnar fracture is the most severe of all and central fracture dislocation is a type of bicolumnar fracture of acetabulum.
- Spur sign—triangular fragment of bone seen in bicolumnar fracture.

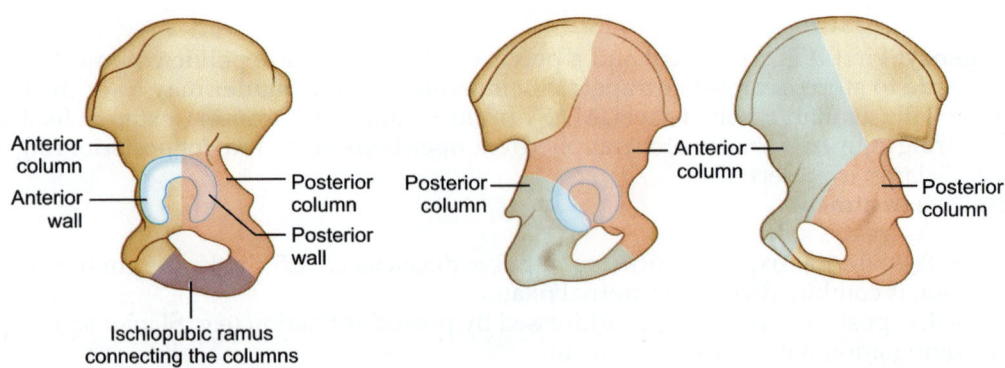

Fig. 7.4: Schematic diagram showing acetabular anatomy and its columns

X-ray—Judet described two oblique views in addition to normal AP view to study walls and column.
- Obturator oblique view—anterior column and posterior wall are better seen (Fig. 7.5B).
- Iliac oblique view—posterior column and anterior wall are better seen (Fig. 7.5A).

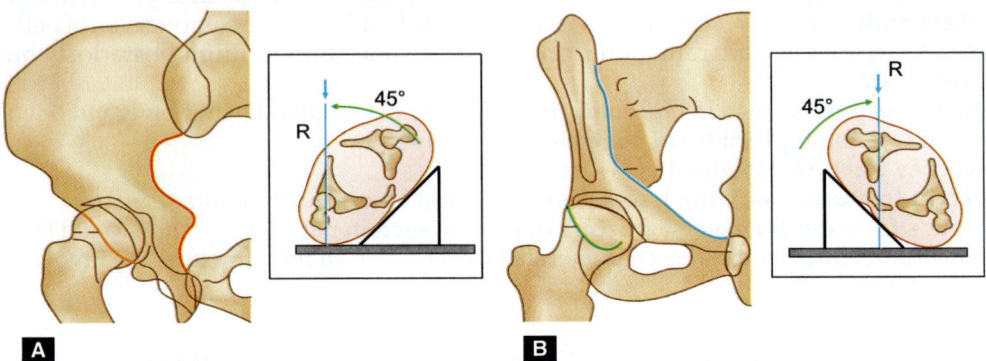

Fig. 7.5: (A) Iliac oblique view, (B) obturator oblique view

Treatment
Aim is to complete anatomical restoration of dome (weight bearing part) of acetabulum with concentric femoral head reduction in the dome. Matta's roof arc angle is the determinant of conservative/surgical treatment. Basically displaced fractures through the weight bearing dome is treated by ORIF. Acetabular fracture surgery is always an elective surgery except in situation like—open injury, neurovascular injury, fracture dislocation where emergency surgery is required.

Complications
- *Early*:
    - Sciatic nerve injury occurs due to both trauma > fracture surgery. Posterior wall fractures and Kocher-Langenbeck approach are most commonly associated with sciatic nerve injury.
    - Iliofemoral vein thrombosis.
- *Late*:
    - Post-traumatic 2° arthritis is the most common late complication.
    - Others—AVN of femoral head, heterotopic ossification, joint stiffness.

HIP DISLOCATION
Hip joint is the most stable joint of the body supported by the strongest ligament (iliofemoral ligament), thus hip dislocation is a high energy trauma. Hip dislocation may occur as pure dislocation or associated with fracture of acetabulum/femoral head. Direction of dislocation depends on position of limb during trauma and direction of force. Types of hip dislocation are posterior (90%) > anterior > central (rare) dislocation. Complication common to all types is AVN of femoral head and joint stiffness. To avoid femoral head AVN, it should be reduced by 6–12 hrs.

Deformities (Fig. 7.6)

- *Ant. dislocation hip (FABER)*: Flexion, abduction → Obturator type–flexion
Pubic type–extension.
- *Post. dislocation hip (FADIR)*: Flexion, adduction, internal rotation (**maximum shortening**).
- *Central fracture dislocation hip*: Abduction/adduction and IR/ER, both are possible depending upon injury mechanism plus there is less shortening.
- *In dislocation a/w fracture classical deformities may not be seen (imp)*.

Posterior Dislocation

Occurs when axial force is applied to a flexed, adducted and internally rotated hip, producing pure posterior dislocation (Fig. 7.6B). If the hip is in neutral/abducted position, then posterior dislocation occurs after fracturing posterior wall, depending on type of fracture of postwall, **Thompson and Epstein** classified posthip dislocation into 5 types.

- Type 4—dislocation with fracture of acetabular floor.
- Type 5—dislocation with fracture of femoral head.
- Thompson and Epstein's type 5 is subdivided by **Pipkin's** into 4:
  - Type II—femoral head fracture cephalad to fovea centralis.
  - Type III—femoral head fracture associated with fracture NOF.
  - Type IV—type I, II or III associated with acetabular fracture.

Dashboard injury—injury in a flexed hip and knee producing posterior fracture dislocation of hip, patella fracture and PCL injury. Since posterior dislocation, it may be associated with sciatic nerve injury and AVN. Normally femoral arterial pulse is felt against femur head, thus in post dislocation femoral pulse is not felt and is known as vascular sign of Narath and femoral head can be palpated posteriorly, producing maximum shortening of limb. CT scan is the investigation of Choice (IOC) in dislocation associated with fractures.

Closed reduction maneuver—should be done within maximum 12 hours to avoid AVN of head.

- Allis maneuver
- Stimpson's gravity method
- Bigelow's maneuver
- East Baltimore maneuver

Indication for open reduction—failed attempt at closed reduction for 1–2 times and associated wall/head fracture.

Complication: Most common dislocation associated with sciatic nerve injury and superior gluteal artery injury (rare).

Anterior Dislocation

Force applied to a hyperabducted and externally rotated hip produces anterior dislocation. The magnitude of hip flexion at the time of injury decides the final position of dislocation: Epstein's—superior (pubic) and inferior (obturator/perineal). Anterior hip dislocations are associated with

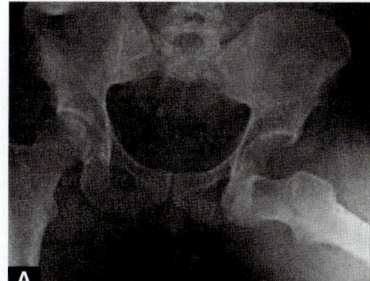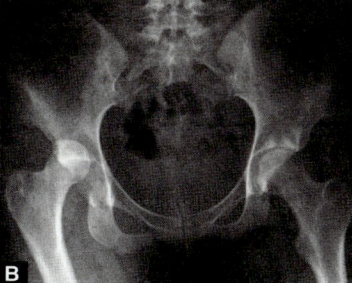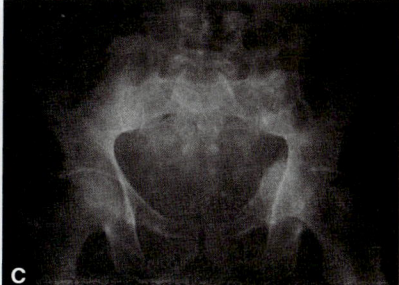

Fig. 7.6: (A) Anterior dislocation (note limb is abducted and LT is more prominent, means hip is ER), (B) Posterior dislocation (note limb is adducted and LT is less prominent means hip is IR), (C) Central fracture dislocation (head medially displaced)

lengthening. The head may be palpable in groin and may injure femoral nerves/vessels (esp. pubic types). Femoral pulses are palpable, thus vascular sign of Narath is not seen (Fig. 7.6A).

Central Fracture Dislocation

Its a rare type and is typical of a fall from height onto the leg with transmission of force through the acetabulum. Extensive degree of concomitant articular injury occurs because head is forced medially through the floor of acetabulum, and head can be palpable in P/R examination. Distal and occassionally, lateral traction of proximal femur may be necessary to effect and maintain reduction of the femoral head (Fig. 7.6C).

FRACTURE NECK OF FEMUR (UNSOLVED FRACTURE)

Fracture NOF is a low energy, intracapsular fracture seen in elderly population (female > male). Fracture NOF is an intracapsular fracture because neck is an intra-articular structure, whereas fracture I/T femur is an extracapsular fracture, as trochanters are extracapsular. Capsule is attached anteriorly along the intertrochanteric line and posteriorly just a finger breadth proximal to the I/T ridge. Prognosis of intracapsular fracture are poor and most common complication is non-union, whereas that of extracapsular fracture is good with most common complication being malunion. There is shortening with external rotation of limb, tenderness in Scarpa's triangle, and loss of active SLRT, while in valgus impacted fracture obvious deformity may be absent.

Classification

- *Anatomic classification* (Fig. 7.7A)
  - Subcapital (worst prognosis)
  - Transcervical
  - Basocervical

	Fracture neck of femur (intracapsular)	Intertrochanteric fracture (extracapsular)
Table 7.1: Comparison between intracapsular and extracapsular fractures of proximal femur		
Mechanism of injury	Most common due to low energy fall (high velocity trauma in young patients)	Same
Clinical features	Moderate pain in Scarpa's triangle, swelling and echymosis are usually absent	Severe pain, swelling and echymoses are usually present around greater trochanter
Deformity	Less due to capsular attachment in distal fracture fragment (shortening <2.5 cm, ER <45°)	More (ER >45° lateral border of foot almost touching the couch, shortening >2.5 cm)
Trochanteric palpation	Normal	Broadening and tenderness
SLRT and walking	May be present in impacted fracture	Not possible
Complications	AVN > non-union > arthritis	Malunion is the most common complication. AVN is not seen

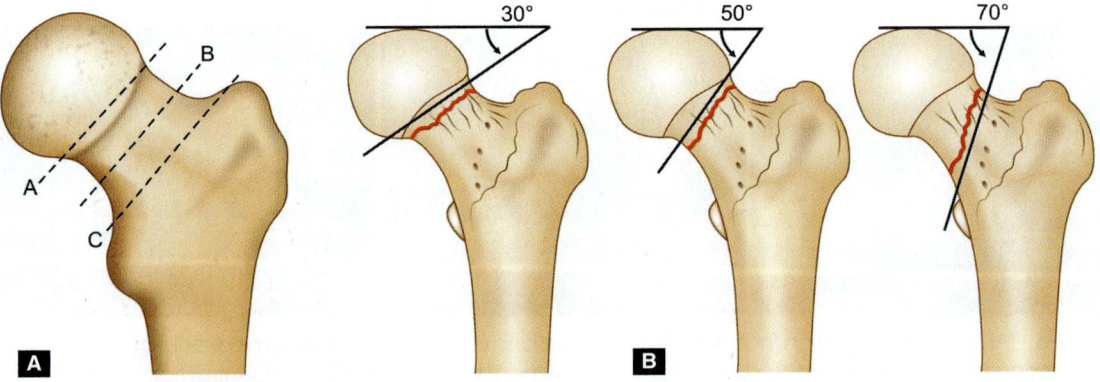

Fig. 7.7: (A) Anatomical classification, (B) Pauwels' classification

- *Pauwels' classification*—depending on angle (Pauwels' angle) formed by the fracture line with the horizontal. More the Pauwels' angle, more unstable is the fracture with poorer prognosis (Fig. 7.7 B).
  - *Type I:* <30°
  - *Type II:* 30–50°
  - *Type III:* >70° (worst prognosis)
- *Garden's classification*—based on the degree of displacement on AP X-ray of hip joint by determining the relation of trabecular lines in the femoral head to those in the acetabulum and neck (Fig. 7.7 C).
  - *Stage I.* Incomplete fracture line (valgus impacted). Normally aligned trabeculae between acetabulum and head. Trabecular bending in neck with respect to head.
  - *Stage II.* Complete fracture line; nondisplaced, with trabeculae alignment maintained in all three structures.
  - *Stage III.* Complete fracture line; **partially** displaced. Trabecular pattern of the femoral head does not line up with that of the acetabulum and that of head not aligned with neck. Head internally rotated and distal fragment externally rotated.
  - *Stage IV.* Complete fracture line; **completely** displaced. Distal fragment gets further externally rotated and head comes in normal position, so trabecular pattern of the head assumes a parallel orientation with that of the acetabulum.
    Stage IV has the worst prognosis.
- **Delbet classification**—used in children
  - Transepiphyseal (rare and worst prognosis)
  - Transcervical (most common)
  - Cervicotrochanteric
  - Intertrochanteric.

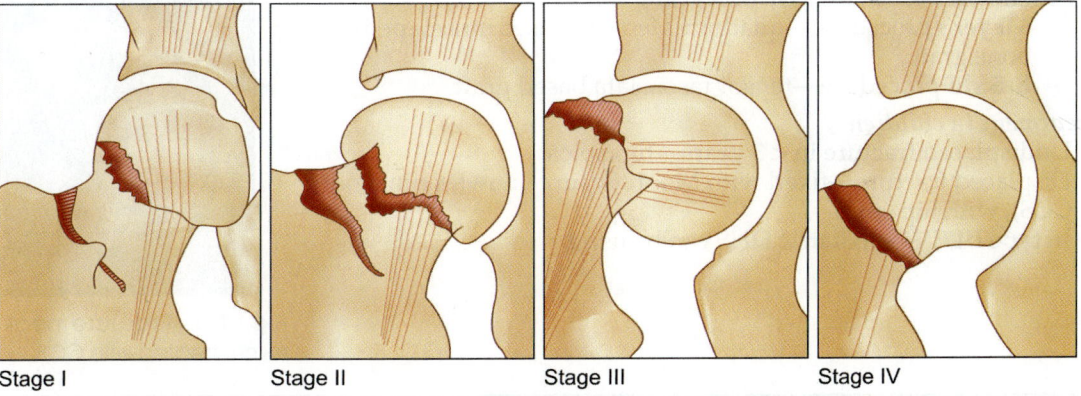

Stage I   Stage II   Stage III   Stage IV

Fig. 7.7: (C) Garden's classification

X-ray

Internal rotation view is the IOC, but in valgus impacted fracture MRI is the IOC.

Treatment

Flowchart 7.1 (adults)

- CRIF with CCS (Fig. 7.8) (3 screws in inverted triangle pattern) is the TOC in fresh cases (<3 weeks) in subcapital/transcervial fracture pattern. In basicervical DHS (dynamic hip screw) can also be used. If closed reduction is unsuccessful, then open reduction and internal fixation is done.
- >60 years/active/long life expectancy/arthritic changes present—TOC is THR
  >60 years/less active/life expectancy is less/no arthritic changes—then a smaller procedure like hemihip arthroplasty can be done.

Flowchart 7.1: Treatment algorithm of fracture neck of femur

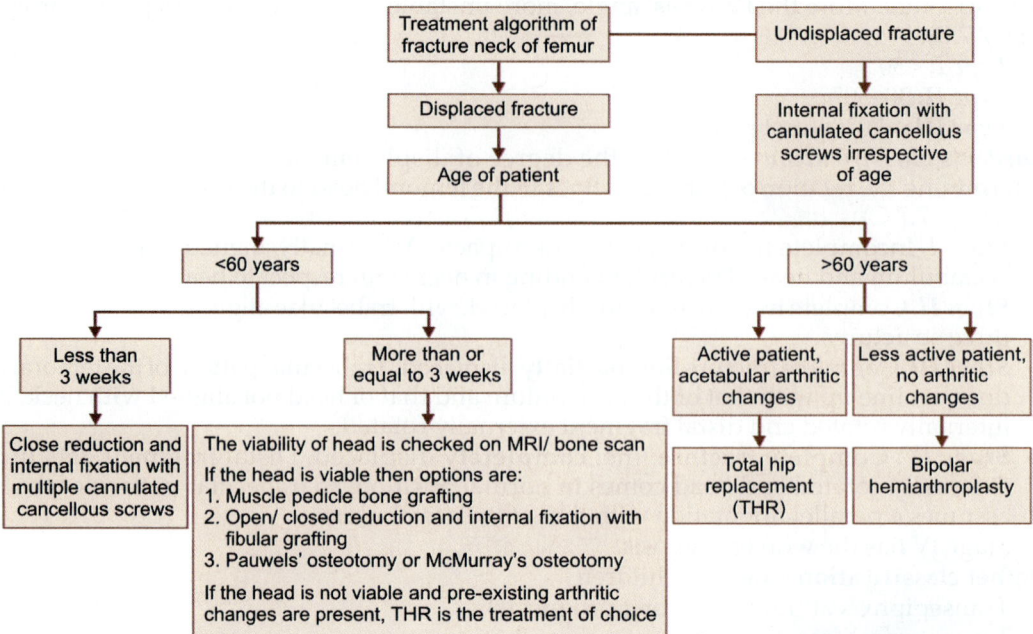

- Late cases (>3 weeks)/nonunion—CCS supplemented by muscle based vascular graft to increase vascularity and increase chances of union and decrease risk of AVN.
  - **Meyer's** procedure—quadratus femoris based muscle pedicle bone graft.
  - **Bakshi** procedure—tensor fascia lata based graft.

Treatment in children
- Undisplaced fracture in < 3 years—hip spica.
- Displaced fracture—fixed with Moore's pin/Knowles pins (not CCS), with hip spica.
- In type III/IV—pediatric DHS can be used.

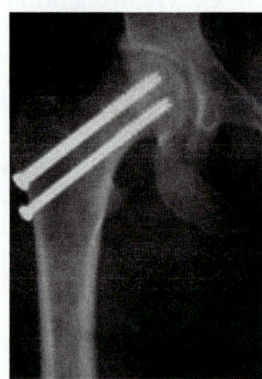

Fig. 7.8: Fracture neck of femur treated with CCS

MULTIPLE CHOICE QUESTIONS

1. Name the test done:

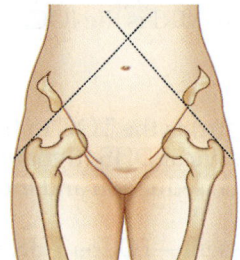

   A. Schoemaker's line B. Nélaton's line
   C. Galeazzi test   D. Thomas test

2. Line jointing anterior superior iliac spine to ischial tuberosity and passes above greater trochanter:
   A. Nélaton's line   B. Schoemaker's line
   C. Chiene's line   D. Perkin's line

3. A patient come with complaint to difficulty in climbing upstairs. When he is made to stand on his right leg, left side of pelvis fell to a lower level. When he stands on left leg, then right side of pelvis can be drawn up. Which of the following nerve of him has got affected?
   A. Right inferior gluteal
   B. Right superior gluteal

C. Left superior gluteal
D. Left inferior gluteal

4. Thomas test helps to detect:
A. Adduction deformity of the hip
B. Integrity of the abductor mechanism
C. Fixed flexion deformity of the hip
D. Apparent shortening at the hip joint

5. Trendelenburg tests would be positive in the following conditions:
A. L 4-L5 PIVD
B. L5-S1 PIVD
C. Synovitis of the hip
D. Femoroacetabular impingement syndrome

6. Identify the test being performed in the image below:

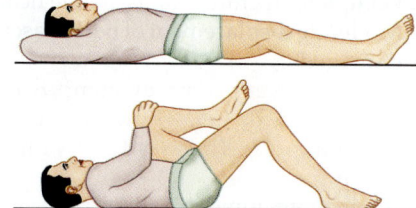

A. Trendelenburg   B. Thomas test
C. Smith   D. Narath

7. Trendelenburg test positive in palsy of:
A. Gluteus maximus   B. Gluteus medius
C. Rectus femoris   D. Vastus medialis

8. Trendelenburg test is mainly for:
A. Gluteus maximus   B. Gluteus medius
C. Gluteus minimus   D. Biceps femoris

9. Trendelenburg's sign is negative in an intertrochanteric fracture because of:
A. Gluteus medius   B. Gluteus maximus
C. Gluteus minimus   D. Tensor fascia lata

10. Trendelenburg's test is positive in all *except*:
A. Posterior dislocation of hip
B. Poliomyelitis
C. Fracture neck of femur
D. Tuberculosis of hip joint

11. Shenton's line is:
A. Line joining ASIS and ischeal tuberosity
B. Line joining ASIS and tip of GT
C. Line joining two ASIS (left and right)
D. Curve formed by neck of femur and obturator foramen

12. All of the following names are associated with tests around the hip joint *except*:
A. Bryant   B. Shenton
C. McMurray   D. Nelaton

13. Telescopic test is useful to diagnosis:
A. Perthes' disease
B. Intracapsular fracture neck of femur
C. Malunited trochanteric fracture
D. Ankylosis of hip joint

14. Spur sign is seen in:
A. Supracondylar fracture humerus
B. Bicolumnar acetabular fracture
C. Fracture neck of femur
D. Radial head fracture

15. Which of the following fractures is associated with high mortality and morbidity?
A. Femur shaft fractures
B. Pelvi acetabular fractures
C. Subtrochanteric fractures
D. Shaft tibia fractures

16. "Judet" view of X-ray is for:
A. Pelvis   B. Calcaneum
C. Scaphoid   D. Shoulder

17. Radiological factors indicating an unstable pelvis are all *except*:
A. Posterior sacroiliac complex displacement by >1 cm
B. Avulsion fracture of sacral or ischial end of the sacrospinous ligament
C. Avulsion fractures of the L5 transverse process
D. Isolated disruption of pubic symphysis with pubic diastasis of 2 cm

18. Pelvic fracture most serious complication is:
A. Hypovolemic shock
B. Neurogenic shock
C. Bladder injury
D. Pelvic instability

19. Morel-Lavallée lesion is seen in:
A. Acetabular fracture
B. Fracture femur neck
C. Fracture SOF
D. Fracture proximal tibia

20. Kocher-Langenbeck approach for emergency acetabular fixation is done in all *except*:
A. Open fracture
B. Progressive sciatic nerve injury
C. Recurrent dislocation in spite of closed reduction and traction
D. Morel-Lavallée lesion

21. Which is not true about Kocher-Langenbeck operation?
A. Adequate exposure of posterior segment
B. Anterior segment is not visualized adequately
C. Superior exposure is limited
D. Sciatic nerve injury in 10 percent in the cases

22. Which is not true about Langenbeck-Kocher operation?
A. Adequate exposure of posterior segment
B. Anterior segment is not visualized adequately
C. Superior exposure is very well exposed
D. Sciatic nerve injury in 10 percent cases

23. True about crescent fracture is:
A. Anteroposterior instability with rotational stability
B. Diastasis of pubis with pubic rami fracture

C. Anteroposterior compression is the mechanism of injury

D. Fracture of the iliac bone with sacroiliac disruption

24. **All of the following areas are commonly involved sites in pelvic fracture *except*:**
    A. Pubic rami
    B. Alae of ileum
    C. Acetabulum
    D. Ischial tuberosities

25. **Open book and bucket handle injuries are seen in:**
    A. Spine
    B. Pelvis
    C. Femur
    D. Humerus

26. **In pelvis fracture, the amount of blood loss is around:**
    A. 1–2 units
    B. 2–4 units
    C. 2–6 units
    C. 4–8 units

27. **A 60-year-old female lands up in emergency with history of fall, the attitude of limb is extension and external rotation, the most probable diagnosis is:**
    A. Intracapsular fracture neck of femur
    B. Posterior dislocation of hip
    C. Intertrochanteric fracture
    D. Acetabulam fracture

28. **The commonest hip injury in the elderly patients is:**
    A. Stress fracture
    B. Extracapsular fracture
    C. Impacted fracture neck of femur
    D. Subcapital capsular fracture neck of femur

29. **A 60-year-old man fell in bathroom and was unable to stand on right buttock region ecchymosis with external rotation of the leg and lateral border of foot touching the bed. The most probable diagnosis is:**
    A. Extracapsular fracture neck of femur
    B. Anterior dislocation of hip
    C. Intracapsular fracture neck of femur
    D. Posterior dislocation of hip

30. **A 80-year-old female after fall developed inability to walk with external rotation deformity on examination SLR is not possible and broadening of trochanter is present. The possible diagnosis is:**
    A. Fracture neck femur
    B. Fracture intertrochanteric femur
    C. Fracture subtrochanteric femur
    D. Fracture greater trochanter

31. **Which of the following fractures of the neck of femur is associated with maximal compromise in blood supply?**
    A. Intertrochanteric fractures
    B. Basicervical fracture
    C. Trans-cervical fracture
    D. Subcapital fractures

32. **Not a complication of fracture neck of femur:**
    A. Non-union
    B. Malunion
    C. AVN
    D. Osteoarthritis

33. **Most common complications of intertrochanteric fracture femur is**
    A. Malunion
    B. Non-union
    C. Osteoarthritis
    D. Nerve injury

34. **Nonunion is common in fracture:**
    A. Scapula
    B. Talus
    C. Neck femur
    D. None

35. **The most common complication of transcervical fracture neck of femur is:**
    A. Avascular necrosis
    B. Malunion
    C. Non union
    D. None

36. **Which of the following describes grade 2 fracture neck femur?**
    A. Incomplete fracture, medial trabeculae intact
    B. Complete fracture with undisplaced neck
    C. Complete fracture with ischemic head
    D. Moderate displacement of neck, vascularity damaged

37. **Nonunion is very common complication of intracapsular fracture of the neck of femur. Which of the following is not a very important cause for the same?**
    A. Inadequate immobilization
    B. Inadequate blood supply
    C. Inhibitory effect synovial fluid
    D. Stress at fracture site due to muscle spasm

38. **The most common type of hip fracture in childhood is:**
    A. Intertrochanteric
    B. Transcervical
    C. Transphyseal (through head)
    D. Subcapital

39. **Garden's classification used for which fracture:**
    A. Surgical neck humerus
    B. Shaft humerus
    C. Neck of femur
    D. Shaft femur

40. **McMurray's osteotomy is done for:**
    A. Malunited intertrochanteric fracture of femur
    B. Nonunion transcervical neck fracture of femur
    C. Nonunion lateral condyle fracture of humerus
    D. Malunited supracondylar fracture of humerus

41. **Fracture neck femur cause of nonunion:**
    A. Injury to blood supply with shearing stress
    B. Poor nutrition of the patient
    C. Smoking
    D. Old age and osteoporosis

42. **Most common fracture in elderly:**
    A. Intertrochanteric fracture
    B. Neck femur fracture
    C. Colles' fracture
    D. Supracondylar fracture

43. **Garden-1 fracture are also known as:**
    A. Complete fracture without displacement
    B. Complete fracture with minimal (partial) displacement

C. Complete fracture with full displacement
D. Valgus impaction fractures

44. Increase in Pauwels' angle indicate:
A. Good prognosis
B. Impaction
C. More chances of displacement
D. Trabecular alignment displacement

45. Name of the type fracture classification used here for fracture neck of femur:
A. Gardens   B. Pauwels
C. Anatomic   D. Delbet

46. Pauwels' angle is:
A. Neck shaft angle of femur
B. The difference between neck shaft angle between two femurs of a patient
C. Formed by joining a line extended from fracture line of femur neck to an arbitrary line depicting the horizontal plane
D. None of the above

47. Postoperative X-ray of a patient is given. Name the injury sustained for which this surgery was done:
A. Fracture neck of femur
B. Fracture I/T femur
C. Fracture head of femur
D. Fracture greater trochanter

48. In fracture neck femur all the trabeculae of pelvis and femur are in alignment in which stage:
A. Stage I   B. Stage II
C. Stage III   D. Stage IV

49. Occult fracture of neck femur are best diagnosed by:
A. Bone scan   B. MRI
C. X-ray   D. CT scan

50. Fracture neck of femur in 80-year-old male sustained 1 week back, the treatment of choice is:
A. Hemiarthroplasty
B. Excision arthroplasty
C. Closed reduction and fixation with three cancellous screws
D. Longitudinal skin traction for 6 weeks

51. A 30-year-old male sustains fracture neck, all the following are possible complications *except*:
A. Avascular necrosis B. Non-union
C. Malunion   D. Arthritis

52. A 40-year-old female with history of fall complaints of pain right hip, inability to walk and on examination tenderness in Scarpa's triangle the X-ray is normal, next investigation is:
A. Aspiration   B. CT scan
C. MRI   D. Bone scan

53. All the following are true *except*:
A. Supracondylar fracture is closed reduced
B. Lateral condyle humerus is open reduced
C. Forearm fracture in children is closed reduced and cast applied

D. Neck femur fracture in geriatrics is treated with open reduction and screw fixation

54. A 65-year-old man presented with fracture neck femur 3 days after injury, treatment of choice is:
A. Multiple screw fixation
B. McMurray osteotomy
C. Hemiarthroplasty
D. Total hip replacement

55. Treatment of choice in fracture neck of femur in a 40-year-old male presenting after 2 days.
A. Hemiarthroplasty
B. Closed reduction and internal fixation by cancellous screws
C. Closed reduction and internal fixation by Austin Moore pins
D. Plaster and rest

56. Femoral neck fracture of 4-week-old in an young adult should be best treated by one of the following:
A. Total hip replacement
B. Reduction of fracture and femoral osteotomy with fixation.
C. Prosthetic replacement of femoral head
D. Reduction of fracture and multiple screw fixation

57. Best treatment for fracture neck femur in a 65-year-old lady is:
A. POP cast
B. Bone grafting and compression
C. THR
D. Hemireplacement arthroplasty

58. McMurray's osteotomy is based on the following principle:
A. Biological   B. Biomechanical
C. Biotechnical   D. Mechanical

59. Trochanteric fracture of femur is best treated by:
A. Dynamic hip screw
B. Inlay plates
C. Plaster in abduction
D. Plaster in abduction and internal rotation

60. A patient presented after RTA with following attitude of the limb. What is the most possible diagnosis?

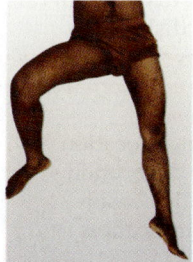

A. Posterior dislocation of hip
B. Anterior dislocation of hip
C. Central dislocation of hip
D. Lateral dislocation of hip

61. **All of the following is true about dashboard injury *except*:**
A. It is associated with posterior dislocation of the hip
B. Sciatic nerve may be involved leading to foot drop
C. Avascular necrosis of the hip could be a late complication
D. The point of impact is on the greater trochanter

62. **Type of injury in this case:**

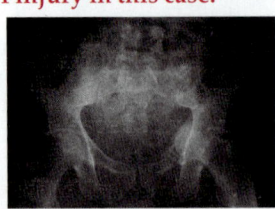

A. Posterior dislocation of hip
B. Anterior dislocation of hip
C. Central dislocation of hip
D. Lateral dislocation of hip

63. **Pipkin's classification system is used for:**
A. Fracture femur head
B. Fracture femur shaft
C. Fracture proximal tibia
D. Fracture calcaneum

64. **Flexion, adduction and internal rotation is characteristic posture in:**
A. Anterior dislocation of hip joint
B. Posterior dislocation of hip joint
C. Fracture of femoral head
D. Fracture shaft of femur

65. **Posterior hip dislocation is characterized by:**
A. Flexion, adduction, external rotation
B. Flexion, adduction, internal rotation
C. Extension, adduction, internal rotation
D. Extension, adduction, external rotation

66. **A patient with hip dislocation with limitation of abduction at hip and flexion and internal rotation deformity at hip and shortening. Diagnosis is:**
A. Central dislocation
B. Anterior dislocation
C. Posterior dislocation
D. Fracture dislocation

67. **A patient presents with lower limb in flexion, abduction and internal rotation with shortening. Diagnosis is:**
A. Posterior dislocation
B. Anterior dislocation
C. Central dislocation
D. Lateral dislocation

68. **Position of limb in posterior dislocation of hip:**
A. Flexion, abduction and external rotation
B. Flexion, adduction and internal rotation
C. Flexion, adduction and external rotation
D. Flexion, abduction and internal rotation

69. **Deformity in anterior dislocation of hip is:**
A. External rotation, abduction, flexion
B. External rotation, adduction, flexion
C. Internal rotation, abduction, flexion
D. Internal rotation, adduction, flexion

70. **Posterior dislocation of hip can damage which nerve?**
A. Superior gluteal   B. Sciatic
C. Inferior gluteal   D. Femoral

71. **Posterior dislocation of hip is characterized by:**
A. Marked shortening of limb
B. Lengthening of limb
C. No change in limb length
D. Extension deformity

72. **Pipkin's classification is for fracture of:**
A. Femur head   B. Femur neck
C. Tibial plateau   D. Hip dislocation

73. **Vascular sign of Narath is positive in:**
A. Anterior hip dislocation
B. Posterior hip dislocation
C. Anterior shoulder dislocation
D. Posterior shoulder dislocation

74. **Sciatic nerve palsy may occur in the following injury:**
A. Posterior dislocation of hip joint
B. Fracture neck of femur
C. Trochanteric fracture
D. Anterior dislocation of hip

75. **Dashboard injury results in:**
A. Anterior dislocation of hip
B. Posterior dislocation of hip
C. Central dislocation of hip
D. Fracture neck femur

76. **Maximum shortening of limbs occurs in:**
A. Intertrochanteric fracture femur
B. Posterior dislocation of hip
C. Fracture neck femur
D. Anterior dislocation of hip

77. **Which is true about dislocation of hip joint?**
A. Posterior dislocation is commoner
B. In posterior dislocation whole lower limb is rotated medially
C. In anterior dislocation whole lower limb is rotated laterally
D. All of the above

78. **Vascular ring of Narath is noticed in:**
A. Fracture neck of femur
B. Perthes disease
C. Posterior dislocation of hip
D. All of the above

79. **Commonest dislocation of the hip is:**
A. Posterior   B. Anterior
B. Central   D. None

80. **In anterior dislocation of hip, the posture of lower limb will be:**
A. Abduction, externally rotated and extension
B. Abduction, externally rotated and flexion
C. Abduction, externally rotated and flexion
D. Abduction, internally rotated and extension

ANSWERS

1. A. Schoemakers line
2. A. Nélaton's line
3. B. Right superior gluteal
4. C. Fixed flexion deformity of the hip
5. A. L4 L5 PIVD
   - Disc prolapse at L4–5 compresses L5 nerve root which supplies gluteus medius and minimus
6. B. Thomas test
7. B. Gluteus medius
8. B. Gluteus medius
9. D. Tensor fascia lata
10. D. Tuberculosis of hip joint
11. D. Curve formed by neck of femur and obturator foramen
12. C. McMurray
13. B. Intracapsular fracture neck of femur
14. B. Subtrochanteic
15. C. Subtrochanteric fractures
16. A. Pelvis
17. D. Isolated disruption of pubic symphysis with pubic diastasis of 2 cm
18. A. Hypovolemic shock
19. A. Acetabular fracture
20. D. Morel-Lavallée lesion
21. D. Sciatic nerve injury in 10 percent in the cases
22. C. Superior exposure is very well exposed
23. D. Fracture of the iliac bone with sacroiliac disruption
24. D. Ischial tuberosities
25. B. Pelvis
26. D. 4–8 units
27. A. Intracapsular fracture neck of femur
28. B. Extracapsular fracture
29. A. Extracapsular fracture neck of femur
30. B. Fracture intertrochanteric femur
31. D. Subcapital fractures
32. B. Malunion
33. A. Malunion
34. C. Neck femur
35. A. Avascular necrosis
36. B. Complete fracture with undisplaced neck
37. D. Stress at fracture site due to muscle spasm
38. B. Transcervical
39. C. Neck of femur
40. B. Nonunion transcervical neck fracture of femur
41. A. Injury to blood supply with shearing stress
42. C. Colles' fracture
43. D. Valgus impaction fractures
44. C. More chances of displacement
45. C. Anatomic
46. C. Formed by joining a line extended from fracture line of femur neck to an arbitrary line depicting the horizontal plane
47. A. Fracture neck of femur
48. B. Stage II
49. B. MRI
50. A. Hemiarthroplasty
51. C. Malunion
52. C. MRI
53. D. Neck femur fracture in geriatrics is treated with open reduction and screw fixation
54. C. Hemiarthroplasty
55. B. Closed reduction and internal fixation by cancellous screws
56. B. Reduction of fracture and femoral osteotomy with fixation
57. D. Hemireplacement arthroplasty
58. B. Biomechanical
59. A. Dynamic hip screw
60. B. Anterior dislocation of hip
61. D. The point of impact is on the greater trochanter
62. C. Central dislocation of hip
63. A. Fracture femur head
64. B. Posterior dislocation of hip joint
65. B. Flexion, adduction, internal rotation
66. C. Posterior dislocation
67. C. Central dislocation
68. B. Flexion, adduction and internal rotation
69. A. External rotation, abduction, flexion
70. B. Sciatic
71. A. Marked shortening of limb
72. A. Femur head
73. B. Posterior hip dislocation
74. A. Posterior dislocation of hip joint
75. B. Posterior dislocation of hip
76. B. Posterior dislocation of hip
77. D. All of the above
78. C. Posterior dislocation of hip
79. A. Posterior
80. B. Abduction, externally rotated and flexion

Lower Limb Fractures

Before going to different fractures let us first understand the anatomy of proximal femur and different deformities.

DEFORMITIES

- *Anterior dislocation hip (FABER)*: Flexion, abduction ⟶ Obturator type—flexion
  Pubic type—extension.
- *Posterior dislocation hip (FADIR)*: Flexion, adduction, internal rotation (**maximum shortening**).
- *Central fracture dislocation hip*: Abduction/adduction and IR/ER both are possible depending upon injury mechanism plus there is less shortening.
- *Fracture NOF (intracapsular) (PDE)*: Shortening, adduction, external rotation.
- *Fracture NOF (extracapsular)/intertrochanteric fracture (PDE)*: But more exaggerated deformities as compared to intracapsular, lateral border of foot can even touch the bed and also there is coxa vara, i.e. reduced femoral neck shaft angle.
- Avascular necrosis head of femur—limitation of internal rotation and abduction.
- TB hip/transient synovitis of hip: In any type of hip synovitis—FABER deformity (because the joint capacity is maximum in this position and thus intracapsular pressure decreases).
- Limitation of abduction and internal rotation and a tendency to increase external rotation as the hip is flexed:
  - Small thin child, constantly running, active and then limping, delayed bone age—Perthes' disease.
  - Adolescence (11–14 years age), during period of rapid growth, overweight, sex immaturity, endocrine disturbances, tenderness at Scarpa's triangle—SCFE.
- *Iliotibial band contracture*: Lumbar scoliosis, pelvic obliquity, hip flexion, external rotation, abduction, triple deformity of knee (knee flexion, posterior and laeral subluxation of tibia, external rotation of tibia), foot in equinus, shortening of limb.
- *Fracture shaft of femur*: Proximal fragment is abducted, flexed and externally rotated.
  Figure 8.1 shows different deformities.

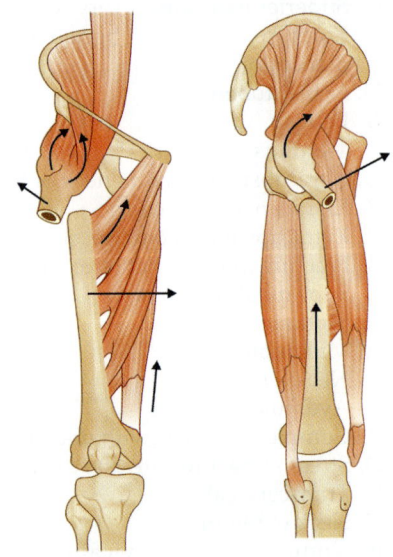

Fig. 8.1: Showing muscular attachment in proximal femur and mechanics behind different deformities

INTERTROCHANTERIC FRACTURE

It is an extracapsular fracture of proximal femur, occurring in older population (low energy trauma) and young patients (high energy trauma). Deformities are same as fracture NOF, but exaggerated, i.e. more shortening with lateral border of foot touching the crouch.

Types: Evans classification
- Type I: Stable (most common)—posteromedial cortex intact
- Type II: Unstable—posteromedial cortex is not intact, thus it collapses in varus.

Treatment
- Type I: Dynamic hip screw (DHS). Name of screw is Richards screw (Fig. 8.2).
- Type II: Intramedullary implant (PFN) to prevent varus collapse.

Role of conservative treatment is less useful. Hamilton Russell traction was used previously for the same. Most important complication is malunion (not nonunion).

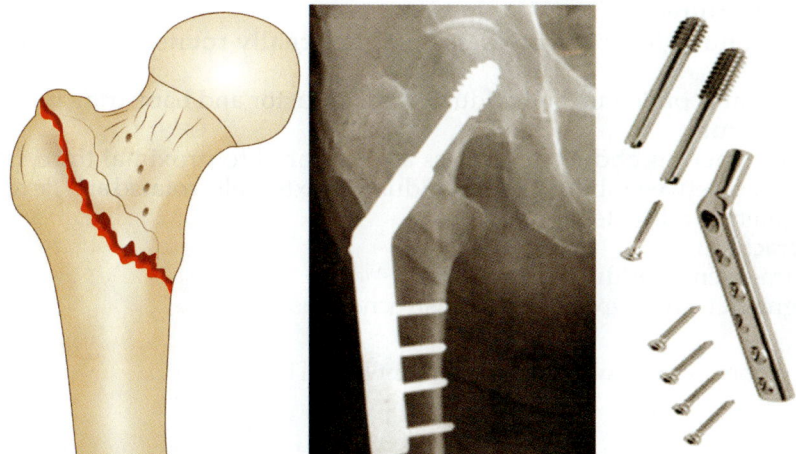

Fig. 8.2: I/T fracture and internally fixed by DHS (*see* screw going into head and implant is extramedullary, i.e. its a plate and fixed by screws to shaft)

SUBTROCHANTERIC FRACTURE

Fractures below lesser trochanter till 5 cm of shaft/isthmus are classified as S/T fracture. They are always due to high energy trauma in adult or low energy in older people. Deformity—proximal fragment is flexed, abducted and externally rotated and distal fragment is adducted.

Classification: Russel Taylor.

Treatment: Intramedullary nail (cephalomedullary)—PFN (proximal femoral nail). PFN has two screws into head, PFN with one screw into head is K/a PFN A2 (Fig. 8.3).

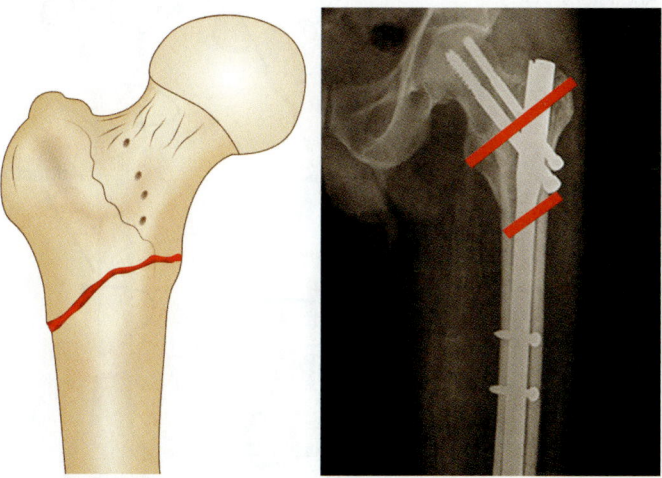

Fig. 8.3: S/T fracture and fixed with PFN (*see* the screw going into head, screw may be one or two, do not confuse and nail is intramedullary. Red line demarcates that fracture may be anywhere of this and treatment is same)

Prognosis of I/T fracture is better than S/T fracture.

Smith Peterson triflanged nail was used earlier for fracture NOF, not S/T fracture.

FRACTURE SHAFT OF FEMUR

Fracture 5 cm distal to lesser trochanter and 5 cm proximal to adductor tubercle is defined as fracture SOF. It is mostly due to high energy trauma. Winquist classified fracture SOF depending upon fracture comminution and helps in deciding treatment. Most common fracture in adults is of middle third and transverse.

Displacement of fragments depends upon the muscular forces (Fig. 8.4)

- **Proximal third fracture:**
  - Proximal fragment is flexed, abducted and externally rotated by gluteus medius and iliopsoas.
  - Distal fragment is pulled up and adducted by adductor and hamstring muscles.
- **Middle third fracture:**
  - Proximal fragment is abducted but less as compared to proximal third fracture due to balancing effect between abductors and adductors, externally rotated and flexed by iliopsoas.
  - Distal fragment is adducted.
- **Distal third fracture:**
  - Proximal fragment is adducted and flexed
  - Distal fragment is hyperextended by gastrocnemius.

Treatment

- In emergency room—1st answer—management by ATLS protocol.
  - Blood loss in fractures
    - Pelvis—4–8 units
    - SOF—2 units
    - Tibia—1 unit
- **Closed fracture**—internal fixation by intramedullary nail (open/closed technique—TOC) or plating. Generally fracture SOF should unite in 100 days , plus minus 20 days (3–4 months).
- **Open fracture**—external fixation (the main aim of external fixation is wound management > maintaining bone length, not bone union).
- **Delayed union**—dynamisation of nail (removing screws from proximal/distal fragment or both) and bone grafting.

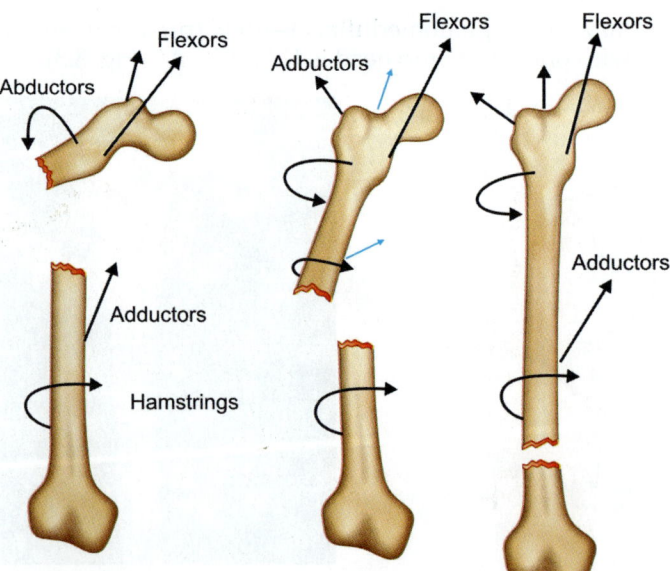

Fig. 8.4: Showing muscular forces acting on fracture SOF at different sites

- **Nonunion**—exchange nailing (removing the previous nail and inserting larger diameter nail after reaming) and bone grafting.

Fracture SOF may be associated with polytrauma and one such triad is—**Waddell's triad**— fracture SOF, intra-abdominal or intrathoracic injury and head injury. Fracture SOF may be associated with hip/knee injuries. In knee most common is cruciate ligament injury and fracture NOF is the most common missed concomitant fracture.

Lower limb fractures are mostly associated with limb shortening (unlike in pediatric fractures), maximum shortening is seen in: Post-hip dislocation > fracture SOF > fracture S/T > fracture I/T > fracture NOF.

Fractures in Children

Most common is proximal 1/3rd fracture. Management is children differ compared to adult. In children after fracture SOF, there may be overgrowth of femur and thus lengthening because of growth stimulation due to fracture.

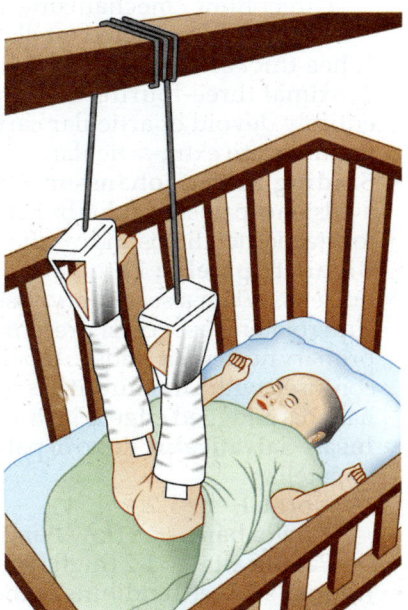

Fig. 8.5: Gallows traction aka overhead Bryant's traction

- **<2 years old:** Gallows traction (or Bryant's traction) for <2 years and who weigh 10–12 kg. Maximum weight used for traction is 2 kg and it should be enough to lift the buttocks off the bed. Traction is applied in both the legs not only in the one which is fractured (Fig. 8.5). After the fracture ends become sticky, it can be replaced by spica cast.
- **<5 years:** Immediate or early spica casting (TOC) in <5 years old. But if the initial shortening is >2–3 cm or unstable fracture pattern or tight swelling in thigh where cast cannot be applied, is managed by initial 3–10 days of skeletal traction and then spica cast.
- **5–10 years:** Flexible intramedullary nail—rush/Ender's/TENS (Titanium Elastic Nailing System). TENS is the TOC and used mainly in stable fracture pattern. If fracture is unstable then plating can be done.
- In 2–10 years old where surgery cannot be done—conservatively managed by 90–90° traction, especially for proximal third fractures (Fig. 8.6).
- **>10 years:** Locked intramedullary nail as per adults.

DISTAL FEMUR FRACTURE

A. *Supracondylar:* Extra-articular fracture involving distal femoral metaphysis.

B. *Unicondylar:* Fracture involving either the medial or lateral femoral condyle. Commonly unicondylar distal femoral fractures occur in the sagittal plane. Fracture of any femoral condyle in coronal plane is called **Hoffa's fracture.**

C. *Intercondylar:* Intra-articular fracture, it can be simple (T or Y type) or complex (comminuted intra-articular fractures).

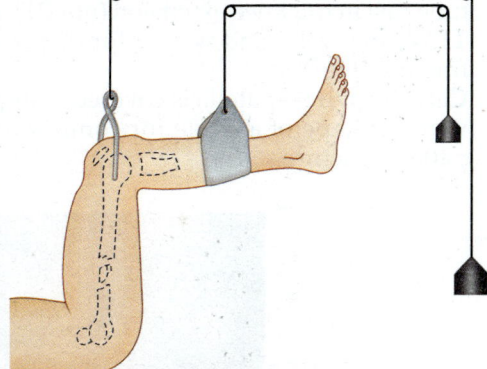

Fig. 8.6: 90–90° traction for proximal 1/3rd fracture

FRACTURE PATELLA

- Patella is the largest sesamoid bone of the body and an important part of extensor apparatus of knee joint. Its fracture is an example of muscular violence. It causes knee extension by increasing the moment of quadriceps contraction.
- **Fracture mechanism:**
  - Indirect mechanism—most common mechanism and leads to transverse fracture (most common type). Occurs following sudden and strong knee flexion against a fully contracted quadriceps muscle.

– Direct blow/mechanism—also known as dashboard injury—comminuted/stellate fracture pattern.
• It has thickest articular cartilage in the body covering proximal three-fourths of the patella. The distal pole is entirely devoid of articular cartilage and thus distal pole fractures are extra-articular.
• **Sinding Larsen Johansson syndrome:** Partial rupture/avulsion of patellar tendon from the lower pole of patella leads to a traction tendinitis and calcification in the patellar ligament.
• **Bipartite patella:** Patella ossifies from a single ossific nucleus. When a secondary ossific nucleus (mostly on the superolateral aspect) is present and fails to unite with the primary nucleus, it leads to bipartite patella. It should not be confused with a fracture, it has rounded edge while fracture has sharp ragged edge (Fig. 8.7).
• **Insall-Salvati ratio:** Ratio of patellar tendon length/length of patella.
  – **Normal**—.8–1.2
  – **Patella baja**—<.8 (low lying patella)
  – **Patella alta**—>1.2 (high lying patella)
• **Jumper's knee:** Tendinitis of the patellar ligament.

Clinical features: Pain and knee effusions which can be graded in size by compressing the supra-patellar pouch and then noting fluid
• Patellar tap
• Bulge sign (10–15 ml)
• Balloon sign
• Ballottement of patella.

Treatment of fracture patella
• **Undisplaced/extra-articular fracture**—cylindrical cast/tube cast in full knee extension (not PTB cast) (Fig. 8.8).
• **TBW**—tension band wiring for displaced transverse fracture (Fig. 8.9).
• **Cerclage wire**—patella is covered at its periphery by a wire in shape of a circle for comminuted or stellate pattern fracture.

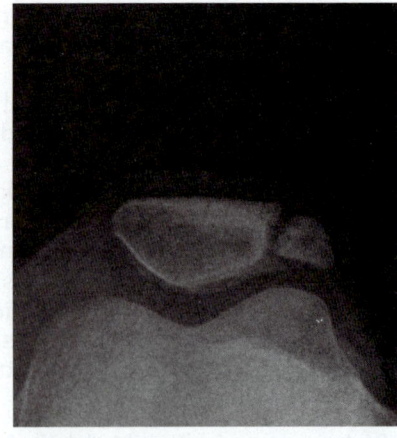

Fig. 8.7: Skyline view of patella showing bipartite patella (note rounded edge of bone, while in fracture its sharp)

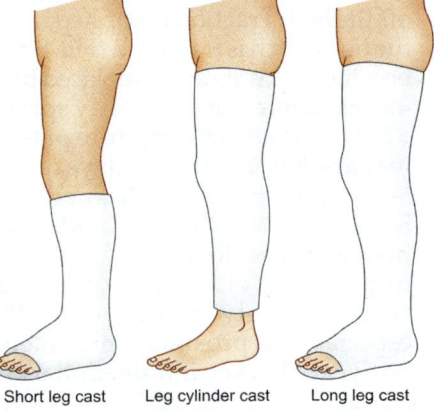

Short leg cast   Leg cylinder cast   Long leg cast

Fig. 8.8: Different types of lower limb cast

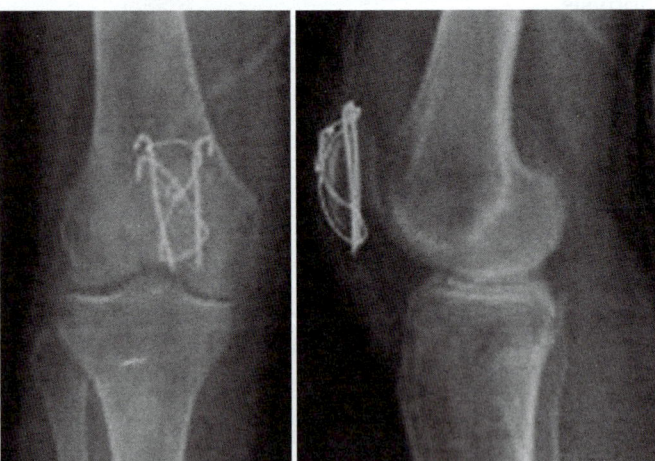

Fig. 8.9: TBW of patella

- **Patellectomy**—every attempt is made to preserve as much patella as possible. In unsalvageable inferior pole comminute fracture, partial pattelectomy is done and proximal part (at least 1/3rd is left intact) or rarely complete patellectomy in severe comminution of whole patella.

FLOATING KNEE
It is a type of flail joint where knee joint is not continuous with femur or tibia. Caused by concomitant fractures of both femur/tibia either at metaphysis or diaphysis.

FAT EMBOLISM SYNDROME
It occurs in polytrauma patients with multiple long bones fracture, most common after fracture SOF (pelvic injury, femur, tibia, arthroplasty). It is more common with closed fractures than open and rarely seen in children. Minimum amount of fat needed to cause FES should be around 100 ml. Fat globules are released into circulation and causes pathophysiology either by mechanical obstruction/ biochemical hydrolysis of fats into free fatty acid.

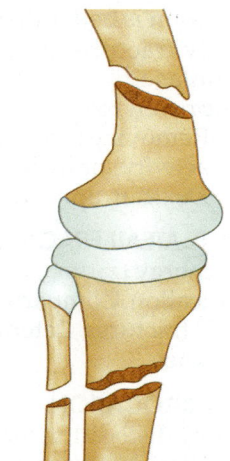

Fig. 8.10: Schematic diagram for floating knee

Clinical features: Develops by 2–3 days of trauma (24–72 hours) and thus fracture SOF are never operated in this window period. **Clinical triad** includes—respiratory dysfunction (earliest manifestation), cerebral dysfunction (transient and reversible) and petechiae (not dt thrombocytopenia). Sites of petechiae—chest, axilla, retina, periumbilical area and palpebral conjunctiva (lower lid). Petechia is the pathognomic feature and is self-limiting.

X-ray: Generally normal initially but later shows the classical multiple flocculent shadows ("snow-storm appearance") due to alveolar hemorrhage and consolidation.

Lung scan: It may show ventilation perfusion mismatch. In the initial phase the V/Q ratio is often high and this phase merges imperceptibly with the stage characterized by low V/Q and fulfilling Gurd's criteria.

Diagnosis is made by **Gurd's criteria**.

Major criteria
Axillary or subconjunctival petechiae
Hypoxaemia PaO_2 <60 mm Hg
CNS depression disproportionate to hypoxaemia
Pulmonary edema

Minor criteria
Tachycardia
Pyrexia
Emboli present in the retina on fundoscopy
Fat globules present in urine
Anemia/thrombocytopenia
Increasing ESR
Fat globules present in the sputum

Treatment: There is no specific therapy for fat embolism syndrome; prevention, early diagnosis, and adequate symptomatic treatment are of paramount importance. It is a self-limiting disease and treatment is mainly supportive. Oxygen is administered in sufficient amount to maintain arterial PO_2 > 80 mm Hg. And O_2 toxicity is avoided by using O_2 conc below 40%. O_2 is administerd by (sequence of increasing severity): Face mask–CPAP (non invasive)–invasive ventilation. If a FIO_2 of >60% and CPAP of >10 cm are required to achieve a PaO_2 >60 mm Hg, then endotracheal intubation, mechanical ventilation with PEEP (positive end expiratory pressure) should be consi-dered. Steroids are of no proven benefit once FES is established, but given to avoid pneumonitis.

Prevention is better than cure:
- Early fracture stabilisation—external fixation in plytrauma patient/floating knee or by splintage.
- Unproven role:
  - Removing fat emboli from circulation by lipolytic agents, e.g. heparin (increase serum lipase activity) or hypertonic glucose (decrease free fatty acid production).
  - Dextran, aprotinin and alcohol.

TIBIAL PLATEAU FRACTURE
High energy trauma, lateral condyle fracture more common than medial. Classified by Schatzker classification. Compartment syndrome is a common complication, and more common in Schatzker type IV fractures. Lateral condylar fracture is by strain on a valgus knee and medial condyle on a varus knee.

KNEE DISLOCATION
Anterior dislocation most common type (tibia displacing anteriorly) followed by posterior knee dislocation. Neurovascular injury is more common with posterior dislocation. Hyperextension is the most common mechanism of injury and most dislocation reduces itself. Ligament injury are very common with knee dislocation and Schenck classified knee dislocation based on ligamentous disruption.

TIBIA FRACTURE
Fracture tibia are one of the most common fractures in emergency. Since subcutaneous, it is also the most common open/compound fracture. Tibial fractures are most commonly associated with fracture fibula, except in children, where isolated fracture tibia is common and is known as toddler fracture.

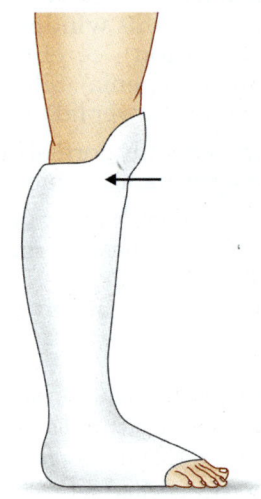

Toddler fracture—seen in children <3 yrs old, minimally displaced spiral/oblique fracture of tibia without fracture of fibula and is also known as CAST (childhood accidental spiral tibial) fracture.

Treatment: Conservative/surgical.

Conservative: After closed reduction, long leg pop cast is applied in 10–20° knee flexion for 3–4 weeks and then changed to PTB cast till union. Patellar tendon bearing (misnomer) cast (Fig. 8.11) is a weight bearing cast and the patient is encouraged to walk with the cast in place. Sarmiento is credited with functional cast (e.g. PTB) and is made of POP (cast)/polyethylene (brace). PTB cast/brace works on hydraulic principle.

Fig. 8.11: PTB cast. Its similar to short leg cast (i.e. below knee cast) but has a proximal extension to include patella (arrow)

Acceptable reduction
- Varus/valgus angulation <5°
- Anterior/posterior angulation <10°
- Rotation <10°
- Shortening <1.5 cm

Surgical: CRIF with locked IMN is the TOC in adult diaphyseal fractures and in children CRIF with TENS is the treatment of choice. In metaphyseal fractures (tibial plateau/distal tibia) ORIF with plating is the TOC. In compound fracture, till Gustillo Anderson type IIIA ORIF can be done and in type IIIB and C, external fixation is the TOC (single best answer for compound fracture).

Xtra edge
- **MIPO:** Minimally invasive plate osteosynthesis is a newer technique for metaphyseal fractures where fracture site is not opened, plate is slided via a small incision under image/C-arm help and fixed with screws.
- Distal third tibia is the most common site for nonunion due to its precarious blood supply (single nutrient artery and less soft tissue cover compared to proximal 2/3rd tibia where two nutrient arteries are present).

- Distal tibia is the most common site for malunion, varus being more common and troublesome than valgus.
- **Pilon fracture:** Tibial plafond is the weight bearing articular portion of tibia in the ankle joint and any fracture of the tibial plafond with proximal extension is known as pilon fracture (also known as distal tibia explosion fracture), except medial/lateral and postmalleolus, where postmalleolus fracture is <1/3rd of the articular surface (Fig. 8.12).

ANKLE INJURIES

Anatomy

Tibial plafond, medial malleolus and lateral malleolus forms the ankle mortise which articulates with talus. Subtalar joint is the articulation between talus (above) and calcaneum (below) and is not a part of ankle joint per se. Ankle joint is stabilised by ligaments:

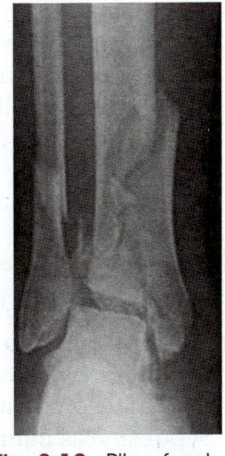

Fig. 8.12: Pilon fracture. See the fracture is involving articular surface (plafond) with proximal extension to shaft

- **Medial collateral ligament**—also known as deltoid ligament with superficial and deep components, with deep component being stronger and the major ankle stabiliser.
- **Lateral collateral ligament**—less stronger and most common involved in ankle sprain/ligament injuries. It has three components:
  - Anterior talofibular ligament—most common ligament to injure in ankle sprain.
  - Middle talofibular ligament—2nd most common to injure.
  - Posterior talofibular ligament—rare and only last to get injured, after the above two in most severe ankle injuries.
- **Ankle syndesmosis**—syndesmosis is defined as a fibrous joint in which two adjacent bones are linked by a strong membrane or ligaments. Ankle syndesmotic joint is formed by two bones and four ligaments. The distal tibia and fibula form the osseous part of the syndesmosis and are linked by the distal anterior tibiofibular ligament, the distal posterior tibiofibular ligament, the transverse ligament and the interosseous ligament.
- **Ankle movements**
  - Plantar flexion (PF)/dorsiflexion—in ankle joint (tibio-talar).
  - Inversion/eversion—inward/outward twisting, i.e. varus/valgus movement occurring at subtalar joint.
  - Supination/pronation—inversion + PF + adduction (tarso-metatarsal joint)/eversion + DF + abduction (tarso-metatarsal joint). Talonavicular and calcaneocuboid joints become parallel in this movement.

Malleolar Fracture

Acronyms
- **Pott's fracture:** Bimalleoli fracture
- **Cotton's fracture:** Trimalleoli fracture
- **Volkmann's fracture:** Posterior malleolus fracture
- **Maisonneuve fracture:** A fracture of the proximal fibula associated with a medial malleolus fracture or deltoid ligament injury.
- **Bosworth fracture:** Fracture of distal fibula with posterior displacement/entrapment of proximal fragment behind tibia.

Lauge-Hansen classification: It employs two words and a number. The first word describes the position of the foot at the time of injury (supination/pronation) and second word, the direction of the deforming force (abduction/adduction/ external rotation/internal rotation). In closed reduction, the direction of manipulation is opposite to the injuring mechanism. Mechanisms described are:
- Supination—adduction (SAD)
- Supination—external rotation (SER)—most common mechanism
- Pronation—abduction (PAB)
- Pronation—external rotation (PER).

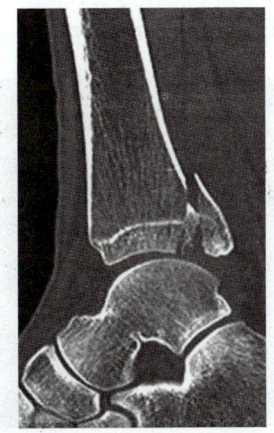

Fig. 8.13: Posterior malleolus fracture

Ottawa ankle rule: Helps physicians decide which patients should have an X-ray following an acute ankle injury. An **ankle X-ray** is only required if:
- There is any pain in the malleolar zone; and,
- Any one of the following:
- Bone tenderness along the distal 6 cm of the posterior edge of the tibia or tip of the medial malleolus, OR
- Bone tenderness along the distal 6 cm of the posterior edge of the fibula or tip of the lateral malleolus, OR
- An inability to bear weight both immediately and in the emergency department for four steps.

X-rays done are—AP, lateral and mortise view (30° internal rotation view).

Treatment: Aim is to maintain articular surface and restore syndesmosis. TOC is ORIF.
- Lat malleolus fracture—1/3rd tubular plate (Fig. 8.14A)
- Med malleolus fracture—TBW/cannulated cancellous screw (CCS) (Fig. 8.14A)
- Syndesmosis injury—syndesmotic screw (Fig. 8.14B)
- Posterior malleolus fracture is operated only if it involves >1/3rd articular surface.

Xtra edge
- Ottawa foot rule—for midfoot injuries, X-rays are ordered if there is pain in midfoot/tenderness at base of 5th metatarsal or navicular tip/inability to bear weight.
- Chronic ankle instability—due to repeated ankle sprains or improperly treated ankle sprain. Treated by Watson-Jone's procedure (reconstruction of ankle ligaments by peronei tendons).

TALUS FRACTURE

2nd largest tarsal bone, mostly covered by articular surface and forms a major weight bearing structure of ankle joint, carrying a greater load per unit area than any other bone in the body. It is divided into head (articulates with navicular), neck and body (articulates with tibia); fracture of neck being the most common. It is the 2nd most common tarsal bone to fracture (1st is calcaneum). Fracture of talar neck leads to AVN of body not head, due to vulnerable retrograde blood supply.

Aviator's fracture: Fracture talar neck due to forced dorsiflexion (most common mechanism).

Canale view: Special view for talar neck.

Chances of AVN of talar body increases with increasing fracture displacement (Hawkins type IV max.). AVN is 1st indicated by increased density of bone (due to necrosis). Hawkins sign (subchondral lucency in talar dome) is an indicator of bone viability and excludes AVN.

Classified by **Hawkins**.

Undisplaced fracture: TOC is POP cast in equinus.

Displaced fracture: ORIF.

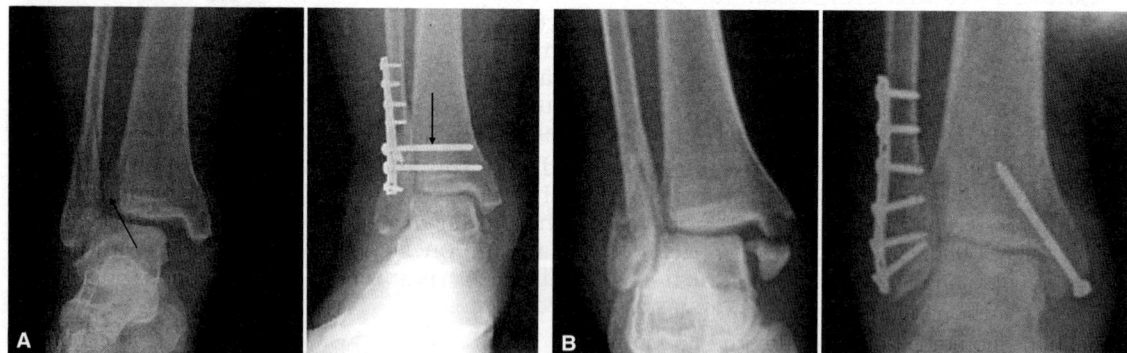

Fig. 8.14: (A) Bimalleoli fracture fixed with 1/3rd tubular plate and CCS, (B) lateral malleoli fracture with syndesmotic injury (arrow) fixed with 1/3rd tubular plate and syndesmotic screw for syndesmosis (arrow)

Xtra edge
- Most common complication of talus fracture is osteoarthritis > AVN. Subtalar joint is the most common site of osteoarthritis not ankle joint.
- Cast in equinus—talus fracture.
- Cast in dorsiflexion—post-malleolus fracture.
- Talus is the only bone without any muscular attachment.

CALCANEUM (HEEL BONE) FRACTURE

The largest and the most common fractured tarsal bone, most common mode of injury is fall from height and thus also known as **Lovers** fracture (Don Juan, a lover, jumped from balcony after getting caught in a love affair).

Fracture may be intra-articular (surgery) > extra-articular (conservative slab). Calcaneum articulates with talus above (subtalar joint) and cuboid. Intra-articular fracture most commonly involves subtalar joint.

X-ray: AP, lateral and **Harris view** (axial view) and **Broden view** (used intraoperatively).

X-ray signs on lateral view (helpful in deciding treatment)
- **Bohler's angle** (normal is 20°–40°): Formed between two lines, one joining the highest point of the anterior process to the highest point of the posterior facet and 2nd line is drawn tangent to the superior edge of the tuberosity. A decrease in Bohler's angle indicates collapse of the weight bearing posterior facet (Fig. 8.15).
- **Gissane's angle** (normal is 100°–145°): It is formed by a line along the lateral margin of the posterior facet and another line extending anterior to the beak of the calcaneus (Fig. 8.15). An increase in this angle represents the collapse of posterior facet.
- **Neutral triangle of calcaneum** (Fig. 8.15): It is an area of sparse trabeculations within the calcaneum trabeculae. This is the weakest area of the calcaneum and fractures usually occur through this area. The triangle is distorted in calcaneal fractures.

Other angles and triangle in orthopedics
- *Southwick's angle*: SCFE
- *Acetabular index*: CDH
- *Alpha and Beta angles*: CDH (on ultrasonography)
- *Kite's angle*: CTEV
- *Ward's triangle*: Femoral neck (significant for osteoporosis grading)
- *Babcock's triangle*: Neck of femur (could be starting point of TB hip)
- *Center edge angle of Wiberg*: CDH
- *Fairbank's triangle*: Congenital coxa vara (classical), Perthes' disease, nonunion neck femur
- *Neck shaft angle*: Normal is 127°
- *Pauwels angle*: Neck of femur fracture
- *Hilgenreiner's epiphyseal angle*: Congenital coxa vara

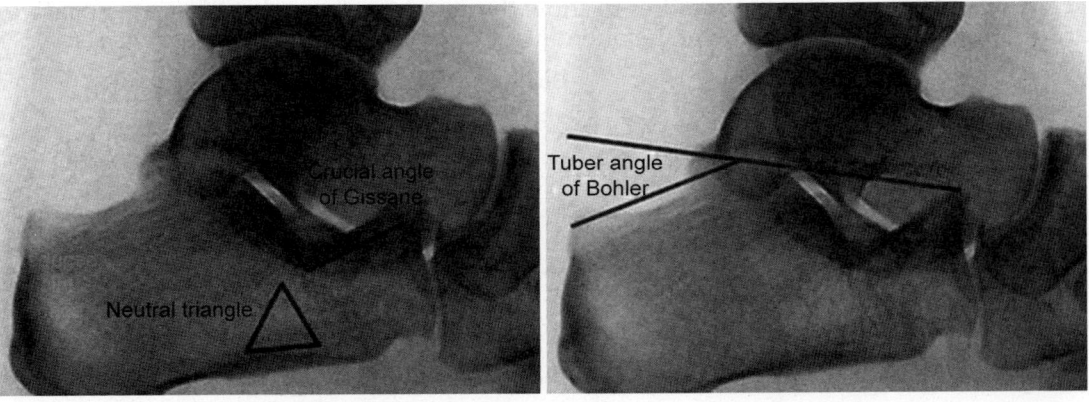

Fig. 8.15: Different angles of calcaneum on lateral view

- *Bohler and Gissane angles*: Calcaneum fractures
- *Neutral triangle*: Calcaneum
- *Meary's angle and calcaneal pitch*: Pes planus and cavus
- *Bauman's angle and anterior humeral line*: Supracondylar humerus fracture
- *Gilula lines*: Congruent arcs in normal wrist X-ray
- *Cobb's angle and Mehta's angle*: Scoliosis
- *Matta's roof arc angle*: Acetabular fractures.

Treatment depends upon duration of injury, degree of displacement, joint dislocation and joint depression.

Xtra edge
- CT scan is the IOC and classified by Saunder's classification.
- Calcaneum fracture is frequently B/L and associated injuries are knee, pelvis, LS and DL spine and thus should always be evaluated in calcaneal fracture.

OTHER FOOT INJURIES

Chopart fracture dislocation: Midtarsal joint (talonavicular and calcaneocuboid) are also known as Chopart joint and their dislocation is known as Chopart fracture dislocation.

Lisfranc fracture dislocation: Fracture dislocation of tarso-metatarsal joint and is the most common fracture dislocation of foot. Compartment syndrome is the most common complication. Basic pathology is disruption of Lisfranc ligament which runs from medial cuneiform to 2nd metatarsal leading to increased space between these two bones (Fleck sign) and the metatarsal bones displace laterally due to avulsion of the ligament. Weight bearing X-ray is the IOC (Fig. 8.16).

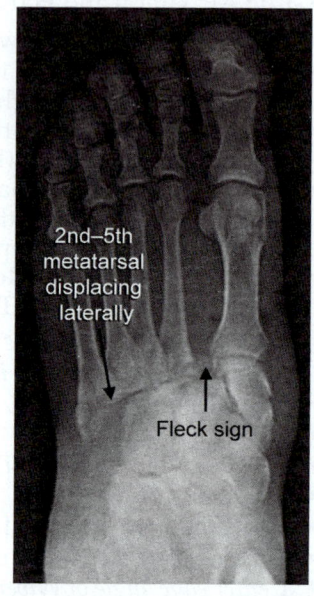

2nd–5th metatarsal displacing laterally

Fleck sign

Fig. 8.16: Weight bearing X-ray of Lisfranc fracture dislocation

Jones Fracture
5th metatarsal is the most common metatarsal to undergo traumatic fracture. Base of 5th metatarsal is divided into three zones:

Zone 1. Avulsion fractures (pseudo Jones fracture/dancer's fracture) of peroneus brevis (not longus) tendon.

Zone 2. Fractures at the metaphyseodiaphyseal junction (Jones fracture).

Zone 3. Stress fractures of the proximal 1.5 cm of the shaft of the fifth metatarsal.

March Fracture
It is a stress fracture (seen in military recruits/dancers, etc.) of the distal part of the **shaft** of the metatarsals (2nd most common > 3rd). Initially X-rays rarely show any sign, MRI (investigation of choice) and bone scan are modalities to show the stress fracture when they are negative on X-rays. Treatment is the cessation of the offending activity with nonweight-bearing cast.

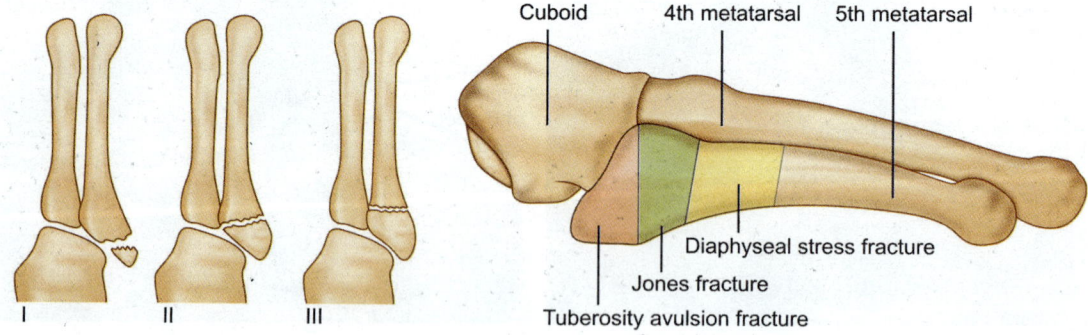

Cuboid   4th metatarsal   5th metatarsal

Diaphyseal stress fracture

Jones fracture

Tuberosity avulsion fracture

I   II   III

Fig. 8.17: Showing different zones of 5th MT base

FALL FROM HEIGHT

Most common injury is that of DL spine and calcaneum is the most common among tarsal bone. Other sites of injury are: Ankle, knee, pelvis, LS spine, atlanto-axial spine. All these area points to an area of stress concentration.

FRACTURE EPONYMS

Dashboard fracture: A fracture of posterior lip of the acetabulum, often associated with posterior dislocation of the hip (other concomitant injuries can involve femoral condyles, patella and posterior cruciate ligament).

Straddle fracture: Bilateral superior and inferior pubic rami fractures.

Pipkin's fracture: Fracture of femoral head associated with posterior dislocation of hip joint.

Open book fracture: A pelvic fracture due to anteroposterior compression of pelvis where the pubic symphysis is disrupted and pelvis opens up like a book.

Malgaigne's fracture: A type of pelvis fracture due to side-to-side compression of pelvis where there is fracture of pubic rami anteriorly and sacroiliac joint or ilium posteriorly but on the same side.

Bucket handle fracture: A type of pelvis fracture due to side-to-side compression of pelvis where there is fracture of pubic rami anteriorly and sacroiliac joint or ilium posteriorly but on the opposite side.

Crescent fracture: Iliac wing fracture in pelvis that enters into SI joint.

Jumper's fracture: Transverse fracture of sacrum seen in patients who have a fall from height during a suicidal attempt. It is characterized by H- or U-shaped fracture line involving upper sacrum (S1 and S2).

Wind swept pelvis: It is a lateral compression injury of ipsilateral hemipelvis and open book or external rotation type injury of contralateral hemipelvis.

Sinding Larson disease: Avulsion injury to lower patellar pole.

Pellagrini Stieda's disease: Injury at femoral attachment of medial collateral ligament with new bone formation.

Segond's fracture: Avulsion fracture of lateral tibial plateau with ACL injury.

Duverney fracture: Isolated iliac wing fracture.

Unresolved fracture: Neck femur fracture.

Underwear fracture: Inter-trochanteric fracture.

Hoffa fracture: Fracture of the condyles of femur in coronal plane.

Bumper fracture: A fracture of the tibial plateau.

Toddler's fracture: A spiral fracture of the tibial shaft seen in toddlers due to twisting injury.

Pott's fracture: Bimalleolar ankle fracture.

Cotton's fracture: Trimalleolar ankle fracture.

Bosworth fracture: A fracture dislocation at ankle where fibula is trapped behind tibia.

Massonaise's fracture: In this an ankle fracture is associated with fracture of the neck of fibula.

Runner's fracture: Stress fracture of the distal fibula.

Pilon fracture: It is a comminuted intra-articular fracture of the distal end of tibia.

Tillaux fracture: This is avulsion of anterior tibial margin by the anterior tibiofibular ligament (Salter Harris type III injury).

LeFort-Wagstaffe fracture: This is fibular avulsion fracture of the anterior tibiofibular ligament (counterpart of Tillaux fracture).

Aviator's fracture: Fracture of neck of talus.

Lover's fracture/Don Juan fracture: Calcaneum fracture when there is fall from height.

Chopart fracture dislocation: A fracture dislocation through inter-tarsal joints.

Lisfranc fracture dislocation: A fracture dislocation through tarsometatarsal joints.

Jones fracture: Avulsion fracture of the base of the 5th metatarsal due to pull of peroneus brevis at the metaphyseodiaphyseal junction.

Pseudo-Jones/dancer's fracture: Avulsion fracture of the tip of 5th metatarsal.

March fracture: Stress fracture of the shafts of 2nd or 3rd metatarsal.

MULTIPLE CHOICE QUESTIONS

1. **True about proximal fragment in supra-trochanteric fracture is:**
   A. Flexion
   B. Abduction
   C. External rotation
   D. All of the above

2. **Subtrochanteric fractures of femur can be treated by all of the following methods *except*:**
   A. Skeletal traction on Thomas splint
   B. Smith-Petersen nail
   C. Condylar blade plate
   D. Ender's nail

3. **What is a floating knee?**
   A. Damage to both anterior and posterior cruciate ligament
   B. Condition of knee due to tear in medial and lateral collateral ligaments
   C. Femoral shaft fracture with proximal tibia metaphyseal fracture
   D. Advanced tuberculosis of knee joint

4. **Name of the injury for which this surgery is done:**

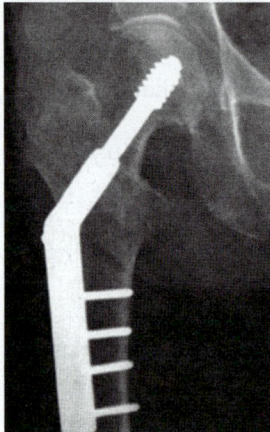

   A. Fracture I/T femur
   B. Fracture S/T femur
   C. Fracture SOF
   D. Fracture head of femur

5. **True supracondylar fracture of femur:**
   A. Type A
   B. Type B
   C. Type C
   D. Type D

6. **A child was given Gallow's traction. What is the diagnosis?**
   A. Fracture shaft femur
   B. Fracture shaft humerus
   C. Fracture ulna
   D. Spine injury

7. **Exsanguinating blood loss in:**
   A. Closed humerus fracture
   B. Closed tibia fracture
   C. Open femur fracture
   D. Open humerus fracture

8. **Blood loss fracture shaft femur:**
   A. 1 unit
   B. 2 unit
   C. 3 unit
   D. 4 unit

9. **In upper one femoral shaft fracture, the displacement of proximal segment is:**
   A. Flexion, adduction and external rotation
   B. Flexion, abduction and external rotation
   C. Flexion, adduction and internal rotation
   D. Flexion, abduction and internal rotation

10. **The femur is fracture at birth at:**
    A. Upper third of shaft
    B. Middle third of shaft
    C. Lower third of shaft
    D. Neck region

11. **Name the type of traction:**

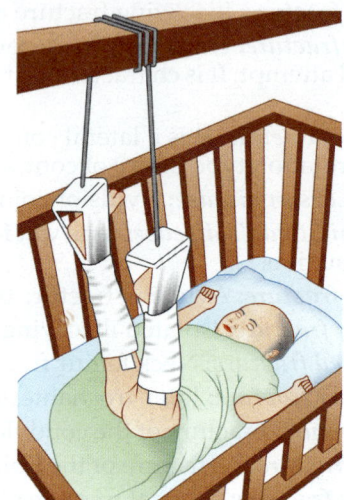

    A. Gallows traction
    B. Bryant's traction
    C. Perkin's traction
    D. Dunlop traction

12. **Gallows traction is most optimum for:**
    A. Fracture shaft femur >2 years of age
    B. Fracture shaft femur <2 years of age
    C. Fracture tibia
    D. Cervical spine injuries

13. **Why fracture shaft femur is early stabilised:**
    A. To prevent blood loss
    B. ARDS
    C. Nonunion
    D. Compartment syndrome

14. **Thomas splint most troubling is:**
    A. Ring
    B. Side bars
    C. Gauze support
    D. Traction attachment

15. **Maximum shortening of lower limb is seen in:**
    A. Fracture shaft femur
    B. Fracture neck femur
    C. Fracture intertrochanteric rotation
    D. Transcervical fracture neck femur

16. **Features of fat embolism:**
    A. Bradycardia   B. Hypoxia
    C. Hypotension   D. Tachypnea
    E. Petechial rash

17. **Regarding Guard's criteria all are correct *except*:**
    A. Diagnostic criteria for fat embolism syndrome
    B. Pulmonary edema is major criterion
    C. Thrombocytopenia is a major criterion
    D. 1 major + 4 minor criteria required to diagnose as fat embolism
    E. $PaO_2 < 60$ is a major criteria

18. **First symptom in fat embolism is:**
    A. Tachypnea   B. Hypoxemia
    C. Rash   D. Drowsiness

19. **A person with multiple injuries develops fever restlessness, tachycardia, tachypnea and subconjunctival rash after 48 hours of injury. The likely diagnosis is:**
    A. Air embolism
    B. Fat embolism
    C. Pulmonary embolism
    D. Bacterial pneumonitis

20. **Fat embolism syndrome is most commonly seen after:**
    A. Femur fracture   B. Acetabular fracture
    C. Pelvis fracture   D. Calcaneal fracture

21. **Fat embolism most common fracture associated is:**
    A. Humerus   B. Tibia
    C. Femur   D. Pelvis

22. **Fat embolism syndrome is characterized by all *except*:**
    A. Tachycardia
    B. Hypoxemia
    C. Fat globules in urine
    D. Thrombocytosis

23. **What is method of fixation of this fracture?**

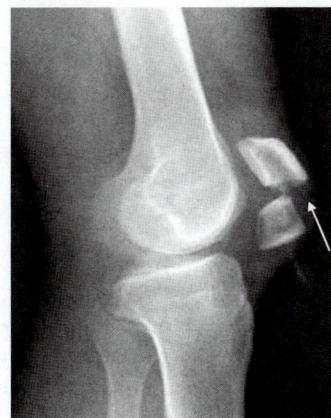

A. Plating   B. Nailing
C. Screws   D. Tension band wiring

24. **Install-Salvati index is used for:**
    A. Olecranon   B. Patella
    C. Talus   D. Scaphoid

25. **Tube (cylinder) cast is applied for the fracture of:**
    A. Shoulder   B. Hip
    C. Pelvis   D. Knee

26. **Transverse fracture of the patella with separation of fragment is best treated by:**
    A. Closed reduction with cylinder cast
    B. Open reduction with screw fixation with Kirschner wire
    C. Blind fixation of the two fragments with Kirschner wire
    D. Open reduction with Kirschner wire fixation of the fragment with tension band wiring

27. **A comminuted fracture of the patella should be treated by:**
    A. Inserting screws and wires
    B. Physiotherapy alone
    C. Patellectomy
    D. Removal of smallest piece only

28. **Bulge sign in knee joint is seen after how much fluid accumulation:**
    A. 100 ml   B. 400 ml
    C. 200 ml   D. <30 ml

29. **Mechanism of injury in lateral condylar fracture of proximal tibia:**
    A. Strain of valgus knee
    B. Strain of varus knee
    C. Strain of valgus knee with axial loading
    D. Rotational injury

30. **Patellar tendon bearing cast is indicated in the following fracture:**
    A. Patella   B. Tibia
    C. Medial malleolus D. Femur

31. **A patient has 2 months POP cast for tibial fracture of left leg. Now he needs mobilisation with a single crutch. You will use this crutch on which side:**
    A. Left side   B. Right side
    C. Any side   D. Both side

32. **Name of this cast is:**

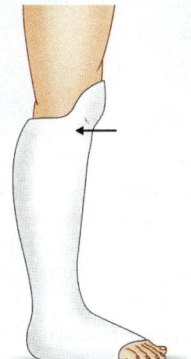

A. PTB cast   B. Below knee cast
C. Above knee cast   D. Cylindrical cast

33. **In posterior compartment syndromes which passive movement causes pain?**
    A. Dorsiflexion of foot
    B. Foot inversion
    C. Toe dorsiflexion
    D. Toe plantar flexion

34. **Pronation of foot the joints that become parallel are:**
    A. Talonavicular and calcaneocuboid
    B. Subtalar and calcaneocuboid
    C. Subtalar and navicular
    D. Subtalar and Lisfranc

35. **Which of the following is a syndesmosis?**
    A. Superior tibiofibular joint
    B. Inferior tibiofibular joint
    C. Talocalcaneal joint
    D. Calcaneocuboid joint

36. **Ottawa ankle rules are used to:**
    A. Diagnose rupture of Achilles tendon
    B. Decide on treatment for CTEV
    C. Decide on need of X-ray for possible fracture
    D. Decide on immediate versus delayed treatment of ankle dislocation

37. **Which muscle is attached to the tuberosity of navicular bone?**
    A. Adductor hallucis
    B. Flexor hallucis brevis
    C. Tibialis anterior
    D. Tibialis posterior

38. **Diagnosis of the X-ray:**

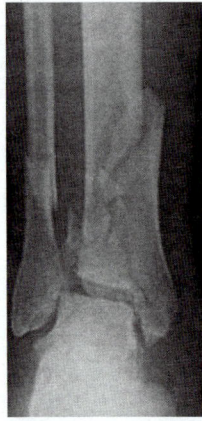

    A. Pilon fracture   B. Aviator's fracture
    C. Pott's fracture   D. Lover's fracture

39. **Runner's fracture involves:**
    A. Tibia   B. Fibula
    C. Metatarsal   D. Talus

40. **Pilon fracture is:**
    A. Intra-articular fracture distal tibia
    B. Intra-articular fracture proximal tibia
    C. Fracture ulna
    D. Fracture radius

41. **Ankle sprain ligament involved is:**
    A. Anterior talofibular ligament
    B. Posterior talofibular ligament
    C. Calcaneofibular ligament
    D. Spring ligament

42. **March fracture involves:**
    A. 1st and 2nd metatarsal
    B. 2nd and 3rd metatarsal
    C. 3rd and 4th metatarsal
    D. 4th and 5th metatarsal

43. **Fracture involving both the malleoli is:**
    A. Cotton's fracture
    B. Pott's fracture
    C. Pirogoff's fracture
    D. Dupuytren's fracture

44. **Fracture of talus without displacement in X-ray would lead to:**
    A. Osteoarthritis of ankle
    B. Osteonecrosis of head of talus
    C. Avascular necrosis of body of talus
    D. Avascular necrosis of neck of talus
    E. Nonunion

45. **MC comp. of fracture talus is:**
    A. Avascular necrosis
    B. Nonunion
    C. Osteoarthritis of ankle joint
    D. Osteoarthritis of subtalar joint

46. **Avascular necrosis is a complication of:**
    A. Fracture of talus
    B. Fracture of medial condyle of femur
    C. Olecranon fracture
    D. Radial head fracture

47. **One of the following fractures required plaster of Paris cast with equines position:**
    A. Distal fracture both bones leg
    B. Distal fracture fibula
    C. Bimalleolar
    D. Fracture talus

48. **Bohler's angle is for:**
    A. Talus
    B. CTEV
    C. Calcaneum
    D. Scaphoid

49. **Bohler's angle is decreased in the fracture:**
    A. Talus
    B. Calcaneum
    C. Navicular
    D. Cuboid

50. **Most commonly injured tarsal bone:**
    A. Talus   B. Navicular
    C. Cuneiform   D. Calcaneum

51. **Long compression is used for which fracture?**
    A. Talus   B. Calcaneum
    C. Fibula   D. Femur

52. **Fracture of calcaneus management depending upon:**
   A. Type of fracture
   B. Subtalar joint dislocation
   C. Duration of presentation
   D. Degree of displacement
   E. All of the above

53. **Gissane's angle in intra-articular fracture of calcaneum:**
   A. Reduced   B. Increased
   C. Not changed   D. Variable

54. **Neutral triangle is seen radiologically in:**
   A. Neck femur   B. Proximal humerus
   C. Calcaneum   D. Talus

55. **Calcaneum is most commonly associated with:**
   A. Fracture rib   B. Fracture vertebrae
   C. Fracture skull   D. Fracture fibula

56. **Least common complication of fall from height is:**
   A. Fracture base of skull
   B. Fracture calcaneum
   C. Fracture fibula
   D. Fracture 12th thoracic vertebra

57. **Watson-Jones approach is done for:**
   A. Neglected club foot
   B. Muscle paralysis
   C. Valgus deformity
   D. Hip replacement

58. **Watson-Jones procedure is done for:**
   A. Polio
   B. Muscle paralysis
   C. Neglected clubfoot
   D. Chronic ankle instability

59. **Which of the following are intra-articular fracture?**
   A. Pilon's fracture   B. Barton's fracture
   C. Ronaldo fracture   D. Hoffa's fracture
   E. Bennett's fracture

60. **Which of the following is an intra-articular fracture?**
   A. Barton's   B. Bennett's fracture
   C. Colles' fracture   D. Pilon fracture
   E. Clay-shoveler's fracture

61. **Chopart fracture involves:**
   A. Midtarsal
   B. Tarsometatarsal joints
   C. Base 5th metacarpal
   D. Fracture neck of talus

62. **Lisfranc fracture is:**
   A. Fracture dislocation at the tarsometatarsal region
   B. Intertarsal dislocation
   C. Avulsion of calcaneal tuberosity
   D. Fracture neck of talus

63. **Diagnosis of the given X-ray:**

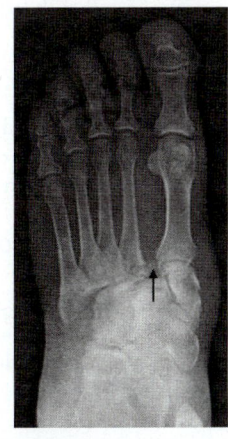

   A. Lisfranc fracture
   B. Fracture base of 2nd MT
   C. Fracture of cuneiform
   D. Metatarsal fracture

64. **Jones fracture is:**
   A. Fracture of base of 5th metatarsal
   B. Fracture of base of 2nd metatarsal
   C. Fracture of base of 1st metacarpal
   D. Fracture of head of 5th metacarpal

65. **Chauffeur's fracture involves the:**
   A. Radial head   B. Radial styloid
   C. Ulnar styloid   D. Base of 1st metacarpal

66. **March fracture:**
   A. 1st metatarsal   B. 2nd metatarsal
   C. 3rd metatarsal   D. 4th metatarsal

67. **Boxer's fracture:**
   A. 1st metacarpal   B. 3rd metacarpal
   C. 4th metacarpal   D. 5th metacarpal

68. **Bennett's fracture:**
   A. Fracture 1st metacarpal
   B. Fracture 2nd metacarpal
   C. Fracture 3rd metacarpal
   D. Fracture 4th metacarpal

69. **Name the type of injury:**

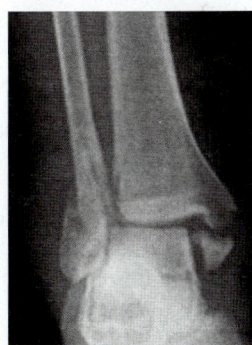

   A. Pott's fracture
   B. Cotton's fracture
   C. Fracture medial malleolus
   D. Pilon fracture

70. Barton's fracture occurs at:
A. Wrist　　　　　B. Elbow
C. Knee　　　　　D. Hip

71. Colles' fracture:
A. Radius　　　　B. Ulna
C. Tibia　　　　　D. Fibula

72. Monteggia fracture:
A. Fracture ulna with dislocation of distal radioulnar joint
B. Fracture ulna with dislocation of proximal radioulnar joint
C. Fracture radius with dislocation of distal radioulnar joint
D. Fracture radius with dislocation of proximal radioulnar joint

73. Tillaux fracture involves:
A. Lower end tibia　　B. Upper end tibia
C. Lower end femur　D. Upper end femur

74. Aviator's fracture involves:
A. Talus　　　　　B. Calcaneum
C. Tibia　　　　　D. Hip

75. Bumper fracture involves:
A. Medial part upper end tibia
B. Lateral part upper end tibia
C. Medial part lower end femur
D. Lateral part lower end femur

76. Bosworth fracture:
A. Fracture distal fibula with posterior dislocation of proximal fragment
B. Fracture distal fibula with dislocation of distal fragment

C. Fracture distal end tibia
D. Fracture distal end femur

77. Cotton's fracture:
A. Bimalleolar fracture
B. Trimalleolar fracture
C. Wrist subluxation
D. Knee subluxation

78. March fracture is:
A. Stress fracture
B. Post-osteomyelitis fracture
C. Involves olecranon
D. Involves tibia

79. Malgaigne's fracture involves:
A. Pelvis
B. Femur head
C. Tibial spine
D. Proximal humerus

80. Pilon fracture is:
A. Intra-articular fracture distal tibia
B. Intra-articular fracture proximal tibia
C. Facture ulna
D. Fracture radius

81. Pellegrini-Stieda disease is:
A. Avulsion of femoral attachment of MCL
B. Avulsion of tibia attachment of MCL
C. Avulsion of femoral attachment of LCL
D. Avulsion of tibial attachment of LCL

82. Toddler fracture involves:
A. Femur
B. Tibia
C. Fibula
D. Talus

ANSWERS

1. D. All of the above
2. B. Smith-Petersen nail
3. C. Femoral shaft fracture with proximal tibia metaphyseal fracture
4. A. Fracture I/T femur
5. A. Type A
6. A. Fracture shaft femur
7. C. Open femur fracture
8. B. 2 unit
9. B. Flexion, abduction and external rotation
10. A. Upper third of shaft
11. A. Gallows traction
12. B. Fracture shaft femur <2 years of age
13. A. To prevent blood loss
14. A. Ring, because it impinges against proximal thigh
15. A. Fracture shaft femur
16. B. Hypoxia; D. Tachypnea and E. Petechial rash
17. C. Thrombocytopenia is a major criterion
18. A. Tachypnea
19. B. Fat embolism

20. A. Femur fracture
21. C. Femur
22. D. Thrombocytosis
23. D. Tension band wiring
24. B. Patella
25. D. Knee
26. D. Open reduction with kirschner-wire fixation of the fragment with tension band wiring
27. C. Patellectomy
28. D. <30 ml
29. C. Strain of valgus knee with axial loading
30. B. Tibia
31. B. Right side
32. A. PTB cast
33. C. Toe dorsiflexion
34. A. Talonavicular and calcaneocuboid
35. B. Inferior tibiofibular joint
36. C. Decide on need of X-ray for possible fracture
37. D. Tibialis posterior
38. A. Pilon fracture

39. B. Fibula
40. A. Intra-articular fracture distal tibia
41. A. Anterior talofibular ligament
42. B. 2nd and 3rd metatarsal
43. B. Pott's fracture
44. A. Osteoarthritis of ankle and C. Avascular necrosis of body of talus
  • In any intra-articular fracture, there's a risk for development of osteoarthritis. The fracture might have been displaced which got reduced on its own or by some else before presenting to the emergency department. Thus an undisplaced fracture must be viewed with suspicion for displacement.
45. D. Osteoarthritis of subtalar joint
46. A. Fracture of talus
47. D. Fracture talus
48. C. Calcaneum
49. B. Calcaneum
50. D. Calcaneum
51. B. Calcaneum
52. E. All of the above
53. B. Increased
54. C. Calcaneum
55. B. Fracture vertebrae
56. C. Fracture fibula
57. D. Hip replacement
58. D. Chronic ankle instability

59. A. Pilon's fracture, B. Barton's fracture, C. Ronaldo fracture, D. Hoffa's fracture and E. Bennett's fracture
60. A. Barton's, B. Bennett's fracture and D. Pilon fracture
61. A. Midtarsal
62. A. Fracture dislocation at the tarsometatarsal region
63. A. Lisfranc fracture
64. A. Fracture or base of 5th metatarsal
65. B. Radial styloid
66. B. 2nd metatarsal
67. D. 5th metacarpal
68. A. Fracture 1st metacarpal
69. A. Pott's fracture
70. A. Wrist
71. A. Radius
72. B. Fracture ulna with dislocation of proximal radioulnar joint
73. A. Lower end tibia
74. A. Talus
75. B. Lateral part upper end tibia
76. A. Fracture distal fibula with posterior dislocation of proximal fragment
77. B. Trimalleolar fracture
78. A. Stress fracture
79. A. Pelvis
80. A. Intra-articular fracture distal tibia
81. A. Avulsion of femoral attachment of MCL
82. B. Tibia

Spine Disorders

ANATOMY OF VERTEBRAL COLUMN

Osteology
- 33 bones in infants and 26 bones in adults
- 5 sections
  - Cervical (7)
  - Thoracic (12)
  - Lumbar (5)
  - Sacral (5-fused bones)
  - Coccygeal (4-fused bones)
- 23 discs in human spine (6 cervical, 12 thoracic, 5 lumbar)
- Spinal cord ends at lower border of L1 vertebrae in adults
- Spinal cord ends at L2–L3 junction in newborns and infants.

Embryology
- Spinal cord arises from neural tube (which arises from ectoderm overlying notochord).
- Nucleus pulposus is a postnatal remnant of notochord.

Blood Supply of Spinal Cord (Fig. 9.1)

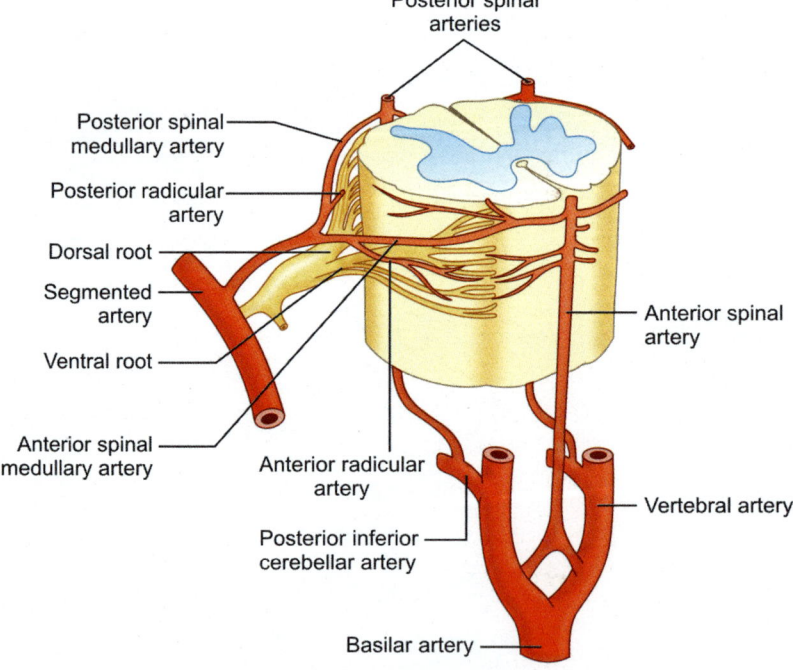

Fig. 9.1: Blood supply of spinal cord

Spinal Tracts (Fig. 9.2)

Dorsal column (which carries deep touch, vibration and proprioception) consists of:
1. Fasciculus gracilis   From lower limbs
2. Fasciculus cuneatus   From upper limbs

Concept of Spinal Stability (Denis' Three Column Theory)

- *Anterior column*: Anterior longitudinal ligament and anterior 2/3 of vertebral body and disc.
- *Middle column*: Posterior 1/3 of vertebral body and disc and posterior longitudinal ligament.
- *Posterior column*: Pedicles, facet joints and supraspinous ligaments.
  If 2 or more columns are involved, it is considered as unstable spinal injury (Fig. 9.3).

Causes of Spinal Injury

- In developing countries (India): Fall from height
- In developed countries: Road traffic accident

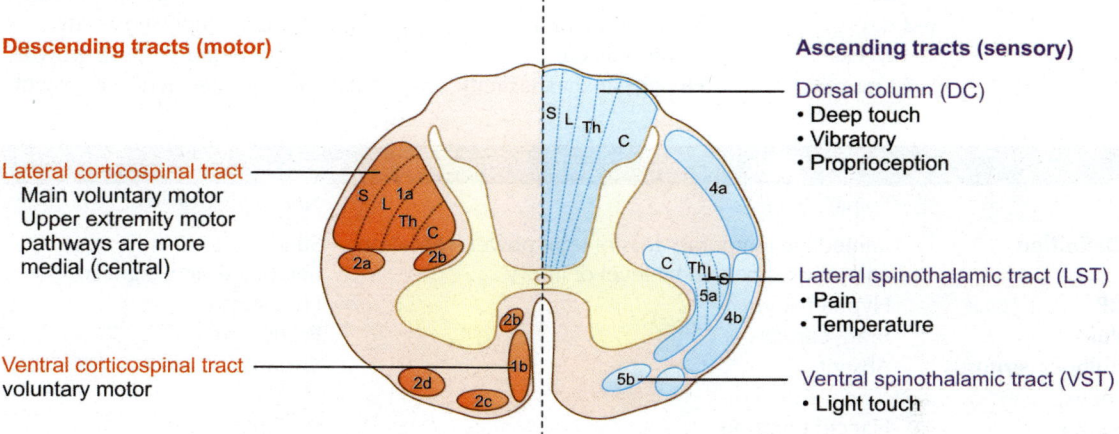

Fig. 9.2: Various tracts of spinal cord

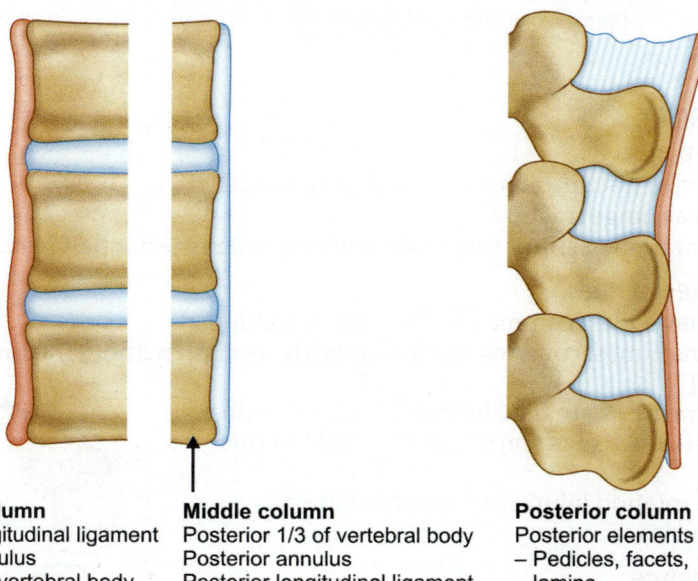

Anterior column
Anterior longitudinal ligament
Anterior annulus
Anterior 2/3 vertebral body

Middle column
Posterior 1/3 of vertebral body
Posterior annulus
Posterior longitudinal ligament

Posterior column
Posterior elements
– Pedicles, facets,
– lamina
– Spinouns process
Posterior ligaments

Fig. 9.3: Denis three column concept

Spinal Shock
- Immediate temporary loss of total power, sensation and reflexes below the level of injury and loss of bulbo-cavernous reflex.
- Usually recovers within 24–48 hours, if does not then its a poor prognostic sign.
- Bulbo-cavernous reflex (S3-S4) is the reflex that returns first, thus marking the end of spinal shock. Thereafter, the upper motor neuron features (features of spinal cord injury) can be appreciated.
- The 'shock' in spinal shock does not refer to circulatory collapse.
- Phases of spinal shock (Table 9.1).
- Spinal shock has to be differentiated from neurogenic shock (Table 9.2).

Table 9.1: Phases of spinal shock			
Phase	*Time*	*Physical examination finding*	*Underlying physiological event*
1	0–1 day	Areflexia	Loss of descending facilitation
2	1–3 days	Initial reflex return	Denervation supersensitivity
3	1–4 weeks	Hyperreflexia	Axon-supported synapse growth
4	1–12 months	Hyperreflexia spasticity	Soma-supported synapse growth

Table 9.2: Spinal shock *vs* neurogenic shock		
	Spinal shock	*Neurogenic shock*
Definition	Immediate temporary loss of total power, sensation and reflexes below the level of injury	Sudden loss of the sympathetic nervous system signals
BP	Hypotension	Hypotension
Pulse	Bradycardia	Bradycardia
Bulbocavernosus reflex	Absent	Variable
Motor	Flaccid paralysis	Variable
Time	48–72 hrs immediate after SCI	
Mechanism	Peripheral neurons become temporarily unresponsiveness to brain stimuli	Disruption of autonomic pathways → loss of sympathetic tone and vasodilation

CRANIAL INJURIES

Motorcyclist's Fracture
- It is a transverse fracture across the floor of the skull
- Also known as hinge fracture
- There is separation of sutures between anterior and posterior half of skull.

CERVICAL SPINE INJURIES
- Cervical spine is most common site for spinal trauma
- Cervical spine is most common site for spinal dislocation without fracture (as facets are aligned in AP plane)
- C1 and C2 fractures are usually not associated with neurological deficits (as spinal canal is wide in this region)
- Flexion and rotation injuries are most common type of spinal injuries.

Jefferson's Fracture
- It is a burst fracture of the ring of C1 vertebra (Fig. 9.4)
- Burst fracture is a type of vertical compression injury

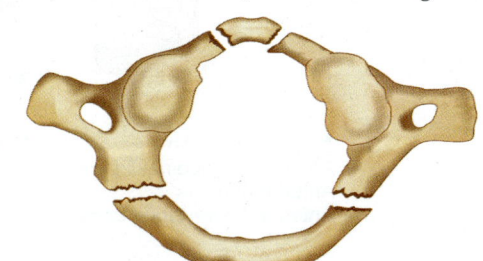
Fig. 9.4: Jefferson's fracture

Hangman's Fracture

It is traumatic fracture (of neural arch—through pars interarticularis) and dislocation (spondylolisthesis) of C2 vertebra over C3 vertebra (Fig. 9.5A).

SCIWORA

- Spinal cord injury without radiological abnormality
- More common in pediatric age group
- X-rays are normal but neurological deficit present
- Cervical spine is most commonly affected
- Is due to lax ligaments permitting traction injuries to cord

Clay-shoveler Fracture

- Fracture of spinous process of lower cervical and upper thoracic vertebrae
- C7 >> T1 (Fig. 9.5B)

Whiplash Injuries

- Hyperextension (main injuring mechanism) followed by flexion (Fig. 9.6)
- Also known as rail road spine

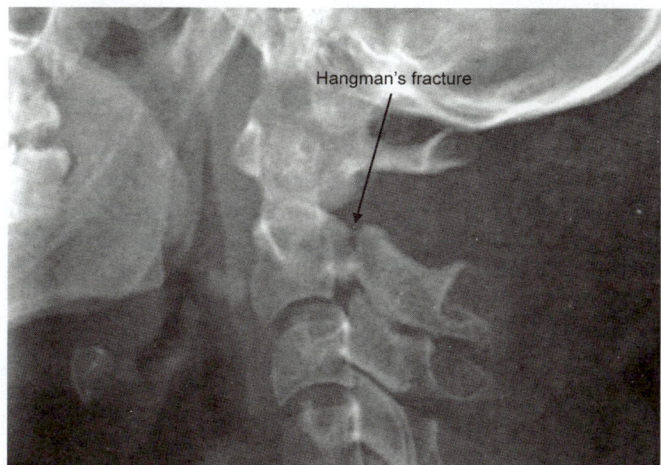

Fig. 9.5A: Hangman's fracture

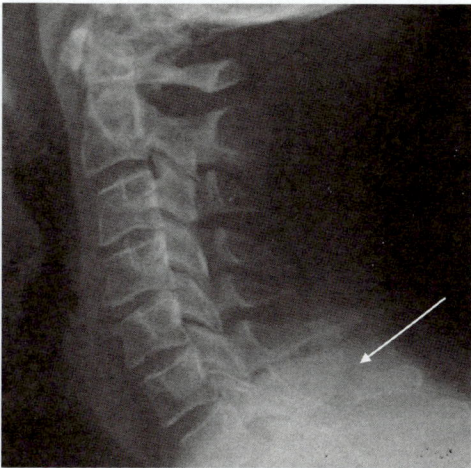

Fig. 9.5B: Clay-shoveler fracture

How whiplash occurs

Motorists involved in rear-end crashes commonly experience whiplash. Injuries to the neck occur as the torso accelerates forward and the neck lags, then the head whips forward.

1. During normal driving, the head and torso move relative to the vehicle

2. As the vehicle is struck from behind, the head tilts backward

3. After the initial impact, the head snaps forward

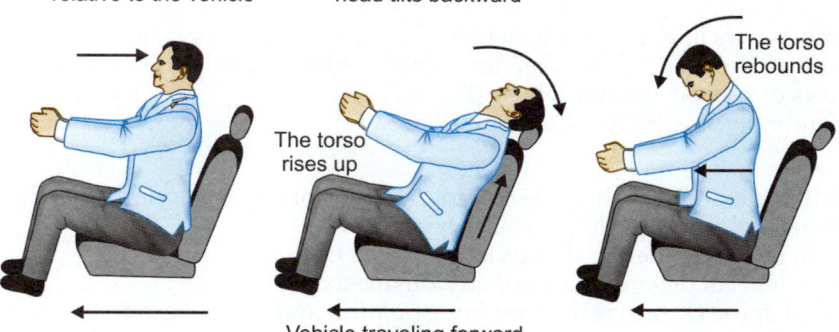

The torso rises up

The torso rebounds

Vehicle traveling forward

Fig. 9.6: Mechanism of Whiplash injury

- Cervical spine is most commonly involved
- Fractures are rare. Most cases have just muscle strain in the neck

Xtra edge
- *Burst fracture*: It is a comminuted fracture of the vertebral body where fragments "burst out" in different directions often entering the canal and injuring cord.
- *Growing fractures*: These are skull fractures seen mainly in infancy and early childhood characterized by progressive diastatic enlargement of the fracture line. A complication can be a cystic mass filled with CSF, called a "leptomeningeal cyst".
- *Undertaker fracture*: It is an artefact related to poor handling of the corpse characterized by subluxation of the lower cervical spine from tearing of the intervertebral disc at C6–C7 vertebral body level. It occurs due to sudden fall of the head over occipital region.

DORSOLUMBAR SPINE INJURIES

Chance Fracture
- Also referred as seat belt fracture
- Flexion distraction type of injury (Jack knife injury)
- Most common in lumbar region
- Associated with abdominal injuries (specially pancreas and duodenum)
- Unstable injury (involves all 3 columns).

MANAGEMENT OF SPINE INJURY

Spinal injury patients are also managed according to ATLS protocol, with primary followed by secondary survey. In the whole process, spine should be taken care of, to prevent any added injury to already injured spine.

Cervical spine is immobilised during primary survey after ascertaining airway patency with Philadelphia collar and dorsal/lumbar spine with a board.
- In spine injury patient, the need of X-ray is evaluated by NEXUS criteria.
- Stability of spine is evaluated by "Denis 3 column concept" or "White and Punjabi criteria".
- In cervical injury patients we immobilise the spine or fracture is reduced by traction, applied by "Crutchfield's tong", but it may cause deterioration of the neurological involvement. Thus, emergency closed reduction by traction is the treatment of choice in alert and co-operative patients. However, it is contraindicated in unconscious/disorientated patient and injuries with unstable spine.
- Surgical treatment
  - Cervical injuries—anterior decompression and fixation by anterior instrumentation.
  - Dorsolumbar injuries—posterior decompression and fixation by posterior instrumentation.
- Role of steroid (debatable)—in acute spinal cord injury/before major spinal surgery. Bolus dose of 30 mg/kg body weight over 15 minutes, then 5.4 mg/kg/hour for next
  - 24 hours, if the bolus dose is given within 3 hours of injury
  - 48 hours, if the bolus dose is given within 8 hours of injury.

SPONDYLOLYSIS AND SPONDYLOLISTHESIS

Spondylolysis
- Spondylolysis is pars interarticularis defect
- Beheaded dog/beheaded Scottish terrier sign/Scottish dog with collar sign is seen best on **oblique views** of spine in spondylolysis (Fig. 9.7)
- Cervical spondylolysis: C5–C6 > C6–C7 > C4–C5.

Spondylolisthesis
- Spondylolisthesis is anterior slippage of superior vertebra over inferior vertebra (Fig. 9.8A)
- Most common level of spondylolisthesis is L5–S1
- Most common level of ischemic spondylolisthesis is L5–S1
- Most common level of degenerative spondylolisthesis is L4–L5
- Lateral view of spine (X-ray) is the first investigation and we can grade the degree of slip in lateral view. AP view of spine is least informative in spondylolisthesis, but in last stages of spondylolisthesis in L5-S1, AP view shows inverted Napoleon hat sign (Fig. 9.8B).

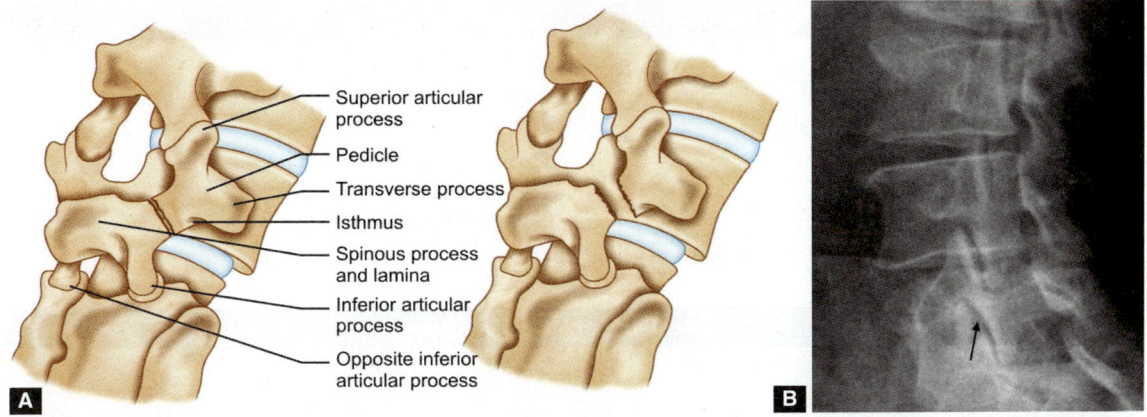

Fig. 9.7: (A) Schematic diagram showing Scottish dog in vertebrae, (B) oblique view of spondylolysis

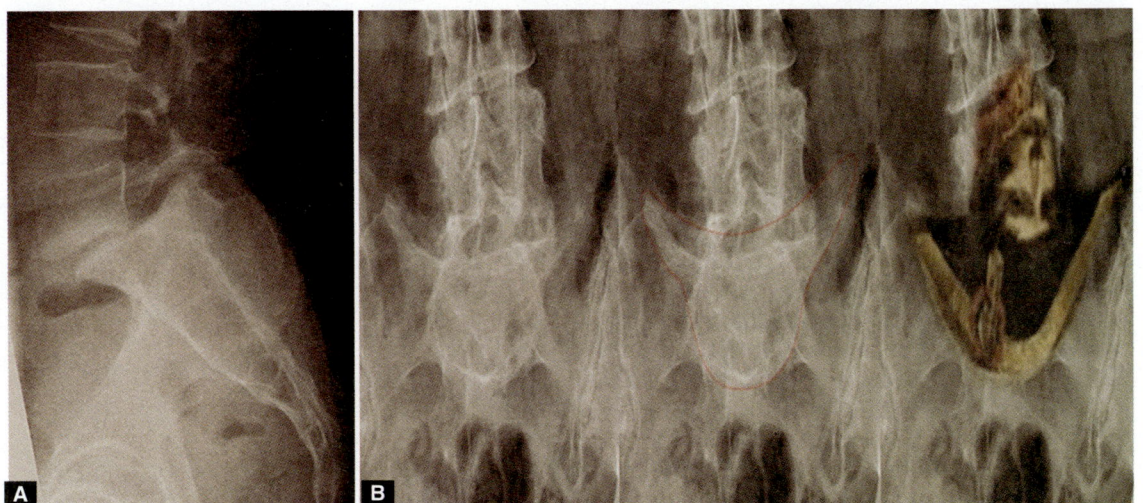

Fig. 9.8: (A) Lateral view of spondylolisthesis, (B) AP view showing "inverted Napoleon hat sign"

LOCALISING LEVEL OF SPINAL CORD INJURY

- Vertebral column is longer than the spinal cord. Spinal cord ends at lower level of L1 vertebra (Fig. 9.9).
- The terminal sacral segments of spinal cord are referred to as 'conus medullaris'.
- Every segment of spinal cord gives rise to a 'spinal nerve' (total 31 pairs). Every nerve exits the spinal canal from its corresponding intervertebral foramina to supply the destined dermatomes and myotomes. Since cord ends at lower border of L1, the remaining nerves descend a fair distance in spinal canal before they can exit. The hanging spinal nerves in the canal are called 'cauda equina'.

Upper Motor vs Lower Motor Neuron Lesion

The term upper motor neuron (UMN) lesion refers to injury to spinal cord while the term lower motor neuron (LMN) refers to injuries to spinal nerves.

Features: In UMN lesion, all functions are absent at the level of transection while all functions (reflexes, muscle tone, etc.) below the level of transection are exaggerated (as lower levels escape from inhibitory cortical control). In LMN lesion, functions are lost only in the distribution of the compressed spinal nerve. The difference is charted in Table 9.3.

Table 9.3: Differentiating features of UMN *vs* LMN lesion

Upper motor neuron	Lower motor neuron
• Weakness is often symmetric	• Often single muscle group (with atrophy)
• Increased DTRs (after spinal shock)	• Decreased DTRs
• Muscle tone increased	• Muscle tone decreased
• No fasciculations	• Fasciculations
• Automatic bladder	• Autonomous bladder

(UMN: Upper motor neuron; LMN: Lower motor neuron; DTR: Deep tendon reflexes)

Table 9.4: Centers for reflexes

Reflex	Center (root value)
Deep tendon reflex	
Biceps jerk	C5 >> C6
Brachioradialis	C6 >> C5
Triceps jerk	C7 >> C6
Knee reflex/patellar reflex	L3–L4
Ankle	S1
Superficial reflex	
Corneal reflex (blink reflex)	5th and 7th cranial nerves
Abdominal reflex	T7–T12
Plantar reflex	L5–S1

Reflex

A 'reflex' is a simple sensory motor pathway that traverses through only the grey matter of a single or couple of spinal segments. No ascending and descending white matter connections are involved.

- In UMN lesions, the level at which spinal cord is transected, reflex function is lost (as affected spinal segment is injured) while the lower level reflexes stay functional (as they are governed by their respective arcs), rather they exhibit exaggeration (owing to loss of cortical inhibition that cannot be relayed down due to spinal cord disruption).
- In LMN lesions, reflexes are lost (absent) only in the distribution of the affected spinal nerves.
- The list of important reflexes has been tabulated in Table 9.4.

Dermatomes and Myotomes

The above terms refer to the distribution of the spinal nerves. While the trunk area is directly supplied by spinal nerves, spinal nerve fibers to the limbs are distributed via the peripheral nerves (that arise from brachial or lumbosacral plexus).

'Dermatome' refers to area of skin supplied by a single spinal nerve (Fig. 9.10) while 'Myotome' refers to the muscle supplied by a single spinal nerve (Table 9.5).

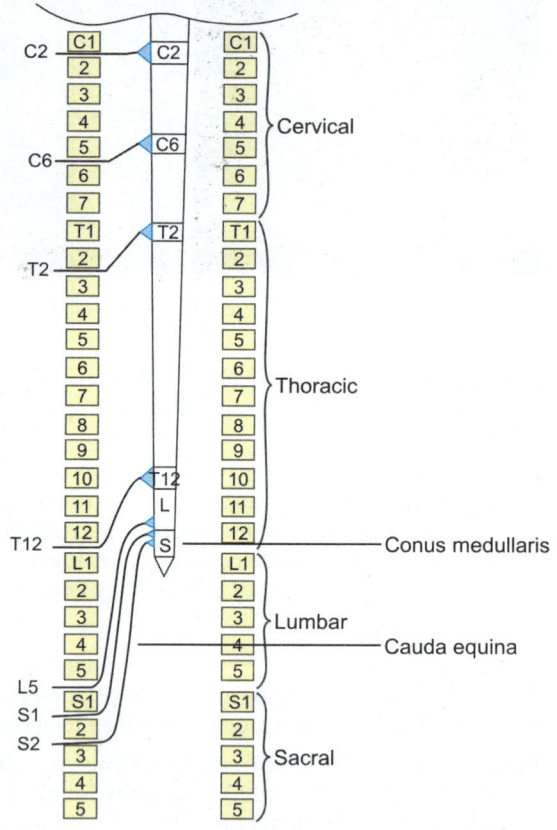

Fig. 9.9: Spinal cord anatomy

Table 9.5: Important dermatomes and myotomes (according to ASIA impairment scale)

Segments	Key muscles (myotomes)	Sensory (dermatomes)	Reflex
C5	Elbow flexors	Lateral proximal arm	Biceps
C6	Wrist extensors	Thumb	Brachioradialis
C7	Elbow extensors	Index and middle finger	Triceps
C8	Finger flexion (distal phalanx of middle finger)	Ring and little finger	
T1	Finger abductors (little finger)	Anteromedial forearm	
L2	Hip flexors	Upper anterior thigh (pocket region)	
L3	Knee extensors	Lower anterior thigh anterior knee	Knee jerk
L4	Ankle dorsiflexors	Medial calf and medial border of foot	Knee jerk
L5	Long toe extensor (EHL)	Dorsal surface of foot (first web space)	
S1	Ankle plantar flexors	Plantar surface of foot lateral aspect foot including 5th toe	Ankle reflex

- In UMN lesions, at the level of transection, the muscles exhibit flaccid paralysis while the muscles below the level of transection exhibit spastic paralysis (owing to loss of cortical inhibition). In LMN lesions, flaccid paralysis results only in muscle groups in distribution of the affected spinal nerve.
- Dermatomes have relatively different manifestation compared from myotomes (muscles). In UMN lesion, since spinal cord is transected at a particular level, no sensory input from lower level is relayed to cortex. Hence, all sensations are lost from the level of transection of cord till the S5 level. In LMN lesion, sensory loss is exhibited only in the distribution of the compressed spinal nerves.

Deciding the Level Involved

- If a patient has exaggerated reflexes and spastic tone; search for a spinal cord injury (UMN). Upper most level in cord lesion can be located by locating the level of absent reflex or myotome having flaccid paralysis.
- If there are only absent reflexes and flaccid paralysis, spinal nerves (LMN) are involved corresponding to the loss in distribution of myotomes and dermatomes.
- Once the level of cord lesion is deduced, one can take out the vertebra that is involved as well by a simple formula mentioned in Table 9.6.

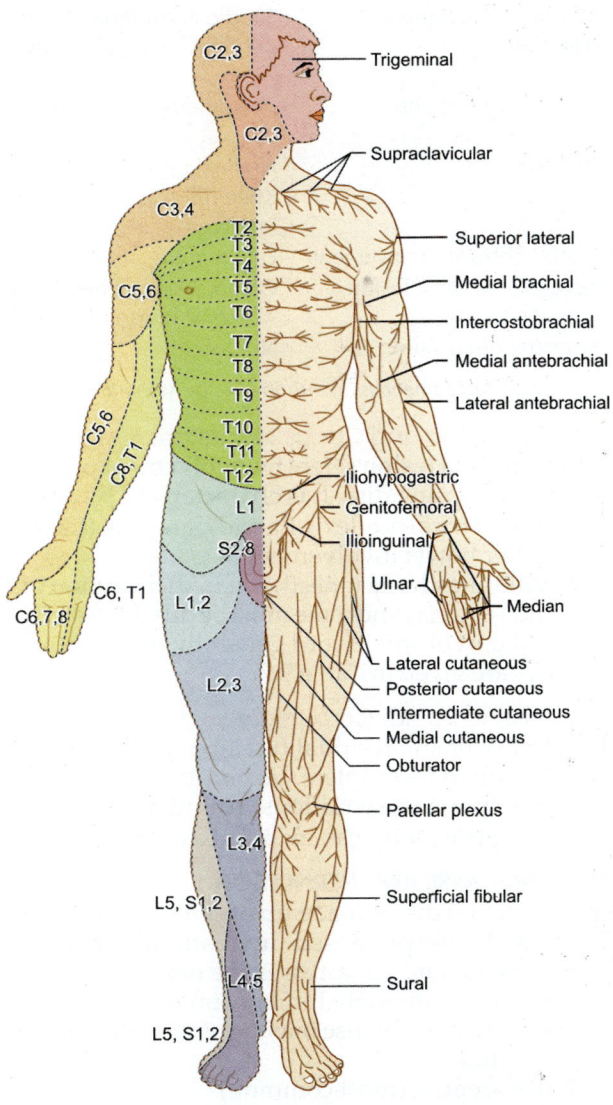

Fig. 9.10: Diagram showing dermatomal distribution

Table 9.6: Deciphering vertebral level from spinal injury level	
Spinal level	*Cord level*
Cervical vertebrae	Add 1 to vertebra level
Upper dorsal (D1 to D6)	Add 2 to vertebra level
Lower dorsal (D7 to D9)	Add 3 to vertebra level
D10	All dorsal segments over
D12	All lumbar segments over
L1	All sacral segments over
Below L1	Cauda equina

Table 9.7: Differences between cauda equina and conus medullaris syndrome		
Features	*Cauda equina syndrome*	*Conus medullaris syndrome*
Presentation	Asymmetric	Symmetric
Radicular pain	Severe	Usually not present
Sensory involvement (Fig. 3.9)	Saddle anesthesia (S2–S4) with perianal sparing initially (S5 sparing)	Perianal anesthesia (S5) as scaral cord compression involves loss of C5 cord segment
Motor involvement	Asymmetric flaccid paralysis	Symmetric usually flaccid sometimes hyper-reflexive paralysis
Reflexes	Areflexia is classical Knee reflex is lost if L3 and L4 roots involved	Knee reflex is always preserved
Bladder bowel involvement	Late feature	Early feature
Level of causative lesion	Compression of nerve roots usually by vertebral lesion L1 vertebra	Compression of conus (sacral part) by D12–L1 vertebral lesions
Sesnsory dissociation	Not found	Sensory dissociation can occur

Taken from Fundamentals of Orthopedics by Mohindra and Jain; 2nd Ed; Jaypee publishers

Cauda Equina and Conus Medullaris Syndrome

Cauda equina lesion refers to involvement of the hanging spinal nerves in the canal generally by a large prolapsing disc. It is characterized by a triad:
1. Asymmetrical areflexic flaccid paralysis (LMN lesion)
2. Bladder bowel involvement
3. Saddle anesthesia (anesthesia in distribution of S2-4; with sparing of S5)

Cauda equina syndrome must be differentiated from **conus medullaris syndrome** (compression of sacral part of spinal cord generally by a fracture, tumor or tuberculous lesion). Differentiating features are given in Table 9.7.

Incomplete Spinal Cord Injury Syndromes

If evidence of any residual function can be ascertained below the level of cord injury, the injury can be termed incomplete. Incomplete injury to the spinal cord at least exhibits 'sacral sparing' (i.e. intact perianal sensations, voluntary rectal motor function and great toe flexor activity).

Incomplete injury can manifest as various important injury syndromes tabulated in Table 9.8.

DISC PROLAPSE AND HERNIATION

Intervertebral disc is made up of central disc (nucleus pulposus) and peripheral fibrous 'annulus fibrosus'. In disc prolapsed/herniation, there is a tear in annulus fibrosus through which nucleus herniates out and compresses the nerve roots (lumbar > cervical spine) or spinal cord (cervical spine). Most commonly lumbar spine (L4–L5 > L5–S1) followed by cervical spine is involved.

Herniation of the disc may be of the following types (Fig. 9.11):
1. Central
2. Paracentral (most common)
3. Far lateral

Table 9.8: Incomplete spinal cord injury syndromes		
Syndrome	*Causes*	*Clinical features*
Complete cord transection	• Trauma, infarction • Transverse myelitis • Abscess, tumor	• Complete loss of sensation below level • Complete paralysis below level
Cord hemisection	• Trauma, MS, tumor • Abscess	• Ipsilateral loss of motor and proprioception • Contralateral loss of pain temperature
Central cord syndrome	• Neck hyperextension • Spinal sterosis/CA • Syringomyelia • Tumor	• Motor impairment > sensory • UL > LL • Distal > proximal • Bladder dysfunction
Anterior cord syndrome	• Hyperflexion • Disc protrusion • Anterior spinal artery occlusion • PostAAA	• Motor function impairment • Pain and temperature loss • Proprioception spared
Cauda equina syndrome	• Disc prolapse • Tumor • Infective	• Bladder/bowel dysfunction • Saddle anesthesia • Sexual dysfunction

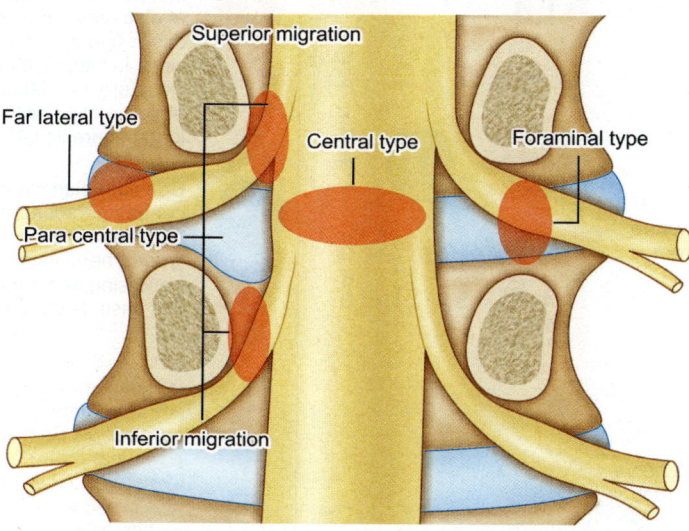

Fig. 9.11: Types of disc herniations

Clinical Features

If disc compresses a nerve root, then there will be radiating pain along that nerve root, most common being sciatica. In disc herniation, **passive straight leg raise test/Laségue's test** is positive, i.e. patient complains of pain along nerve root on straight leg elevation before 90° hip flexion (normally patient can raise till 90). Other tests: Bragard sign, Bowstring sign of McNab, well leg SLR (contralateral SLR).

Nerve root involved in a prolapsing disc (Fig. 9.12A and B)
• For any cervical disc: Always lower nerve root is affected, e.g.: Any C6–C7 disc (central/para-central/far-lateral/foraminal disc) will lead to C7 nerve root symptoms.
• For Lumbar disc (e.g. of L4–L5 disc herniation)
  – Central/para-central Lumbar disc (e.g. L4–L5 disc): Cause traversing nerve root symptoms, i.e. the one below (e.g. L5 nerve root).
  – Far lateral/foraminal disc (e.g. L4–L5 disc): Causes exiting nerve root compression symptoms (e.g. L4 nerve root)

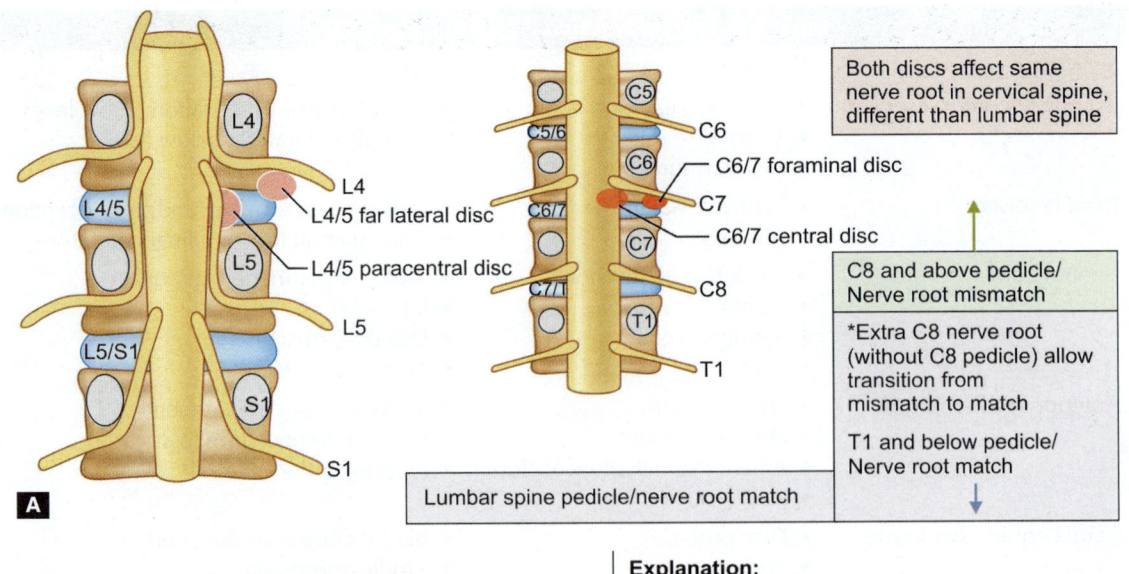

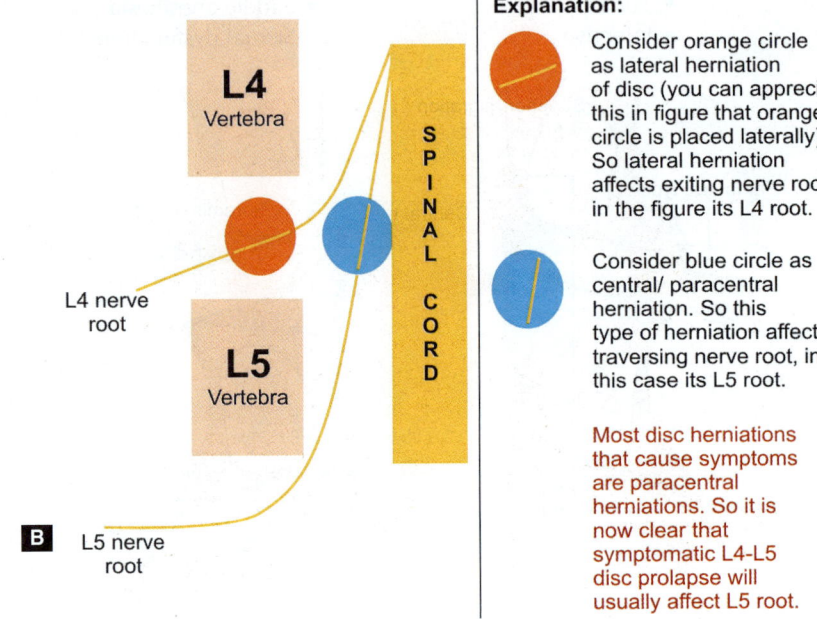

Fig. 9.12A and B: Diagrammatic depiction of nerves involved by a prolapsing disc

Investigations
X-ray may be done to rule out other pathology not for disc herniation per se. MRI is the investigation of choice.

Treatment
- Bedrest is the best therapy, but not given for long periods (maximum 3 days usually).
- Back strengthening exercise after pain relief.
- If not relieved, then: NSAIDs → centrally acting neurogenic pain killer → epidural injection of steroids/LA to the nerve root → surgery.
- Surgery indication: Start of neurological deficit or increasing neurodeficit > persistent pain or failure of conservative method (at least 6 weeks).
- During surgery lamina is opened (laminectomy/laminotomy) to approach the disc. Following exposure herniated disc is removed (discectomy).

Xtra edge
- Newer surgical methods—microscopic/endoscopic disc removal.
- Chemonucleolysis—percutaneous injection of proteolytic enzymes (papain) to dissolve the disc.

SPINAL CANAL STENOSIS
- Spinal canal stenosis (lumbar > cervical) term is used when lumbar canal diameter is <10 mm.
- The causes may be congenital or acquired. The latter is more common and etiology in most cases is primarily degenerative.
  Discs desiccate with age → micro-instability in facet joints → facet joint osteophytes and ligamentum flavum hypertrophy → canal stenosis → symptoms
- Neurogenic claudication (pain radiating down the leg) is the most common symptom. Pain worsens on prolonged standing and walking and can be reproduced on walking for some distance (claudication distance). Flexed postures give relief (positive shopping cart sign).
- Surgical treatment is needed in those not responding to conservative management. Decompression via laminectomy or preferably laminoplasty (lamina swung open not cut open, to decompress spinal cord) is performed.

VERTEBROPLASTY AND KYPHOPLASTY
Vertebroplasty and kyphoplasty (Fig. 9.13, Table 9.9) are interventional radiological procedures done for the treatment of intense pain refractory to other managements caused by vertebral compression fractures due to osteoporosis, tumors and trauma. Recently it has also been used in treatment of vertebral hemangiomas.

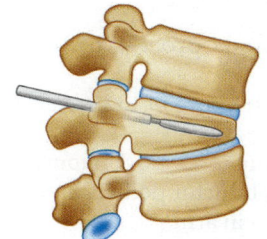 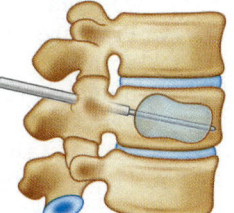 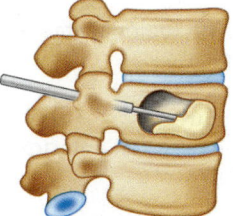 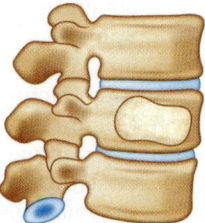

| Balloon inserted into fractured vertebra | Balloon inflated inside damaged vertebra | Special material injected into fractured vertebra | Special material hardens, stabilizing vertebra |

Fig. 9.13: Diagrammatic representation of kyphoplasty

Table 9.9: Vertebroplasty and kyphoplasty

Kyphoplasty	Vertebroplasty
• Uses balloon temp to restore vertebral height and followed by insertion of bone cement • Used in vertebral compression fractures • Substance used is (bone cement) polymethyl methacrylate **Contraindications:** • Infections (tuberculosis)	• Just insert bone cement • Does not use balloon temp (so vertebral height is not restored as much as in kyphoplasty)

MULTIPLE CHOICE QUESTIONS

1. **Denis gave how many theory to define stability of spine:**
   A. 1
   B. 2
   C. 3
   D. 4

2. **The commonest cause of spinal cord injuries in our country is:**
   A. Road traffic accident
   B. Fall from a height
   C. Fall into well
   D. House collapse

3. **Return of bulbocavernous reflex in spinal shock:**
   A. Sign of recovery from spinal shock
   B. Partial lesion of spinal cord
   C. Complete transection of spinal
   D. Incomplete transection of spinal cord A

4. **Spinal injury with no radiological finding is commonly seen in:**
   A. Children   B. Older men
   C. Older women   D. In middle age

5. **Earliest reflex to reappear after shock:**
   A. Knee jerk
   B. Ankle jerk
   C. Bulbocavernous reflex
   D. Abdominal reflex

6. **Full from of SCIWORA:**
   A. Stellate fracture across base of skull
   B. Spinal cord injury without radiological abnormality
   C. Spinal cord involvement with radiological abnormality
   D. Spinal cord injury without radiological abnormity
   E. Spinal cord injury with regional ataxia

7. **Motorcyclist fracture:**
   A. Ring fracture
   B. Communicated fracture
   C. Separation of suture between anterior and posterior half of skull
   D. Fracture base of skull

8. **Dislocation without fracture is seen is:**
   A. Sacral spine   B. Lumbar spine
   C. Cervical spine   D. Thoracic

9. **In a patient with head injury, unexplained hypertension warrants evaluation of:**
   A. Upper cervical spine
   B. Lower cervical spine
   C. Thoracic spine
   D. Lumbar spine

10. **The compression fracture is commonest in:**
    A. Cervical spine
    B. Upper thoracic spine
    C. Lower thoracic spine
    D. Lumbosacral region

11. **Tear drop fracture of lower cervical spine implies:**
    A. Wedge compression fracture
    B. Axial compression fracture
    C. Flexion–rotation injury with failure of anterior body
    D. Flexion compression failure of body

12. **All the following are true about fracture of the atlas vertebra, *except*:**
    A. Jefferson fracture is the most common of atlas
    B. Quardriplegia is seen in 80% cases

C. Atlanto-ocipital fusion may sometimes be needed
D. CT scan's should be done for diagnosis

13. **Regarding hangman's fracture true is:**
    A. High post-admission mortality
    B. Most common axis is necessary
    C. Surgical treatment is necessary
    D. Union almost always occurs

14. **'Whiplash' injury is caused due to:**
    A. A fall from a height
    B. Acute hyperextension of the spine
    C. A Blow on top head
    D. Acute hyperflexion of the spine.

15. **Mechanism underlying burst fracture is:**
    A. Avulsion fracture
    B. Wedge compression
    C. Vertical compression injury
    D. Whiplash injury

16. **Clay-schoveler's fracture is:**
    A. Fracture of spinous process of lower cervical verterbrae
    B. Fracture of spinous process of midthoracic vertebra
    C. Fracture of spinous process of lumbar vertebra
    D. Spinous process fracture of lower cervical vertebrae

17. **Which is not a feature of cervical syringomyelia?**
    A. Hypertrophy of abductor pollicis brevis
    B. Burning sensation in arm
    C. Biceps reflex absent
    D. Extensor plantar

18. **The following X-ray was taken of a 50-year-old female with chronic backache. What is the most likely diagnosis?**

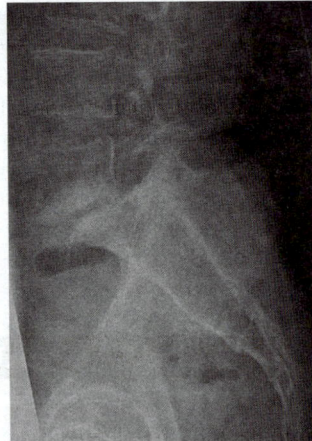

    A. Spondylolysis
    B. Spondylosis
    C. Spondylolisthesis
    D. Prolapsed intervertebral disc

19. In Sponylolisthesis, which of the following is NOT useful investigation?
A. Anteroposterior X-ray
B. Lateral view X-ray
C. CT
D. MRI

20. Spot the X-ray sign shown here:

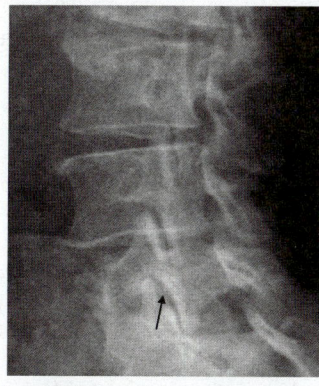

A. Beheaded Scottish terrier dog sign
B. Inverted Napoleon hat sign
C. Dumb bell sign
D. None

21. Partial anterior dislocation of one segment of the spine over another is:
A. Spondylosis
B. Spondylolisthesis
C. Kyphosis
D. Scoliosis

22. A patient with chronic backache has come with the following X-ray, diagnosis:

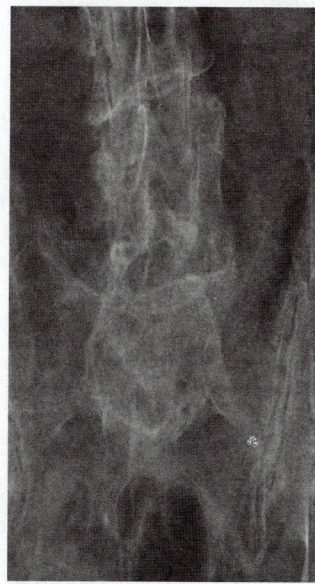

A. Spondylolisthesis
B. TB spine
C. Disc herniation
D. Fracture of L5 vertebrae

23. Spondylolisthesis most common level:
A. L4–L5
B. L5–S1
C. C5–C6
D. C6–C7

24. For spondylolisthesis which is least preferred?
A. MRI
B. CT
C. X-ray lateral view
D. X-ray AP view

25. In spondylolisthesis, there is fracture of vertebra in:
A. Spinous process
B. Neural arch pars interarticularis
C. Transverse process
D. Body

26. True about spondylolisthesis is/are:
A. Congenital defect of posterior arch
B. Slipping of L5 over S1
C. Progressive slipping
D. Abnormal congenital development

27. Ankle reflex nerve root:
A. L4
B. L5
C. S1
D. S2

28. Root value of sensory supply of thumb and middle finger:
A. C6 C6
B. C7 C7
C. C7 C8
D. C6 C7

29. A patient involved in a road traffic accident present with quadriparesis, sphincter disturbance, sensory level up to the border of sternum and respiratory rate of 35/minute. The level of lesion is:
A. C1-C2
B. C4-C5
C. T1-T2
D. T3-T4

30. A 40-year-old male after RTA, attains spinal injury. His lower limb power is greater than that of upper limb and sacral sensation are present. Type of spinal cord lesion is:
A. Central cord syndrome
B. Anterior cord syndrome
C. Posterior cord syndrome
D. Complete cord syndrome

31. Complete transection of the spinal cord at the C7 level produces all of the following effects *except*:
A. Hypotension
B. Limited respiratory effort
C. Anesthesia below the level of the lesion
D. Areflexia below the level of the lesion

32. A patient presented with saddle anesthesia, bladder and bowel are normal and muscle power is normal, the diagnosis is:
A. Cauda equina syndrome
B. L3–L4 root involvement
C. Conus medullan's syndrome
D. L4–L5 disc prolapsed

33. Symmetrical areflexic bladder bowel and lower limb occur in:
A. Cauda equina syndrome
B. Conus medullaris syndrome
C. Nerve root damage
D. Brown secured syndrome

34. All of the following are red flag sign of back pain *except*:
A. Previous history of malignancy
B. Previous history of steroid use
C. Saddle anesthesia
D. Age between 35 and 50 years

35. The investigation of choice to select a prolapsed intervertebral disc is:
A. CT scan   B. MRI
C. Myelography   D. Radiograph

36. Straight leg raising test is/are positive in:
A. Spinal stenosis
B. Spinal abscess
C. Also called Trendelenburg test
D. Prolapsed intervertebral disc
E. Sciatica

37. Removal of vertebral disc is by all these methods *except*:
A. Laminotomy
B. Laminectomy
C. Laminoplasty
D. Hemilaminectomy

38. When do you operate for prolapsed disc:
A. Busy executive needs quick surgery
B. Only with weakness no pain
C. Severe pain interfering with activity and not relieved by rest and treatment of 8 weeks
D. Patient of PID with difficulty in ambulation

39. Test used for prolapsed lumbar intervertebral disc is:
A. Active straight leg raising test
B. Laségue test
C. Thomas test
D. Apley's grinding test

40. Lumbar canal stenosis presents as:
A. Claudication
B. Scoliotic deformity
C. Kyphotic deformity
D. Radiculopathy

41. H reflex on electromyography is seen in:
A. L1 radiculopathy
B. L4 radiculopathy
C. L5 radiculopathy
D. S1 radiculopathy

42. Disc prolapsed is common at all site *except*:
A. L4–L5   B. L5–S1
C. C6–C7   D. T3–T4

43. Most common nerve used for conduction study in H reflex:
A. Median nerve   B. Ulnar nerve
C. Tibial nerve   D. Peroneal nerve

44. Investigation of choice for lumbar prolapsed disc:
A. X-rat   B. CT sacn
C. MRI   D. Myelogram

45. L5–S1 nerve involved:
A. L4   B. L5
C. S1   D. S2

46. A patient has decreased sensation on tip of middle finger and decreased triceps reflex. This presentation can be linked to disc prolapsed at:
A. C5-C6   B. C6-C7
C. C8-T1   D. T1-T2

47. Disc prolapsed is M/C in lumbar spine, due to:
A. Less hydrated
B. Posterior nucleus pulposus
C. Weak ligamentum flavum
D. More degenerative forces

48. Most common site for lumbar disc prolapsed:
A. L4–L5   B. L5–S1
C. L1–L2   D. L3–L4

49. A 44-year-old man presented with acute onset of low backache radiating to the right lower limb. Examination revealed SLRT <40 degrees on the right side, weakness of extensor hallucis longus on the right side, sensory loss in the first web space of the right foot and brisk knee jerk. Which of the following is the most likely diagnosis:
A. Prolapsed intervertebral disc L4–5
B. Spondylolysis L5–S1
C. Lumbar canal stenosis
D. Spondylolisthesis L4–5

50. Which one of the following is not recommended in the treatment of chronic low back pain?
A. NSAIDs
B. Bedrest for 3 months
C. Exercises
D. Epidural steroid injection

51. A previously healthy 45 years old laborer suddenly develop acute lower back pain with right leg pain and weakness of dorsiflexion of the right great toe. Which of the following is true?
A. Immediate treatment should include analgesics muscle relaxants and back strengthening exercises.
B. The appearance of the foot drop indicate early surgical intervention.
C. If the neurological sign resolves within 2–3 weeks but low back pain persists, the proper treatment would include fusion of affected lumbar vertebra.
D. If the neurological sign fails to resolve within 1 week, lumbar laminectomy and excision of any

52. A patient is diagnosed with disc prolapse. Examination reveals paralysis of extensor hallucis longus. Which nerve root is affected?
A. L3   B. L4
C. L5   D. S1

53. L4–L5 disc prolapse compresses commonly:
A. L3   B. L4
C. L5   D. S1

54. Substance that is used for vertebroplasty is:
A. Polymethyl methacrylate
B. Polyethyl methacrylate
C. Polymethylethacrylate
D. Polyethylethacrylate

56. What is vertebroplasty?
A. Stabilization of verterbral compression fracture
B. Replacement of verterbral body only
C. Replacement of verterbral body with intervertebral disc
D. Fusion of the adjacent vertebrae

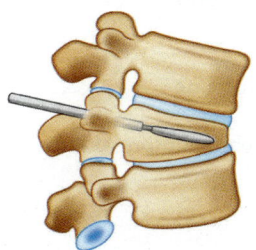
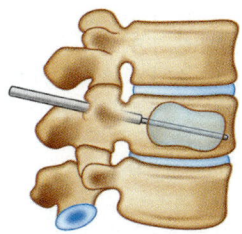

Balloon inserted into fractured vertebra

Balloon inflated inside damaged vertebra

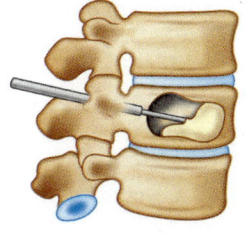
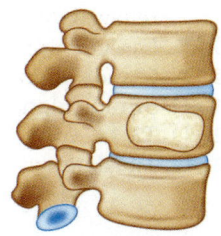

Special material injected into fractured vertebra

Special material hardens, stabilizing vertebra

55. Name the procedure done here:
A. Vertebroplasty   B. Kyphoplasty
C. Both correct   D. None

57. Percutaneous vertebroplasty is not done for:
A. TB   B. Osteoporosis
C. Hemangioma   D. Metastasis

ANSWERS

1. C. 3
2. B. Fall from a height
3. A. Sign of recovery from spinal shock
4. A. Children
5. C. Bulbocavernous reflex
6. B. Spinal cord injury without radiological abnormality
7. C. Separation of suture between anterior and posterior half of skull
8. C. Cervical spine
9. A. Lower cervical spine > C. thoracic spine
10. C. Lower thoracic spine
11. D. Flexion compression failure of body
12. B. Quardriplegia is seen in 80% cases
    • Spinal canal being very wide in C1-C2 region, fracture in this region rarely results in quadriplegia
13. D. Union almost always occurs
14. B. Acute hyperextension of the spine
15. C. Vertical compression injury
16. A. Fracture of spinous process of lower cervical verterbrae
17. A. Hypertrophy of abductor pollicis brevis
18. C. Spondylolisthesis
19. A. Anteroposterior X-ray
20. A. Beheaded Scottish terrier dog sign
21. B. Spondylolisthesis
22. A. Spondylolisthesis
    • Note the inverted Napoleon hat sign

23. B. L5-S1
24. D. X-ray AP view
25. B. Neural arch pars interarticularis
26. A. Congenital defect of posterior arch, B. Slipping of L5 over S1, C. Progressive slipping and D. Abnormal congenital development
27. C. S1
28. D. C6 C7
29. B. C4-C5
    • C3: Sensory supply to lower part of neck, till clavicle
    • C4: Sensory supply to subclavicular region/upper part of sternum
    • Phrenic nerve (C3–5) supplies diaphragm.
    • Thus lesion at C4–5 will cause above mentioned symptoms.
30. A. Central cord syndrome
31. D. Areflexia below the level of the lesion
    • Limited respiratory effort because diaphragm is supplied by phrenic nerves (C3-5) with major contribution coming from C4, which is spared in this case and other respiratory muscles supplied from thoracic nerve roots are involved. Deep tendon reflex below the level of lesion will be exaggerated not absent.
32. C. Conus medullaris syndrome
    • It is characterized by bilateral saddle anesthesia with the preservation of muscle strength largely.

33. B. Conusmedullaris syndrome
34. D. Age between 35 and 50 years
35. B. MRI
36. D. Prolapsed intervertebral disc and E. Sciatica
37. C. Laminoplasty
    - Lamina is either removed (laminectomy) or opened (laminotomy) to approach the intervertebral disc
38. C. Severe pain interfering with activity and not relieved by rest and treatment of 8 weeks
39. B. Laségue test
40. A. Claudication
41. D. S1 radiculopathy
42. D. T3-T4
43. C. Tibial nerve
44. C. MRI
45. C. S1
46. B. C6–C7
47. A. Less hydrated
48. A. L4–L5
49. A. Prolapsed intervertebral disc L4–5
50. B. Bedrest for 3 months
51. B. The appearance of the foot drop indicate early surgical intervention
52. C. L5 root
53. C. L5
54. A. Polymethyl methacrylate
55. A. Vertebroplasty
56. A. Stabilization of vertebral compression fracture
57. A. TB

10

Sports Injuries and Cumulative Soft Tissue Trauma Disorders

SHOULDER JOINT

Adhesive Capsulitis (Frozen Shoulder/Periarthritis Shoulder)

- A condition of uncertain etiology characterised by significant restriction of both active and passive shoulder motion in all directions, that occurs in absence of a known intrinsic shoulder disorder (i.e. stable joint with normal articular surface).
- *Order of affected movements*: Rotations (external > internal rotation) followed by abduction.
- Diabetes mellitus, hyperlipidemia, hyperthyroidism, Dupuytren's disease, hemiplegia, etc. are independent risk factors.
- Rotator interval > anterior capsule of joint is primarily affected.
- Stages of periarthritis are given in Table 10.1.

Painful Arc Syndrome/Impingement Syndrome

- Clinical syndrome in which there is pain in the shoulder and upper arm during mid-range of abduction (60–120 degrees of abduction).
- *Causes*: Subacute supraspinatus tendinitis >> calcification of supraspinatus tendon, subacromial bursitis, greater tuberosity fracture and partial (not complete) tear of supraspinatus tendon.
- Clinical examination may reveal tenderness along the acromion. Neer's test and Hawkins-Kennedy test are the clinical tests commonly useful for diagnosing the condition.
- *Differential diagnosis*: Frozen shoulder, biceps tendinitis.

Rotator Cuff Arthropathy

Rotator cuff consists of several muscles/tendons (Table 10.2), which blend with the joint capsule forming a musculotendinous cuff around anterior/posterior and superior aspects of shoulder joint (thus inferior part of shoulder joint is the weakest area) and its tendinosis or partial/complete tear may lead to group of symptoms which if neglected/unmanaged can lead to arthropathy of shoulder known as rotator cuff arthropathy.

Treatment: NSAIDs and physiotherapies, steroid injection for pain and arthroscopic surgery (TOC) for—impingement syndrome, partial/complete tear. Irreparable tears in less than 70 years old

Table 10.1: Stages of periarthritis	
Stage	*Symptoms*
Stage 1: Freezing (painful)	Shoulder pain is hallmark. It starts gradually and progressively worsens (it may last up to 9 months)
Stage 2: Frozen (stiffening)	Pain may reduce in this stage, although shoulder stiffness and restriction increases. Shoulder range of motion is dramatically reduced (persists for 4 to 20 months)
Stage 3: Thawing/resolution	Characterised by spontaneous thawing. Shoulder range of motion gradually increases and shoulder will be more responsive to stretching exercises and treatment (5 to 26 months)

Table 10.2: Muscles of rotator cuff	
Rotator cuff muscle	*Test*
Subscapularis	• Lift off test/Gerber's test (Fig. 10.1) • Belly press test • Napoleon sign
Supraspinatus	• Jobe's test • Drop arm test
Teres minor	• Horn blowers test
Infraspinatus	• External rotation lag sign

are managed by tendon transfers while in elderly (>70 years old) are treated with reverse shoulder arthroplasty.

Xtra edge
- Rotator interval—interval between leading edge of supraspinatus tendon and superior edge of subscapularis muscle. Contents: Long head of biceps tendon, coracohumeral ligament and superior glenohumeral ligament.
- Spaces around shoulder joint
  - Quadrangular space: Contains axillary nerve and posterior circumflex vessels.
  - Upper triangular space: Contains scapular circumflex vessels.
  - Lower triangular space/interval: Radial nerve with profunda brachii artery.

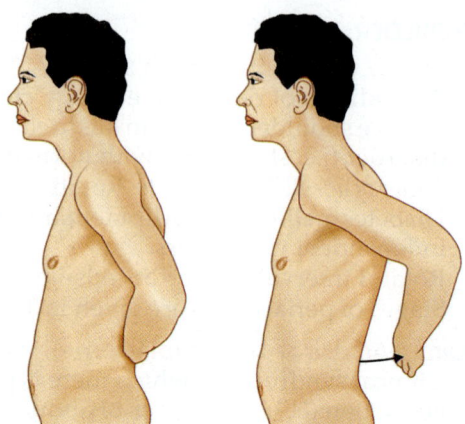

Fig. 10.1: Lift off test for subscapularis muscle

- Treatment for shoulder arthritis is shoulder replacement (total shoulder arthroplasty) but for rotator cuff arthropathy (where rotator cuff is deficient) surgery of choice is "reverse shoulder replacement". The latter shifts the center of rotation of shoulder down and medially allowing deltoid to overtake the function of supraspinatous.

SLAP Lesions
- SLAP stands for 'superior labral tear from anterior to posterior'.
- It is basically a tear of superior labrum that leads to painful shoulder in throwing athletes.
- Etiology involves posterior capsular contracture owing to repeated throwing. Partial articular sided supraspinatous (rotator cuff) tears are commonly found in association.
- Treatment involves arthroscopic reapir.
- Test for SLAP lesions
  - O'Brien's test
  - Crank test

Recurrent Shoulder Dislocation
Recurrent dislocation occurs due to intrinsic problem in bone/soft tissue or labrum. Shoulder joint is the most common joint for recurrent dislocation followed by patella. Ankle joint is the rarest followed by knee. Recurrent dislocation occurs with minimal trauma and rarely associated with nerve/vessel injury. Joint capsule may be lax while in traumatic dislocation, capsule is ruptured at the time of dislocation. Lesions associated with recurrent shoulder dislocation:

Anterior shoulder instability/dislocations
- AKA TUBS—traumatic unilateral dislocation with a Bankart lesion requiring surgery.
- Bankart lesion—an avulsion of the anterior fibrocartilaginous labrum from the anterior rim of glenoid cavity and anterior band of the inferior glenohumeral ligament from the anterior inferior glenoid rim. (B = below)

- Bony Bankart lesion—fracture of the anterior inferior glenoid (Fig. 10.2).
- Hill-Sachs lesion—a chondral impaction injury in the posterosuperior and lateral humeral head (Fig. 10.3) secondary to contact with the glenoid rim in anterior dislocation. If this impaction fracture is large (>20% surface area of glenoid) then shoulder joint becomes unstable leading to recurrent instability/dislocation (Hill = high = superior).

Posterior shoulder instability/dislocation
- Reverse Hill-Sachs lesion—also called a **McLaughlin lesion**, is defined as an impaction fracture of anteromedial aspect of the humeral head specially following non-reducible and difficult to reduce posterior dislocation of the humerus.
- Posterior/reverse Bankart lesions—characterised by detachment of posterior inferior capsulolabral complex.

Multidirectional shoulder instability (MDI)
Also referred to as AMBRI
- Atraumatic
- Multidirectional
- Bilateral (frequently)
- Rehabilitation (often respond to)
- Inferior capsular shift (best alternative to nonoperative management).

Tests for glenohumeral instability in recurrent dislocation: Positions producing dislocation are tried to reproduce or force applied from posterior (anterior instability) or anterior (for posterior instability) and the patient becomes apprehensive in fear of dislocation and tries to stop the maneuver.
- **Anterior instability:** Anterior apprehension test, Jobe's relocation test, Andrews test, fulcrum test, Crank test and surprise test (most accurate). (Mnemonic—*Andrews surprised* his friend *Jobes* by hitting from behind, so hard with a *fulcrum* that, it produced a *crank* sound dislocating shoulder anteriorly).
- **Posterior instability:** Posterior apprehension test, posterior Clunk test, Jahnke test, Jerk (provocative) test, push pull test, circumduction test. (Pneumonic—typical scene in a bus: piche se (*posterior*) *janke jerk* and *push pullkia* and last main *circumduction* hi kardia).
- **Inferior instability:** Sulcus test/sign.

Surgical procedures for recurrent dislocation of shoulder:
- **Bankart's operation:** Performed for a Bankart's lesion. Anterior structures which were detached are re-attached to the glenoid rim with sutures.

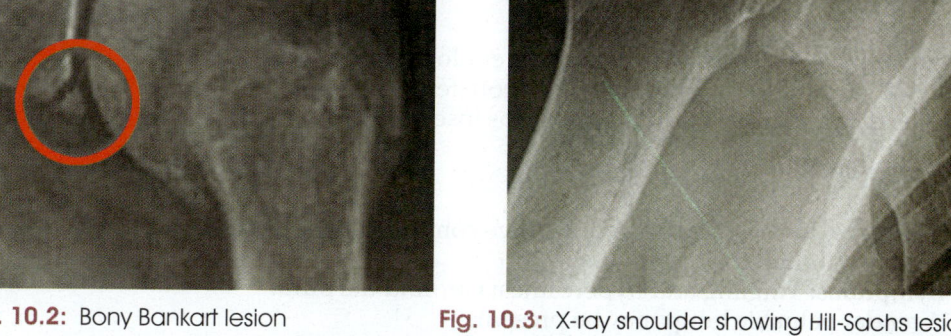

Fig. 10.2: Bony Bankart lesion   **Fig. 10.3:** X-ray shoulder showing Hill-Sachs lesion

- **Putti-Platt's technique:** Joint is reinforced by overlapping and tightening subscapularis tendon with the capsule. Prevents a Hill-Sachs lesion from engaging.
- Neer capsular shift for multidirectional instability.
- **Bone defects:** When glenoid has large bony deficiency, i.e. >25% bone loss, it may be reconstructed with iliac crest or coracoid (Latarjet procedure) bone graft. When humeral head has bone defect (Hill-Sachs lesion), up to 10% loss may be neglected; 10–30% loss may need infraspinatous tacking in the defect (Remplissage) while >30–40% may need bone grafting or Latarjet procedure. Defects larger than 40% on humeral side are best managed with prosthetic replacements.
- Neglected shoulder dislocation (most common posterior)—surgically reduced.

ELBOW

Tennis Elbow

Lateral epicondylitis/chronic tendinitis of common extensor origin, associated with activities that require repeated supination and pronation of the forearm with the elbow in near full extension.

Pathology: Microtear in origin of extensor carpi radialis brevis mainly (may also involve tendons of ECRL or extensor digitorum communis).

Microscopic finding: Immature reparative tissue resembling angiofibroblastic hyperplasia.

Clinical signs and tests:
- Occurs more frequently in non-athletes than athletes.
- Peak incidence: Early 5th decade.
- Tenderness at lateral epicondyle.
- Cozen's test: Pain in region of lateral epicondyle on wrist extension against resistance.
- Maudsley's test: Middle finger extension against resistance.
- Mill's test

X-ray: Normal or calcification near lateral epicondyle.

D/D: Radial tunnel syndrome, i.e. compressive neuropathy of posterior interosseous nerve (tenderness is more distal as opposed to that in tennis elbow), osteochondritis dissecans of capitellum, lateral compartment arthrosis, etc.

Management: 95% responds to conservative management. If not relieved, then steroid injection at site of maximum tenderness, autologous blood injection to promote fibrosis and PRP (platelet rich plasma) injections to promote healing. Operative management which includes debridement of degenerated origin of ECRB or release of its origin.

Golfer's Elbow

- Chronic overuse tendinitis of the common flexor pronator origin (especially flexor carpi radialis).
- Tenderness localized to the medial epicondyle.
- This condition is much less common and more difficult to treat than tennis elbow.
- Frequently occurs with repetitive overhead motion and racket sports.
- Pain at medial elbow on resisted forearm pronation or wrist flexion.
- Even in golfers, tennis elbow is more common.

Baseball Pitchers' Elbow/Little Leaguer's Elbow

Medial epicondylar apophysitis seen in young players before or around the age of puberty.

Javelin Throwers' Elbow

Painful elbow in a Javelin thrower. Two etiologies are described:
- Round arm action: A sprain of ulnar collateral ligament of the elbow or.
- Over arm action: A tendinitis of triceps insertion at olecranon/avulsion of tip of olecranon.

WRIST AND HAND

Bowler's Thumb

- Perineural fibrosis caused by repetitive compression of ulnar digital nerve (branch of median nerve) of thumb due to bowling.
- **Symptoms:** Tingling and hyperesthesia around the pulp.
- A tender palpable lump may be present.

- **Management:** Splinting, padding and rest from bowling. Neurolysis and dorsal transfer of nerve become necessary occasionally.

Skier's Thumb/Gamekeeper's Thumb

- Injury to thumb metacarpophalangeal joint ulnar collateral ligament.
- **Mechanism of injury:** Snow skiing accident and fall on outstretched hand with forceful abduction of thumb.
- **Signs and symptoms:** Painful swelling and ecchymosis around MCP joint along with tenderness.
- **Stener lesion:** Adductor aponeurosis interposed between the ruptured thumb MCP joint ulnar collateral ligament and its site of insertion at base of proximal phalanx. This prevents healing necessitating surgical repair.
- It is important to differentiate between partial and complete tear as later requires surgery while partial is managed conservatively.
- **Management:**
  - *Incomplete tear*: Protection in thumb spica cast/brace for 4–6 weeks.
  - *Complete tear*: Acute cases need repair while > 6 weeks old cases are managed with ligament reconstruction (replacement of torn ligament with a tendon graft).

Mallet Finger/Baseball Finger

- Disruption of terminal extensor tendon (**extensor digitorum communis**) resulting in distal interphalangeal joint extension lag, is called mallet/baseball finger.
- It is due to avulsion of extensor tendon from the base of dorsum of distal phalanx with or without a chip of bone.
- **Mechanism of injury:** Forceful blow to tip of finger causing sudden flexion of DIP joint
- Patient is unable to actively extend DIP joint, but passive extension is possible.
- Proximal IP joint hyperextension may occur giving rise to a swan neck deformity.
- **Management:** In acute cases—splinting with DIP in extension for 6–8 weeks.

Jersey Finger

- Disruption of flexor digitorum profundus (FDP) tendon from its insertion at the volar aspect of the distal phalanx is called jersey finger.
- Usually caused by sudden hyperextension of an actively flexed finger.
- Most commonly affects 4th digit as FDP insertion into ring finger is weaker.

Trigger Finger

It is a stenosing tenovaginitis of flexor tendon of the affected finger which may lead to entrapment of the tendon at A1 pulley at the level of MCP joint. Ring and middle fingers are most commonly affected. It may be due to thickening of fibrous tendon sheath or constriction of mouth/exit of tendon (A1 pulley) and a tender nodule can be palpated at MCP joint. Catching/locking of the affected finger is present after forceful flexion and is extended with an audible click/trigger.

Causes: Trauma, rheumatoid arthritis, gout, diabetes, etc.

Ganglion

- Most common cause of focal hand masses.
- **Unilocular** cystic swelling filled with mucinous fluid arising from synovium or tendon sheaths but **without** a synovial or epithelial lining.
- Dorsal wrist ganglion arises from scapholunate interosseous ligament.
- It communicates with tendon sheath/joint cavity and stalk can be identified communicating between cyst and adjacent joint or tendon sheath.
- **Most common:** Dorsal wrist ganglion, but also common on volar surface.
- **Management:** It is reported that 50% ganglions subside by themselves.
  - *Non-operative*: NSAIDs for pain and aspiration with injecting steroid or sclerosing agent.
  - Recurrence rate is higher with aspiration and injection in comparison to excision.
  - *Operative*: Open or arthroscopic excision.
- Compound palmar ganglion is chronic inflammation of common sheath of flexor tendons above and below flexor retinaculum leading to an hour glass swelling. Rheumatoid arthritis and TB are common etiological factors.

de Quervain's Disease

- Stenosing tenosynovitis of the abductor pollicis longus (APL) and extensor pollicis brevis (EPB) tendon (1st dorsal compartment of wrist).
- **Age:** 30–50 years.
- Females >> males.
- **Etiology:** Overuse, rheumatoid arthritis.
- **Presenting symptom:** Pain and tenderness near radial styloid.
- **Finkelstein's test** is positive. Patient's thumb is grasped and hand is quickly abducted ulnar ward. This causes pain over styloid tip.
- **Intersection syndrome:** Inflammation at intersection where APL and EPB crosses ECRL and ECRB.
- **Management:** Analgesics, rest on a splint and injection of steroid preparation.
  If above methods fail, surgery may be required. Surgery involves splitting the thickened tendon sheath and releasing tendons.

Dupuytren's Contracture

- It is proliferative fibroplasia of subcutaneous palmar tissue (palmar aponeurosis) in form of nodules and cord that may result in flexion contractures in fingers and palm.
- Increased fibroblast proliferation and deposition of **collagen type 3** and dominant cell type: Myofibroblast.
- **Age:** 40s to 60s with male > female (10 times).
- Presents earlier in males (mean 55 years) than females (mean 65 years).
- Higher incidence in epileptics receiving phenytoin, diabetics, alcoholics, smokers and liver cirrhosis patients. Hereditary predisposition plays a role too.
- Usually begins on ulnar side of hand at distal palmar crease and involves ring finger > little finger > middle > index.
- Causes contracture of MCP > PIP joints. DIP joint is spared.
- Pain is present but never the most important feature.
- Ectopic Dupuytren disease deposits:
  - *Ledderhose disease*—similar lesion in medial plantar fascia of feet
  - *Garrod nodules (Knuckle pads)*—dorsum of PIP joint
  - *Peyronie disease*
- Type of collagen deposited: Type 3
- Cleland ligament and transverse ligaments are spared.
- **Management**
  - Initially, conservative management in the form of range of motion and stretching exercises are done.
  - Percutaneous needle aponeurotomy.
  - Partial or complete fasciectomy with z plasties/skin transplantation.

ZONES OF HAND

Zones of Flexor Tendon (Fig. 10.4)

Zone 1: Distal to insertion of flexor digitorum superficialis (FDS).

Zone 2: Between distal palmar crease and insertion of FDS (**Bunnel's no man's land).**

Zone 3: Between distal margin of transverse carpal ligament (carpal tunnel) and beginning of critical area of pulley's or 1st annulus (area of lumbrical origin).

Zone 4: Zone covered by transverse carpal ligament (within carpal tunnel).

Zone 5: Proximal to carpal tunnel.

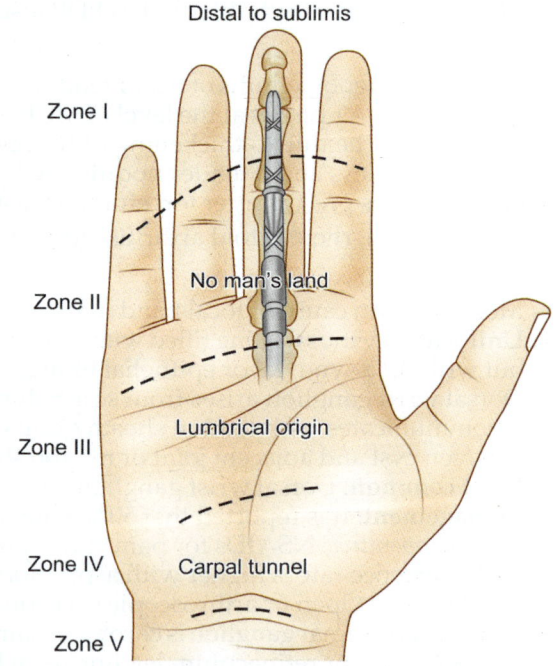

Fig. 10.4: Zones of hand

Pulleys

Tendons are bound to bones by special fibrous structures called pulleys. They can be *annular* or *cruciate*.

Annular pulleys/ligaments: Numbered from A1 to A5
- A2 and A4—opposite proximal and distal phalanx respectively, prevent bowstringing.
- A1, A3 and A5 overlie at MP, PIP and DIP joints respectively.
- Pulley involved in trigger finger: A1.
- A5 pulley is thinnest.
- Most crucial pulleys: A2 and A4 (A2 > A4).

KNEE JOINT

Anatomy of Knee Joint

Knee joint is the **largest joint** of the body. It is a **compound synovial joint** comprising of tibio-femoral and patella-femoral articulations. Tibio-femoral joint is a modified hinge joint (in addition to flexion and extension its motion has a rotary component also) and the patello-femoral joint is a saddle joint. The articular surface of medial condyle is longer than that of lateral condyle. The articular surfaces of knee are not congruent. Pes-anserinus is a group of tendons inserting (in a "J/hockey" shaped manner) in anteromedial side of tibia: Sartorius, gracialis and semitendinosus.

Integral to the knee joint is the ligaments and menisci (Fig. 10.5) which stabilise it:
- Two cruciate ligaments: Anterior (ACL) and posterior (PCL)
- Two collateral ligaments: Medial and lateral
- Two Menisci: Medial and lateral.

Cruciate Ligaments

Intra-articular, extra-synovial (they have their own synovial sheath), principally provide antero-posterior stability, although also have their role in rotational stability.

ACL

It starts anteriorly from intercondylar area of tibia, runs upward, backward and laterally to insert on posterior part of medial surface of lateral femoral condyle.
- Tibial attachment site is larger and more secure than femoral attachment
- Blood supply: Middle genicular artery (primary)

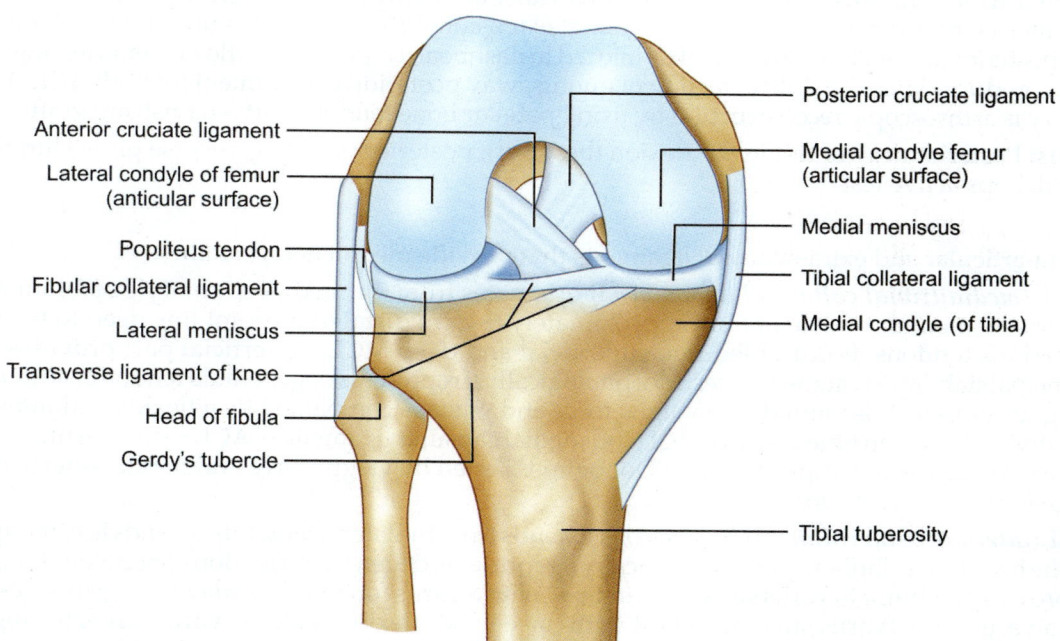

Fig. 10.5: Anatomy of the knee joint

- Nerve supply: Posterior articular nerve (branch of tibial nerve)
- Have Mechano-receptors (proprioception)

ACL has two bundles: Anteromedial—tight in flexion and posterolateral (bulky), which is tight in extension. (Provides principal resistance to hyperextension).

Function: Restricts anterior tibial gliding/hyperextension of tibia on femur. It also stabilises internal rotation of tibia and lateral stability. Tension in ACL is least at 30–40 degree of flexion. Length of ACL is maximum in the direction of movement which it restricts/stabilises and thus gets injured when that limit is exceeded. When one walks downhill, hyperextension of tibia occurs and ACL becomes taut and thus stabilises the movement. Injured ACL produces knee instability/feeling of giving away anteriorly.

Segond fracture: Avulsion fracture of lateral tibial plateau (capsular avulsion). It is frequently associated with ACL tear.

Tests

Anterior drawer test—done in knee flexed to 90°. A tight hamstring or abutment of posterior horn of medial meniscus against medial femoral condyle (known as door step effect) may lead to false negative anterior drawer test by resisting anterior displacement of tibia on femur.

Lachman test—more sensitive and done with knee flexed 20° instead of 90°. More useful in acute painful/swollen situations where knee is difficult to flex 90°. In less degree of flexion, the doorstep effect of posterior horn of menisci is negated.

Tests in decreasing order of sensitivity and specificity: Lachman's test > flexion rotation drawer test > anterior drawer test > Pivot shift test.

PCL

It starts proximally from lateral surface of medial femoral condyle and courses posteriorly and laterally to insert on an area that is around 1.5 cm posterior and inferior to the posterior articular margin of the tibia. It is bulkier and stronger than ACL and has two bundles: Anterolateral (major part) and posteromedial.

Function: Limits posterior displacement/glide of tibia on femur and restricts hyperextension only after ACL is ruptured. It is active in almost all knee movements and checks hyperextension when ACL is injured. It forms the axis around which rotation of knee occurs. It guides the "screw home" mechanism on internal rotation of femur during terminal extension. When one walks uphill, PCL stabilises the posterior glide of tibia on femur. It is injured in dashboard injury/hyperflexion injuries. Injured PCL produces knee instability/feeling of giving away posteriorly. Treatment for both ACL/PCL injury is arthroscopic reconstruction by using patellar bone tendon graft > hamstring graft.

Tests: Posterior drawer test in 90° flexion (best test), posterior tibial sag, reverse pivot shift test, quadriceps active test.

Collateral Ligaments

Extra-articular and extra-synovial ligaments that provide mediolateral stability.

MCL (medial/tibial collateral ligament): It originates from the medial epicondyle of femur and inserts on medial condyle of tibia approximately 6–7 cm distal to the joint line deep to the pes anserinus tendons. It is divided into superficial and deep MCL. Superficial part provides the principal stability to valgus stresses. Morphologically it represents degenerated tendon of adductor magnus muscle. It is injured by a valgus force and when accompanied by a flexion and internal rotation of femur on tibia leads to: MCL and medial capsular ligament → ACL → medial meniscus injury, known as unhappy triad of O'Donoghue. Tested by valgus force (valgus stress test), best with knee in 30° of flexion.

LCL (lateral/fibular collateral ligament): It extends from the lateral femoral epicondyle to the apex of the head of the fibula and morphologically it represents degenerated tendon of peroneus longus. It provides restraint to varus stress. It is injured with a varus force and ligament integrity is tested by a varus force (varus stress test) best with knee in 30° flexion. Valgus/varus stress testing in extension that reveals significant instability suggests cruciate ligament and posterior capsule disruption in addition to collateral ligament disruption.

Rotatory Instabilities of Knee

Posterolateral instability: Posterolateral complex (PLC) consists of LCL, popliteus tendon, fabellofibular ligament, arcuate ligament and popliteofibular ligament. Posterolateral corner of the knee is also sometimes referred to as the 'dark corner' of the knee, as missing these ligament injuries is often the foremost cause of failure in treatment of other major ligament injuries. It is tested by dial test in 30° flexion/tibia external rotation test (best) and reverse pivot shift test.

Anterolateral instability (commonest combined instability) consists of failure of ACL + LCL + lateral half of joint capsule. Tested by anterior drawer test with foot internally rotated 30° and pivot shift phenomena.

Anteromedial instability consists of failure of ACL + MCL + medial knee joint capsule (posterior oblique ligament). Tested by anterior drawer test with externally rotated 15°.

Xtra Edge

- Fabella is a sesamoid bone present in the tendon of the lateral head of the gastrocnemius muscle. The ligament that extends from the fabella to the fibular head (fabello-fibular ligament) is called the ligament of valloise.

Menisci

The menisci are the wedge-shaped fibro-cartilaginous discs made primarily of type I collagen (type II collagen in articular cartilage) lying between the opposing femoral and tibial condyles. These are intra-articular and intra-synovial structures that derive their nutrition, primarily from synovial fluid. Menisci are largely avascular (maximum 30% part is vascular) except near there periphery. Inferior surface is flat while superior surface is concave corresponding to the contour of underlying tibial plateau and overlying femoral condyles. Menisci move with knee movements. They move forward in extension of the knee and move backward during flexion of the knee. Each meniscus has an anterior horn, body and a posterior horn.

Functions of the menisci:

1. They act as a joint filler so that flat tibial condyles articulate well with the femoral condyles.
2. Shock absorbers in the knee on axial loading.
3. Aid in joint lubrication, distribution of synovial fluid and nutrition of articular.
4. Protect the articular cartilage.
5. Contribute to stability.

Medial Meniscus

- C-shaped (semilunar), larger in radius and narrower in body than the lateral meniscus.
- Posterior horn wider than anterior horn and bears more weight.
- It covers less tibial articular surface than lateral meniscus.
- Entire peripheral border attached firmly to medial capsule and through the **coronary ligament** to the upper border of tibia.
- Outer aspect of meniscus is attached to posterior deep fibres of MCL.
- Since it is more firmly attached, it is less mobile and more prone to injury.

Lateral Meniscus

- Semi-circular in shape (more circular) with smaller diameter and wider body as compared to medial.
- Both horns are of equal size and cover larger portion of tibial articular surface (nearly 2/3rd).
- Posterior horn attached to medial femoral condyle through menisco-femoral ligaments called ligament of Humphrey (anterior to PCL) and ligament of Wrisberg (posterior to PCL).
- Tendon of popliteus (intra-articular tendon) separates posterolateral periphery of lateral meniscus from capsule and LCL, and prevents it from injury by drawing it posterolaterally during knee flexion.
- It is more mobile than medial meniscus due to its less firm attachment to capsule and thus less prone to injury.

Injury occurs most commonly to medial meniscus, causing a complete vertical longitudinal tear known as bucket handle tear. Mechanism of injury is a twisting force on knee. In adults only 10–25% of lateral and 10–30% of medial meniscus are vascular and the supply is by medial and lateral genicular arteries (inferior and superior). Implications: Healing potential is maximum for tears in periphery. On the basis of vascularity, tears are classified into three zones: Red, red-white and white.

Symptoms: Pain, joint line tenderness, popping, catching and pathological locking (inability to extend knee for last few degrees), and knee instability (feeling of giving away). Squatting, crossed leg position is very painful.

Tests for menisci:
1. McMurray's test
2. Apley's grinding test
3. Thessaly test
4. Steinman's test
5. Ege's test (McMurray test done in weight bearing position).
6. Difficult squatting/crossed legged position (Payr's sign)
7. *Bounce home test*—knee is suddenly extended from flexed position and checked for the end point of extension. Normally it has hard (bony) or firm (cartilaginous) feel but in ACL/ meniscal injury is rubbery feel.

Arthroscopy is the gold standard and MRI is the IOC for diagnosing meniscal tear. Arthroscopic excision (total/partial meniscectomy) is the treatment of choice as avascular menisci seldom heal. Repair can be done when tears involve the peripheral vascular zone of the meniscus.

Xtra edge
- Meniscal injury: Medial > lateral.
- Meniscal cyst: Lateral > medial.
- Discoid meniscus: Lateral > medial.
- **Screw home mechanism:** Physiological locking/unlocking. It is due to the specific bony anatomy of the knee (condyles are unequal) and relative differences in lengths of the two cruciate ligaments.
  - *Open chain*: When the foot is off the ground and knee extends from flexion, tibia rotates externally while on flexion tibia rotates internally.
  - *Closed chain*: When the foot is on the ground, on knee extension femur rotates medially and thus tibial tuberosity moves towards lateral border of patella. Physiological locking of knee occurs as a result of medial rotation of femur during last 30° of extension (quadriceps muscle) and unlocking is by lateral rotation of femur over tibia in initial phase of flexion (popliteus muscle).
- **Causes of pathological locking:** Meniscal injury, loose bodies in knee, osteochondral fracture, fractures tibial spine, OA knee with fracture of osteophytes.
- **Pirani sign:** Meniscal cysts disappear on knee joint flexion.
- Q angle is the angle between quadriceps and patellar tendon with knee in 30° flexion. Normal values is more in females than males and this lateral force is countered by vastus medialis pull. If the angle increases, it overloads the patella laterally leading to chondromalacia patellae, recurrent patella subluxation/dislocation.
- Table 10.3 gives differentiating features in injuries to various knee ligaments.
- **Cruciate or collateral ligament injury:** Causes hemarthrosis and immediate swelling (within 2 hours).
- **Meniscal injury:** Causes effusion and delayed swelling. If involving peripheral part, it may also cause hemarthrosis.

Table 10.3: Differentiating different knee injuries		
Structure	*Injury mechanism*	*Test*
1. MCL	Valgus force	Valgus stress, knee 30° flexed
2. LCL	Varus force	Varus force, knee 30° flexed
3. ACL	Anterior force	Lachman, anterior drawer
4. PCL	Posterior force	Posterior drawer
5. Meniscus	Twisting force with leg weight bearing	Twisting force (McMurray's test)

- **Causes of hemarthrosis:**
  - Cruciate ligaments injury (commonest cause)
  - Osteochondral fracture
  - Peripheral meniscal injury
  - Tear in deep portion of joint capsule.

BURSITIS

Knee joint has many bursa in its surrounding and its inflammation leads to swelling.
- Anteriorly—prepatellar (housemaid's knee—most common); infrapatellar bursitis (Clergyman's knee).
- Medially—bursa between pes-anserinus and MCL.
- Posteriorly—semimembranosus bursa.
- Bursa comminucating with knee joint—suprapatellar, popliteus bursa, gastrocnemius bursa, pes-anserinus bursa.
- Popliteal cyst (Morrant-Baker cyst)—synovial outpouching due to OA/RA between medial head of gastrocnemius and semimembranosus and can be compressed. Prominent on knee flexion and disappear with knee extension. Soft, fluctuant and no transillumination.
- TB bursitis—most commonly involves trochanteric bursa > pes-anserinus bursa.
- Eponyms (Table 10.4)

Table 10.4: Eponyms for various bursitis	
Weavers bottom	*Ischial bursitis*
Bunion	1st metatarsal head bursitis
Student's elbow/miner's elbow	Olecranon bursitis
Tailor's ankle	Lateral malleolus bursitis
Bunionette	5th metatarsal head bursitis

Plica Syndrome

Plica are phylogenetical remnants of synovial folds which divides knee in different compartments. If they undergo inflammation after repeated trauma, they may cause pain and knee swelling/locking. Most common is that of suprapatellar plica and diagnosed by arthroscopy and best treated by arthroscopic excision.

MISCELLANEOUS

Athletic pubalgia: Chronic pain in the inguinal or pubic region due to pull of rectus abdominis muscle on pubis. Primarily seen in athletes and occur after exertion, also known as "sportman's hernia" or "Gilmore's groin".

Ankle sprain: Ligament injury is most common in ankle joint and is popularly called ankle sprain. Most common mechanism is inversion of plantar flexed foot and most common ligament to injured is anterior talofibular ligament.

Achilles tendon (TA) injury: Strongest tendon in the body named after a warrior (Achilles). Its distal 5–6 cm is avascular (watershed area—most common site of tendinitis and tendon rupture) and may be inflamed in overuse/exertion.
- Insertional tendinitis—inflammation at the insertion site on calcaneum, due to overuse. Risk factors are bursitis/osteophytes near its insertion—retrocalcaneal bursitis, Haglund deformity (pump-bump), i.e. exostosis on calcaneum near its insertion site.
- Non-insertional tendinitis—most common and often seen in runners and jumpers. Involves the watershed area.
- TA rupture—mostly occurs in watershed area due to repeated microtrauma which makes it weaker. Mechanism is sudden violent dorsiflexion of plantar flexed foot >> sudden forced plantar flexion of foot. Clinical test: Thompson's test, O'Brien needle test.

Plantar fasciitis: Inflammation of plantar fascia associated with long periods of weight bearing and overweight patients. Pain is mainly on undersurface of sole and increases on prolonged weight bearing. Due to stretch/pull of plantar fascia, a bony spur (Fig. 10.6) may be seen in calcaneum, at the site where it inserts. Diagnosis is mainly clinical and may be supported by X-ray visualisation of spur. Treatment: Conservative (KL splint with rest, cold and NSAIDs → steroid injection) and if not relieved then surgery (plantar fascia release).

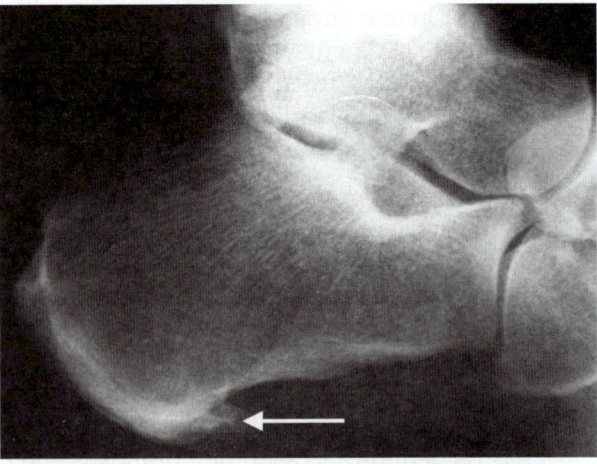

Fig. 10.6: X-ray showing calcaneal spur

Toe deformities
- Hammer toe (Fig. 10.7A)—plantar flexion deformity of PIP joint frequently associated with hyperextension of MTP joint.
- Hallux valgus (Fig. 10.7B)—most common foot deformity where the great toe points laterally, and may cause overriding/underriding of 2nd toe. Due to its lateral deviation, 1st MTP joint/MT head becomes prominent medially and prone to bursitis/bunion/and later osteoarthritis. It may be congenital due to varus angulation of 1st MT known as metatarsus primary varus. Mostly managed conservatively by toe filler/spacers and surgery is reserved for painful cases/cosmetic reason. Outcomes of surgery are not very good (Chevron osteotomy).

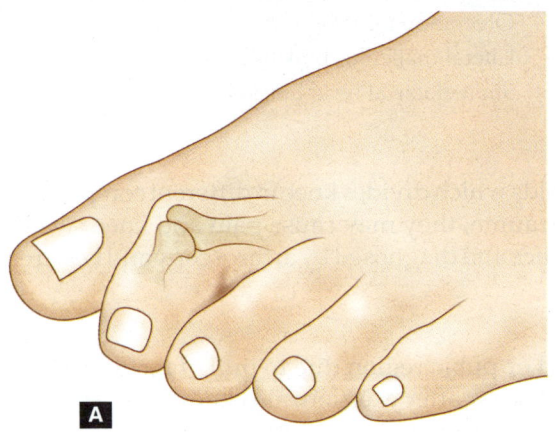
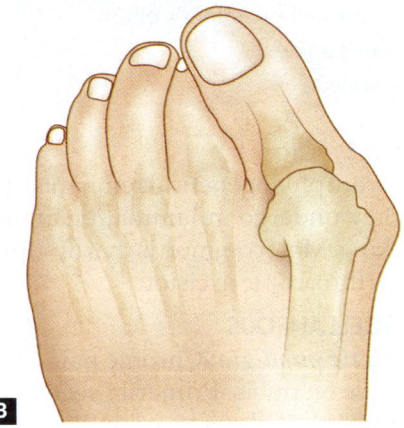

Fig. 10.7: (A) Hammer toe, (B) Hallux valgus

MULTIPLE CHOICE QUESTIONS

1. **Dynamic stabilisers of shoulder joint:**
   A. Glenoidal labrum
   B. Rotator cuff muscles
   C. Glenohumeral ligament
   D. Coracohumeral ligament

2. **For long the muscle was not given its due importance and was called forgotten muscle of rotator cuff. Which one is the muscle?**
   A. Subscapularis   B. Supraspinatus
   C. Infraspinatus   D. Teres minor

3. **Rotator interval is between:**
   A. Supraspinatus and teres minor
   B. Teres major and teres minor
   C. Supraspinatus and subscapularis
   D. Subscapularis and infraspinatus

4. **Muscle crossing through the shoulder join is:**
   A. Biceps short head
   B. Biceps long head
   C. Triceps long head
   D. Coracobrachialis

5. **Gradual painful limitation of shoulder movement in an elderly suggest that the most probable diagnosis is:**
   A. Arthritis
   B. Osteoarthritis
   C. Periarthritis
   D. Myositis ossifications
   E. Fracture–dislocation

6. **All of the following associated with frozen shoulder except:**
   A. Diabetes   B. Hyperthyroidism
   C. Psoriasis   D. Hemiplegia

7. **Which of the following movements is restricted in frozen shoulder?**
   A. Abduction and internal rotation
   B. Abduction and external rotation
   C. All range of movement
   D. Only abduction

8. **First movement to be restricted in frozen shoulder is:**
   A. Flexion   B. Extension
   C. Internal rotation   D. External rotation

9. **Causes of painful arc syndrome is/are:**
   A. Supraspinatus tendinitis
   B. Subacromial bursitis
   C. Frature of greater tuberosity
   D. All of the above

10. **The following are true regarding rotator cuff tendinitis except:**
    A. Injection of local anesthetic helps in diagnosis
    B. Steroid injection are contraindicated
    C. Painful arc movement causes secondary weakness
    D. Acromial beak of bone appears with age

11. **Painful arc syndrome is seen in all except:**
    A. Complete tear of supraspinatus
    B. Fracture greater tuberosity
    C. Subacromial bursitis
    D. Supraspinatus tendinitis

12. **Bankart's lesion is seen in:**
    A. Recurrent anterior shoulder dislocation
    B. Posterior shoulder dislocation
    C. Rotator cuff tear
    D. Interior shoulder dislocation

13. **Which of the following structure passes through the quadrangular space?**
    A. Axillary nerve
    B. Radial nerve
    C. Median nerve
    D. Brachial artery

14. **The posterolateral lesion in the head of humerus in cases of recurrent anterior shoulder dislocation is:**
    A. Bankart's lesion
    B. Hill-Sachs lesion

C. Reverse Hill-Sachs lesion
D. Greater tuberosity avulsion

15. **A 42-year-man is diagnosed to have irreparable tear of the rotator cuff. Treatment of choice will be:**
    A. Tendon transfer
    B. Total shoulder replacement
    C. Reverse shoulder replacement
    D. Acromioplasty

16. **Bankart's lesion involves the _____ of the glenoid labrum:**
    A. Anterior lip
    B. Superior lip
    C. Anterior lip
    D. Anteroinferior lip

17. **Most common muscle damaged in rotator cuff:**
    A. Supraspinatus
    B. Infraspinatus
    C. Subscapularis
    D. Teres minor

18. **Painful arc syndrome is caused by impingement of:**
    A. Subacromial bursa
    B. Subdeltoid bursa
    C. Rotator cuff tendon
    D. Biceps tendon

19. **Rotator cuff muscle, all are true except:**
    A. Supraspinatus
    B. Subscapularis
    C. Teres minor
    D. Subscapularis

20. **A patient of recurrent anterior dislocation presents with the following X-ray, diagnosis is:**

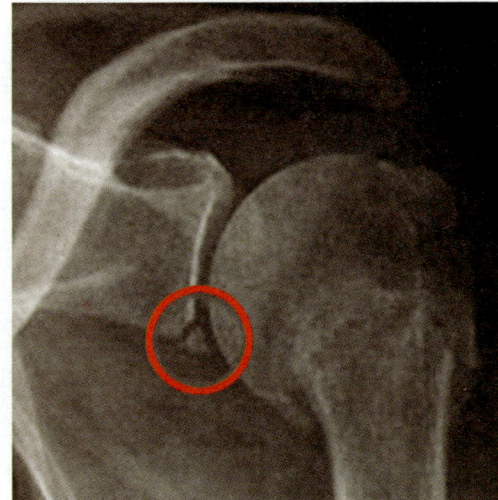

A. Bankart lesion
B. Hill-Sachs lesion
C. Fracture scapula
D. Reverse Hill-Sachs lesion

21. **Lift off test is done for:**
    A. Supraspinatus   B. Infraspinatus
    C. Teres minor   D. Subscapularis
22. **A patient of rotator cuff injury evaluated by the following test, muscle tested is:**

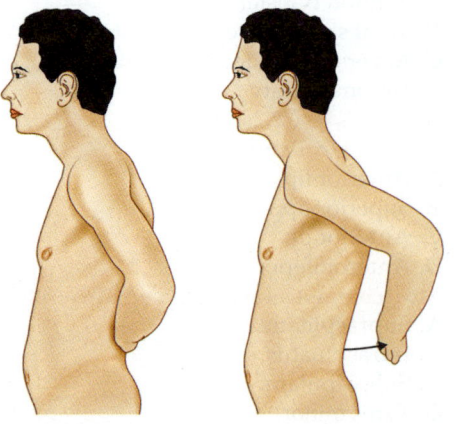

    A. Subscapularis   B. Supraspinatus
    C. Biceps brachii   D. Infraspinatus
23. **Weakest portion of shoulder join capsule is:**
    A. Anterior   B. Posterior
    C. Inferior   D. Superior
24. **Hill-Sachs lesion in recurrent shoulder dislocation is:**
    A. Injury to humeral head
    B. Rupture of tendon of supraspinatus muscle
    C. Avulsion of glenoid labrum
    D. None of the above
25. **Shoulder dislocation false is:**
    A. Most common early complication of anterior dislocation shoulder is nerve injury
    B. Hill-Sachs is seen in recurrent anterior shoulder dislocation
    C. Rotator cuff injury is a common cause of recurrent dislocation
    D. Posterior dislocation presents with difficulty in external rotation of shoulder
26. **Putti-Platt's operation involves tightening of which muscles?**
    A. Supraspinatus   B. Subscapularis
    C. Infraspinatus   D. Deltoid
27. **Which of the following is true about anterior shoulder dislocation?**
    A. It is most common type of shoulder dislocation
    B. It is most commonly subclavicular
    C. Patient keeps his arm in saluting position
    D. Injury to brachial plexus may occur
28. **Following defect (lesion) is NOT responsible for recurrent anterior dislocation of shoulder:**
    A. Bankart's lesion
    B. Hill-Sachs lesion

C. Bristow's lesion
D. A defect in the anterior-inferior capsule
29. **Putti-Platt's operation is done for:**
    A. Elbow instability
    B. Shoulder instability
    C. Rotator cuff tear
    D. Biceps tendinitis
30. **Neglected shoulder dislocation in a young laborer is:**
    A. Medically managed
    B. Surgically managed
    C. Neglected
    D. Counselled
31. **In recurrent anterior dislocation of shoulder, the movement that causes dislocation is:**
    A. Flexion and internal rotation
    B. Abduction and external rotation
    C. Abduction and internal rotation
    D. Extension
32. **Recurrent dislocations are least commonly seen in:**
    A. Ankle   B. Hip
    C. Shoulder   D. Patella
33. **All are related to recurrent shoulder dislocation *except*:**
    A. Hill-Sachs defect   B. Bankart lesion
    C. Lax capsule   D. Rotator cuff injury
34. **Traumatic glenohumeral instability in one direction with Bankart's lesion is treated by:**
    A. Conervative methods
    B. Surgery
    C. Rehabilitation
    D. Inferior capsule shift
35. **Following anterior dislocation of the shoulder, a patient develops weakness of flexion at elbow and lack of sensation over the lateral aspect forearm: Nerve injured is:**
    A. Radial nerve
    B. Musculocutaneous nerve
    C. Axillary nerve
    D. Ulnar nerve
36. **In posterior dislocation of shoulder Hill-Sachs lesion is seen in:**
    A. Anterior   B. Anteromedial
    C. Posterior   D. Posteromedial
37. **Which is true regarding shoulder dislocation?**
    A. Posterior dislocation is often overlooked
    B. Pain is severe in anterior dislocation
    C. Radiography may be misleading in posterior dislocation
    D. All of the above
38. **Which of the following is test of posterior glenohumeral instability?**
    A. Fulcrum   B. Sulcus test
    C. Jerk test   D. Crank test

39. A 6-year-old boy a history of recurrent dislocation of the right shoulder. On examination, the orthopedician puts the patient in the supine position and abducts his arm to 90° with the bed as the fulcrum and then externally rotates it but the boy does not allow the test to be performed. The test done by the orthopedician:
    A. Apprehension test
    B. Sulcus test
    C. Dugas test
    D. McMurray's test

40. Tennis elbow, is characterized by:
    A. Tenderness over the medial epicondyle
    B. Tendinitis of common extensor origin
    C. Tendinitis of common flexor origin
    D. Painful flexion and extension

41. Lateral epicondylitis elbow begins in:
    A. Flexor digitorum superficialis
    B. Flexor digitorum profundus
    C. Extensor carpi radialis longus
    D. Extensor carpi radialis brevis

42. Cozen's test is used for the diagnosis of:
    A. Tennis elbow
    B. Golfer's elbow
    C. Base bailer's pitcher elbow
    D. Carpal tunnel syndrome

43. A 40-year-old man was repairing his wooden shed on Sunday morning. By afternoon, he felt that the hammer was becoming heavier and heavier. He felt pain in lateral side of elbow and also found that squeezing water out of sponge hurt his elbow. Which of the muscles are most likely involved?
    A. Biceps brachii and supinator
    B. Flexor digitorum superficialis
    C. Extensor carpii radialis brevis
    D. Triceps brachii and anconeus

44. de Quevian's tenovaginitis involves tendons of:
    A. 1st dorsal compartment
    B. 2nd dorsal compartment
    C. 3rd dorsal compartment
    D. 4th dorsal compartment

45. de Quervain's tenovaginitis involves:
    A. Abductor pollicis longus
    B. Extensor pollicis brevis
    C. Both of the above
    D. None of the above

46. Finkelstein's test is used for:
    A. Golfer's elbow
    B. de Quervain's tenovaginitis
    C. Trigger linger
    D. Tennis elbow

47. Dupuytren's contracture is fibrosis of:
    A. Palmar fascia   B. Firearm muscles
    C. Sartorius fascia   D. None of the above

48. Which of the following is true regarding Dupuytren's contracture?
    A. It is nodular hypertrophy and contracture of superficial palmar fascia
    B. Inherited as autosomal recessive trait
    C. Pathology as proliferation of myelo-fibroblasts
    D. Most commonly affected is radial nerve
    E. Pain is predominant feature throughout disease process

49. The best treatment for Dupuytren's contracture is:
    A. Fasciotomy
    B. Fasciectomy
    C. Incision and release
    D. Subtotal fasciectomy + skin transplantation

50. Dupuytren's contracture can be caused by:
    A. Eptoin
    B. Alcoholism
    C. Diabetes
    D. All of the above

51. A 50-year-old diabetic/alcoholic patient, presented with 15 degree flexion deformity of the little finger, what is the most appropriate management?
    A. Wait and watch
    B. Subtotal fasciectomy
    C. Total fasciectomy
    D. Percutaneous fasciectomy

52. Dupuytren's contracture occurs in:
    A. Diabetes mellitus
    B. Alcohol
    C. Epilepsy
    D. Rheumatoid arthritis
    E. Chronic pulmonary disease

53. Trigger finger is:
    A. A feature of carpal tunnel syndrome
    B. Injury to fingers while operating a gun
    C. Stenosis tenovaginitis of flexor tendon of affected finger
    D. Any of the above

54. Most common cause of trigger finger:
    A. Trauma   B. Alcohol
    C. Smoking   D. Drug abuse

55. In trigger finger level of tendon sheath constriction is found at the level of:
    A. Middle phalanx
    B. Proximal interphalangeal joint
    C. Proximal phalanx
    D. Metacarpophalangeal joint

56. Trigger finger occurs in:
    A. Rheumatoid arthritis
    B. Trauma
    C. Osteosarcoma
    D. Osteoarthritis

57. Cause of trigger finger is:
A. Thickening of the fibrous tendon sheath
B. Following local trauma
C. Unaccustomed activity
D. All of the above

58. Pulley involved in trigger finger:
A. A1   B. A2
C. A3   D. A4

59. True about ganglion is A/E :
A. Cystic tumor of hand
B. Solid tumor of head
C. Treated by enucleation
D. Unilocular
E. Filed with mucinous fluid

60. True about ganglion:
A. Common in volar aspect
B. Seen adjacent to tendon sheath
C. Communicates with joints cavity and tendon sheath
D. It is unilocular

61. Compound palmar ganglion is:
A. Tuberculosis affection of ulnar bursa
B. Pyogenic affection of ulnar bursa
C. Non-specific of ulnar bursa
D. Ulnar bursitis due to compound injury

62. Jersey finger is caused by rupture of:
A. Flexor digitorum profundus
B. Extensor digiti minimi
C. Flexor digitorum superficialis
D. Extensor indicis

63. Mallet finger is due to rupture of:
A. Central extensor slip of finger
B. Distal end of index extensor
C. Distal end of flexor digitorum profundus
D. None of the above

64. Mallet finger is:
A. Facture of proximal phalanx
B. Avulsion of extensor tendon
C. Rupture of flexor tendon
D. Capsular rupture of PIP joint

65. Mallet finger is caused by injury to extensor tendon insertion at:
A. Distal phalanx
B. Middle phalanx
C. Proximal phalanx
D. Second metacarpal bone

66. Mallet finger treatment is:
A. Observe   B. Surgery
C. Antibiotic   D. Splint

67. A 30-year-old man involved in a fight, injured his middle finger and noticed slight flexion of DIP joint. X-rays were normal. The most appropriate management at this stage is:
A. Ignore
B. Splint the finger in hyperextension
C. Surgical repair of the flexor tendon
D. Buddy strapping

68. Game keepers thumb is:
A. Thumb metacarpophalangeal joint ulnar collateral ligament rupture
B. Thumb metacarpophalangeal joint radial collateral ligament rupture
C. Thumb interphalangeal joint ulnar collateral ligament rupture
D. Thumb interphalangeal joint radial collateral ligament rupture

69. Game keeper's thumb is:
A. Ulnar collateral ligament injury of MCP joint
B. Radial collateral ligament injury of MCP joint
C. Radial collateral ligament injury of CMC joint
D. Ulnar collateral ligament injury of CMC joint

70. Cricketer while catching a ball gets hit on thumb. Which damage should be looked for specifically?
A. Ulnar collateral ligament
B. Volar plate
C. Abductor pollicis
D. Extensor pollicis brevis

71. No Man's land in hand surgery all are true *except*:
A. Results of flexor tendon repair are satisfactory in this area
B. Comprises zone II
C. Extends from distal palmar crease and flexor crease of PIP
D. Extends from distal palmar crease and insertion of flexor superficialis

72. All of the following are true about ACL *except*:
A. Prevents anterior motion of femur over tibia
B. Also provides secondary varus-valgus stability
C. Is taught in extension of knee

73. Regarding anterior cruciate ligament all are true *except*:
A. Lachman's test is the most sensitive test for ACL tear
B. Non-contact pivoting injury causes ACL damage
C. Posterolateral bundle becomes taut in flexion
D. Almost always associated with meniscal tear
E. Is pathognomic of Segond's fracture

74. In complete ACL rupture the tibia move over the femur in which direction?
A. Forward
B. Backward
C. Lateral
D. Medial

75. **Muscle with intra-articular tendon:**
    A. Popliteus   B. Semimembranosus
    C. Sartorius   D. Triceps
76. **Posterior gliding of tibia on femur is prevented by:**
    A. Anterior cruciate ligament
    B. Posterior cruciate ligament
    C. Medial collateral ligament
    D. Lateral collateral ligament
77. **Lachman's test is used for:**
    A. ACL injury   B. PCL injury
    C. MCL injury   D. LCL injury
78. **Which of the following is the SAFEST test to be performed in a patient with acutely injured knee joint?**
    A. Lachman's test   B. Pivot shift test
    C. McMurray's test   D. Apley's grinding test
79. **In "bounce home" test of knee 'end feels' are interference, all are 'end feels' *except*:**
    A. Firm   B. Sponge block
    C. Empty   D. Bony
80. **Lateral blow to knee with fracture in inter-condylar area structured injured is:**
    A. MCL   B. ACL
    C. LCL   D. Menisci
81. **Snapping knee syndrome is due to involvement of:**
    A. Pes anserinus
    B. Quadriceps tendon
    C. Gastrocnemius origin
    D. Lateral collateral ligament
82. **Injury from lateral side of knee causes damage to:**
    A. MCL   B. LCL
    C. ACL   D. PCL
83. **Anterior drawer test is for:**
    A. ACL   B. PCL
    C. Medial meniscus   D. Lateral meniscus
84. **A patient met with road traffic accident and developed knee pain. DIAL test was positive. Structure injured is:**
    A. Medial collateral ligament injury
    B. Medial meniscal injury
    C. Lateral meniscus tear
    D. Posterolateral corner injury
85. **Posterior cruciate ligament, true statement is:**
    A. Attached to the lateral femoral condyle
    B. Intrasynovial
    C. Prevents posterior dislocation of tibia
    D. Relaxed in full flexion
86. **Which one of the following tests will you adopt while examining a knee joint where you suspect an old tear of anterior cruciate ligament?**
    A. Posterior drawer   B. McMurray's test
    C. Lachman's test   D. Pivot shift test

87. **Which activity will be difficult to perform for a patient with an anterior cruciate deficient knee joint?**
    A. Walk downhill
    B. Walk uphill
    C. Sit cross leg
    D. Getting up from sitting
88. **Positive pivot shift test in knee is because of injury to:**
    A. Anterior cruciate ligament
    B. Posterior cruciate ligament
    C. Medial meniscus
    D. Lateral meniscus
89. **A patient sustained injury to his knee with a twisting force. On examination pain is felt more on medial femoral side of knee than tibial side. Injured structure might be:**
    A. Anterior cruciate ligament
    B. Posterior cruciate ligament
    C. Medial collateral ligament
    D. Lateral collateral ligament
90. **Which among the following is not a feature of Unhappy triad of O' Donoghue?**
    A. ACL injury
    B. Medial meniscus injury
    C. Medial collateral ligament injury
    D. Fibular collateral ligament injury
91. **A twisting injury of knee in flexion position would result in injury to all *except*:**
    A. Meniscal tear
    B. Capsular tear
    C. Anterior cruciate ligament
    D. Fibular collateral ligament
92. **Structural integrity of collateral ligaments are tested by:**
    A. Varus/valgus stress test in full flexion
    B. Varus/valgus stress test in full extension
    C. Varus/valgus stress test in 30 degree of flexion
    D. Varus/valgus stress test in 90 degree of flexion
93. **All are true about menisci of knee joint *except*:**
    A. Lateral meniscus covers more articular surface of tibia
    B. Lateral meniscus is more mobile
    C. Lateral meniscus is more prone to injury
    D. Lateral meniscus is semicircular
94. **The tests done for medial meniscal tear:**
    A. McMurray's test
    B. Lachman test
    C. Apley's grinding test
    D. Ege's test
95. **Torsion of knee results in injury most commonly to:**
    A. Anterior cruciate ligament
    B. Medial meniscus
    C. Fibular collateral ligament
    D. Tibial collateral ligament

96. A young boy presents with swollen knee, on getting hit over lateral aspect of knee and there was a twist while playing. Joint line tenderness was present. Anterior drawer test done was negative. X-ray shows no fracture. Which structure is most likely to be damaged in the person?
A. ACL
B. Medial meniscus
C. PCL
D. Lateral meniscus

97. A young boy presents with swollen knee, on getting hit over lateral aspect of knee. Anterior Drawer test done was negative. X-ray shows no fracture. Which structure is most likely to be damaged in the person?
A. ACL
B. MM
C. MCL
D. LM

98. Patient presents with knee problem. He gives history of injury during playing hockey 3 months back. On testing knee was unstable anteriorly in extension but was stable in 90° of flexion. Probably injury involves:
A. ACL anteromedial fiber
B. ACL posterolateral fiber
C. PCL
D. Anterior posterolateral fiber

99. Unlocking of knee is caused by:
A. Rectus femoris
B. Quadriceps
C. Hamstrings
D. Popliteus

100. Menisci to tibia connection is:
A. Coronary ligaments
B. Wrisberg ligaments
C. Arcuate ligaments
D. Oblique ligaments

101. Q angle is used for:
A. Knee
B. Hip
C. Elbow
D. Wrist

102. Locking of knee can be due to:
A. Menisci
B. Loose body
C. Both
D. None

103. Which of the following statements about 'Menisci' is not true?
A. Medial meniscus is more mobile than lateral.
B. Lateral meniscus covers more tibial articular surface than lateral
C. Medial meniscus is more commonly injured that lateral
D. Menisci are predominantly made up of type I collagen

104. It is wise to keep and repair the meniscus rather than removing it when the injury is to which of the following?
A. Medial part of meniscus
B. Mid part of meniscus
C. Peripheral part of meniscus
D. Associated with collateral ligament injury

105. An athlete is sitting on the edge of table with knees flexed at 90 degree. When he extends his knee fully, what will happen to the tibial tuberosity in relation to patella?
A. No change
B. Movement of TT towards medial border of patella
C. Movement of TT towards lateral border of patella
D. Movement of TT towards center of patella

106. Physiological locking involves:
A. Internal rotation of femur over stabilized tibia
B. Internal rotation of tibia stabilized femur
C. External rotation of tibia over stabilized femur
D. External rotation of femur over stabilized tibia

107. Locking of knee joint can be caused by:
A. Osgood-Schlatter
B. Loose body in knee joint
C. Tuberculosis of knee
D. Medial meniscal partial tear

108. McMurray's test is positive in injury of:
A. Anterior cruciate ligament
B. Posterior cruciate ligament
C. Medial cruciate ligament
D. Lateral cruciate ligament
E. Popliteal bursitis

109. An 18-year-old boy was playing football, when he suddenly twisted his knee on the ankle and he fell down. He got up after 10 min and again started playing, but next day his knee was swollen and he could not move it. The most probable cause is:
A. Medial meniscus tear
B. Anterior cruciate ligament injury
C. Medical collateral ligament
D. Posterior cruciate ligament

110. Athlete sustained an injury around the knee joint suspecting cartilage damage, which of the following is an investigation of choice?
A. Pain X-ray
B. Clinical examination
C. Arthroscopy
D. Arthrotomy

111. Which type of injury causes more damage to the semilunar cartilage in the knee?
A. Flexion arid extension at the ankle
B. Rotation on a flexed knee
C. Rotation on an extended knee
D. Squatting position

112. Commonest dangerous complication of posterior dislocation of knee is:
A. Popliteal artery injury
B. Sciatic nerve injury
C. Ischemia of lower leg compartment
D. Femoral artery injury

113. A patient gives a history of twisting stair and locking of the knee joint, the most likely diagnosis is:
- A. Avulsion of tibial tubercle
- B. Meniscal tear
- C. Tearing of lateral collateral ligament
- D. Tear of anterior cruciate ligament

114. Which is the investigation of choice for a sport injury of the knee?
- A. Ultrasonography
- B. Plain radiography
- C. Arthrography
- D. Arthroscopy

115. Bucket handle tear at knee joint is due to:
- A. Injury to medial collateral ligament
- B. Injury to lateral collateral ligament
- C. Injury to ligamentum patellae
- D. Injury to menisci

116. Olecranon bursitis:
- A. Tennis elbow
- B. Golfer's elbow
- C. Student's elbow
- D. Lesser leagues elbow

117. Bursa involved in Clergyman's knee:
- A. Prepatellar bursa
- B. Infrapatellar bursa
- C. Olecranon bursa
- D. Ischial bursa

118. Bunion is commonly seen at:
- A. Greater toe MTP joint
- B. Medial malleolus
- C. Lateral malleolus
- D. Shin of tibia

119. Housemaid's knee is bursitis of:
- A. Prepatellar bursa
- B. Infrapatellar bursa
- C. Olecranon
- D. Ischial bursa

120. Ischial bursitis is also known as:
- A. Clergyman's knee
- B. Housemaid's knee
- C. Weaver's bottom
- D. Student's elbow

121. Site of TB bursitis:
- A. Prepatellar
- B. Subacromial
- C. Subdeltoid
- D. Subpatellar
- E. Trochanteric

122. Which of the following cysts is medially situated?
- A. Housemaid's knee
- B. Clergyman's knee
- C. Bursa anserine
- D. Morrant Baker's cyst

123. The primary pathology in Athletic Pubalgia is:
- A. Abdominal muscle strain
- B. Recuts femoris strain
- C. Gluteus medius strain
- D. Hamstring strain

124. Commonest ligament injured in ankle injury:
- A. Anterior talofibular ligament
- B. Calcaneofibular ligament
- C. Posterior talofibular ligament
- D. Spring ligament

125. A 23-year-old professional footballer suffered a twisting injury to his right ankle. On examination there is a lot of swelling around the medial malleolus but X-ray does not show any fracture. The structure injured could be:
- A. Deltoid ligament
- B. Anterior talofibular ligament
- C. Spring ligament
- D. Tendo Achillis

126. When the foot is in plantar flexed position, if it is suddenly inverted which of the ligament will be injured?
- A. Ant talofibular
- B. Post-tibiofibular
- C. Calcaneocuboid
- D. Calceneofibular

127. Injury around the ankle joint occurs due to:
- A. Inversion of foot
- B. Eversion of foot
- C. Internal rotation of foot
- D. External rotation of foot

128. Sudden dorsiflexion of foot may lead to which of the following injuries?
- A. Anterior talofibular ligament injury
- B. Tendo Achillis avulsion injury
- C. Rupture of deltoid ligament
- D. Tarsal tunnel syndrome

129. The most common site for ligamentous injuries are those of the:
- A. Shoulder joint
- B. Elbow
- C. Knee joint
- D. Ankle joint

130. All are the common sites of tendon rupture *except*:
- A. Supraspinatus tendon
- B. Long head of biceps brachii
- C. Achilles tendon
- D. Extenson Hallucis longus tendon

131. Ruptured tendon is most commonly seen in:
- A. Stab injury
- B. Soft tissue tumor
- C. Athletes
- D. Congenital defect

132. Identify the abnormality shown in the following picture:

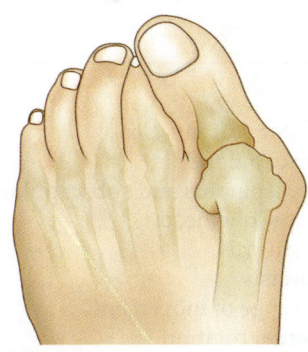

- A. Hallux valgus
- B. Hallux varus
- C. Rheumatoid valgus
- D. Subcutaneous nodule

133. A patient complains of pain in sole of pro-longed standing with the following X-ray, diagnosis is:

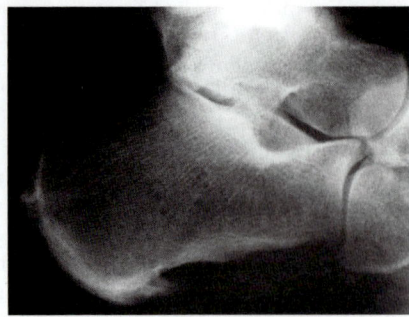

  A. Plantar fasciitis
  B. Tarsal coalition
  C. Ankylosing spondylitis
  D. Calcaneal old healed fracture

134. Which of the following is true about hallux valgus?
  A. Great toe points laterally
  B. Great toe point medially
  C. Lateral angulation of the 1st metatarso-phalangeal joint
  D. Dorsal angulation of the 1st metatarso-phalangeal joint

135. Hallux valgus means:
  A. Outward deviation of great toe
  B. Inward deviation of great toe
  C. Outward deviation of fifth toe
  D. Inward deviation of fifth toe

136. Hallux valgus is associated with all *except*:
  A. An exostosis on the medial side of the head of the first metatarsal
  B. A bunion
  C. Osteoarthritis of the metatarsophalangeal joint
  D. Over-riding or under-riding of the second toe by the third

137. In hallux valgus surgery, the patients who are likely to be most satisfied are:
  A. Those with pain
  B. Those with hammer toe
  C. Those with metatarsus primus varus
  D. Young age

138. KL splint is used for:
  A. Fracture tibia
  B. Plantar fasciitis
  C. de Quervain's tenosynovitis
  D. Tennis elbow

139. Impingement syndrome refers to:
  A. Nerve entrapped in closed space
  B. Soft tissues entrapment
  C. Arterial injury
  D. Venous engorgement

140. Identify the abnormality shown in the following picture:

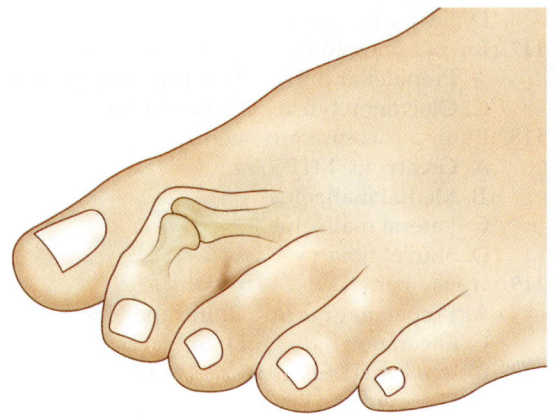

  A. Hallux valgus
  B. Hallux varus
  C. Rheumatoid valgus
  D. Hammer toe

ANSWERS

1. B. Rotator cuff muscles	**13.** A. Axillary nerve
2. A. Subscapularis	**14.** B. Hill-Sachs lesion
3. C. Supraspinatus and subscapularis	**15.** A. Tendon transfer
4. B. Biceps long head	**16.** A. Anterior lip
5. C. Periathritis	**17.** A. Supraspinatus
6. C. Psoriasis	**18.** C. Rotator cuff tendon
7. C. All range of movement	**19.** D. Teres minor
8. C. Internal rotation	**20.** A. Bankart lesion
9. D. All of the above	**21.** D. Subscapularis
10. B. Steroid injection are contraindicated	**22.** A. Subscapularis
11. A. Complete tear of supraspinatus	**23.** C. Inferior
12. A. Recurrent anterior shoulder dislocation	**24.** A. Injury to humeral head

25. C. Rotator cuff injury is a common cause of recurrent dislocation
26. B. Subscapularis
27. A. It is most common type of shoulder dislocation
28. C. Bristow's lesion
29. B. Shoulder instability
30. B. Surgically managed
31. B. Abduction and external rotation
32. A. Ankle
33. D. Rotator cuff injury
34. B. Surgery
35. B. Musculocutaneous nerve
36. B. Anteromedial
37. D. All of the above
38. C. Jerk test
39. A. Apprehension test
40. B. Tendinitis of common extensor origin
41. C. Extensor carpi radialis brevis
42. A. Tennis elbow
43. C. Extensor carpiirtadialis brevis
44. A. 1st dorsal compartment
45. C. Both of the above
46. B. de Quervain's tenovaginitis
47. A. Palmar fascia
48. A. It is nodular hypertrophy and contracture of superficial palmar fascia and C. Pathology as proliferation of myelofibroblasts
49. D. Subtotal fasciectomy + skin transplantation
50. D. All of the above
51. A. Wait and watch
    - Diagnosis is Dupuytren's contracture. Surgical management is recommended when more than 30° contracture is produced
52. A. Diabetes mellitus, B. Alcohol, C. Epilepsy, and E. Chronic pulmonary disease
53. C. Stenosis tenovaginitis of flexor tendon of affected finger
54. A. Trauma
55. D. Metacarpophalangeal joint
56. A. Rheumatoid arthritis; B. Trauma
57. D. All of the above
58. A. A1
59. B. Solid tumor of head and C. Treated by enucleation
60. ALL
61. A. Tuberculosis affection of ulnar bursa
62. A. Flexor digitorum profundus
63. B. Distal end of index extensor
64. B. Avulsion of extensor tendon
65. A. Distal phalanx
66. D. Splint
67. B. Splint the finger in hyperextension
68. A. Thumb metacarpophalangeal joint ulnar collateral ligament rupture

69. A. Ulnar collateral ligament injury of MCP joint
70. A. Ulnar collateral ligament
71. A. Results of flexor tendon repair are satisfactory in this area
72. A. Prevents anterior motion of femur over tibia
73. C. Posterolateral bundle becomes taut in flexion
74. A. Forward
75. A. Popliteus
76. B. Posterior cruciate ligament
77. A. ACL injury
78. A. Lachman's test
79. C. Empty
80. B. ACL
    - Fracture at intercondylar which is the site insertion points towards ACL injury
81. A. Pes anserinus
82. A. MCL
83. A. ACL
84. D. Posterolateral corner injury
85. C. Prevents posterior dislocation of tibia: PCL prevents posterior gliding (subluxation) of tibia over femur
86. C. Lachman's test
87. A. Walk downhill
88. A. Anterior cruciate ligament
89. C. Medial collateral ligament
90. D. Fibular collateral ligament injury
91. D. Fibular collateral ligament
92. C. Varus/valgus stress test in 30 degree of flexion
93. C. Lateral meniscus is more prone to injury
94. A. McMurray's test
95. B. Medial meniscus
96. B. Medial meniscus
    - Joint line tenderness is a good clue to medial meniscus injury
97. C. MCL
98. B. ACL posterolateral fiber
99. D. Popliteus
100. A. Coronary ligaments
101. A. Knee
102. C. Both
103. A. Medial meniscus is more mobile than lateral
104. C. Peripheral part of meniscus
105. C. Movement of TT towards lateral border of patella
106. A. Internal rotation of femur over stabilized tibia
107. B. Loose body in knee joint, D. Medial meniscal partial tear
108. C > D. Medial meniscus injury > Lateral meniscus injury
109. A. Medial meniscus tear
110. C. Arthroscopy is investigation of choice for damage to the structures of knee

111. B. Rotation on a flexed knee
112. A. Popliteal artery injury
113. B. Meniscal tear
114. D. Arthroscopy
115. D. Injury to menisci
116. C. Student's elbow
117. B. Infrapatellar bursa
118. A. Greater toe MTP joint
119. A. Prepatellar bursa
120. C. Weaver's bottom
121. E. Trochanteric
122. C. Bursa anserine
123. A. Abdominal muscle strain
124. A. Anterior talofibular ligament
125. A. Deltoid ligament

126. A. Ant talofibular
127. A. Inversion of foot
128. B. Tendo Achillis avulsion injury
129. D. Ankle joint
130. D. Extenson Hallucis longus tendon
131. C. Athletes
132. A. Hallux valgus
133. A. Plantar fasciitis
134. —
135. A. Outward deviation of great toe
136. A. An exostosis on the medial side of the head of the first metatarsal
137. A. Those with pain
138. B. Plantar fasciitis
139. B. Soft tissues entrapment
140. D. Hammer toe

Peripheral Nerve Injuries and Entrapment Syndromes

INTRODUCTION
- Every segment of spinal cord gives rise to a nerve called spinal nerve (total being 31 pairs). Each spinal nerve is a mixed nerve, formed at the intervertebral foramen by the union of its dorsal or sensory root with its ventral or motor root.
- Myelin sheath is an insulating membrane.
- Nodes of Ranvier (myelin deficient) are rich in ion channels and action potential jumps from one node to another node of Ranvier (length 1–1.8 mm).
- Vessels supplying nerves are called vasa nervorum. They enter through the mesoneurium, which is loose connective tissue extending from the epineurium to the surrounding tissues.
- Internal topography (complex network of branching and intermingling of fascicles) constantly changes throughout the course of the nerve and its complexity diminishes distally (Fig. 11.2).

Neuronal Degeneration and Regeneration
When an axon is detached from its cell body **degeneration** begins in both the:

Proximal k/a Wallerian degeneration   Distal k/a retrograde/primary/traumatic
- Histologically both degenerations are identical.
- Detached axons remain excitable and can transmit nerve signals for several days following injury.

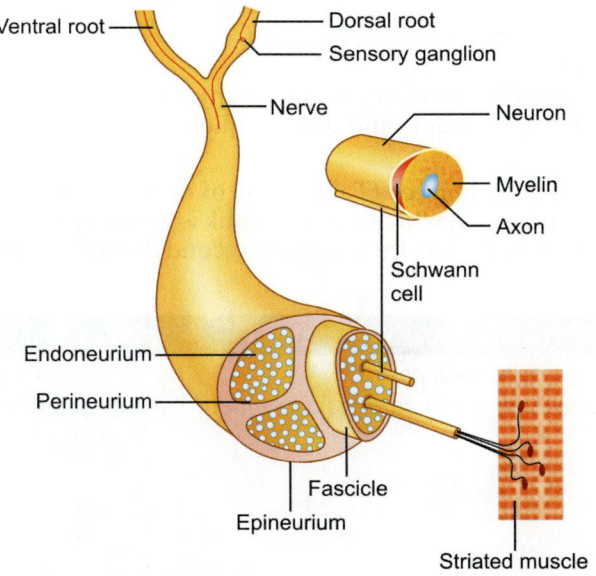

Fig. 11.1: Microscopic anatomy of a nerve

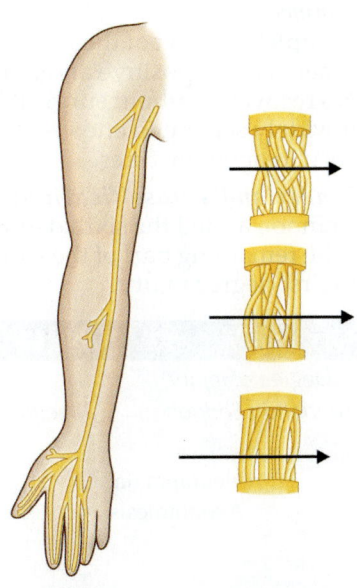

Fig. 11.2: Internal topography

- Depending on the proximity to cell body and severity of injury retrograde degeneration can be limited to next node of Ranvier or extensive involving the entire segment up to the cell body.
- Wallerian degeneration is also seen in several degenerative neurological diseases like- Parkinson's disease, Alzheimer's disease, amyotrophic lateral sclerosis (ALS).
- Nerve regenerates at the rate of 1 mm /day (or 1 inch/month).
- End neuroma forms when there is complete cut of the peripheral nerve with widely separated ends while a partial cut with similar situation ends up in "neuroma in continuity".
- Motor march—the muscles nearest to the site of injury are re-innervated first followed by others. It is an evidence of recovery.
- **Tinel's sign** aka **Hoffman's sign:** A positive sign indicates axonal regeneration.
  - On percussion tingling sensation is felt only distally along the course of the nerve and not at the percussion site (law of projection).
  - With progressive regeneration, Tinel's sign moves distally and is a favorable sign.
  - Positive Tinel's sign indicates sensory recovery and with progressive axonal regeneration, it fades proximally (it disappears as myelinisation takes place) and moves distally.
  - It is positive in axonotmesis and Sunderland (*read below*) types 2 and 3. Sunderland type 4 and 5 would not show a positive Tinel's sign unless repaired.

Classifications

1. *Seddon's classification*: Nerve injury in increasing severity of damage → Neuro**p**raxia > **A**xonotmesis > **N**eurotmesis (**PANT**).

Neuropraxia
- Temporary physiological disruption of nerve impulse conduction.
- Loss of function is incomplete and complete recovery is the rule. Complete recovery takes place in one go.
- No Wallerian degeneration/Tinel's sign negative.
- *For example*: Crutch palsy (radial nerve/brachial plexus), Saturday night palsy, tourniquet palsy.

Axonotmesis
- Distal Wallerian degeneration is seen.
- Tinel's sign positive and progressive.
- Motor march is seen.
- Recovery is never complete.
- *For example*: Closed fractures and dislocations.

Neurotmesis
- Complete section of the nerve.
- Tinel's sign is positive and nonprogressive.
- No recovery without surgical intervention and full recovery is never achieved.
- If widely separated ends—it forms: Proximally neuroma and distally glioma.
- Seen in open fractures.

2. *Sunderland's classification*: He described five degrees (Table 11.1) of nerve injuries and Mackinnon added the sixth degree, i.e. mixed injury, in which a nerve trunk is partially severed, and the remaining part of the trunk sustains fourth degree, third degree, second degree, or rarely even first degree injury.

Table 11.1: Sunderland classification of nerve injuries								
Degree of injury		*Histopathological changes*					*Tinel sign*	
Sunderland	*Seddon*	*Myelin*	*Axon*	*Endoneurium*	*Perineurium*	*Epineurium*	*Present*	*progresses distally*
I	Neurapraxia	±	−				−	−
II	Axonotmesis	+	+	−			+	+
III		+	+	+			+	+
IV		+	+	+	+		+	−
V	Neurotmesis	+	+	+	+	+	+	−

Xtra Edge

- Usually, motor function is more profoundly affected than sensory function. Sensory modalities are affected in order of decreasing frequency as follows: Proprioception, touch, temperature, and pain. Sympathetic fibers are the most resistant to this type of injury.
- Nerve recovery is in the reverse order—1st to recover is pain and temperature.
- Autonomic dysfunction after peripheral nerve injury—loss of sweating and pilomotor response, vasomotor paralysis and anhidrosis.
- Postinjection palsies are neurotmesis.
- Osteoporosis often follow peripheral nerve injuries. It is more likely to be pronounced in incomplete lesions associated with pain.
- Table 11.2 depicts the commonest nerves involved in different fractures.

High vs Low Nerve Palsy

By convention, the major nerve injuries of upper limb are divided into high and low types depending on whether the injury site is proximal to elbow (high injury) or distal to elbow (low injury).

Autonomous zone: After severance of a peripheral nerve, only a small area of complete sensory loss is found. This area is supplied exclusively by the severed nerve and is called the *autonomous zone* or *isolated zone*.

- Median nerve—tip of index finger and middle finger
- Ulnar nerve—tip of little finger
- Radial nerve—1st web space of the dorsum of hand
- Deep PN—dorsum of 1st web space of foot.

Maximal zone: When a nerve is intact, and the adjacent nerves are blocked or sectioned, an area of sensibility exceeds the gross anatomical distribution of the nerve; this area is known as the *maximal zone*.

Investigations

- Autonomic function—starch iodine test, ninhydrin printing test, skin resistance test by Richter dynamometer and wrinkle test. In autonomous area presence of sweat, rules out complete injury as sweat fibres are most resistant to compression.
- EMG—denervation fibrillation potentials appear at 2–3 weeks. It is the earliest indicator of nerve recovery and useful in detecting more subtle nerve injury. It may be helpful in workers compensation or litigation cases and differentiate between myopathy and neuropathy.

Table 11.2: Common nerves involved in various fractures	
Injury	*M/C nerve involved*
Shoulder dislocation (Ant./ Inf.)	Axillary nerve
Fracture surgical neck of humerus	Axillary nerve
Fracture shaft of humerus (lower 1/3rd)	Radial nerve
Fracture supracondylar humerus	In flexion—radial nerve
	In extension—anterior
	Interosseous nerve
	Overall—anterior interosseous nerve
Fracture medial condyle of humerus	Ulnar nerve
Monteggia fracture dislocation	Posterior interosseous nerve
VIC lunate dislocation	Median nerve
Hip dislocation (posterior)	Sciatic nerve
Acetabulum fracture	Sciatic nerve
Knee dislocation	CPN
Fracture neck of fibula	CPN
Cubitus valgus (lateral condyle humerus fracture)	Tardy ulnar nerve palsy

- NCV—when stimulated proximal to the site of injury there is no response but on distal stimulation normal conduction is recorded, as nerves are electrically excitable immediately after injury. After ten days post injury, due to Wallerian degeneration in axonotmesis and neurotmesis there is no response distally, but it cannot differentiate between the two. Best time to do NCV test is 10–14 days post-injury.
- MRI—value in spinal cord study, spinal root avulsion.

General Principles of Management

- When closed fractures are complicated by peripheral nerve deficits, awaiting reinnervation seems reasonable, and early surgical exploration is usually avoided.
- Conversely, if the nerve deficit follows manipulation or casting of a closed fracture in the absence of a prior nerve deficit, early exploration of the nerve is favored.
- An associated fracture does not delay nerve regeneration while an associated vascular injury may delay the same due to tissue ischemia.
- In closed injury splints are used awaiting nerve regeneration:
  - Axillary nerve—shoulder abduction splint
  - Brachial plexus—aeroplane splint
  - Median nerve—knuckle bender splint
  - Radial nerve—cock up splint (dynamic splint better than static)
  - CPN—foot drop splint.
- In open injuries/fractures:
  - Primary repair—within 6–8 hours
  - Delayed primary repair—7–18 days
  - Secondary repair—after 18 days.
- Prognosis for repair is better for pure nerves (motor > sensory), e.g. radial nerve, a pure motor nerve heals better than mixed nerves.
  Order: Radial > median > ulnar (worst prognosis in upper limb) > peroneal > sciatic (worst prognosis)
- The more proximal the injury, the more incomplete the overall return of motor and sensory function, especially in the more distal structures. Conditions are more favorable for recovery in the more proximal muscles.
- Gaps between nerve ends can be brought close by (1) nerve mobilization, (2) nerve transposition, (3) joint flexion, (4) nerve grafts, and (5) bone shortening (it should be used as last resort).
- Nerve grafting is advised if, after the nerve is mobilized, the gap cannot be closed by flexing the main joint of the limb 90 degrees.
- Nerve grafts—most commonly harvested from sural nerve.
- Nerve suturing is done by 8–0, 9–0, 10–0 monofilament nylon.
- Neurotization—transfer of fibres of an intact nerve to a damaged nerve to augment its function.
- If nerve recovery does not take place, tendon transfer can be carried out, m/c used tendon for transfer is palmaris longus.
- Some important tendon transfers are given in Table 11.3.

Table 11.3: Some important tendon transfers
Omer's transfer: Ulnar nerve palsy
Jones transfer: Radial nerve palsy
Saha's transfer (trapezius to deltoid): Deltoid paralysis in polio or brachial plexus palsy
Camitz transfer (palmaris longus to abductor pollicis brevis): Carpal tunnel syndrome
Zancolli tenodesis: Claw hand
Sharad/mustard transfer (iliopsoas to greater trochanter): Gluteus medius paralysis (poliomyelitis)
Kaufer (tibialis posterior to peroneus brevis): Equinovarus deformity at foot
Hoffer (tibialis anterior to medial cuneiform): Equinovarus deformity at foot
Perry (peroneus brevis to tibialis posterior): Equinovalgus deformity of foot

BRACHIAL PLEXUS INJURY

Anatomy

- Anatomy of brachial plexus is given in Fig. 11.3.
- Prefixed (C4) origin is more common than postfixed (T2) origin.
- Pectoralis muscle is the only muscle of upper limb that receives nerve supply from all the roots of brachial plexus.

Mechanisms of Brachial Plexus Injury (BPI) (Fig. 11.4A and B)

1. Traction injury—commonest cause and affects the supraclavicular portion of brachial plexus
2. Contusion/bruise
3. Compression
4. Ischemia
5. Radiation induced

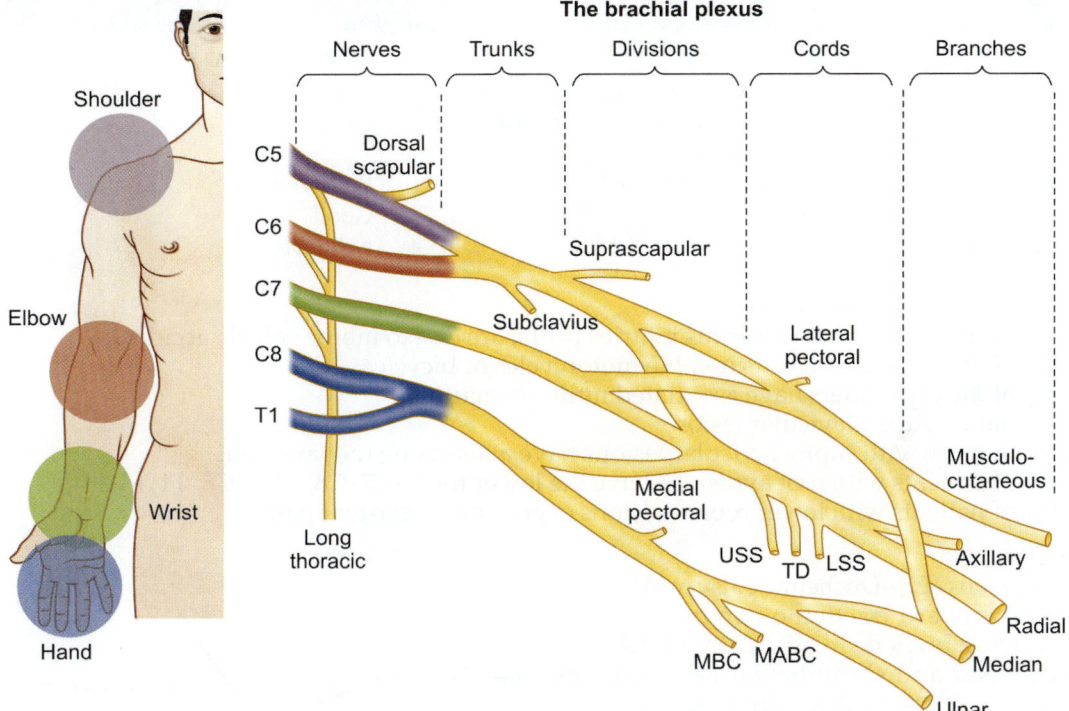

Fig. 11.3: Formation of brachial plexus from anterior rami of C5–8 and T1

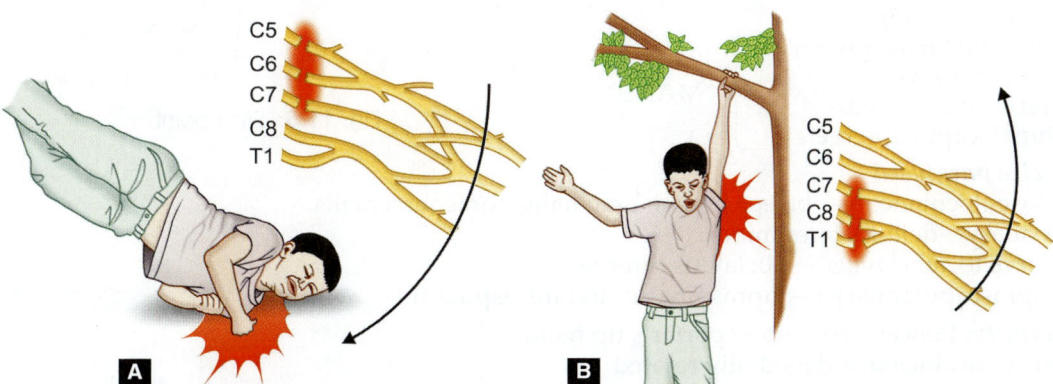

Fig. 11.4A and B: Mechanism of supraclavicular and infraclavicular BPI

Traction injuries are generally classified as supraclavicular (most common), infraclavicular and combined (rare).

- Supraclavicular injuries are seen in motor cycle accidents when the head and neck are violently moved away from the ipsilateral shoulder and places upper roots at risk (Fig. 11.4A) and may be associated with subclavian artery injury. In RTA helmet may prevent from brain damage but due to increased kinetic energy places more risk of BPI.
- Infraclavicular lesions are seen with forced separation of arm from torso (Fig. 11.4B) and usually associated with fractures and dislocations of shoulder and axillary artery injury. Penetrating injuries are usually infraclavicular.
- Roots C5, 6, 7/upper trunk/lateral cord are commonest to be injured by stretching mechanism.
- Roots C8, T1 (lower brachial plexus) are most sensitive to root avulsion.

Preganglionic *vs* Postganglionic Lesions

	Preganglionic lesion	Postganglionic lesion
Table 11.4: Differentiating features of preganglionic vs postganglionic lesions		
Site	Injury is proximal to dorsal root ganglion (avulsion of nerve root from spinal cord)	Disruption of nerve distal to dorsal root ganglion
Treatment	Surgically irreparable	Reparable
Prognosis	Poor	Good
Histamine test	Positive	Negative

NARAKUS' "Law of Seven Seventies"

- 70% of traumatic brachial plexus injuries (BPIs) are due to motor vehicle accidents.
- 70% of the vehicle accidents involve motorcycles or bicycles.
- 70% of the cycle riders have associated multiple injuries.
- 70% have a supraclavicular lesion.
- 70% of those with supraclavicular lesions have at least one root avulsed.
- 70% of patients with root avulsions have the lower roots (C7, C8, T1 or C8, T1) avulsed.
- 70% of patients with lower root avulsions experience persistent pain.

ERB'S PALSY

Upper plexus/Erb-Duchenne palsy results from downward traction on an infant's arm during birth or in adults in a RTA where head and shoulder move apart generating stress at Erb's point (Fig. 11.5).

It is a point where 6 nerves meet:
1. C5 nerve root (main)
2. C6 nerve root (partly)
3. **M**usculocutaneous nerve ⎫
4. **A**xillary nerve   ⎬ "MANS"
5. **N**erve to subclavius   ⎪
6. **S**uprascapular nerve   ⎭

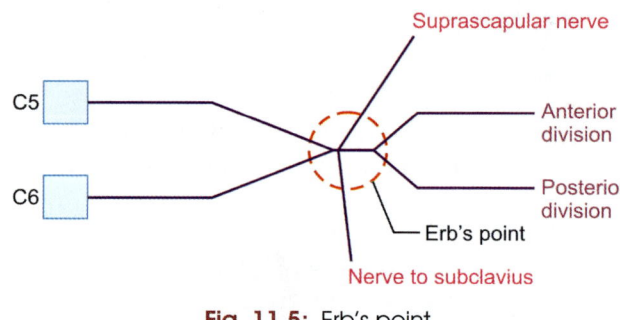

Fig. 11.5: Erb's point

Muscles paralysed
- Musculocutaneous—biceps brachi, brachialis, coracobrachialis.
- Axillary—deltoid, teres minor.
- Nerve to subclavius—subclavius muscle.
- Suprascapular nerve—supraspinatus and infraspinatus.

Deformity: Policeman/waiter/porter's tip hand.
1. Arm—adducted and medially rotated
2. Forearm—extended and pronated
3. Arm hangs simply by the side

Klumpke's Paralysis

- Lower plexus / Klumpke's paralysis results from upward traction on arm (e.g. in forcible breech delivery).
- Although less common than Erb's palsy, but it is more severe.
- Injury occurs to lower trunk (mainly T1 and partly C8) of brachial plexus leading to
  - Horner syndrome
  - Claw hand
  - Cutaneous anesthesia in narrow zone along ulnar nerve
  - All small muscles of hand are paralysed
- A complete BPI, i.e. C5-T1 leads to a flail limb.

Obstetric BPI

- Upper part of the brachial plexus, i.e. Erb's point is involved most commonly as it is a traction injury.
- A prefixed brachial plexus is more susceptible to BPI and a post-fixed type is rarely seen in obstetric BPI.
- The lesion may vary from mild stretching with resultant edema and temporary loss of conductivity to actual complete tear and loss of continuity.
- Lower part of plexus is less often involved and is most commonly an avulsion injury leading to Horner's syndrome.

AXILLARY NERVE INJURY

Axillary nerve, a branch of posterior cord (C5, 6) is injured in fracture surgical neck of humerus and shoulder dislocation (anterior/inferior) and sometimes by I/M injections in the deltoid region. The nerve is most commonly injured just proximal to the quadrangular space.

Clinical findings

Motor

- Deltoid muscle palsy leads to
  - loss of rounded contour of shoulder
  - weakness of abduction (15–90°)
- Teres minor palsy hardly causes any symptoms

Sensory

- Lateral cutaneous nerve of arm
- Sensory loss over lower half of deltoid (regimental batch sign)

MUSCULOCUTANEOUS NERVE INJURY

- Supplies biceps brachii (supinates forearm and in supinated position flexes forearm), brachialis (flexes forearm in all positions) and coracobrachialis (assists anterior deltoid and pectoralis major in flexing and adducting arm).
- Continues in forearm as lateral cutaneous nerve of forearm.
- Lesions of nerve produce weakness of elbow flexion and supination.

RADIAL NERVE INJURY

Anatomy

- It is the largest branch of brachial plexus and is actually the continuation of posterior cord (C5–8, T1).
- It descends behind the 3rd part of the axillary artery and lies anterior to the posterior axillary wall.
- It passes through the lower triangular space with profunda brachii artery.
- Wartenberg's syndrome is radial sensory nerve entrapment (superficial branch) beneath the edge of brachioradialis about 6 cm above radial styloid.
- In the wrist it passes through the 4th dorsal compartment of extensor retinaculum.
- The course of the nerve has been depicted in Fig. 11.6.

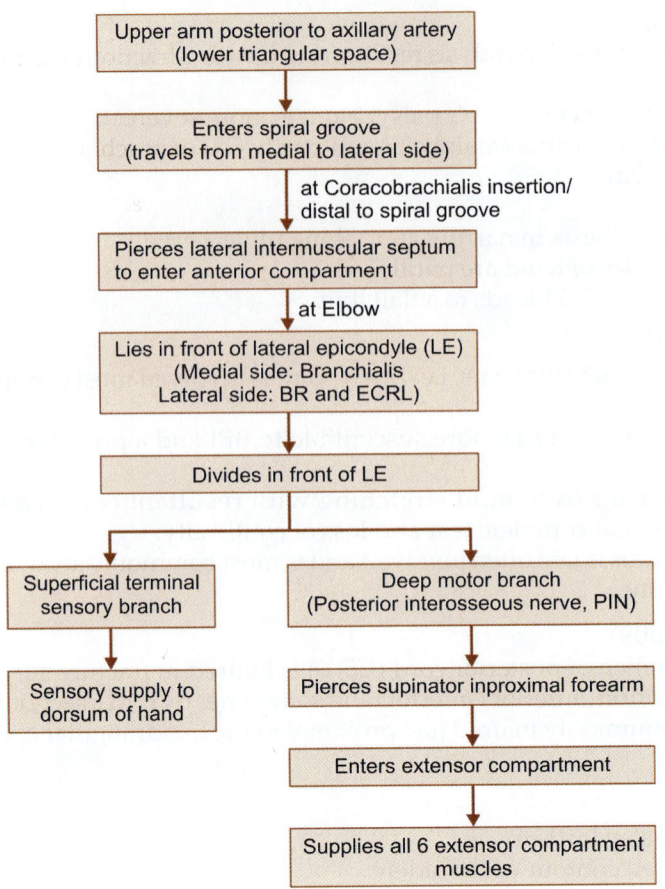

Fig. 11.6: Course of radial nerve

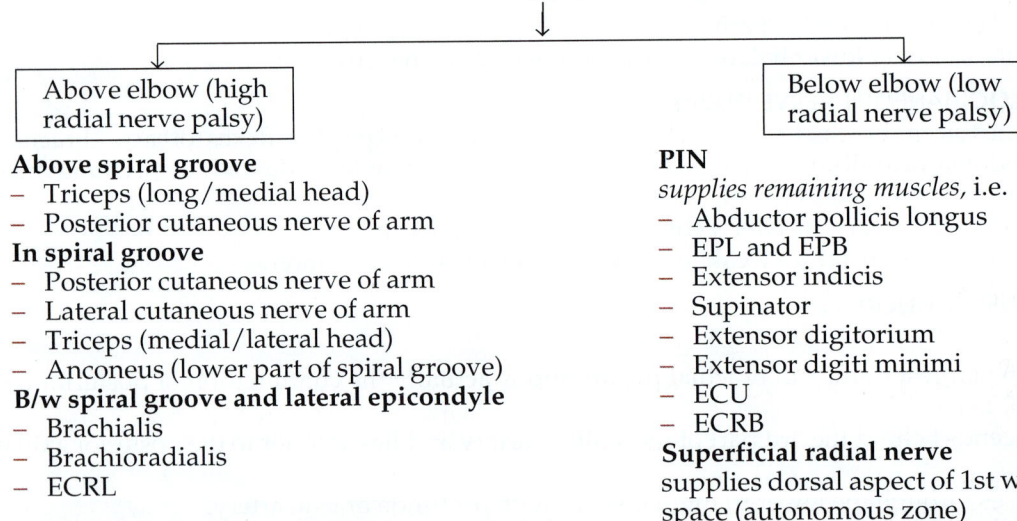

- Nerve to medial head of triceps (above spiral groove) is called ulnar collateral nerve.
- ECRB may receive branches from the main trunk of radial nerve or from proximal part of PIN. After supplying ECRB, PIN passes through supinator and gives additional branches to the muscle and then supplies other muscles.

Common sites of compression
- *Arm (most common site)*: Compression high up in axilla above the spiral groove by an axillary crutch (crutch palsy), in the spiral groove (Saturday night palsy) or in or below the groove as in injury during fractures of the shaft humerus (most common cause—**Holstein Lewis fracture**) and elbow region and intramuscular injections of the arm.
- *Forearm*: PIN can be injured either in fracture dislocations in the area (e.g. Monteggia fractures) or by compression from various structures in the vicinity (*see* radial tunnel syndrome).

Types of Radial Nerve Lesions
1. Very high (above spiral groove)
   - Total paralysis (elbow, wrist, thumb, finger)
   - Loss of sensation
2. High (between spiral groove and lateral epicondyle)
   - Elbow extension spared (triceps—long/medial head) that differentiates it from very high palsy.
   - Lost—wrist, thumb, finger extension.
   - Sensation lost.
   - Brachioradialis (BR) is also involved (differentiates it from low palsy)
3. Low (below elbow)
   - Elbow (triceps) and wrist extension spared (ECRL)
   - BR spared
   - Lost-thumb and finger extension
   - Loss of sensation
4. Posterior interosseous nerve (PIN) palsy (pure motor nerve)
   - Elbow (triceps) and wrist extension spared (ECRL, supplied by main radial nerve)
   - Sensations spared
   - Loss of MCP joint extension (thumb/finger drop)
   - PIN supplies all extensor muscles of wrist and hand except ECRL (radial nerve) and lumbricals/interossei (median/ulnar nerve).
   - PIN palsy presents with only loss of extension of MCP joint without loss of extension of wrist and IP joint (lumbricals/interossei) and there is no sensory loss.
   - Radial nerve/PIN palsy weakens (affects) abduction and extension movements of thumb and spares flexion, adduction and opposition.

Treatment
- Nerve repair is the treatment of choice (if patient presents early) and cock up slab during recovery (external splint) is given to prevent contractures.
- Internal splint—pronator teres can be transferred to ECRB at the time of nerve repair eliminating the need of wearing an external splint during recovery.
- Tendon transfer—the tendon transferred looses power by 1 grade, so for useful postoperative movements, preoperative 4/5 power is a must in the donor muscle.
- **Jones** transfer
  - Pronator teres to ECRL/ECRB → wrist extensors
  - FCU to EDC → finger extensors
  - FCR to EPL → thumb extension
- Others: **Brand** transfer and **Boyes** transfer.

MEDIAN NERVE (LABORER'S NERVE) INJURY
Anatomy
- Formed by union of terminal branches of medial (C8, T1) and (main) lateral (C5, C6) cords of the brachial plexus.
- The axillary artery (3rd part) is clasped between the two roots, the median root crossing in front of vessel and the main median nerve is lateral or anterior to axillary artery.
- It passes to forearm between the two heads of pronator teres and then descends in forearm between FDS (above) and FDP (below).
- The course of the nerve has been depicted in Fig. 11.7.

Common sites of compression
- *Distal arm*
  Supracondylar humerus fracture
- *Proximal forearm*
  The nerve may be compressed as it passes between two heads of PT (pronator syndrome). The anterior interosseous branch (AIN) may be compressed by the deep head of pronator teres, edge of laceratus fibrosus or by the tendinous FDS arch (*see* AIN syndrome/Kiloh-Nevin syndrome)
- *Wrist (most common site)*
  Compression may be there in the carpal tunnel (*see* carpal tunnel syndrome), fracture of distal end radius, lunate dislocations.

Supply
- No supply in axilla and arm
- Near elbow
  - Articular branch to elbow joint.
  - Muscular branches to all superficial flexors muscles except FCU (ulnar nerve), i.e.
    - Pronator teres (highest and 1st branch)
    - FCR
    - Palmaris longus
    - FDS
- Anterior interosseous nerve (AIN)
  - FPL (flexes IP joint of thumb)
  - Lateral half of FDP (index and middle finger) (medial half is by ulnar nerve)
  - Pronator quadrates
  - Articular branch to wrist joint.
- Hand
  - 1st two lumbricals (index and middle finger)
  - Thenar muscles (except adductor pollicis which is supplied by ulnar nerve)
    - Abductor pollicis brevis
    - Flexor pollicis brevis (deep head by ulnar nerve)
    - Opponens pollicis
- Sensory
  - Palmar—lateral half of palm, lateral 3 and a half finger
  - Dorsal—distal part of lateral 3 and a half finger

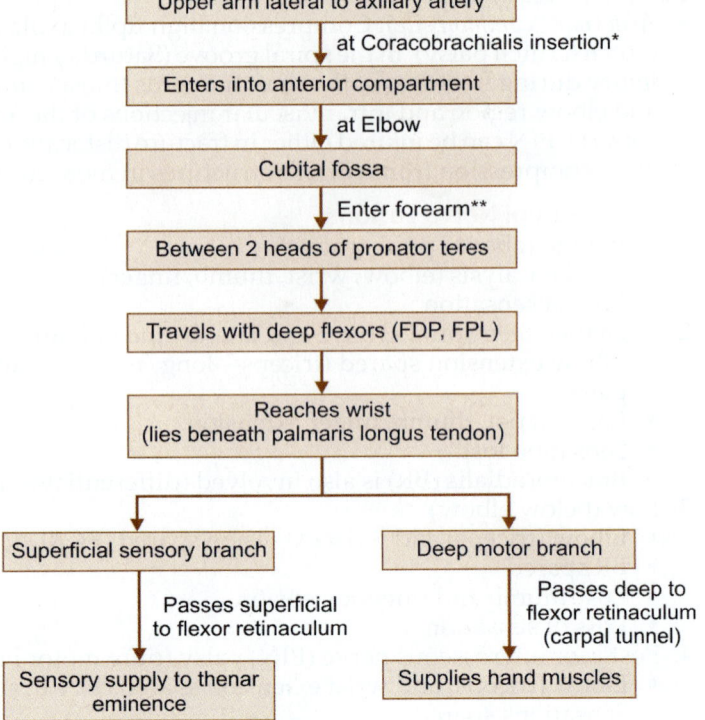

Fig. 11.7: Course of the median nerve

Clinical findings in Common Lesions*
1. Injury at wrist level
   - **Ape thumb** deformity due to paralysis of abductor pollicis brevis. The thumb is adducted and laterally rotated and lies in the same plane as palm due to unopposed action of EPL (radial nerve) and adductor pollicis (ulnar nerve).
   - **Loss of opposition and abduction.**

---

*Even though lateral lumbricals are paralysed; no clawing is seen. The lumbricals have a complex interconnection and the medial lumbricals (supplied by ulnar nerve) take over the function in median nerve palsy.

- **Pen test**—paralysis of abductor pollicis brevis. The patient is unable to touch the object/pen, held at right angle to palm by thumb abduction.
- Sensory loss.
2. Injury at elbow
   - All the above features plus below mentioned ones.
   - Pronators → paralysed → forearm kept in supine position.
   - Long flexors → paralysed (except FCU and FDP medial ½) → weak wrist flexion with ulnar deviation (intact FCU).
   - FPL → paralysed → flexion of terminal phalanx of thumb is lost.
   - Flexion of IP joints of index and middle finger is lost so, there is **pointing index/positive Oschner's clasp/ Benediction or Pope sign.**
   - **AIN injury** test– Kiloh-Nevin sign.
     The pinch of thumb (FPL) and index finger (FDP lateral ½) is strong if AIN is intact, and the weak pinch is called **Kiloh-Nevin sign.**
   - AIN palsy causes weakness of pinch grip (FPL and FDP of index finger) and no sensory symptoms (differentiating feature from pronator syndrome, *see later*).

ULNAR NERVE (MUSICIAN'S NERVE) INJURY

- Ulnar nerve (C7, 8 and T1) is the largest branch and direct continuation of medial cord of brachial plexus.
- It runs through axilla medial to axillary artery and has no branch in arm.
- It enters the forearm by passing between the two heads of FCU and compression at this site (basically behind the medial epicondyle by a fibrous arch that connects the two heads of FCU) is called cubital tunnel syndrome (most common site of compression).
- It descends on forearm lying between FCU (above) and FDP (below).
- It continues in hand lying anterior to flexor retinaculum (but travels deep to pisohamate ligament in an area called Guyon's canal, second commonest site of compression).
- The course of the nerve has been depicted in Fig. 11.8.

Supply

- Forearm
  - Near elbow branch to FCU and medial ½ of FDP.
  - Palmar cutaneous branch arises in mid-forearm which supplies hypothenar area.
  - Dorsal cutaneous branch arises about 5 cm proximal to the wrist.
- Hand—the deep branch of nerve enters the hand by passing through Guyon's canal (area under the pisohamate ligament) and supplies:
  - Medial 1½ digits (palmar digital branch)
  - Palmaris brevis
  - Hypothenar muscles
  - 3rd/4th lumbricals and all interossei
  - Ends by supplying adductor pollicis, 1st palmar interossei and usually deep head of flexor pollicis brevis.

Clinical Findings in Palsy

- Wrist flexion weak and wrist radially deviated (intact FCR) on attempted flexion.
- **Positive card test**—due to weakness of palmar interossei (mnemonic: PAD—palmar interossei are adductors of fingers).
- **Positive book test/frommet sign**—due to weakness of adductor pollicis patient holds book between thumb and index finger by flexing the thumb (using FPL) rather than by adducting the thumb.
- **Positive Egawa's test**—patient unable to fan the fingers due to weakness of dorsal interossei (mnemonic: DAB—dorsal interossei are abductors of fingers).
- **Wartenburg sign**—weakness of little finger adduction that is held in abducted position at rest.
- Loss/weakness of extension of PIP/DIP joint of medial two fingers due to weakness of interossei and lumbricals (3rd and 4th).
- Grip is weak due to paralysis of intrinsic muscles.

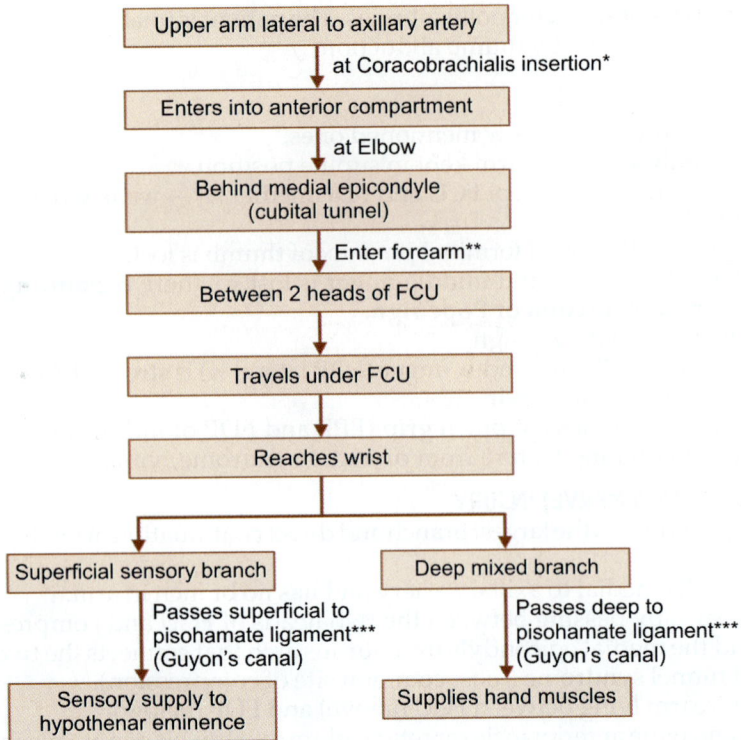

* Every nerve changes its compartment at the level of insertion of coracobrachialis (CB)

** Every nerve enters the forearm between two heads of a muscle

*** Pisohamate ligament is the degenerated tendon of flexor carpi ulnaris (FCU) area under the ligament is Guyon's canal.

Fig. 11.8: Course of ulnar nerve

- Atrophy of hypothenar area.
- **Ulnar claw hand (intrinsic minus hand)**—clawing of ring and little finger, i.e. hyperextension at MCP joint and flexion at IP joint.
- **Ulnar paradox**—in low ulnar nerve palsy forearm muscles are spared but the clawing is more (as compared to high ulnar nerve palsy) because in low ulnar nerve palsy finger flexors are spared which adds on to the deformity by flexing IP joints.
- **Partial claw hand**—only ulnar nerve palsy.
- **Complete claw hand**—combined ulnar nerve and median nerve palsy.
- Treatment for tardy ulnar nerve palsy is night elbow extension splint because elbow flexion increases the symptoms.
- Anastomosis between median and ulnar nerve.
    - In forearm—**Martin-Gruber anastomosis**.
    - In palm—**Riche-Cannieu anastomosis**.
  Because of these anomalous innervations, an ulnar nerve lesion may fail to produce the classical claw hand!

SCIATIC NERVE

Anatomy
- Thickest/largest nerve in the body.
- Arises from lumbosacral plexus and has two components
    - Common peroneal nerve (CPN) (L4-S2)—peripherally arranged.
    - Tibial nerve (L4-S3)—centrally arranged.

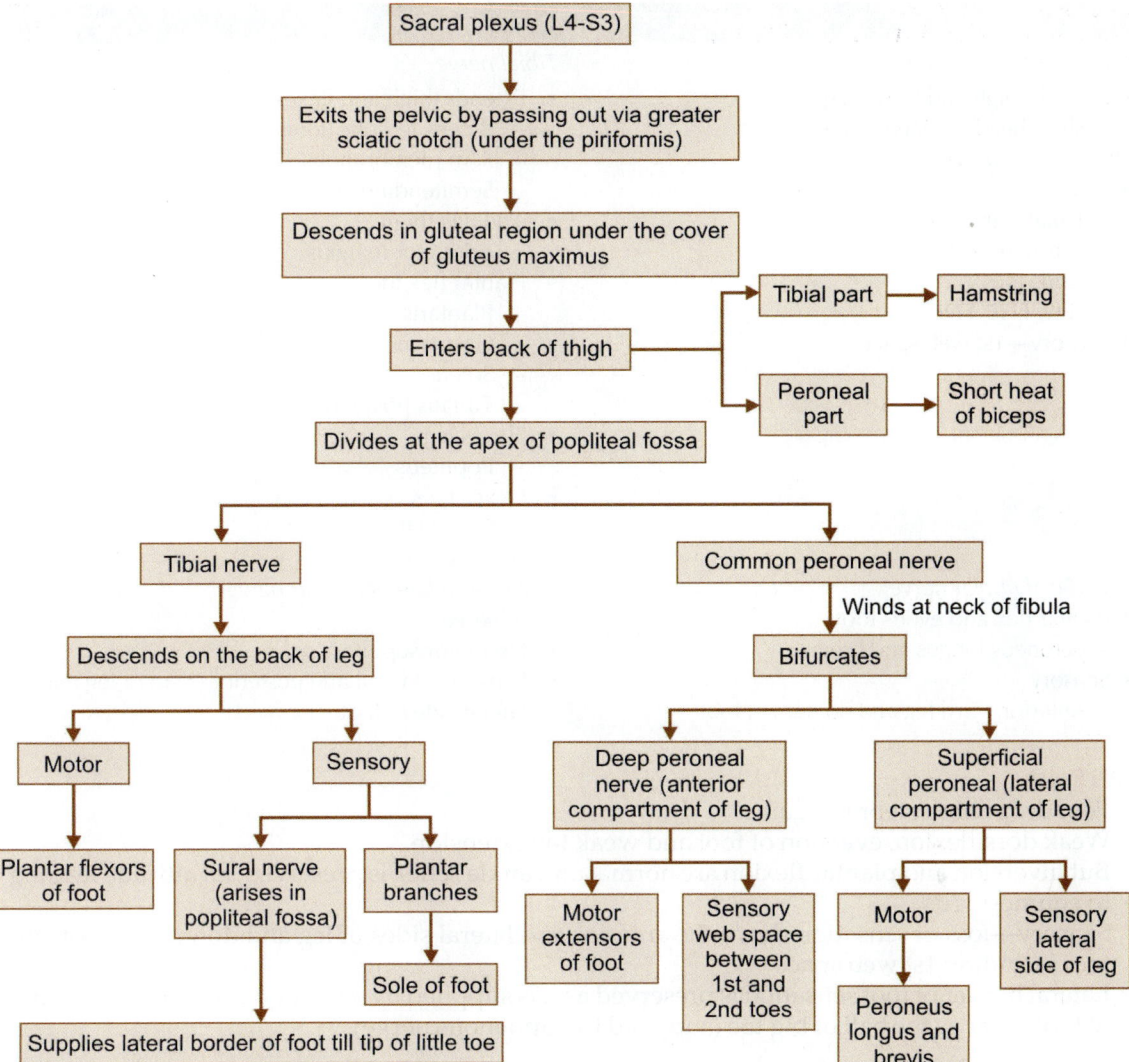

Saphenous nerve: Branch of femoral nerve given in femoral triangle.
Supplies medical leg and foot till ball of great toe

Fig. 11.9: Course of the sciatic nerve

- Injury to sciatic nerve can present injury to only CPN component as it is more vulnerable due to its peripheral arrangement and fixed and superficial nature as it winds around neck of fibula where it is prone to external pressure.
- The course of the nerve has been depicted in Fig. 11.9.

Causes of Compression
- The commonest cause of sciatic nerve injury is iatrogenic. Other causes include gunshot injury (most common cause for complete division), hip dislocations, intramuscular gluteal injections and acute compression (coma, drug overdose, intensive care unit, prolonged sitting), etc.
- Sciatic nerve is also the commonest nerve injured in total hip arthroplasty.

Supply
Motor and sensory supply of sciatic nerve has been summarized in Table 11.5.

Table 11.5: Supply of Sciatic nerve	

Common fibular nerve
• Extends thigh and flexes leg
  – Short head of biceps femoris
Deep fibular nerve
• Dorsiflexes foot
  – Tibialis anterior
  – Peroneus tertius
• Extends toes
  – EDL, EHL, EDB
• Sensory—1st web space
	Tibial nerve
	• Extends thigh and flexes leg
	  – Biceps femoris (long head)
	  – Semimembranous
	  – Semitendinosus
	• Adducts thigh
	  – Adductor magnus
	• Plantar flex foot
	  – Plantaris
	  – Gastrocnemius
	  – Soleus
	  – Tibialis posterior
	• Flexes leg
	  – Popliteus
	• Flexes toes
	  – FDL, FHL
	  Sensory—none
	Medial and lateral plantar nerves

Superficial fibular nerve
• Plantar flex and everts foot
  – peroneus longus and brevis
• Sensory
  – Anterior 1/3rd leg and dorsum of foot
	Sural nerve
	• No motor supply
	• Sensory—lateral and posterior 1/3rd of leg and lateral side of foot

CPN Palsy

- Foot drop/high stepping gait.
- Weak dorsiflexion, eversion of foot and weak toe extension.
- But inversion and plantar flexion are normal and ankle reflex is preserved, an attitude leading to equino-varus.
- Sensory—loss of sensation down the anterior and lateral sides of leg and dorsum of foot and toes including 1st web space.
- Lateral border of foot sensation is preserved as it is supplied by sural nerve and medial border of foot as far as the ball of big toe (supplied by saphenous nerve).

Xtra Edge

- Most common PNI is radial nerve. Most common nerve injury in athletes is stingers (mild traction injuries of brachial plexus in sports person).
- Most common cause of radial nerve palsy (leading to wrist drop) is fracture shaft humerus.
- Most common cause of neurological deficit in upper limb is Erb's palsy.
- Most common nerve injury involved in intramuscular injection injury is sciatic nerve > radial nerve.
- Fig 11.10 gives the contribution of various nerves in nerve supply of foot.

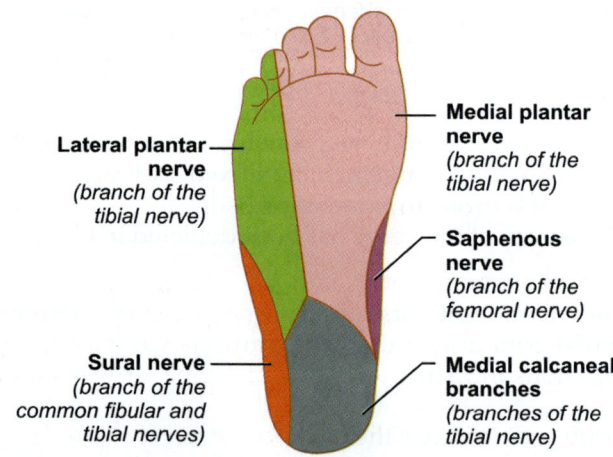

Fig. 11.10: Contributions of various nerves in supplying the foot

NERVE ENTRAPMENT SYNDROMES (Table 11.6)

Cheiralgia Paresthetica

Entrapment of superficial radial nerve in the area of anatomical snuff box, mostly due to tight wrist watch/band/'hatkadi'.

Carpal Tunnel Syndrome

- Commonest entrapment neuropathy
- Median nerve compression occurs below flexor retinaculum
- Etiology—idiopathic (most common), hypothyroidism (2nd most common), rheumatoid arthritis, acromegaly, pregnancy, diabetes, amylodosis, gout, malunited Colles' fracture, etc.
- Women >> men
- Age: 30–60 years
- Burning pain, paraesthesia, tingling, numbness in the median nerve distribution (lateral 3½ fingers)
- Pain characteristically occurs at night and awakens patient from sleep and relieved by hanging the arm over the side of the bed. Pain is increased by activities
- Examination:
  - Tinel's sign positive
  - Phalen's test—wrist fully flexed for a minute reproduces the pain
  - Reverse Phalen's test
  - Durkan test (best)—pain reproduced by compression over the flexor retinaculum
  - Positive hand diagram and Semmes Weinstein test
- NCV is the IOC
- Treatment: NSAIDs, steroid injection in carpal tunnel and surgical decompression by incising flexor retinaculum completely which is formed by
  - Deep forearm fascia proximally
  - Transverse carpal ligament over the wrist
  - Aponeurosis between the thenar and hypothenar muscle distally.

Cubital Tunnel Syndrome

Entrapment or compression of the ulnar nerve also may occur at the supracondylar process of the humerus medially (also associated with median nerve compression), at the arcade of Struthers near the medial intermuscular septum, between the heads of origin of the flexor carpi ulnaris, and at the wrist in the Guyon's canal.

In cubital tunnel ulnar nerve is first bordered by the medial epicondyle anteriorly, then by the elbow joint laterally, and finally by the two heads of the flexor carpi ulnaris medially. Pain in cubital tunnel syndrome is increased by elbow flexion.

Table 11.6: Some common entrapment syndromes*

	Compression neuropathies
Entrapment syndrome	**Nerve involved**
Carpal tunnel syndrome (M/C)	Median nerve at wrist
Pronator syndrome	Median nerve between two heads of pronator teres
Kiloh-Nevin syndrome	AIN branch of median nerve
Radial tunnel syndrome	PIN branch of radial nerve
Cubital tunnel syndrome	Ulnar nerve behind the medial epicondyle
Guyon's canal	Ulnar nerve at wrist below pisohamate ligament
Piriformis syndrome	Sciatic nerve compression
Meralgia paresthetica	Lateral cutaneous nerve of thigh (branch of femoral nerve)
Cheiralgia paresthetica	Superficial sensory branch of radial nerve
Tarsal tunnel syndrome	Posterior tibial nerve (behind and below medial malleolus)
Morton's metatarsalgia	Interdigital nerve compression

*Least common nerve involved in entrapment is femoral nerve.

Guyon's Canal

At the wrist, ulnar nerve passes along with the ulnar artery deep to the superficial part of the flexor retinaculum in Guyon's canal:

- **Roof:** Palmar carpal ligament, palmaris brevis muscle and hypothenar connective tissue.
- **Floor:** Transverse carpal ligament, pisohamate ligament.
- **Lateral wall:** Hook of hamate, transverse carpal ligament.
- **Medial wall:** Pisiform bone, flexor carpi ulnaris tendon.

In the Guyon's canal ulnar nerve divides into terminal superficial and deep branches with the ulnar artery.

Radial Tunnel Syndrome

- Entrapment of the posterior interosseous nerve can cause chronic and refractory tennis elbow. Such entrapment is called radial tunnel syndrome and can occur at four potentially compressive anatomical structures:
    1. The origin of the extensor carpi radialis brevis
    2. Adhesions around the radial head
    3. The radial recurrent arterial fan, and
    4. The arcade of Frohse as the posterior interosseous nerve enters the supinator
- Pain is 5 cm distal to the lateral epicondyle.
- Radial tunnel syndrome (RTS) can be differentiated from supinator/PIN syndrome (compression of PIN by supinator muscle) by the fact that patients with PIN syndrome have a loss of motor function, whereas patients with RTS have only lateral forearm pain without motor involvement. The difference in clinical presentation may be due to differences in the degree of compression.

Pronator Syndrome

Entrapment neuropathy of the median nerve in elbow at the following sites:
- Ligament of Struthers
- Bicipital aponeurosis
- Compression at deep head of pronator teres—PT may be hypertrophic/high origin/fibrous band within the muscle may be causing compression.
- Radial attachment of FDS.

Anterior Interosseous Syndrome (Kiloh-Nevin Syndrome)

- It refers to compression of the AIN branch of median nerve. Typically, these patients have only motor deficits and they fail to make an 'OK' sign (Kiloh-Nevin sign), as flexion of the interphalangeal joint of the thumb (FPL) and the distal interphalangeal joint of the index finger (FDP) is impaired.
- **Parsonage-Turner syndrome** is a variant where there are bilateral AIN signs caused by viral induced brachial plexus neuritis.
- Nonsurgical treatment is same as above but surgical decompression may be needed in non-responding cases.

Morton's Neuroma/Morton's Metatarsalgia

It is a benign neuroma of an intermetatarsal plantar nerve, most commonly of the second and third intermetatarsal spaces. It presents with pain and numbness or paresthesias, particularly on weight bearing. On examination, one may find Mudler's click (a click on squeezing the two metatarsal heads).

Meralgia Paresthetica

This chronic neurological disorder involves entrapment or compression of the lateral cutaneous nerve of thigh where it passes between the iliac crest and the inguinal ligament near the attachment at the anterior superior iliac spine. Injury to the nerve can also occur after performing McRobert's maneuver for delivering a child.

Tarsal Tunnel Syndrome

- Analogous to carpal tunnel syndrome in the upper limb.
- The nerve involved is the posterior tibial nerve at the flexor retinaculum or the laciniate ligament.

- *Causes*: Idiopathic, rheumatoid arthritis (most common), ankylosing spondylitis, ganglion or tumors encroaching the tarsal tunnel or in talar and calcaneal fractures.
- The patient presents with burning pain or paresthesias over plantar aspect of the foot more at night and on bearing weight.
- Release of the flexor retinaculum is not as effective in tarsal tunnel syndrome as release of transverse carpal ligament in carpal tunnel syndrome.

THORACIC OUTLET SYNDROME (TOS)

Anatomy

The outlet is basically bounded by the clavicle above, the first rib below, the scalenus anterior in front and scalenus medius behind. The structures mainly involved are the brachial plexus, the subclavian vein, and rarely, the subclavian artery. The outlet comprises three narrow passages:

- *Interscalene triangle*: Its boundaries are the scalenus anterior anteriorly, the scalenus medius muscle posteriorly and the medial surface of the first rib inferiorly. The triangle becomes even narrower with certain provocative maneuvers. Important pathologies causing constriction in this area are fibrous bands, cervical ribs and anomalous muscles.
- *Costoclavicular triangle*: It is bounded by the clavicle anteriorly, the first rib posteromedially and the upper border of scapula posterolaterally.
- Subcoracoid space which lies beneath the coracoid process deep to the pectoralis minor tendon.

Etiology

TOS results due to decreased outlet space due to abnormal posturing, hypertrophy of scalenus muscles (scalenus anticus syndrome), by compression from the cervical rib (fibrous/bony) or fractures/anomalies of nearby bones and shoulder girdle on arm movement, pancoast tumor, etc.

Clinical Features

Depend on the structures involved. Pain and paresthesia in ulnar nerve distribution are the most common symptoms.

- *Neurological presentation*: This is the most common presentation and account for more than 95% cases of TOS. Most patients complain of pain and paresthesias travelling down the arm from base of the neck that are aggravated by postural changes especially abduction of arm and neck hyperextension. True motor weakness is rare.
- *Arterial presentation*: It is least common subtype (< 1% cases) and symptoms mimic neurologic type, although cause here is ischemia.
- *Venous presentation*: It accounts for 2–3% cases of TOS. A painful, swollen and blue arm, particularly after strenuous physical activity, could be the first sign of a subclavian vein compression.

Tests

Adson's test, Wright test, Halstead test, costoclavicular maneuver/military posturing, Roos stress test, Spurling test.

Diagnosis

Mainly clinical supplemented by X-ray, CT/MRI and NCV.

Treatment

- Conservative—rest, physiotherapy, etc.
- Surgery—cervical rib or 1st thoracic rib excision in nonresponders.

MULTIPLE CHOICE QUESTIONS

1. **Obstetric nerve palsy associated with puerperium:**
   A. Median
   B. Facial
   C. Radial nerve
   D. Femoral nerve

2. **Most common nerve used for monitoring in anesthesia response:**
   A. Ulnar
   B. Median
   C. Radial
   D. Musculocutaneous

3. **What is the action of muscle on MCP joint as shown in image?**

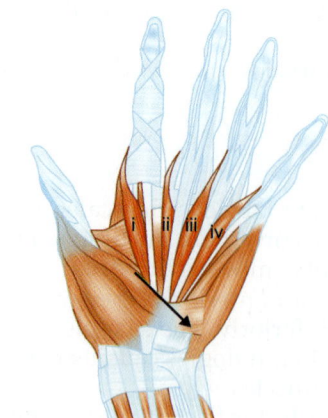

A. Flexion
B. Extension
C. Adduction
D. Abduction

4. **Following nerve injury, the injured nerve regenerates at a rate of:**
   A. 0.001 cm/day
   B. 0.1 cm/day
   B. 10 mm/day
   D. 0.0001 cm/day

5. **A politician was shot by a gun in back in political rally at T8 level, after which he developed paraplegia. The fact that the injured nerve is not able to regenerate is due to all the reasons** *except*:
   A. No endoneurial tube
   B. Glial scar formation
   C. Absence of growth factor
   D. Lack of myelin inhibitors

6. **Tinel's sign is positive and progressive in:**
   A. Axonotmesis
   B. Neurotmesis
   C. Neuropraxia
   D. All of the above

7. **Postinjection palsy is:**
   A. Neurotmesis
   B. Neuropraxia
   C. Axonotmesis
   D. None

8. **Seddon's classification all are true** *except*:
   A. Complete anatomic division of nerve is classified neurotmesis
   B. Axonotmesis has Tinel's sign positive and progressive
   C. Neurotmesis has complete recovery with/ without surgical intervention
   D. Saturday night palsy involves radial nerve

9. **Nerve biopsy in leprosy is usually taken from:**
   A. Ulnar
   B. Median
   C. Lateral popliteal
   D. Sural

10. **Tendon most commonly used for tendon transfer:**
    A. Palmaris longus
    B. Flexor carpi ulnaris
    C. Patellofemoral tendon
    D. Gracilis

11. **Tinel's sign is used for:**
    A. To assess the severity of damage of nerve
    B. To classify the type of nerve injury
    C. To locate the site of nerve injury
    D. To assess the recovery

12. **Sunderland classification is used for:**
    A. Nerve injury
    B. Muscle injury
    D. Tendon injury
    D. Ligament injury

13. **While performing flexor tendon graft repair, graft is taken from:**
    A. Plantaris
    B. Palmaris longus
    C. Extensor digitorum
    D. Extensor indicis

14. **A patient woke up in the morning with inability to extend digits, rest sensory and motor examination of hand was normal. What is nerve involved in this patient?**
    A. C8T1 nerve roots
    B. Posterior interosseous nerve
    C. Radial nerve
    D. Lower brachial plexus

15. **Saturday night palsy is which type of nerve injury?**
    A. Neuropraxia
    B. Axonotmesis
    B. Neurotmesis
    D. Complete section

16. **Which of the following is true about nerve injury?**
    A. In all cases of open wound with clinical signs of nerve injury, nerve exploration should always be done
    B. Nerve conduction velocity is best predictor within 48 hours of injury
    C. Positive Tinel's sign indicates the accurate location of lesion
    D. Traction nerve injury should be repaired immediately

17. **Tinel's sign is seen for:**
    A. Nerve injury
    B. Fascial injury
    C. Fracture
    D. Tumors

18. **Foot drop is due to palsy of:**
    A. Superficial peroneal nerve
    B. Deep peroneal nerve
    C. Femoral nerve
    D. Obturator nerve

19. **Nerve with best recovery:**
    A. Ulnar
    B. Median
    C. Sciatic
    D. Radial

20. **Motor march is seen in:**
    A. Axonotmesis
    B. Neuropraxia
    C. Neurotmesis
    D. All of the above

21. **Prognosis after secondary nerve suturing is better in pure than in mixed ones. Based on this criterion, which one of the following nerves should be given the best result after suturing in identical conditions?**
    A. Common peroneal nerve
    B. Radial nerve
    C. Ulnar nerve
    D. Median nerve

22. A pole vaulter had a fall during pole vaulting and had paralysis of the arm. Which of the following investigations gives the best recovery prognosis?
    A. Electromyography
    B. Muscle biopsy
    C. Strength duration curve
    D. Creatine phosphokinase levels

23. A patient after sleeping on chair with arm hanging whole night, presents with weakness in muscles supplied by ulnar nerve, causing claw hand. It is managed by:
    A. Electrophysiological studies
    B. Knuckle bender splint and wait and watch
    C. Exploration of the nerve
    D. Tendon transfer

24. Which of the following deformity is evident in case of Erb's palsy?
    A. Policeman tip deformity
    B. Winging of scapula
    C. Claw hand
    D. Wrist drop

25. Aeroplane splint is used in:
    A. Radial nerve injury
    B. Ulnar nerve injury
    C. Brachial plexus injury
    D. Scoliosis

26. All are true regarding brachial plexus injury, *except*:
    A. Preganglionic lesions have a better prognosis than postganglionic lesions
    B. Erb's palsy causes paralysis of the abductors and external rotators of the shoulder
    C. In Klumpke's palsy, Homer's syndrome may be present on the ipsilateral side
    D. Histamine test is useful to differentiate between the preganglionic and postganglionic lesions.

27. Erb's paralysis involves:
    A. C5-C6   B. CT1
    C. T1-T2   D. None

28. Klumpke's paralysis involves:
    A. C1-C2   B. C4-C5
    C. C5-C6   D. C8-T1

29. All of the following are features of musculocutaneous nerve injury at axilla *except*:
    A. Loss of flexion of shoulder
    B. Loss of flexion at elbow
    C. Loss of supination of forearm
    D. Loss of sensation of radial side of forearm

30. Erb's palsy lesion is at:
    A. Upper trunk
    B. Lower trunk
    C. Whole plexus
    D. C5-C6

31. In Erb's palsy all the movements are lost *except*:
    A. Supination
    B. External rotation at shoulder
    C. Abduction at shoulder
    D. Pronation

32. Muscles paralysed in Erb's palsy are all *except*:
    A. Biceps
    B. Triceps
    C. Brachioradialis
    D. Brachialis

33. A 45-year-old male with abrupt onset, pain, weakness, loss of contour of shoulder and wasting of muscle of arm on 5th day of tetanus toxoid immunization in deltoid. Likely cause is:
    A. Radial nerve entrapment
    B. Thoracic outlet syndrome
    C. Brachial neuritis
    D. Hysteria

34. All of the following muscles undergo paralysis after injury to C5 and C6 spinal nerves *except*:
    A. Biceps
    B. Coracobrachialis
    C. Brachialis
    D. Brachioradialis

35. Most common cause of neurological deficit in upper limb is:
    A. Polio
    B. Erb's palsy
    C. C1-C2 dislocation
    D. Fracture dislocation of cervical spine

36. Which of the following muscle is supplied by axillary nerve?
    A. Teres minor   B. Teres major
    C. Supraspinatus   D. Infraspinatus

37. Axillary nerve injury likely to be seen in:
    A. Shoulder dislocation
    B. Coracoid process fracture
    C. Humerus shaft fracture
    D. Brachial plexus injury

38. Axillary nerve injury is least likely in:
    A. Shoulder dislocation
    B. Fracture proximal humerus
    C. Intramuscular injection
    D. Improper use of crutch

39. A 21-year-old male with fracture surgical neck humerus presented with regimental badge sign and difficulty in abduction nerve most likely to be injured is:
    A. Axillary nerve injury
    B. Suprascapular nerve injury
    C. Erb's palsy injury
    D. Musculocutaneous nerve

40. Child after a motor vehicle trauma is unable to abduct his arm. X-ray shows fracture around surgical neck humerus. Nerve likely to be injured:
A. Musculocutaneous nerve
B. Axillary nerve
C. Radial nerve
D. Ulnar nerve

41. In axillary nerve paralysis, all of the following are true *except*:
A. Deltoid muscle is wasted
B. Extension of shoulder with arm abducted to 90 degree is impossible
C. Small area of numbness is present over the shoulder region
D. Patient cannot initiate abduction

42. All of the following features can be observed after the injury to axillary nerve, *except*:
A. Loss of rounded contour of shoulder
B. Loss of sensation along lateral side of upper arm
C. Loss of overhead abduction
D. Atrophy of deltoid muscle

43. Which of the following nerve injury is most commonly associated with a humerus shaft fracture?
A. Radial nerve   B. Median nerve
C. Axillary nerve   D. Ulnar nerve

44. Radial nerve is a branch of:
A. Posterior cord   B. Anterior cord
C. Medial cord   D. Lateral cord

45. Radial nerve related to:
A. Radius   B. Ulna
C. Humerus   D. Clavicle

46. Martin-Gruber anastomosis is between:
A. Median and ulnar nerves
B. Ulnar and radial nerves
C. Radial and median nerves
D. None

47. Wrist drop is a feature of:
A. Superficial radial nerve
B. Posterior interosseous nerve palsy
C. High radial nerve palsy
D. Avulsion of triceps tendon

48. Dorsum of 1st web space of hand is an autonomas zone for:
A. Radial nerve   B. AIN
C. PIN   D. Median nerve

49. Saturday night palsy involves which nerve?
A. Radial   B. Median
C. Axillary   D. Musculocutaneous

50. A 24-year-old male presents with a humerus fracture as shown in the figure. Which is the nerve likely to be involved by the fracture?

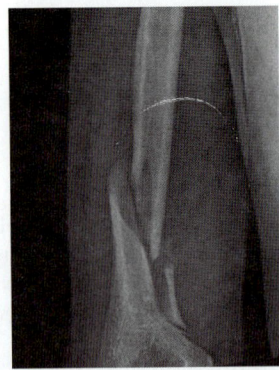

A. Ulnar   B. Radial
C. Medial   D. Musculocutaneous

51. A 45-year-old carpenter with a blunt trauma to his arm sustained a fracture following which he developed wrist drop, loss of extension at fingers and loss of sensations on the lateral aspect of the wrist joint. Which of the following is true?
A. Patient has an injury to the median nerve
B. He should have also lost extension of the forearm
C. Patient has injured the radial nerve in the spiral groove
D. There is combined involvement of the radial nerve and median nerve

52. A patient cannot extend his wrist after he has met with an accident. He has no sensory loss. Level at which the affected nerve is injured:
A. Spiral groove of humerus
B. Head of radius
C. Near medial epicondyle
D. Surgical neck of humerus

53. In a patient with history of trauma of forearm and X-ray showing fracture of proximal part of medial bone with dislocation of proximal part of lateral bone. The muscles which may be paralysed?
A. Flexor carpi ulnaris
B. Adductor pollicis
C. Extensor pollicis longus
D. Opponens pollicis

54. Extensor carpi radialis longus is:
A. Extensor and ulnar deviator of the wrist
B. Extensor and radial deviator of the wrist
C. Injured in posterior interosseous nerve injury
D. Weak extensor of the wrist

55. Extension of metacarpophalangeal joint of the hand is lost in injury to:
A. Median nerve
B. Ulnar nerve
C. Anterior interosseous nerve
D. Posterior interosseous nerve

56. **Which of the following is used as a substitute for wrist extensors in radial nerve palsy?**
    A. Pronator teres
    B. Palmaris longus
    C. Flexor digitorum superficialis
    D. Flexor digitorum profundus

57. **Cock up splint is used in treatment of:**
    A. Radial nerve palsy
    B. Ulnar nerve palsy
    C. Median nerve palsy
    D. Posterior interosseous nerve palsy

58. **Wrist drop is seen with:**
    A. Radial nerve palsy
    B. Median nerve palsy
    C. Ulnar nerve palsy
    D. Posterior interosseous nerve palsy

59. **Which of the following statements about low radial nerve palsy is not true?**
    A. Loss of nerve supply to brachioradialis
    B. Loss of nerve supply to extensor carpi radialis brevis
    C. Loss of nerve supply to extensor pollicis brevis
    D. Loss of sensation over first dorsal web space

60. **A person is not able to extend his metacarpophalangeal joint. This is due to injury to which nerve?**
    A. Ulnar nerve
    B. Radial nerve injury
    C. Median nerve injury
    D. Postinterosseous nerve injury

61. **Commonest cause of "wrist drop" is:**
    A. Intramuscular injection
    B. Fracture humerus
    C. Dislocation of elbow
    D. Dislocation of shoulder

62. **Wartenburg sign is seen in palsy of:**
    A. Ulnar nerve   B. Median nerve
    C. Radial nerve   D. Axillary nerve

63. **Palmar interossei are involved in:**
    A. Ulnar nerve injury
    B. Radial nerve injury
    C. Median nerve injury
    D. Erb's palsy

64. **Wrist drop is caused by palsy of:**
    A. PIN   B. Radial nerve
    C. Median nerve   D. Ulnar nerve

65. **A 30-year-old male underwent excision of the right radial head. Following surgery, the patient developed inability to extend the fingers and thumb of the right hand. He did not have any sensory deficit. Which one of the following is the most likely cause?**
    A. Injury to posterior interosseous nerve
    B. Iatrogenic injury to common extensor origin
    C. Injury to anterior interosseous nerve
    D. High radial nerve palsy

66. **Injury to radial nerve in lower part of spiral groove:**
    A. Spares nerve supply to extensor carpi radialis longus
    B. Results in paralysis of anconeus muscle
    C. Leaves extensions at elbow joint intact
    D. Weakens pronation movement

67. **Labourer's nerve:**
    A. Ulnar nerve
    B. Median nerve
    C. Radial nerve
    D. Musculocutaneous nerve

68. **In fracture of distal half of humerus, the nerve injured is:**
    A. Axillary   B. Median
    C. Radial   D. Ulnar

69. **Cock-up splint is used in management of:**
    A. Ulnar nerve palsy
    B. Brachial plexus palsy
    C. Radial nerve palsy
    D. Combined ulnar and median nerve palsy

70. **A patient sustains injury in his arm following which he develops loss of sensation on dorsum of hand and inability to extend wrist and fingers:**
    A. C7 neuropathy
    B. Radial nerve injury
    C. PIN injury
    D. Brachial plexus injury

71. **Nail bed of index finger is supplied by:**
    A. Median nerve
    B. Ulnar
    C. Palmar branch of median nerve
    D. Palmar branch of ulnar nerve

72. **Commonest cause of wrist drop is:**
    A. Intramuscular injection
    B. Fracture humerus
    C. Dislocation of elbow
    D. Dislocation of shoulder

73. **Saturday night palsy involves nerve:**
    A. Radial   B. Ulnar
    C. Median   D. Axillary

74. **Musician nerve:**
    A. Ulnar nerve   B. Median nerve
    C. Mallet finger   D. Hammer toe

75. **A patient can make his fist but unable to flex his index finger. Which nerve is affected in him?**
    A. Radial nerve
    B. Ulnar nerve
    C. Musculocutaneous nerve
    D. Median nerve

76. **Damage to median nerve produces:**
    A. Claw hand   B. Winging of scapula
    C. Ape thumb   D. Wrist drop

77. **Compression of a nerve within the carpal tunnel produces inability to:**
   A. Abduct the thumb
   B. Adduct the thumb
   C. Flex the distal phalanx of the thumb
   D. Oppose the thumb

78. **Median nerve is injured during:**
   A. Elbow dislocation
   B. Fracture lateral epicondyle of humerus
   C. Fracture medial epicondyle of humerus
   D. Supracondylar fracture of humerus

79. **Adductor pollicis is supplied by:**
   A. Deep branch of ulnar nerve
   B. Median nerve
   C. Superficial branch of ulnar nerve
   D. AIN branch of median nerve

80. **A patient complaints of flexion of interphalangeal joints and hyperextension of MCP of hands. He is most likely suffering from:**
   A. PIN palsy
   B. Dupuytren's contracture
   C. Claw hand
   D. Erb's palsy

81. **Claw hand is also known as:**
   A. Intrinsic minus hand
   B. Intrinsic plus hand
   C. Extrinsic plus hand
   D. Extrinsic minus hand

82. **A patient came with complaints of difficulty in adducting his fingers and flexion of extended metacarpophalangeal joint. Muscles that are paralysed are:**
   A. Interossei
   B. Lumbricals
   C. Flexor digitorum profundus
   D. Flexor carpi radialis

83. **Pointing index sign is seen in ...... nerve palsy.**
   A. Ulnar   B. Radial
   C. Median   D. Axillary

84. **Ulnar paradox is seen in:**
   A. High ulnar nerve palsy
   B. Low ulnar nerve palsy
   C. Combined median and ulnar nerve palsy
   D. Guyon's canal entrapment of ulnar nerve

85. **Froment's sign is seen in:**
   A. Ulnar nerve palsy
   B. Median nerve palsy
   C. Musculocutaneous nerve palsy
   D. Posterior interosseous nerve palsy

86. **Card test is done for testing:**
   A. Lumbricals   B. Palmar interossei
   C. Dorsal interossei   D. Adductor pollicis

87. **Froment's sign is positive in cases of weakness of:**
   A. Thumb adduction   B. Thumb abduction
   C. Thumb flexion   D. Thumb extension

88. **A patient presents with loss of sensation of ring and little finger with wasting of hypothenar muscles. Where is the lesion?**
   A. Deep branch of ulnar nerve
   B. Superficial branch of ulnar nerve
   C. Ulnar nerve before division into deep and superficial
   D. Median nerve

89. **"Ulnar paradox" is seen in:**
   A. High ulnar lesion   B. Low ulnar lesion
   C. Triple nerve disease D. Radial nerve disease

90. **Tardy ulnar nerve palsy:**
   A. Early onset
   B. Late onset
   C. Caused by shoulder dislocation
   D. None

91. **Knuckle bender splint is for:**
   A. Median nerve injury B. Radial nerve injury
   C. Ulnar nerve injury D. None

92. **Which of the following will not take place in a patient with ulnar nerve injury in arm?**
   A. Claw hand
   B. Thumb adduction
   C. Sensory loss over medial aspect of hand
   D. Weakness of flexor carpi ulnaris

93. **In axillary nerve paralysis, all the following are true _except_:**
   A. Deltoid muscle is wasted
   B. Extension of shoulder with arm abducted to 90 degree is impossible
   C. Small area of numbness is present over the shoulder region
   D. Patient cannot initiate abduction

94. **A patient can make his first but unable to flex his index finger. Which nerve is affected in him?**
   A. Radial nerve
   B. Ulnar nerve
   C. Musculocutaneous nerve
   D. Median nerve

95. **Nail bed of index finger is supplied by:**
   A. Median nerve
   B. Ulnar
   C. Palmar branch of median nerve
   D. Palmar branch of ulnar nerve

96. **Damage to median nerve produces:**
   A. Claw hand   B. Winging of scapula
   C. Ape thumb   D. Wrist drop

97. **All of the following features can be observed after the injury to axillary nerve, _except_:**
   A. Loss of rounded contour of shoulder
   B. Loss of sensation along lateral side of upper arm
   C. Loss of overhead abduction
   D. Atrophy of deltoid muscle

98. Following an incised wound in the front of wrist, the subject is unable to oppose the tips of the little finger and the thumb. The nerve(s) involved is/are:
A. Ulnar nerve alone
B. Median nerve alone
C. Median and ulnar nerves
D. Radial and ulnar nerves

99. A patient with leprosy presents with clumsiness of hand. His ulnar nerve is affected. Clumsiness is due to palsy of which muscle?
A. Extensor carpi ulnaris
B. Abductor pollicis brevis
C. Opponens pollicis
D. Interosseous muscle

100. "Ulnar paradox" is related with the following:
A. Lumbricals   B. Intrinsic muscle
C. EPL   D. Ulnar half of FDP

101. High stepping gait is seen in:
A. CTEV
B. Common peroneal nerve palsy
C. Polio
D. Cerebral palsy

102. The "Card test" tests the function of:
A. Median nerve   B. Ulnar nerve
C. Axillary nerve   D. Radial nerve

103. Road traffic accident, a patient lying in right lateral position with bruise on face, elbow and lateral side of knee. Which nerve injury has maximum chances in this position of the victim?
A. Trigeminal nerve
B. Ulnar nerve
C. Common peroneal nerve
D. Tibial nerve

104. Common peroneal nerve is related to:
A. Shaft of tibia
B. Neck of fibula
C. Lower tibiofibular joint
D. Shaft of fibula

105. A 25-year-old lady sustained a lacerated wound on the back of right thigh by a horn of a bull. The wound was sutured. Two months later she developed foot drop and an ulcer on the dorsum of the foot. The most likely diagnosis is:
A. Chronic ischemia to limbs due to popliteal artery injury
B. Partial injury to sciatic nerve
C. Complete division of sciatic nerve
D. Injury to hamstring muscles

106. Foot drop results because of injury to:
A. Superficial peroneal nerve
B. Deep peroneal nerve
C. Posterior tibial nerve
D. Anterior tibial nerve

107. Injury to the common peroneal nerve at the lateral aspect of head of fibula results in all of the following *except*:
A. Weakness of ankle dorsiflexion
B. Foot drop
C. Loss of ankle reflex
D. Sensory impairment on lateral aspect of leg extending to the dorsum of foot

108. Tinel's sign is seen in:
A. Avascular necrosis of scaphoid
B. Kienböck's disease
C. 1st carpometacarpal joint arthritis
D. Carpal tunnel syndrome

109. Most common cause of carpal tunnel syndrome:
A. Pregnancy
B. Idiopathic
C. Alcoholism
D. Occupational—excessive use of vibration instruments

110. A person came with symptoms of tingling and burning sensation over his palm near base of his thumb. He will also have which symptoms?
A. Atrophy of hypothenar muscles
B. Paresthesia over lateral 3 fingers
C. Loss of adduction of thumb
D. Loss of opposition of thumb

111. Which of the following nerve is involved in 'pronator teres syndrome'?
A. Median nerve
B. Ulnar nerve
C. Radius nerve
D. Anterior interosseous nerve

112. Investigation of choice for entrapment neuropathy is:
A. CT scan   B. Clinical examination
C. Ultrasonography   D. EMG NCV

113. Durkan test is used in clinical diagnosis of:
A. Carpal tunnel syndrome
B. Radial tunnel syndrome
C. Pronator syndrome
D. Any nerve injury

114. Carpal tunnel syndrome test used is:
A. Phalen's test   B. Finkelstein test
C. Cozen's test   D. Thompson test

115. Kiloh-Nevin syndrome is entrapment neuropathy of:
A. Median nerve   B. Ulnar nerve
C. AIN   D. PIN

116. Meralgia paresthetica is due to involvement of:
A. Lateral cutaneous nerve of thigh
B. Ilioinguinal nerve
C. Genitofemoral nerve
D. Saphenous nerve

117. Causes of carpal tunnel syndrome are all *except*:
   A. DM   B. RA
   C. Leprosy   D. Gout
118. Meralgia paresthetica is due to involvement of:
   A. Lateral thoracic nerve
   B. Lateral cutaneous nerve of thigh
   C. Anterior femoral nerve
   D. Gluteal nerve
119. In carpal tunnel syndrome all are present *except*:
   A. Ulnar nerve dysfunction
   B. Tinel's sign
   C. Phalen's sign
   D. Pain and paresthesia of wrist
120. Cubital tunnel syndrome involves:
   A. Median nerve
   B. Ulnar nerve
   C. Tibial nerve
   D. Common peroneal nerve
121. Carpal tunnel syndrome is due to compression of:
   A. Radial nerve
   B. Ulnar nerve
   C. Palmar branch of the ulnar nerve
   D. Median nerve
122. Carpal tunnel syndrome nerve compressed is:
   A. Median nerve
   B. Ulnar nerve
   C. Superficial radial nerve
   D. Musculocutaneous nerve
123. Tarsal tunnel syndrome involves:
   A. Lateral cutaneous nerve of thigh
   B. Posterior tibial nerve
   C. Common peroneal nerve
   D. Sciatic nerve
124. Morton's neuroma is entrapment neuropathy of:
   A. Plantar intermetatarsal nerve
   B. Posterior tibial nerve
   C. Superficial peroneal nerve
   D. Calcaneal nerve
125. Compression neuropathy is:
   A. Nerve entrapped in closed space
   B. Muscle entrapped in closed space
   C. Vein entrapped in closed space
   D. Artery entrapped in closed space
126. Guyon's canal nerve is:
   A. Median nerve
   B. Ulnar nerve
   C. Radial nerve
   D. Musculocutaneous nerve
127. Cheiralgia paresthetica involves:
   A. Ulnar nerve
   B. Median nerve
   C. Superficial radial nerve
   D. Musculocutaneous nerve

128. The root value of the long thoracic nerve is:
   A. C3, 4, 5   B. C4, 5, 6
   C. C5, 6, 7   D. C6, 7, T1
129. Sciatic nerve palsy most common cause is:
   A. Fractures   B. Injections
   C. Idiopathic   D. Lumbar plexus injury
130. Most common cause of tarsal tunnel syndrome:
   A. Osteoarthritis
   B. Ankylosing spondylitis
   C. Psoriatic arthritis
   D. Rheumatoid arthritis
131. Winging of scapula is due to palsy of:
   A. Long thoracic nerve
   B. Nerve to latissimus dorsi
   C. Spinal accessory nerve
   D. Nerve to rhomboid
132. A 45-year-old man presents with weakness, pain and fatigue in both lower limbs. He gives history of both limb paralysis 20 years back. What is the most probable diagnosis?
   A. Polymyositis
   B. Muscular dystrophy
   C. Post-polio syndrome
   D. Neuropathy
133. A 35-year-old female hypothyroid on treatment complaints of heaviness and tingling in left index and middle finger, the pain often increases in night and she often has to get up. Which of the following is not a clinical test for this condition?
   A. Finkelstein test   B. Phalen's test
   C. Tinel's sign   D. Tourniquet test
134. Meralgia paresthetica involves:
   A. Axillary nerve
   B. Sural nerve
   C. Median nerve
   D. Lateral cutaneous nerve of thigh
135. Thoracic outlet syndrome is best diagnosed by:
   A. CT scan
   B. MRI
   C. Digital subtraction angiography
   D. Clinical examination
136. In a 3-year-old child with polio paralysis, tendon transfer operation is done at:
   A. 2 months after the disease
   B. 2 years after the disease
   C. 6–12 months after the disease
   D. After skeleton maturation
137. Entrapment neuropathies commonly affect the following nerves *except*:
   A. Tibial
   B. Femoral
   C. Lateral cutaneous nerve of thigh
   D. Common digital nerve

138. **Sudden hyperflexion of thigh over abdomen (McRobert's procedure), which of the following nerve is commonly involved?**
     A. Common peroneal nerve
     B. Obturator nerve
     C. Lumbosacral trunk
     D. Lateral cutaneous nerve of thigh

139. **In a patient with a history of burning pain localized to the plantar aspect of the foot, the differential diagnosis must include:**
     A. Peripheral vascular disease
     B. Tarsal coalition
     C. Tarsal tunnel syndrome
     D. Plantar fibromatosis

140. **The commonest cause for neuralgic pain in foot is:**
     A. Compression of communication between medial and lateral plantar nerves
     B. Exaggeration of longitudinal arches
     C. Injury to deltoid ligament
     D. Shortening of planter aponeurosis

141. **You have treated the simple and undisplaced fracture of shaft of right tibia in a nine-year-old girl with above knee plaster cast. Parents want to know the prognosis of union of the fractured limb which was affected by poliomyelitis four years ago. What is the best possible advice will you offer to the parents?**
     A. Fracture will unite slowly
     B. Fracture will not unite
     C. Fracture will unite normally
     D. Fracture will unite on attaining puberty

142. **Test for tight iliotibial band is:**
     A. Ober's test
     B. Osber's test
     C. Simmand's test
     D. Charnley's test

143. **Which of the following does not predispose to carpal tunnel syndrome?**
     A. Hypertension   B. Hypothyroidism
     C. Pregnancy   D. Acromegaly

ANSWERS

1. D. Femoral nerve (Ref: Kelly M Scott. Musculoskeletal Health in Pregnancy and Postpartum, pp 93–114. Neural Injury During Pregnancy and Childbirth)
   Lower extremity nerves are mostly affected during childbirth. Lateral femoral cutaneous nerve is the commonest nerve damaged during delivery and child birth process causing meralgia paresthetica. Foot drop is also very common as both sciatic nerve and CPN can be injured as well owing to the lithotomy position in obstetric procedures.

2. A. Ulnar (Ref: Recommendations for standards of monitoring during anaesthesia and recovery 2015: Association of Anaesthetists of Great Britain and Ireland Anaesthesia. 2016 Jan; 71(1): 85–93. Published online 2015 Nov 19. doi: 10.1111/anae.13316)
   Adductor pollicis supplied by 'Ulnar nerve' is the most commonly used to monitor anesthesia response.

3. A. Flexion (function of lumbricals is to flex MCP joint and extend interphalangeal joints).

4. B. 0.1 cm/day

5. D. Lack of myelin inhibitors

6. A. Axonotmesis

7. A. Neurotmesis

8. C. Neurotmesis has complete recovery with/ without surgical intervention

9. D. Sural

10. A. Palmaris longus

11. D. To assess the recovery

12. A. Nerve injury

13. B. Palmaris longus

14. B. Posterior interosseous nerve

15. A. Neuropraxia

16. A. In all cases of open wound with clinical signs of nerve injury, nerve exploration should always be done

17. A. Nerve injury

18. B. Deep peroneal nerve

19. D. Radial

20. A. Axonotmesis

21. B. Radial nerve

22. A. Electromyography

23. B. Knuckle bender splint and wait and watch

24. A. Policeman tip deformity

25. C. Brachial plexus injury

26. A. Preganglionic lesions have a better prognosis than postganglionic lesions

27. A. C5-C6

28. D. C8T1

29. A. Loss of flexion of shoulder

30. A. Upper trunk

31. D. Pronation

32. B. Triceps

33. C. Brachial neuritis

34. B. Coracobrachialis

35. B. Erb's palsy

36. A. Teres minor

37. A. Shoulder dislocation

38. D. Improper use of crutch

39. A. Axillary nerve injury

40. B. Axillary nerve

41. D. Patient cannot initiate abduction

42. C. Loss of overhead abduction

43. A. Radial nerve

44. A. Posterior cord

45. C. Humerus
46. A. Median and ulnar nerves
47. C. High radial nerve palsy
48. A. Radial nerve
49. A. Radial
50. B. Radial
51. C. Patient has injured the radial nerve in the spiral groove
52. A. Spiral groove of humerus
53. C. Extensor pollicis longus
54. B. Extensor and radial deviator of the wrist
55. D. Posterior interosseous nerve
56. A. Pronator teres
57. A. Radial nerve palsy
58. A. Radial nerve palsy
59. A. Loss of nerve supply to brachioradialis
60. D. > B. Post interosseous nerve injury > radial nerve injury
61. B. Fracture humerus
62. A. Ulnar nerve
63. A. Ulnar nerve injury
64. B. Radial nerve
65. A. Injury to posterior interosseous nerve
66. C. Leaves extensions at elbow joint intact
67. B. Median nerve
68. C. Radial
69. C. Radial nerve palsy
70. B. Radial nerve injury
71. A. Median nerve
72. B. > A. Fracture humerus > intramuscular injection
73. A. Radial
74. A. Ulnar nerve
75. D. Median nerve
76. A. Ape thumb
77. D. Oppose the thumb
78. A. Elbow dislocation and D. Supracondylar fracture of humerus
79. A. Deep branch of ulnar nerve
80. C. Claw hand
81. A. Intrinsic minus hand
82. A. Interossei
83. C. Median
84. A. High ulnar nerve palsy
85. A. Ulnar nerve palsy
86. B. Palmar interossei
87. A. Thumb adduction
88. C. Ulnar nerve before division into deep and Superficial
89. A. High ulnar lesion
90. B. Late onset
91. C. Ulnar nerve injury
92. B. Thumb adduction
93. D. Patient cannot initiate abduction
94. D. Median nerve
95. A. Median nerve
96. C. Ape thumb
97. C. Loss of overhead abduction
98. C. Median and ulnar nerves
99. D. Interosseous muscle
100. D. Ulnar half of FDP
101. B. Common peroneal nerve palsy
102. B. Ulnar nerve
103. C. Common peroneal nerve
104. B. Neck of fibula
105. B. Partial injury to sciatic nerve
106. B. Deep peroneal nerve; D. Anterior tibial nerve
107. C. Loss of ankle reflex
108. D. Carpal tunnel syndrome
109. B. Idiopathic
110. B. Paresthesia over lateral 3 fingers
111. A. Median nerve
112. D. EMG NCV
113. A. Carpal tunnel syndrome
114. A. Phalen's test
115. C. AIN
116. A. Lateral cutaneous nerve of thigh
117. C. Leprosy
118. B. Lateral cutaneous nerve of thigh
119. A. Ulnar nerve dysfunction
120. B. Ulnar nerve
121. D. Median nerve
122. A. Median nerve
123. B. Posterior tibial nerve
124. A. Plantar intermetatarsal nerve
125. A. Nerve entrapped in closed space
126. B. Ulnar nerve
127. C. Superficial radial nerve
128. C. C5, 6, 7
129. A. Fractures
130. A. Osteoarthritis
131. A. Long thoracic nerve
132. C. Post-polio syndrome
133. A. Finkelstein test
134. D. Lateral cutaneous nerve of thigh
135. D. Clinical examination
136. B. 2 years after the disease
     • Tendon transfers are ideally done after 5 years of age, so that they can have compliance with physiotherapy exercises. As the child is 3 years old, tendon transfer should be done after 2 years (at 5 years of age).
137. B. Femoral
138. D. Lateral cutaneous nerve of thigh
     • McRoberts maneuver—femoral nerve > lateral cutaneous nerve of thigh
139. C. Tarsal tunnel syndrome
140. A. Compression of communication between medial and lateral plantar nerves
141. A. Fracture will unite slowly
142. A. Ober's test
143. A. Hypertension

12

Infection of Bone and Joints

OSTEOMYELITIS
General facts of bone infections
- Osteomyelitis is defined as an inflammation of the bone and marrow caused by an infecting organism.
- The infection is generally due to a single organism but in diabetes there may be polymicrobial infection.
- Osteomyelitis starts from metaphysis of bone because
    - Relative absence of phagocytic cells
    - Stasis of blood/hair pin arrangement of blood vessels
    - Sluggish blood flow
    - Dead and degenerating cartilage cells from physeal plate in children
    - Microfractures and local hematoma are common in metaphyseal area
- The classic triad is—fever, swelling and tenderness.
- Classification of osteomyelitis:

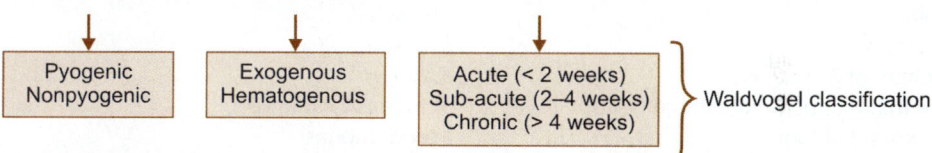

| Pyogenic Nonpyogenic | Exogenous Hematogenous | Acute (< 2 weeks) Sub-acute (2–4 weeks) Chronic (> 4 weeks) | Waldvogel classification |

Acute Osteomyelitis
- Acute hematogenous osteomyelitis is the most common type of bone infection and usually seen in children.
- The most common site is metaphysis of the rapidly growing long bones (lower end of femur > upper end of tibia).
- In adults most common site of bone infection is the thoracolumbar spine.
- The age distribution in children is bimodal—< 2 yrs age and 8–12 yrs age.

Pathology
Metaphyseal infection → metaphyseal abscess → increased intramedullary pressure → pus escapes through the Volkmann's canal to the subperiosteal space → periosteum lifted up (due to its loose attachment in children) → leading to periosteal reaction (seen 7–10 days after onset of symptoms).
- Thus the sequence is inflammation, suppuration, necrosis, reactive new bone formation, resolution and healing.
- The diaphysis is rarely involved in children
- Exception—in adults metaphyseal cortex is thick and periosteum is not loosely attached and thus the diaphysis is at greater risk in these patients.

Conditions when osteomyelitis can lead to septic arthritis (i.e. joint infection):
- <2 yrs of age—there is a common metaphyseal and epiphyseal blood supply, thus can allow spread of a metaphyseal abscess into the epiphysis and leading to joint infection.
    - Thus these patients are also susceptible to limb shortening and angular deformity.
    - Hip joint is the most commonly affected joint in young patients.

- Physis (do not confuse physis, i.e. growth plate with epiphysis) which are intra-articular:
  - Proximal humerus
  - Radial neck
  - Distal fibula.
- After the physis is closed, infection can directly spread from metaphysis to epiphysis and involve the joint.

  Causes of diaphyseal osteomyelitis:
  - Salmonella
  - Tubercular
  - Drug abusers/immunocompromised
  - Long standing osteomyelitis in children
  - Post-traumatic
  - Implant related

Absent periosteal reaction: Tubercular (bone destruction more than bone formation) osteomyelitis, long standing resolving osteomyelitis.

Organism: Most common cause is *Staph. aureus.*

Most common in all age groups	*S. aureus*
Sickle cell anaemia	Salmonella
I/V drug addicts	Pseudomonas
HIV, Immunocompromised	*S. aureus*
In open fractures and post traumatic cases	*S. aureus*
Post surgical cases	*S. aureus*
Sexually active	*Neisseria gonorrhoeae*
Animal bite	Pasteurella
Human bite	Eikenella
Diabetic ulcers	*S. aureus*
Healthy infant of 2–4 weeks	*S.aureus*
Premature infant under treatment in N-ICU	*S. aureus*/Gram –ve
Puncture wound of foot	Pseudomonas

- There is increased incidence of Gram –ve infection in vertebral bodies.
- *H. influenzae* infections were once very common in 6 months to 4 years aged children, the number having gone down significantly after introduction of Hib vaccine.

Clinical Features
Fever, swelling, pain, tenderness, systemic symptoms, increased ESR, CRP (systemic signs like fever may be absent in neonates and immunocompromised).

Absent movements of a limb (pseudoparalysis) after ruling out trauma in pediatric population—osteomyelitis >> scurvy.

The only clinical sign that may suggest the diagnosis is metaphyseal tenderness.

Investigations
1. Increased ESR, CRP, TLC.
   Peak elevation of ESR occurs at 3–5 days after infection and returns to normal approximately 3 weeks after treatment is begun. The CRP increases within 6 hours of infection, reaches a peak elevation 2 days after infection and returns to normal within 1 week after adequate treatment is begun. Thus CRP is a better indicator of recovery/better investigation during follow-up.
2. Serum procalcitonin (>0.4 ng/ml) is a sensitive and specific marker for acute osteomyelitis (and also septic arthritis).
3. X-ray
   - Normal in < 24 hours.
   - 1st change on X-ray is loss of soft tissue planes/haziness due to increased blood flow seen after 48 hours.
   - 1st bony change is periosteal reaction and seen after 7–10 days.

4. MRI: It can identify the marrow edema (within 6 hours) and soft tissue edema at the earliest and hence can diagnose osteomyelitis at the earliest and is the best diagnostic modality (IOC).
5. Tc99, Ga-67 or Indium 111 labelled leucocytes (best out of three) are the 2 bd best radiological investigation and can show changes within 24–48 hours.
6. Gold standard for diagnosis—tissue diagnosis, i.e. isolation/culture of the organism from the lesion.
7. Order/sequence of investigation: X-ray → MRI → Bone scan but the order of investigation that show positive changes are: MRI → Bone scan → X-ray.

Differential Diagnosis
- Acute septic arthritis
- Ewing's sarcoma
- Acute rheumatic arthritis and JRA
- Scurvy
- Osteosarcoma
- Sickle cell crisis

Criteria for Diagnosis
- Morrey and Peterson's criteria
- Peltola and Valvanen's criteria

Management
- Acute osteomyelitis, an emergency and clinical suspicion, is the most important indication for treatment. Treatment should be started immediately without waiting for the confirmation of diagnosis.
- General principles: Rest and elevation of the affected part, splintage, IV fluids, analgesics, etc.
- Antibiotics: Broad spectrum I/V antibiotics are started (3rd gen. Cephalosporin) and continued until condition begins to improve or CRP values return to normal, usually for 2 weeks. Thereafter oral antibiotics are given for another 4 weeks. Antibiotics are changed according to culture and sensitivity report.
- Antibiotic therapy are effective only before pus formation which generally forms by 2–3rd day and hence if the patient presents late, i.e. after 24 hours or there is failure to improve despite antibiotic treatment for 72 hours, the patient is undertaken for surgery.
- Surgery—pus drainage. If no pus found in soft tissue planes then drill holes are made in the metaphysis to decompress the bone of pressure. If pus comes out on making drill holes, then, cortical window is made to drain out pus.

Complications
1. Chronic osteomyelitis—most common complication
2. Septicemia/pyemia
3. Septic arthritis
4. Metastatic abscess
5. Pathological fracture
6. Altered growth due to epiphyseal involvement—limb length/angular deformity
7. Recurrence.

Subacute Osteomyelitis

Brodie's Abscess
- This is a long standing localized form of osteomyelitis seen in cases where either the virulence of the infective organism is low or the immunity of the host is good (i.e. immuno-competent host), such that the host is able to localize the infection within the metaphysis.
- Proximal tibia is the most common site of affection and most affected patients are 10–20 years old (slightly older as compared to patients with acute osteomyelitis).
- Indolent clinical course and ESR, CRP.
- X-ray—lytic cavity in epi-metaphyseal area with sclerotic margins and no periosteal reaction (Fig. 12.1)

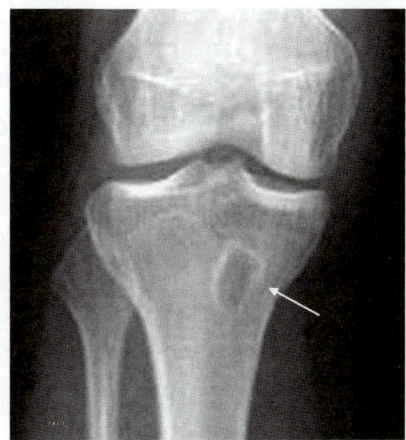

Fig. 12.1: Brodie's abscess. D/D of the X-ray: Brodie's abscess, osteoid osteoma, intracortical hemangioma

- *S. aureus* is the most common isolate although most cultures are negative.
- Treatment—trial of antibiotics → If failed, then curettage and bone grafting with antibiotics.

Chronic Osteomyelitis
- Chronic osteomyelitis is defined as the presence of ongoing bone infection for longer than 1 month in the presence of devitalized/necrotic bone.
- Chronic osteomyelitis occurs as a sequel of acute osteomyelitis because of delay in its diagnosis or when acute osteomyelitis is inadequately treated.
- Most common causative organism again is *S. aureus.*
- Most common bone involved is tibia followed by femur and humerus.
- There are usually no systemic symptoms.
- Discharging sinus (especially with history of discharge of bony chips) is the clinical hallmark and the most common presenting symptom.
- **Pathology:** When acute osteomyelitis starts entering into a chronic phase, periosteum is lifted, blood supply to underlying bone is damaged, so a part of the bone is rendered avascular. This avascular segment becomes dead, gets surrounded by infected granulation tissue and segregates from viable parent bone to form "sequestrum" (sequestrum means separated).
  - Pathognomic of chronic osteomyelitis
  - Sequestrum formation generally takes around 3 months postinfection.
  - It acts as a nidus for infection and is the m/c cause of non-healing sinus in chronic osteomyelitis.
  - It is denser than surrounding bone
  - If this piece is placed in water, it sinks and if it is examined on histopathology, one finds a closed haversian system.
  - May be absent in infants.

Lack of blood supply to involved area makes it difficult for body to halt infection, so the body tries to wall off sequestrum by forming reactive new bone around it, which is referred to as "involucrum".

But the organisms in the sequestrum have proteolytic enzymes and create openings in the involucrum that are called cloaca. Pus travels out from these cloacae, out of the bone and finally out of the tissues and skin thereby creating openings in the skin, called 'sinuses', the clinical hallmark of chronic osteomyelitis.

Tubercular sinus/osteomyelitis:
- Sinus has bluish undermined margins
- Skin surrounding the sinus is anesthetic/paresthetic
- Serous discharge unless there is superadded bacterial infection.

Classification—Cierny and Madar

Investigations
- X-ray: Sequestrum
- Involucrum
- Focal cortical defects—cloaca
- Loss of corticomedullary differentiation
- Local irregular cortical thickening
- Multiple lytic and sclerotic areas, called honeycomb pattern/moth eaten appearance (late cases)
- MRI: MRI may reveal a well-defined rim of high signal intensity surrounding the focus of active disease (Penumbra/Rim sign)
- Bone scan—not much useful in chronic cases as X-ray often clinches diagnosis
- Sinogram—to localise the source of pus
- Gold standard is biopsy and culture.

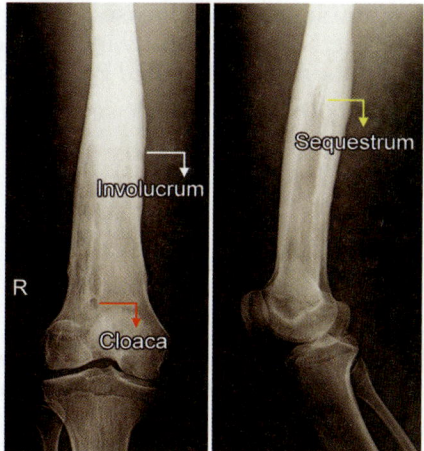

Fig. 12.2: Chronic osteomyelitis (label as shown)

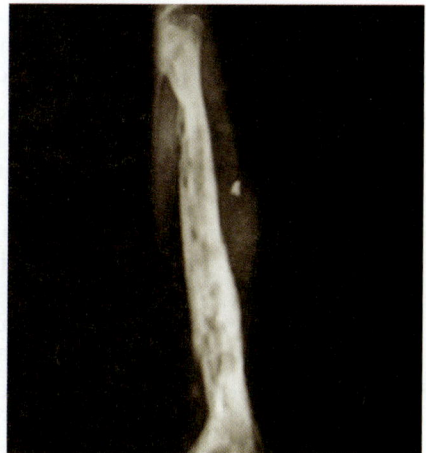

Fig. 12.3: Moth eaten appearance in chronic osteomyelitis of humerus

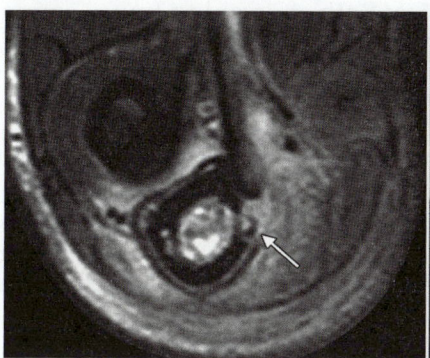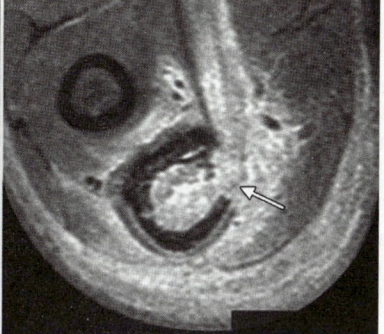

Fig. 12.4: Penumbra/Rim sign

Table 12.1: Different types of sequestrum	
Ring sequestrum	Amputation stumps
	Around pin tracts
Conical sequestrum	Amputation stump
Pencil-like sequestrum	Infants
Coralliform	Perthes' disease
Rice grain sequestrum	
Coke-shaped sequestrum	
Sand type sequestrum	Tuberculosis
Kissing sequestrum	Paradiscal tuberculosis of spine
Feathery sequestrum	Tuberculosis > Syphilis
Ivory sequestrum	Syphilis
Tubular sequestrum	Hematogenous osteomyelitis
	Segmental fractures (middle segment)
Button sequestrum	Pheochromocytoma
Bombay sequestrum	On the exposed surface of bone due to hydrogen sulphide deposition
Colored sequestrum	Fungal
Black sequestrum	Gunshot
	Actinomycosis
Linear/flake sequestrum	Only one cortex involved
Muscle	Volkmann's ischemic contracture

Treatment: Since the source of persistent infection is sequestrum surgery involves sequestrectomy (removal of the sequestrum), curettage of the walls of cavity, creating the cavity into shape of a saucer (saucerization). The bone is debrided till bleeding points are visible called **Paprika sign**.

Pre-requisite—well formed involucrum surrounding the discretely visible sequestrum
adequately at least 2/3rd diameter of bone
(3 walls intact on two X-ray views).
↓
The dead space that is created is managed by bone graft/
bone cement/**Papineau** technique of bone grafting.
↓
Skin/bone coverage is managed by local skin closure, myoplasty,
composite graft of bone, muscle and skin.

Instillation suction technique—may be used after debridement where 2 pipes are used, one for continuous antibiotic irrigation and other for continuous suction.

Complications
- Acute on chronic osteomyelitis: Acute exacerbation is the most common complication of chronic osteomyelitis.
- Growth disturbances and limb deformities: Both shortening (more common) and limb lengthening (due to increased blood flow) may result.
- Pathological fractures
- Restricted joint movements leading to joint stiffness
- Amyloidosis
- Marjolin's ulcer, i.e. squamous cell carcinoma in the sinus tract (rarely sarcoma of bone).

Osteomyelitis in HIV patients: After septic arthritis the next most common musculoskeletal infection in HIV patients is osteomyelitis. The disease in HIV patients also is mostly caused by *Staph. aureus*, although in one-third cases the infection is polymicrobial. The pathology is absolutely similar with necrosis of bone and a periosteal reaction. However, involvement may at times be bilateral. The bone most commonly involved is tibia.

Salmonella osteomyelitis: Salmonella infection is mostly seen in children with sickle cell disease. It occurs during the convalescent phase of the disease. Usual sites of involvement are diaphysis of long bones (most commonly tibia and forearm bones). Sometimes involvement may be multifocal or bilateral symmetrical. The radiological hallmark is marked diaphyseal sclerosis.

Sclerosing Osteomyelitis of Garré
- This is a non-suppurative (i.e. no pus formation) chronic osteomyelitis characterized by marked bony sclerosis (whitening of bone) and cortical thickening and absence of sequestra.
- It is thought to be caused due to low grade possibly anaerobic bacteria.
- Typically affects mandible followed by diaphysis of a tubular bone (mostly tibia).
- There are no discharging sinuses.
- Treatment is largely supportive and broad spectrum antibiotics may be given.

Chronic Recurrent Multifocal Osteomyelitis (CRMO)
- Autoimmune disease with recurrent and relapsing course of bone inflammation
- No discharging sinus present
- No micro-organism isolated
- Associated with skin lesions
- Diagnosis of exclusion

SEPTIC ARTHRITIS
The term septic arthritis refers to infection of the joint caused by pyogenic bacteria with the exception of tuberculosis. Knee is the commonest joint involved, followed by the hip (commonest in infants) and shoulder.
- Septic arthritis is more common in children, with males more commonly affected than females.
- The most common route of infection is hematogenous.

- Infection through contiguous sites like a nearby site of osteomyelitis (hip is commonly involved by this mode from a focus in proximal femur).
- *Etiology: S. aureus* is the most common causative organism in all age groups.

Table 12.2: Common organisms isolated in some special situations
• Prosthetic joints coagulase –ve staphylococci (*S. epidermidis*) closely followed by *S. aureus* and *Propionibacterium acnes* are the common isolates.
• Patients with SLE—Salmonella.
• Intravenous drug abusers—Pseudomonas infection.
• Sexually active young adults—*Neisseria gonorrhoeae*.
• Patients on TNF inhibitors (e.g. RA patients)—Mycobacterial infections.
• Pneumococcus is more common in alcoholics and in patients with hemoglobinopathies.

Clinical Features
- Toxic child with signs and symptoms of knee inflammation.
- Severe limitation of joint movements in all directions (in osteomyelitis relative limitation of joint movements).
- Joint kept in position of ease
  - Flx + Abd + ER → hip
  - Flexion → elbow and knee
  - Palmar flexion → wrist
- Psoas abscess mimic hip septic arthritis in position of ease—psoas abscess presents with pseudo hip flexion deformity and may be differentiated by Cope's Psoas test, hip rotation in flexion is less painful in case of psoas abscess.
- Absent movements of a joint after ruling out trauma in pediatric population is septic arthritis till proved otherwise.

Investigation
- Blood—increased WBC count with predominant neutrophilia.
- Blood culture may show causative organism in 60% of cases.
- X-ray—normal → increased joint space → joint space narrowing due to cartilage destruction → bony ankylosis. (Note in TB fibrous ankylosis is the rule except in spine where bony ankylosis is the rule.)
- USG—effusion and synovial thickening and aspiration can be done for isolation of the organism.
- MRI—effusion, synovitis and cartilage destruction and can differentiate from transient synovitis.
- Joint aspiration decreases intra-articular pressure and reduces chances of AVN of femoral head.
  - Fluid for analysis: >50,000 cells/ml and >75% PMNs
  Culture of the aspirate is the gold standard for diagnosis.
- Order of investigation: X-ray → MRI → Aspiration (invasive).
- Septic arthritis with negative cultures, diagnostic criteria by **Morrey et al,** 5 out of 6 should be present to label as septic arthritis
  1. Temperature 38.3°C
  2. Systemic symptoms present
  3. Swelling of affected joint
  4. Painful range of movement
  5. Absence of other pathological process that could be attributed
  6. Satisfactory response to antibiotic treatment.

Treatment
- Arthrotomy + drainage of pus (decompression of joint) + synovectomy + antibiotics (2 weeks I/V and 4 weeks oral).
- Septic arthritis is an emergency and non-operative treatment has no role.

Complications
- Septicemia
- Secondary osteoarthritis

- Pathological dislocation
- Ankylosis—septic arthritis results in bony ankylosis and is the m/c cause of bony ankylosis.
  1. Fibrous ankylosis—two articular surfaces are fused by fibrous tissue.
     - Some movement of the joint is possible
     - Painful movement
     - Most common site: TB arthritis of hip and knee.
  2. Bony ankylosis- bony union between two articular surfaces
     - no movements possible
     - joint is painless
     - most common cause: Acute septic/pyogenic arthritis >Pott's spine.

TOM SMITH ARTHRITIS

- Tom Smith arthritis is the septic arthritis of the hip in infants
- Peculiarity of this condition is that in a child of less than 1 year of age, the head of the femur is largely cartilaginous, which gets easily and rapidly destroyed by the bacteria, l/t features of hip instability, as the head is either completely or partially absent/absorbed.
- Many a times initial diagnosis is missed and patient present with the following deformity (as the head is destroyed/absorbed):
  - Painless limp with shortening
  - Unstable Trendelenburg gait
  - Hip is externally rotated
  - Motion of the hip is increased in all directions
  - Telescopy sign is positive.

Extra Edge

- Septic arthritis in farmers due to brucella infection and m/c joint is hip joint.
- Gonococcal arthritis
  - Joint infection usually manifests after 2 weeks of urethral discharge.
  - Involvement can be polyarticular (although the knee is the most common joint involved) and the condition is often associated with a papular rash.
  - Joint cultures are usually negative, but cultures from pharynx and urethra may be positive.
  - Gonococcal arthritis has generally good prognosis if treated with appropriate antibiotics (drug of choice is penicillin) and drainage is not required.

TRANSIENT (TOXIC) SYNOVITIS OF HIP

- Aka irritable hip, observational hip, coxitis serosa.
- It is a self-limiting, inflammatory condition of synovium and is the commonest cause of hip pain and limping in children in 6–12 yrs age (septic arthritis is most common cause in 0–5 years age)
- Boys are most commonly affected and condition is mostly unilateral.
- A recent history of URTI/viral infection is usually present.
- Hip attitude—flexed, abducted and externally rotated.
- Guarded hip rotation (i.e. less than septic arthritis) and pain at extremes of rotation.
- Patient is nontoxic and blood investigations are normal.
- X-ray—normal > widened joint space medially.
- USG—mild effusion and widened joint space.
- Joint aspirate—<15,000 cells/ml and <25% PMNs.
- Treatment—self limiting
  - Bedrest, light traction, oral NSAIDs.
  - After pain decreases joint is mobilised.
- USG guided aspiration and fluid analysis with isolation of the organism is the best way to differentiate it from septic arthritis.

MADURA FOOT

- Mycetoma (Madura foot) is a chronic granulomatous infection of skin and underlying tissues caused by bacteria (actinomycetes) or fungi (eumycetomas) that can extend to the underlying bone.
- It is characterized by the triad—swelling (painless) of the affected area, multiple sinus tracts and discharge of (seroanguinous fluid) granules that contain the causative agent.

- The disease was first described in the Indian town of Madura in South India, and hence the name.
- It mainly affects agricultural workers who walk barefoot in the ground and foot is m/c involved.
- Cutaneous sinus tract frequently develops which may spontaneously resolve and recur.
- X-ray—calcification, sunray appearance, Codman's triangle.
- MRI—dot in circle sign.
- HPE and culture is the gold standard for diagnosis.

Treatment
- Actinomycetoma—usually medically managed.
- Eumycetoma—surgically managed.
- Actinomycosis—most commonly involves orocervicofacial region
  - Overall most common site is mandible.
  - X-ray—cystic areas of bone destruction with concomitant bone formation and bone formation.

SYPHILIS
- Joints may be affected in secondary or tertiary stage of the disease.
- In secondary stage, there are transient polyarthralgias that generally involve large joints.
- In the tertiary stage, gummatous arthritis (synovial and osseous forms) is the characteristic manifestation.
- An indirect consequence that may occur in the tertiary stage (tabes dorsalis) is Charcot's arthropathy

Orthopedic Manifestations in Congenital Syphilis
- Frontal bossing/Olympian brow
- Higoumenaki sign: Bilateral enlargement of the sternal end of clavicle due to periostitis.
- Saber shin: Anterior bowing of mid-portion of the tibia.
- Parrot joints: Syphilitic osteochondritis in children.
- Clutton joints: Painless, symmetrical synovitis most commonly involving knee in children near puberty.
- Bilateral symmetrical metaphyseal erosions most commonly seen in the tibia

HAND INFECTIONS
The fascia and fascial septae in the hand form many spaces. The anatomy of these spaces is important because these spaces may get infected and infection from one space may reach the other space. The important spaces of hand are:
- Palmar spaces:
  - Pulp space of fingers
  - Web space
    - Deep palmar spaces
    - Mid-palmar space
    - Thenar space
- Dorsal spaces:
  - Dorsal subcutaneous space
  - Dorsal subaponeurotic space
- The forearm space of Parona

Acute Paronychia
Paronychia is the infection of soft tissue fold around the finger nail (eponychium) most commonly caused by *S. aureus* associated with poor nail hygiene.

Treatment
- When there is no pus point visible, infection is controlled by oral or IV antibiotics.
- In late stages when there is abscess only on one side of the nail, incision and drainage are done.
- If pus is extended to opposite side and under the nail, a second incision is made and proximal third of the nail is removed.

Felon
- A felon is the infection of the subcutaneous tissue of the distal pulp of a digit, the most common site being thumb followed by the index finger.
- *S. aureus* is the most common causative organism. Throbbing pain, swelling and redness of the terminal pulp are the presenting symptoms. Abscess formation may follow rapidly.
- An abscess can extend into underlying bone and may cause osteomyelitis of the distal phalanx (osteomyelitis > tenosynovitis).
- Treatment consists of antibiotics and incision and drainage.

Whitlow
- Whitlow is an infection of the pulp space of digit usually caused by Herpes simplex type I virus.
- The distinction between "felon" and "whitlow" is made primarily on the basis of:
  - Herpetic whitlow usually presents with a prodromal phase of 24–72 hours of burning pain prior to the development of the classical skin changes. First, there is erythema and swelling, then the formation of clear vesicles. The vesicles coalesce, often around the nail fold. The fluid within the vesicles is turbid, but not frankly purulent. The pulp of the affected digit is not tense as in a felon. The disease persists over approximately 2 weeks and then resolves over the next 1 week.

Web Space Infection (Collar Button Abscess)
- Web space is a fat-filled triangular interdigital space at the level of metacarpophalangeal (MCP) joints.
- This infection usually seen in laborers, begins beneath palmar creases.
- Abscess, if undrained, may spread through the lumbrical canal into the mid-palmar space.

Thenar space infection: It results from index finger or thumb.

Mid-palmar space infection: It results from middle and ring finger.

Infections of the Forearm Space of Parona
Rectangular space situated deep to the lower part of the forearm just above the wrist. It is bordered by the pronator quadratus dorsally, flexor pollicis longus laterally, flexor carpi ulnaris medially and long flexor tendons on the palmar aspect. Inferiorly, it extends up to flexor retinaculum and communicates with the mid-palmar space and superiorly it may extend up to the oblique origin of flexor digitorum superficialis. Infections in this space generally are related to infections of the digital synovial sheaths, especially the ulnar bursa.

TENOSYNOVITIS
The flexor tendons of the fingers are surrounded by their own synovial sheaths.
- The digital synovial sheaths of the second, third and fourth digits are independent and terminate proximally at the level of the MCP joints.
- The digital synovial sheath of the little finger continues proximally in the palm as the ulnar bursa while that of the thumb as radial bursa (Fig. 12.5).
- The two bursas extend proximally for 2–3 cm above the wrist and communicate with each other and may communicate with the "Forearm space of Parona".
- Acute suppurative tenosynovitis is a purulent infection of the digital tendon sheaths.
- Most commonly affected are the ring, middle and index fingers and
- *S. aureus* is the most common infective organism.
- **Kanavel's signs**
  1. Fusiform swelling of the finger,
  2. Partially flexed posture of the digit,
  3. Tenderness over the entire flexor tendon sheath and
  4. Disproportionate pain on passive extension.

The last sign is the most constant and typically the first being present in early cases.

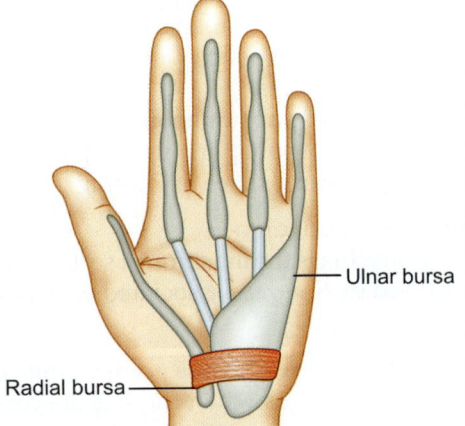

Fig. 12.5: Synovial sheath of flexor tendons and their relation

Compound Palmar Ganglion

Infections of one bursa can spread to other resulting in an hour glass swelling both proximal and distal to the wrist (flexor retinaculum) producing the "Compound palmar ganglion" (Fig. 12.6), a clinical picture more commonly seen in patients with rheumatoid arthritis and tuberculosis.

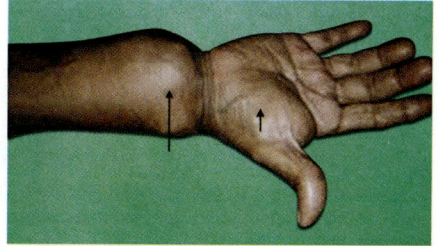

Fig. 12.6: Compound palmar ganglion showing two swellings with the arrow

MULTIPLE CHOICE QUESTIONS

1. **Tom Smith arthritis most commonly affects:**
   A. Capital epiphysis of femur
   B. Acetabulum
   C. Neck of femur
   D. Greater trochanter

2. **Multifocal osteomyelitis is associated with:**
   A. SAPHO syndrome B. Multiple myeloma
   C. Thalassemia   D. Salmonella

3. **25 years old male having pain and deformity of the tibia. What is the most probable diagnosis?**
   A. Ewing's sarcoma
   B. Chronic osteomyelitis
   C. Osteosarcoma
   D. Stress fracture

4. **Investigation for rapid diagnosis of osteomyelitis:**
   A. X-ray   B. CT scan
   C. MRI   D. Isotope scanning

5. **Most common cause of osteomyelitis in sickle cell disease is:**
   A. Salmonella
   B. Staph. aureus
   C. Pseudomonas
   D. Streptococcus pyogenes

6. **Kanavel's sign are seen in:**
   A. Tenosynovitis
   B. Trigger finger
   C. Carpal tunnel syndrome
   D. Dupuytren's contracture

7. **Compound palmar ganglion is:**
   A. Pyogenic affection of ulnar bursa
   B. Tuberculosis affection of ulnar bursa
   C. Nonspecific affection of ulnar bursa
   D. Ulnar bursitis due to compound injury

8. **Brodie's abscess is:**
   A. Acute osteomyelitis
   B. Subacute osteomyelitis
   C. Chronic osteomyelitis
   D. Septic arthritis

9. **Most common organism causing infection after open fractures:**
   A. Staphylococcus aureus
   B. Pseudomonas
   C. Klebsiella
   D. Gonococcus

10. **True about HIV osteomyelitis is all *except*:**
    A. Bilateral
    B. Necrosis is absent
    C. Periosteal new bone formation
    D. Most common cause is Staph. aureus

11. **Earliest change of osteomyelitis on X-ray:**
    A. Lytic defects
    B. Loss of soft tissue planes
    C. Sequestrum
    D. Periosteal reaction

12. **Most common joint involved in septic arthritis:**
    A. Knee   B. Shoulder
    C. Hip   D. Elbow

13. **A 7-year-old boy presented with abrupt onset of pain in right hip with the hip held in abduction. Hemogram and X-ray are normal but the ESR is raised. Appropriate line of management is from here would be**
    A. Hospitalise and observe
    B. Intravenous antibiotics
    C. Ambulatory observation
    D. USG guided aspiration of hip

14. **Tom Smith arthritis manifests as**
    A. Hip stiffness
    B. Ankylosis
    C. Lengthening of limb
    D. Increased hip mobility and instability

15. **A 30-year-old male, HIV positive, on antiretroviral therapy, has pain in right hip region. There is flexion, abduction and external rotation deformity of right hip since 2 months. Most likely diagnosis is:**
    A. TB hip   B. Avascular necrosis
    C. Septic arthritis   D. Transient synovitis

16. **Most common site of actinomycosis amongst the following is**
    A. Femur   B. Mandible
    C. Tibia   D. Rib

17. **Most common finger infected by felon is**
    A. Thumb   B. Index finger
    C. Middle finger D. Ring finger

18. **Ring sequestrum is seen in**
    A. Typhoid osteomyelitis
    B. Chronic osteomyelitis
    C. Amputation stump
    D. Tuberculosis osteomyelitis

19. **The common cause of limp in a child of seven years is:**
    A. TB hip
    B. CDH
    C. Perthes' disease
    D. Slipped capital femoral epiphysis

20. **Most common cause of monoarthritis in children in India is:**
    A. Septic arthritis
    B. Osteoarthritis
    C. Tuberculous arthritis
    D. RA

21. **Osteomyelitis most commonly starts at:**
    A. Epiphysis   B. Metaphysis
    C. Diaphysis   D. None

22. **X-ray knee of the patient with following image shows:**

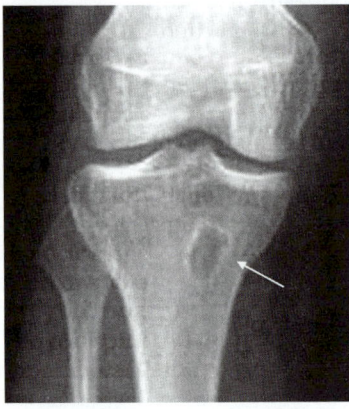

    A. Ewing's sarcoma
    B. Osteosarcoma
    C. Callus
    D. Brodie's abscess

23. **An 18-year-old male presents with a draining sinus on his left leg with pus discharge and discharge of bony pieces since 3 months. The diagnosis is:**
    A. Chronic osteomyelitis
    B. Ewing's sarcoma
    C. Osteoid osteoma
    D. Cellulitis

24. **Total duration of antibiotics in acute osteomyelitis is:**
    A. 4 weeks   B. 2 weeks
    C. 6 weeks   D. 8 weeks

25. **The diagnosis for the following image in a 15-year-old girl with sinus in the thigh and old healed scar:**

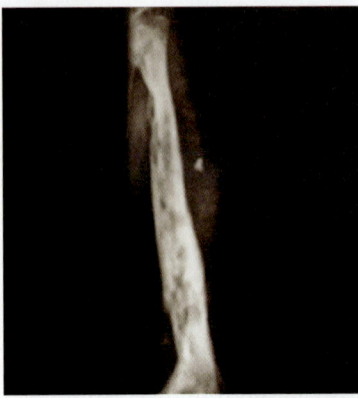

    A. Ewing's sarcoma   B. Chronic osteomyelitis
    C. Osteosarcoma   D. Brodie's abscess

26. **True regarding osteomyelitis in newborn:**
    A. Most common in diaphysis
    B. The infection is unifocal
    C. Organisms are derived from maternal genital tract
    D. Most common organism is *E. coli*

27. **The diagnosis for the following image (MRI) in a 15-year-old girl with sinus in the thigh and old healed scar:**

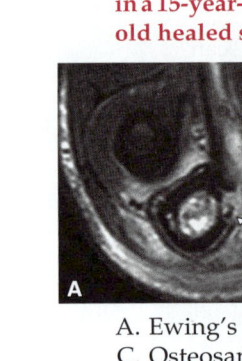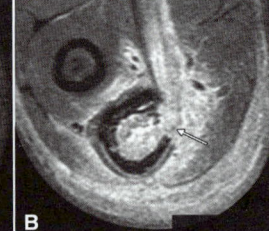

    A. Ewing's sarcoma   B. Chronic osteomyelitis
    C. Osteosarcoma   D. Brodie's abscess

28. **All are true about septic arthritis *except*:**
    A. *Staph. aureus* is most common causative organisms
    B. Common in children
    C. Affect growth plate
    D. *E. coli* is the commonest causative organisms
    E. Aspiration of joint fluid is used for diagnosis

29. **Brodie's abscess is a terminology for:**
    A. Subungual infection
    B. Chronic osteomyelitis
    C. Web space infection
    D. Infected hematoma

30. Commonest cause of acute osteomyelitis:
    A. Trauma
    B. Surgery
    C. Fungal infection
    D. Hematogenous route
    E. Tubercular infection

31. Post-traumatic osteomyelitis causing organism is:
    A. *Staphylococcus aureus*
    B. *Staphylococcus pyogenes*
    C. *E. coli*
    D. Pseudomonas

32. Osteomyelitis of spine most common organism is:
    A. *Staphylococcus aureus*
    B. Pseudomonas
    C. Tuberculosis
    D. Streptococcus

33. All are about chronic osteomyelitis *except*:
    A. Reactive new bone formation
    B. Cloaca is an opening in involucrum
    C. Sequestrum is dead bone
    D. Sequestrum is heavy bone

34. Brodie's abscess is:
    A. Acute osteomyelitis
    B. Subacute osteomyelitis
    C. Chronic osteomyelitis
    D. Septic arthritis

35. Chronic persistent neutrophilic discharged is seen in:
    A. Chronic osteomyelitis
    B. Acute osteomyelitis
    C. Septic arthritis
    D. None

36. Cloacae are best present in:
    A. Sequestrum   B. Involucrum
    C. Septic arthritis   D. Myositis

37. Sequestrum is best defined as:
    A. A piece of dead bone
    B. A piece of bone with poor vascularity
    C. A piece of dead bone surrounded by infected tissue
    D. None

38. Postsurgical osteomyelitis most common organism is:
    A. Steaphylococcus
    B. Pseudomonas
    C. Streptococcus
    D. *E. coli*

39. Brodie's abscess at upper end tibia is:
    A. Acute osteomyelitis
    B. Subacute osteomyelitis
    C. *Nocardia asteroides*
    D. *Borrelia vincentii*

40. A 16-year-old male has history of surgical drainage of left thigh and he now has a discharging sinus along the lateral aspect of thigh, femoral bone is irregular and tender. On X-ray there is lamellated appearance of periosteal reaction, has sclerosed fragment in centre and reactive new bone around the sclerosed bone:
    A. Sclerosed bone is sequestrum
    B. Reactive bone is involucrum
    C. Both correct
    D. Both wrong

41. Acute osteomyelitis is most commonly caused by:
    A. *Staphylococcus aureus*
    B. *Actinomyces bovis*
    C. *Nocardia asteroides*
    D. *Septic vincentii*

42. Acute osteomyelitis of long bones commonly affect the:
    A. Epiphysis   B. Diaphysis
    C. Metaphysis   D. Articular surface

43. Chronic osteomyelitis is diagnosed mainly by:
    A. Sequestrum   B. Bone fracture
    C. Deformity   D. Brodie's abscess

44. Which of the following is Not True regarding tubercular osteomyelitis:
    A. It is a secondary TB
    B. Periosteal reaction is seen
    C. Sequestration is uncommon
    D. Inflammation is minimum

45. Complication of acute osteomyelitis: (multiple options may be correct)
    A. Malignancy
    B. Fracture of the affected bone
    C. Septic
    D. Chronicity

46. True regarding acute osteomyelitis in a child: (multiple options may be correct)
    A. Diagnosis by X-ray shows periosteal reaction in 0–10 days after onset
    B. There is tenderness at the site
    C. Antibiotic therapy should be at least for 6 weeks
    D. Salmonella is the most common cause

47. An 8-year-old boy present with a gradually progressing swelling and pain since 6 months over the upper tibia. On X-ray, there is a lytic lesion with sclerotic margin in the upper-tibial metaphysis. The diagnosis is:
    A. Osteogenic sarcoma B. Osteoclastoma
    C. Ewing's sarcoma   D. Brodie's abscess

48. All are associated with chronic osteomyelitis *except*:
    A. Amyloidosis   B. Sequestrum
    C. Carcinoma   D. Myositis ossificans

49. True about HIV, osteomyelitis is all *except*:
A. Necrosis absent
B. Often bilateral
C. Periosteal new bone formation
D. Most common cause is *Staphylococcus aureus*

50. The most common organism causing osteo-myelitis in drug abusers is:
A. *E. coli*
B. Pesudomonas
C. Klebsiella
D. *Staphylococcus aureus*

51. The most common source of bone and joint infection is:
A. Direct spread   B. Percutaneous
C. Lymphatic   D. Hematogenous

52. Installation treatment in osteomyelitis is:
A. Continuous suction + continuous drainage
B. Intermittent suction + continues drainage
C. Continuous suction + intermittent drainage
D. Intermittent suction + intermittent drainage

53. The ideal treatment for acute osteomyelitis of long bones is:
A. Antibiotics only
B. Drilling of bone
C. Decompression
D. Antibiotics and if indicated decompression

54. What is Brodie's abscess?
A. Long standing localizes pyogenic abscess in the bone
B. Cold abscess
C. Subperiosteal abscess
D. Soft tissue abscess

55. When does the bony lesion of osteomyelitis appear on X-ray?
A. 2 hours   B. 24 hours
C. 1 week   D. 2 weeks

56. Non-healing sinus is a common clinical feature is chronic osteomyelitis. The most common frequent cause for this presentation is:
A. Resistant organisms
B. Retained foreign body
C. Presence of sequestrum
D. Intraosseous cavity

57. Tom Smith arthritis is:
A. Tuberculosis involvement of hip joint
B. Tuberculosis involvement of knee joint
C. Syphilitic arthritis of hip joint
D. Septic arthritis of hip joint infants

58. In case of suspected septic arthritis, best way to confirm the diagnosis is by:
A. Aspiration of joint
B. CT (computerized tomography) scan
C. MRI (magnetic resonance imaging) scan
D. Blood investigations

59. Which of the following is an orthopedic emergency?
A. Intra-articular fracture
B. Septic arthritis
C. Fracture lateral condyle humours
D. Fracture neck femur

60. Most common joint involved in septic arthritis:
A. Knee   B. Flip
C. Shoulder   D. Elbow

61. Aspirated synovial fluid in septic arthritis will have:
A. Clear color
B. High viscosity
C. Markedly increased polymorph/neutrophil
D. None of the above

62. Identify the disease:

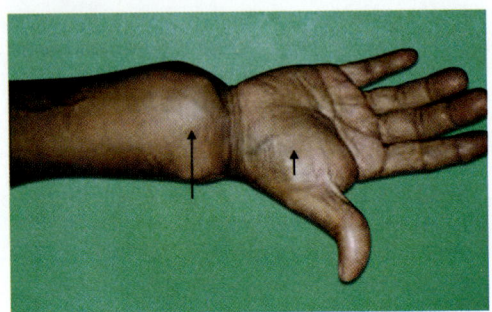

A. Compound palmar ganglion
B. Malunited fracture distal radius
C. Madura foot
D. Madelung deformity.

63. Which is false regarding acute osteomyelitis?
A. Staphylococcus is the usual organism
B. Rest and elevation relieves pain
C. Parenteral antibiotics are given
D. Surgery is the only treatment

64. When osteomyelitis spreads by hematogenous way the most affected part of bone is:
A. Metaphysis   B. Epiphysis
C. Diaphysis   D. Any of the above

65. Bony ankylosis results from:
A. Pyogenic arthritis
B. Tuberculosis arthritis
C. Osteoarthritis
D. Rheumatic arthritis

66. Brodies abscess usually involves:
A. Long bones   B. Short bones
C. Pelvic bones   D. Flat bones

67. What Brodie's abscess?
A. Long standing localized pyogenic abscess in the bone
B. Cold abscess
C. Subperiosteal abscess
D. Soft tissue abscess

68. **Actinomycosis is commonly seen in:**
    A. Tibia   B. Mandible
    C. Scapula   D. Femur
69. **Sclerosis of a long bone may suggest:**
    A. Osteoid osteorna
    B. Sclerosing osteomyelitis
    C. Both are correct
    D. None of the above
70. **Which of the following terms is inappropriate to the condition of osteomyelitis?**
    A. Cloacae   B. Involucrum
    C. Sequestrum   D. Myelocoele
71. **Acute suppurative arthritis is associated with all *except*:**
    A. May be caused by a penetrating wound
    B. May be caused by a compound fracture involving a joint
    C. May be due to bloodborne infection
    D. Causes the joint to be held in the position of ease
    E. Tends to end with the formation of a fibrous ankylosis
72. **Involucrum means**
    A. Fragment of dead bone
    B. Hole formed in the bone during the formation of a draining sinus
    C. Osteomyelitis of spine
    D. Periosteal new bone formation around necrotic sequestrum

73. **About sequestrum not true is**
    A. Infection nidus
    B. Lighter than live bone
    C. Dead piece of bone
    D. Heavier than live bone and trabeculated
74. **Involucrum is found**
    A. Underneath sequestrum
    B. Around the sequestrum
    C. At metaphysis
    D. Beneath the periosteum
75. **All are associated with chronic osteomyelitis *except*:**
    A. Amyloidosis
    B. Sequestrum
    C. Metastatic abnormality
    D. Myositis ossificans
76. **A patient with swelling foot, pus discharge, multiple sinuses. KOH smear shares filamentous structures. Diagnosis is:**
    A. Osteomyelitis   B. Madura mycosis
    C. Anthrax   D. Tetanus unilateral
77. **Sabre tibia seen in A/E:**
    A. Tuberculous osteomyelitis
    B. Syphilitic osteitis
    C. Rickets
    D. Paget's disese
78. **Arthritis of tertiary syphilis most frequently involves:**
    A. Shoulder joint   B. Elbow joint
    C. Knee joint   D. All of these

ANSWERS

1. A. Capital epiphysis of femur
2. A. SAPHO syndrome
   An entity initially known as CRMO was first described in 1972 and subsequently, several cases of CRMO were associated with blisters on the palms and soles (palmoplantar pustulosis). The term SAPHO (synovitis, acne, pustulosis, hyperostosis, osteitis) was coined to represent this spectrum of inflammatory bone disorders that may or may not be associated with dermatologic pathology.
3. B. Chronic osteomyelitis
   Ewing's sarcoma and osteosarcoma would be common between 10–20 years age. Stress fractures would generally not have a deformity. Considering the age group and site (tibia), chronic osteomyelitis seems to be best pick. However, the information given in the question is too less to conclude.
4. C. MRI
5. A. Salmonella
6. A. Tenosynovitis
7. B. Tuberculosis affection of ulnar bursa
8. B. Subacute osteomyelitis
9. A. *Staphylococcus aureus*
10. B. Necrosis is absent
11. B. Loss of soft tissue planes
12. A. Knee
13. D. USG guided aspiration of hip
14. D. Increased hip mobility and instability
15. A. TB hip
    In HIV patients TB is more common than AVN. When arthritis sets in, the deformity is generally FADIR (flexion, adduction and IR). But, in initial stage, deformity in TB hip is FABER (as in any infective pathology of hip) while in AVN is limitation of abduction and IR.
16. B. Mandible
17. A. Thumb
18. C. Amputation stump
19. C. Perthes' disease
    7–10 years: Perthes
    10–14 years: SCFE

20. C. Tuberculous arthritis
21. B. Metaphysis
22. D. Brodie's abscess
23. A. Chronic osteomyelitis
    The history given in the que are "the diagnostic" features of chronic osteomyelitis
24. C. 6 weeks
25. B. Chronic osteomyelitis
26. C. Organisms are derived from maternal genital tract
27. B. Chronic osteomyelitis.
    In chronic osteomyelitis MRI may reveal a well-defined rim of high signal intensity surrounding the focus of active disease (Penumbra/Rim sign)
28. D. *E. coli* is the commonest causative organisms
29. B. Chronic osteomyelitis (better answer would have been subacute osteomyelitis but since it is not mentioned second best answer is chronic osteomyelitis).
30. D. Hematogenous route
31. A. *Staphylococcus aureus*
32. C. Tuberculosis
33. D. Sequestrum is heavy bone
34. B. Subacute osteomyelitis
35. A. Chronic osteomyelitis
36. B. Involucrum
37. C. A piece of dead bone surrounded by infected tissue. (Sequestrum is defined as a piece of dead bone surrounded by infected tissue. Both options A and C include dead bone, but option C is complete definition of sequestrum, thus the best answer of choice).
38. A. Staphylococcus
39. B. Subacute osteomyelitis
40. C. Both correct
41. A. *Staphylococcus aureus*
42. C. Metaphysis
43. A. Sequestrum (pathognomic of chronic osteomyelitis)
44. B. Periosteal reaction is seen (periosteal reaction is usually not seen in tubercular osteomyelitis)
45. B. Fracture of the affected bone; C. Septic; D. Chronicity (Malignancy is not seen in acute osteomyelitis, but can be seen in chronic osteomyelitis)
46. A. Diagnosis by X-ray shows periosteal reaction in 0–10 days after onset, B. There is tenderness at the site, C. Antibiotic therapy should be at least for 6 weeks.
47. D. Brodie's abscess
    D/D of lytic lesions with sclerotic margins:
    1. Simple bone cyst
    2. Brodie's abscess
    3. Osteoblastoma
    4. Chondroblastoma

48. D. Myositis ossificans
49. A. Necrosis absent
    After septic arthritis the next m/c musculo skeletal infection in HIV patients is osteomyelitis. The disease in HIV patients also is mostly caused by *Staph. aureus*, although in one-third cases the infection is polymicrobial. The pathology is absolutely similar with necrosis of bone and a periosteal reaction. However, involvement may at times be bilateral, the bone m/c involved is tibia.
50. B. Pesudomonas
51. D. Hematogenous
52. A. Continuous suction + continuous drainage
53. D. Antibiotics and if indicated decompression (decompression is done by making drill holes in the bone, to relieve the intramedullary pressure. If pus escapes out of holes, then a window is created for continuous drainage of the pus).
54. A. Long standing localizes pyogenic abscess in the bone
55. D. 2 weeks
56. C. Presence of sequestrum
57. D. Septic arthritis of hip joint infants
58. A. Aspiration of joint (invasive investigation, although the best, but should never be the 1st investigative modality)
59. B. Septic arthritis
60. A. Knee
61. C. Markedly increased polymorph/neutrophil
62. A. Compound palmar ganglion
63. D. Surgery is the only treatment (surgery is the last treatment in acute osteomyelitis, and the only treatment when abscess is produced)
64. A. Metaphysis
65. A. Pyogenic arthritis
66. A. Long bones
67. A. Long standing localized pyogenic abscess in the bone
68. B. Mandible
69. C. Both are correct
70. D. Myelocoele
71. E. Tends to end with the formation of a fibrous ankylosis
72. D. Periosteal new bone formation around necrotic sequestrum
73. D. Heavier than live bone and trabeculated
74. B. Around the sequestrum
75. D. Myositis ossificans
76. B. Madura mycosis
77. A. Tuberculous osteomyelitis
78. C. Knee joint

Tuberculosis of Bone

SKELETAL TUBERCULOSIS

History

- Tuberculosis (TB) has been known to mankind since time immemorial and the Vedas recognized the disease as "Yakshma".
- The basic microscopic lesion of tuberculosis, 'the tubercle', was discovered by Laennec (inventor of stethoscope). It was an irony of fate that he himself succumbed to the disease at an early age of 45.
- Percival Pott first described the TB of spinal column.

Sites

- After the lungs and lymph nodes, the bones and joints are the third most common site of tuberculosis.
- Amongst skeletal system, spine is the most common site of involvement, followed by the hip, knee, foot, elbow, hand and shoulder in order of frequency.
- The least common bone/joint to be involved are the mandible and the temporomandibular joint.
- However, the least common orthopedic site for tuberculosis is a bursa (out of which the trochanteric bursa is most commonly involved).

Terms

- Spinaventosa is tuberculosis of short bones of hand.
- Tuberculosis of shoulder is dry TB (no effusion) and is k/a caries sicca. An important differential of the condition is frozen shoulder.
- Tuberculosis with polyarthritis is called Poncet's disease.
- Implantation TB that occurs after implant surgery.

Pathology

- Infection is paucibacillary (bacterial load in skeletal lesion is 10^5 as compared to pulmonary lesion where its $10^7–10^9$) and is mostly secondary to lung infection (50–75% patients have concomitant pulmonary lesion).
- In cases where smear results are positive, the minimum load of TB bacilli is >10000/ml.
- Bacilli reach the bone via hematogenous route (more common) or by direct extension from a neighboring focus.
- Microscopically, the lesions are of two types: Granular (dry type) and exudative (wet type). In clinical practice both types of TB (granular and exudative) co-exist, one predominant over other.
- Lesion starts in the metaphysis in children and in the epiphysis in adults.

  Insidious onset dull aching pain with night cry (relaxation in muscle tone causes loading of lesion and hence pain during sleep) is diagnostic of TB.

Investigations

In a clinically suspected case of TB one needs to investigate for *M. tuberculosis*, atypical mycobacteria, pyogenic organisms and fungi (total 4). X-rays are the first line of investigation but isolation of the organisms from tissue remains the confirmatory method.

The material for isolating the organisms is obtained from curetting/scrapping walls of the tubercular cavities in bone or linings of the sinus tracts. The material thereafter is sent for:

- ZN stain
- Löwenstein-Jensen media/automated liquid culture system (BACTEC MGIT 960)— sensitivity and specificity low, culture may take 6–8 weeks to show growth.

- Nucleid acid amplification technique (NAAT) are PCR-based assays that amplify the target nucleid acid that are specific to TB. They can detect bacilli as low as 10–50 from the sample and results can be obtained within hours. Drug resistant strains can also be identified from NAAT.

Quanti-feron-TB Gold assay-blood test to detect a latent or active TB infection. It detects cell mediated inflammatory response to TB infection by measuring interferon gamma levels in patients who has been exposed to *M. tuberculosis* antigen *in vitro*.

X-ray Findings

- Changes are seen in routine X-rays 2–4 months after the onset of disease.
- In tuberculous arthritis, localized osteoporosis is the first radiological sign of active disease.
- The articular margins and bony cortices become irregular and hazy with no periosteal reaction/ new bone formation.
- Bony destruction in the absence of periosteal new bone formation is pathognomonic of tuberculosis.
- The synovial fluid, thickened synovium and pericapsular tissues may cause a soft tissue swelling.
- With the destruction of articular cartilage, the joint space is reduced. In later stages, there is bone destruction with collapse, subluxation/dislocation and deformity of the joint.
- Healing: Remineralisation and reappearance of bony trabeculae and sharpening of cortical and articular margins.

Treatment Principles

- ATT drugs are the hallmark of treatment. 9–12 months of therapy with daily based regime is recommended.
- Rest/traction helps in the earlier stage.
- The joints should be given rest in the position of function.
- Later gradual mobilisation/ physiotherapy is started.

Xtra Edge

- Common opportunistic infection in HIV infected individuals is tuberculosis. Treatment of tuberculosis in patients with HIV follows the same principles as treatment of uninfected patients. However, it is important to consider the potential for drug interactions particularly between rifampicin and anti-retroviral agents.
- All ATT drugs (except streptomycin) are safe during pregnancy. Prophylactic pyridoxine (10 mg/day) must be added along with ATT.
- With atypical mycobacterial infection human to human transmission generally does not occur.
- Synovial sheath infections are more common with atypical mycobacteria than infection of osseous tissues.
- Osseous TB lesions are relatively more resistant than synovial lesions.
- With prolonged ATT therapy histological appearances loose their characteristic form.
- Under the influence of ATT most of the TB sinus heals within 3–4 months without surgical intervention.
- A negative Mantoux test rules out the disease.
- After the start of treatment X-ray may show deterioration as X-ray/radio pictures lag behind the clinic—physiological response, thus it should not cause unnecessary alarm.
- A patient on ATT may have arthralgia (especially due to pyrazinamide). Generally, serum uric acid levels are raised and uricosuric drugs would relieve the pain.
- The great Madras experiment established the efficacy and supremacy of ATT drugs beyond any doubt.
- Halothane like anesthetic should be avoided in patients on ATT drugs.

Immunomodulation: Drugs given to increase the immune response of the patient

- Levamisole
- BCG
  - The protection afforded by BCG in the control of TB is approximately 80%.
  - BCG vaccination—0.1 ml of vaccine injected intradermally proximal to the insertion of deltoid or in the lateral aspect of thigh.
  - BCG osteitis runs a benign course and m/c location is the epiphysis and metaphysis of long bones.
- DPT

Ankylosis: Intubercular arthritis—generally the outcome is fibrous ankylosis (i.e. dense fibrosis occurs around joint, limiting its movements), but if superadded infection is also present, then the outcome may be bony ankylosis. However, in spinal TB the outcome is often bony ankylosis rather than fibrous (owing to contact between adjacent cancellous bones of vertebrae due to erosion of end plates with further compression added by weight bearing forces).

SPINAL TUBERCULOSIS (CARIES SPINE)
- Spine is the most common site of skeletal TB and the most common infective pathology of spine in India is TB.
- Acute pyogenic infection of spine is uncommon and is mostly caused by *S. aureus.*
- Commonest part of vertebral column to be involved in TB: Lower dorsal > upper lumbar > dorsolumbar (D12-L1)*>upper dorsal, cervical and sacral. Cervical TB is commonly seen in children.
- Repeated mechanical strain/trauma in these parts of the spine which are mobile is the reason of its frequent involvement.

Types
TB bacilli reach the spine via hematogenous route through the artery or Bateson paravertrebal plexus of veins (valveless venous system).

Types in decreasing order of incidence:
1. *Paradiscal:* M/C type. Contiguous areas of 2 adjacent vertebrae with the intervening disc are involved. It occurs because they develop from the same sclerotome with the common blood supply.
2. *Central type:* Only vertebrae is involved without involvement of disc space. It occurs when infection spreads by intraosseous venous system (not Bateson plexus). Later vertebral body collapses (concertina collapse/vertebra plana).
3. *Anterior:* Infection starts anteriorly beneath the ALL and infection spreads under ALL up and down. Pus that accumulates give a shadow on X-ray which simulate an aneurysm of aorta thus k/a "aneurysmal phenomena".
4. *Posterior:* Posterior involvement is very rare and involves the posterior elements (pedicles, laminae, transverse process, facet joints and spinous process). Facet joints followed by spinous processes are the least commonly involved structures in posterior type.

Clinical Picture
Pain is the earliest symptom and tenderness is the earliest sign. Stiff spine (due to paraspinal muscle spasm), deformity and paraplegia may be seen as disease progresses. The term 'Pott's spine' refers to tuberculosis with presence of neurological deficit (paraplegia/quadriplegia).
- Types of spinal deformities:
  - Knuckle–single vertebra involved—not seen in Pott's spine
  - Angular kyphus: 2 or 3 vertebrae involved (gibbus was an older term for the same)—most commonly in Pott's spine
  - Rounded kyphus: > 3 vertebrae involved. Seen is osteoporotic collapse/Pott's spine.
- Pott's spine is the most common cause of kyphotic deformity in males.
- In the thoracic region kyphosis is most marked because of its normal kyphotic curvature.
- Maximum deformity is seen in dorsal > lumbar > cervical spine.

Cold abscess: TB is the most common cause of cold abscess. Psoas abscess can give rise to pseudo-hip flexion deformity which is confirmed by Cope's psoas test.

Tubercular Paraplegia (Pott's Spine)
Paraplegia most commonly occurs in Pott's spine of upper thoracic region because of its normal anatomy (spinal canal is narrow, spinal cord is large and kyphosis is most acute).

Early onset (good prognosis)
Occurs during the active stage of the disease usually within 2 years of disease onset.

Late onset (bad prognosis)
Occurs after 2 years of the persistence of disease. It may be associated with recrudescence of the disease or due to mechanical pressure on the cord.

---

*Dorsolumbar region is the most common, not the dorsolumbar junction (D12-L1).

Causes
- Inflammatory edema,
- Granulation tissue,
- Abscess,
- Caseous tissue,
- Ischemic lesion of the cord
- Caseous tissue
- Tubercular debris
- Sequestra
- Internal gibbus
- Canal stenosis severe kyphosis

Although the commonest cause is compression by pus and tubercular granulation tissue, sudden onset paraplegia may result from ischemia of the cord due to thromboembolic phenomena, or cord transection due to pathological dislocation or a rapidly accumulated epidural abscess.

Order of neurological deficit: The motor system is almost always affected before the sensory system because the diseased area in the spine (i.e. vertebral body) lies anterior to the cord near the motor tracts. As motor tracts are compressed, the first neurological sign that appears is ankle clonus followed by plantar extensor. The sensations carried by lateral spinothalamic tract—pain, crude touch and temperature are affected first, followed by sensations carried by dorsal column—vibration and proprioception. Stages of tubercular paraplegia are given in Table 13.1.

Table 13.1*: Stages of tubercular paraplegia
Stage 1: Patient is unaware of neural deficit, physician detects plantar extensor and/or clonus.
Stage 2: Patient is aware of neural deficit, presents with complaints of clumsiness or incoordination while walking, but is able to manage to walk with or without support.
Stage 3: Nonambulatory patient due to paraplegia in extension; sensory loss is less than 50%.
Stage 4: Stage 3 plus flexor spasms/paraplegia in flexion/flaccid paraplegia/sensory loss more than 50%/bladder-bowel involvement.

*Incoordination is the earliest symptom and ankle clonus is the earliest sign.

Diagnosis

X-Rays

The classic radiographic triad of TB spine is disk space reduction (disc space is intact in uncommon anterior, posterior and central types), lysis of the vertebra and paravertebral soft tissue abscesses

- Osteopenia followed by loss of definition of paradiscal margins and disc space reduction are the earliest findings, seen in the commoner paradiscal type of tuberculosis.
- Thereafter, the contiguous parts of the affected vertebrae get eroded and osseous destruction becomes evident. However, it is not until 2–4 months that osteopenia manifests, as 30–40% of calcium must be lost from any bone to show up as radiolucent area on X-ray.
- Anterior wedging of vertebra leading to kyphotic deformity.
- On the contrary, central TB lesions present with a concertina collapse (vertebra plana) while anterior lesions can be identified by the aneurysmal sign. Diminution of disk space is minimal in these cases.
- Posterior disease:
  - Beakless owl sign—spinous process involvement.
  - Winking owl sign—single pedicle involvement.
- In thoracic disease paraspinal abscess may cast a shadow leading to a fusiform appearance/globular appearance/bird's nest appearance (Fig. 13.1).
- In cervical TB a retropharyngeal abscess may be seen on lateral X-ray (Fig. 13.2). It is identified when the space between the pharynx and the spine is more than 0.5 cm (if above cricoid cartilage) or more than 1.5 cm (if below cricoid cartilage).
- Kyphus angle is measured by Dickson's method (Fig. 13.3).

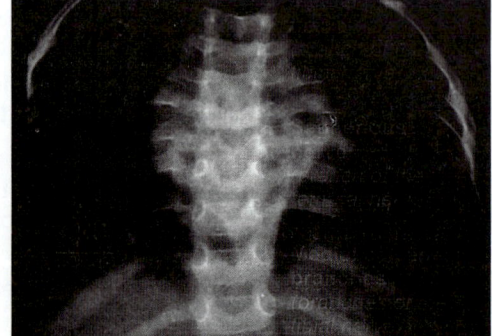

Fig. 13.1: Paravertebral abscess in TB thoracic spine

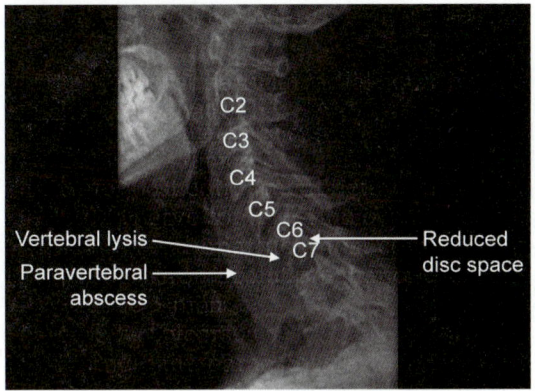

Fig. 13.2: Retropharyngeal abscess

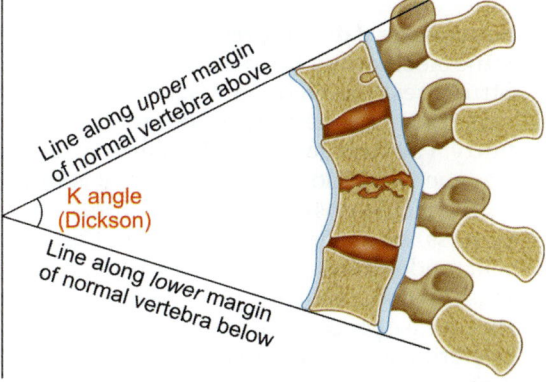

Fig 13.3: Kyphus angle measurements in TB spine

- Prof Rajasekaran has described the radiographic signs of spine at risk. X-ray signs in tuberculosis to caution against a progression of the tuberculous deformity. These include:
  - Subluxation of the facet joint at the apex of the kyphus deformity
  - Presence of retropulsion (posterior displacement) of the vertebra
  - Posterior toppling of the vertebra
  - Lateral translation of the vertebra

MRI
This is the best investigation, provides earliest diagnosis and is the IOC. Can also evaluate the status of spinal cord and evaluate sites like craniovertebral, cervicodorsal and sacrococcygeal which are difficult to image on X-ray. On gadolinium contrast study there is peripheral enhancement.

Biopsy
CT guided transpedicular (biopsy needle enters into vertebral body via pedicle, under CT guidance) vertebral biopsy is considered the gold standard for establishing the diagnosis.

Differential Diagnosis
Tumor: It is the most important differential, especially in older individuals where the metastasis is to be ruled out. Preservation of disk space and absence of para-vertebral shadow provide the diagnosis. Mostly tumors tend to involve pedicles, an infrequently involved area in tuberculosis.

Spinal tumor syndrome: The name is a misnomer as it is not a tumor of the spine. It refers to a condition when an extra dural mass (a granuloma over dura mater/tuberculoma) compresses the cord. On X-ray, there are no osseous changes, but the patient may present with neurological deficit. MRI is the investigation of choice. Since vertebra is not eroded, surgical management involves decompression via laminectomy unlike Pott's spine where laminectomy is contraindicated and anterolateral decompression is the treatment of choice.

Treatment
Middle path regimen: It means nonoperative treatment (i.e. ATT) for all cases of caries spine and operative treatment in cases of failure of conservative therapy and development of complications. DOTS regimen is not followed in skeletal TB and ATT is continued for minimum 9–12 months and may be continued for 18–24 months depending on response.

Taylor's brace is given in Pott's spine of dorsal region to prevent kyphotic deformity formation.

Indications for Surgery
- Indicated in cases where there is deterioration in clinical/neural status when patient is on ATT or when there is no improvement after conservative trial for 3 weeks.
- Stage 4 (Table 13.1) paraplegia.
- Cold abscesses heal with ATT. However, they are aspirated when they lead to symptoms, e.g. in paravertebral abscess leading to dyspnea or dysphagia, aspiration of abscess is indicated. Abscess as such is not an indication for surgery.

Surgery

- **Anterolateral decompression (ALD):** ALD (Fig. 13.4) is the most commonly performed surgical procedure. Structures removed are: Part of rib, one side transverse process, one pedicle and small part of vertebral body (posterolateral). Incision used is called Capener's incision and the surgery is carried out in right lateral position. Laminectomy and spinous process removal are contraindicated as their removal will render the spine unstable in an already compromised spine. As the spine is destroyed anteriorly by the disease process only anterior structures are removed in surgery to decompress the cord and posterior structures are preserved for stability.

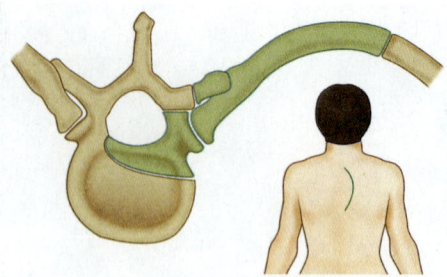

Fig. 13.4: Anterolateral decompression

- **Anterior decompression:** This involves removal of the diseased vertebral body and is the ideal procedure. However, owing to difficulty going through the anterior approach, this is not performed routinely.
- **Laminectomy:** Removal of posterior structures (and hence laminectomy) is contraindicated in Pott's spine. However, it remains the surgical procedure of choice in spinal tumour syndrome and posterior spinal disease.
- **Hong Kong procedure:** This involves radical anterior decompression followed by spinal fusion. It is mostly performed in tuberculosis of cervical spine where anterior approach is relatively easier and allows anterior decompression with less morbidity.

Prognostic factors

Factors	Good	Bad
1. Age	Young	Old
2. Onset	Early onset	Late onset
3. Duration	Shorter	Longer
4. Progression	Slow	Rapid
5. Lesion type	Wet (exudative)	Dry
6. Severity	Stages 1 and 2	Stages 3 and 4
7. General condition	Good	Poor
8. Vertebral disease	Active	Healed
9. Kyphosis	<60°	>60°
10. Cord status on MRI	Normal	Myelomalacic changes

Taken from tuberculosis of skeletal system (by Dr SM Tuli)

TUBERCULOSIS OF HIP

- The most common orthopedic site of extraspinal TB is the hip joint.
- The initial focus may start in the acetabular roof (most common), femur (an area of watershed between obturator and femoral circulation called Babcock's triangle) or greater trochanter.

Clinical Picture

Painful limp is the commonest and the earliest symptom. As stage progresses (Table 13.2) movements become painful, limb shortens and deformities develop.

Table 13.2: Stages of TB of hip		
Stage	Clinical findings	
Synovitis	Flexion, abduction, external rotation, apparent lengthening	FABER, apparent lengthening
Early arthritis	Flexion, adduction, internal rotation, apparent shortening	FADIR + <1 cm true shortening
Advanced arthritis	Flexion, adduction, internal rotation, shortening	FADIR + >1 cm true shortening
Advanced arthritis with	Flexion, adduction, internal rotation with subluxations/dislocation	FADIR, wandering acetabulum/ mortar and pestle appearance

X-ray Findings
- Haziness of the articular margins is the earliest radiological sign.
- Phemister's triad is diagnostic:
    - juxta-articular osteopenia
    - periarticular erosions
    - reduced joint space
- Pestle and mortar appearance (Fig. 13.5A) and wandering acetabulum (Fig. 13.5B) are classical.
- Shanmugasundaram classification of TB hip (Fig. 13.6).

Treatment
- ATT, rest and traction are the initial management.
- Operative—if there is no response to conservative therapy and in stage 3/4 of disease.
    - Wilkinson's joint debridement (in early stages)
    - Girdlestone excisional arthroplasty (in late stages)
        - Head and neck of femur are removed.
        - Postoperatively shortening and instability are present.
    - Arthrodesis
    - Total hip replacement (under cover of ATT).

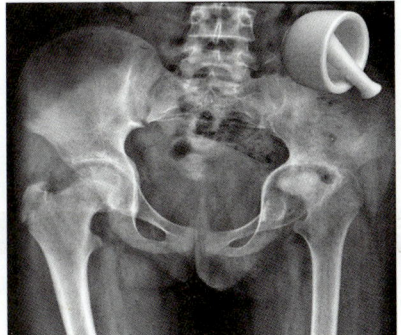

Fig. 13.5A: Pestle and mortar appearance

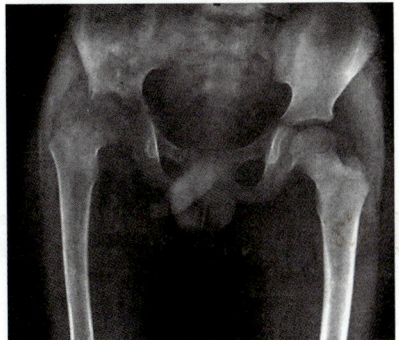

Fig. 13.5B: Wandering acetabulum (with false acetabulum)

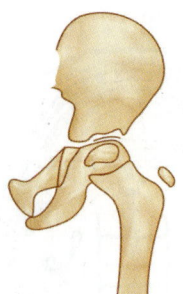

Type 1. 'Normal'

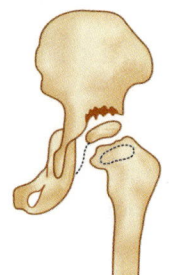

Type 2. Travelling acetabulum

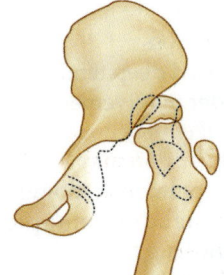

Type 3. Dislocating

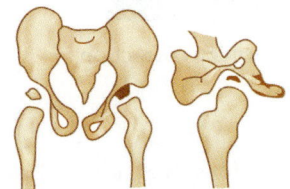

Type 4. Perthes

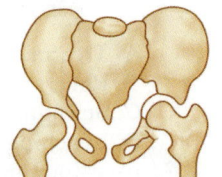

Type 5. Protrusio acetabuli

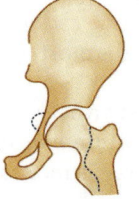

Type 6. Atrophic

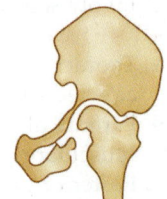

Type 7. Mortar and pestle

Fig. 13.6: Shanmugasundaram classification of TB hip

TUBERCULOSIS OF KNEE

- The knee is the third most common site for skeletal tuberculosis.
- TB arthritis is insidious in onset and often monoarticular in involvement. It is the most common cause of monoarticular arthritis in children.
- The origin of tuberculosis in the knee can be:
  - Synovial (most common)
  - Osseous, involving articular surfaces
  - Osseous but involving nonarticular parts of the tibia or femur

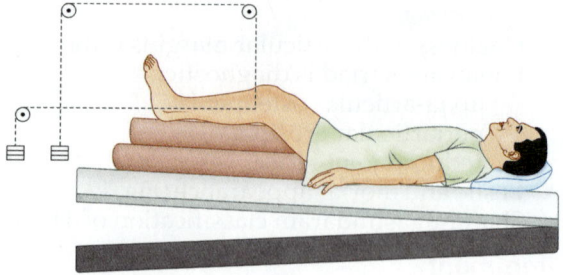

Fig. 13.7: 90–90 traction used to neutralize triple deformity of knee

- Since TB arthritis in knee is mostly a synovial origin, peripheral destruction of joint (by pannus) occurs earlier than the central part and movements are lost gradually.
- Kissing arthritis—when both sides of the joint are involved simultaneously.
- In advanced stage, triple deformity results due to ilio-tibial band contracture.
  - Flexion
  - Posterior subluxation of tibia   } D/D: TB, polio, rheumatic arthritis, ITB contracture,
  - External rotation   hemophilic arthropathy
- Treatment:
  - ATT and rest in functional position
  - Joint debridement: Wilkinson joint clearance surgery
  - In late stages: Arthrodesis/TKR
  - For triple deformity: 90–90 traction

MULTIPLE CHOICE QUESTIONS

1. **Most common site of TB:**
   A. Spine   B. Knee
   C. Hip   D. Shoulder

2. **A patient with tuberculosis of spine first neurological sign is:**
   A. Motor loss
   B. Sensory loss
   C. Increased deep tendon reflexes
   D. Bladder involvement

3. **About TB spine choose the correct statement: (Muliple option may be correct)**
   A. Most common in thoracic spine
   B. Long standing paraplegia carries poor prognosis
   C. Has hematogenous spread
   D. Middle path regime is used for treatment in our country
   E. Involves posterior complex commonly

4. **All are true about Pott's spine** *except*:
   A. Thoracic vertebrae T6–T8 is most commonly affected site
   B. Paradiscal is commonest variety
   C. Muscular rigidity and stiffness is common
   D. Posterior part of vertebrae is more affected than anterior part
   E. Back pain is the commonest presenting symptom

5. **The earliest radiological sign in Pott's disease is:**
   A. Erosion of vertebral bodies
   B. Collapse and destruction of vertebral
   C. Narrowing of intervertebral disc space
   D. Paraspinal soft tissue shadow

6. **Identify the maneuver**

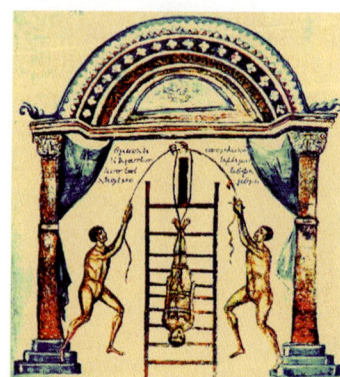

   A. Treatment for deformity correction
   B. Reverse hanging
   C. Strangulation
   D. Lynching

7. **Investigation of choice for spinal tuberculosis usually is:**
   A. X-ray   B. CT-scan
   C. Open biopsy   D. MRI

8. **Identify the procedure:**

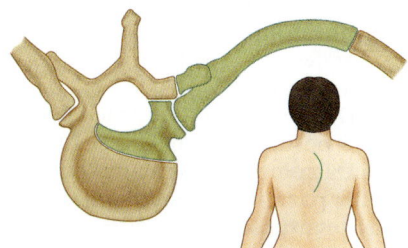

A. Anterolateral decompression
B. Posterolateral decompression
C. Surgery for scoliosis
D. Surgery for PIVD

9. **Carries sicca is seen in:**
A. Hip
B. Shoulder
C. Knee
D. None of the above

10. **Poor prognosis indicator of Pott's paraplegia:**
A. Early onset
B. Active disease
C. Healed disease
D. Wet lesion

11. **All are true about spinal tuberculosis** *except*:
A. Back pain earliest symptom
B. Dorsolumbar spine commonest site
C. Exaggerated lumbar lordosis
D. Secondary to lung injection

12. **False about Pott's spine:**
A. Commonest at dorsolumbar junction
B. Always heals by chemotherapy
C. Back pain is an early symptom
D. There is disk space narrowing on X-ray

13. **TB hand:**
A. Spina ventosa
B. Caries sicca
C. Pott's disease
D. None

14. **Most common site of TB:**
A. Spine
B. Knee
C. Hip
D. Shoulder

15. **Anterolateral decompression is done for:**
A. Sacral
B. Cervical
C. Dorsolumbar
D. Lumbosacral

16. **Anterolateral decompression is done for:**
A. Spinal tuberculosis
B. Chest TB
C. Hand TB
D. Foot TB

17. **Tuberculosis with polyarthritis is called:**
A. Poncet's disease
B. Barton's disease
C. von Gierke's disease
D. Gordon's disease

18. **Indication of steroids in Pott's spine:**
A. Pain
B. Deformity
C. Meningitis
D. Fever

19. **Hong Kong's operation is done for:**
A. Tuberculosis
B. Leprosy
C. Septic arthritis
D. Osteomyelitis

20. **Tuberculosis of spine best diagnostic modality is:**
A. Clinical
B. X-ray
C. MRI
D. CT guided biopsy

21. **Tuberculosis in bone is due to:**
A. Paucibacillary and hematogenous
B. Multibacillary and hematogenous
C. Paucibacillary and lymphatic
D. Multibacillary and lymphatic

22. **A 35-year-old lady with chronic backache. On X-ray she had a D12 collapse. But inter vertebral disk spine maintained. All are possible** *except*:
A. Multiple myeloma
B. Osteoporosis
C. Metastasis
D. Tuberculosis

23. **Poor prognostic factors in Pott's paraplegia (PGI type):**
A. Acute onset of paraplegia
B. Sudden progression of paraplegia
C. Motor paralysis alone
D. Long standing paraplegia
E. Paraplegia in children

24. **Earliest feature of spinal tuberculosis:**
A. Gibbus
B. Muscle spasm
C. Pain
D. Psoas abscess

25. **The most common sequelae of tuberculous spondylitis in an adolescent is:**
A. Fibrous ankylosis
B. Bony ankylosis
C. Pathological dislocation
D. Chronic osteomyelitis

26. **Tuberculosis of the spine commonly affects all of the following parts of the vertebra** *except*:
A. Body
B. Lamina spinous process
C. Pedicle

27. **A 46-year-old, know alcoholic, presented with pain in the dorsal spine. On examination there is tenderness at the dorsal lumbar junction. Radiograph shows destruction of the 12th dorsal vertebra and L2 vertebra with loss of disk space between D12 and L1 vertebra. The most probable diagnosis is:**
A. Metastatic spine disease
B. Pott's spine
C. Missed trauma
D. Multiple myeloma

28. **In tuberculosis of spine, which one of the following is not a cause for paraplegia?**
A. Stretching of spinal cord in gibbus deformity
B. Spinal artery compression
C. Compression by granulation tissue
D. Edema of spine cord

29. **The 1st sign of TB is:**
A. Narrowing of intervertebral space
B. Rarefaction of vertebral bodies
C. Destruction of laminae
D. Fusion of spinous processes

30. **Cold abscess in chest wall is most common due to:**
A. TB spine
B. TB rib
C. TB pelvis
D. TB pleura

31. **Tuberculosis of the spine starts in:**
    A. Vertebral body   B. Nucleous pulposus
    C. Annulus fibrosis D. Paravertebral fascia

32. **The most common type of spinal tuberculosis is:**
    A. Anterior   B. Posterior
    C. Central   D. Paradiscal

33. **Commonest site for tuberculous spondylilis is:**
    A. T12/L1   B. C6-7
    C. L4-5   D. S1-2

34. **The most common cause of kyphosis in a male is:**
    A. Congenital   B. Tuberculosis
    C. Trauma   D. Secondaries

35. **The commonest infective lesion of the spine in India is:**
    A. Pyogenic infection B. Fungal
    C. TB   D. Typhoid

36. **The ideal surgical treatment for Pott's paraplegia is:**
    A. Laminectomy and decompression
    B. Anterior decompression and bone grafting
    C. Anterolateral decompression
    D. Costotransversectomy

37. **The most common cause of paraplegia of early onset of tuberculosis of spine is?**
    A. Spinal artery thrombosis
    B. Sudden collapse of vertebra
    C. Sequestrum pressing on cord
    D. Cold abscess pressing on the cord

38. **Surgical treatment in Pott's spine is indicated if there is:**
    A. Progressive loss of function in spite of medical treatment
    B. No improvement in motor power in spite of 3 months of treatment
    C. There is no improvement in fever in 3 months of treatment
    D. Patient who is an adult or middle age

39. **Short long bones of hand and foot are commonly infected by the following organism:**
    A. Pyogenic   B. Tuberculosis
    C. Fungal   D. All of the above

40. **In bony ankylosis, there is:**
    A. Painless, no movement
    B. Painful complete movement
    C. Painless complete movement
    D. Painful incomplete movement

41. **A 25-year-old male complaints of pain in lower back region for three months. Has history of slipping of bathroom slippers. Mild weakness of both lower limbs but can walk without support. There is 30% sensory loss and has bladder symptoms. D12-L1 is tender. X-ray shows paradiscal destruction of vertebrae and MRI shows destruction with indentation of thecal sac. Management is:**
    A. Wait and watch
    B. Domiciliary ATT
    C. Admit and ATT
    D. ATT and decompression

42. **Anterolateral decompression (ALD) and anterior decompression (AD) for Pott's spine all are true *except*:**
    A. ALD and AD results are the same
    B. ALD position of patient is right lateral
    C. ALD laminectomy is always a part
    D. ALD part of ribs is removed and spinal nerves exposed

43. **Identify the procedure:**

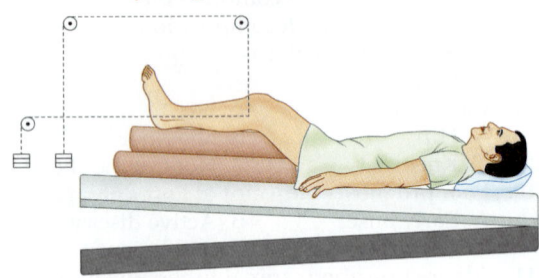

    A. 90–90 traction
    B. Bryant's traction
    C. Gallow's traction
    D. Perkin's traction

44. **Wandering acetabulum is seen in:**
    A. Fracture of acetabulum
    B. Hip dislocation
    C. Rheumatoid arthritis
    D. TB of hip

45. **Apparent lengthening of limb is seen in which TB hip stage of:**
    A. 1   B. 2
    C. 3   D. 4

46. **Girdlestone arthroplasty is carried out for:**
    A. Chronic elbow infections
    B. Acute elbow infections
    C. Chronic hip infection
    D. Acute hip infection

47. **Identify the X-ray in a case of late TB hip:**

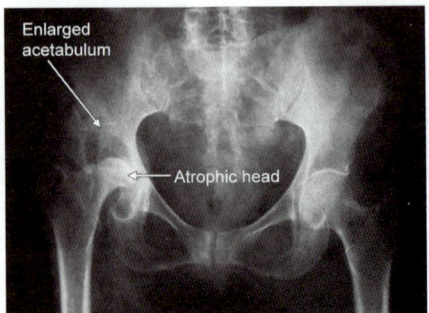

Enlarged acetabulum

Atrophic head

    A. Atrophic
    B. Wandering acetabulum
    C. Mortar and pestle acetabulum
    D. Perthes type acetabulum

48. A 30-year-old male HIV positive on anti-retroviral therapy has pain in right hip region. Flexion, abduction and external rotation deformity of right hip for 2 months, what is the most likely diagnosis?
    A. Avascular necrosis
    B. TB hip
    C. Transient synovities
    D. Septic arthritis

49. Which of the following is a feature of triple deformity of the knee joint?
    A. Posterior subluxation of tibia
    B. Internal rotation of tibia
    C. Medial angulation of tibia
    D. Recurvatum

50. Complication of join TB:
    A. Fibrous ankylosis
    B. Bony ankylosis
    C. Normal ankylosis
    D. None

51. Treatment of triple deformity is:
    A. ATT
    B. ATT+ immobilization
    C. ATT + immobilization + debridement
    D. ATT + replacement

52. Triple deformity of knee is classically seen in:
    A. Fracture patella
    B. Tuberculosis
    C. Rheumatic arthritis
    D. Cervical spine

53. The most common site of skeletal tuberculosis is:
    A. Hip + spine
    B. Knee + hip joint
    C. Knee joint
    D. Cervical spine

54. The most common cause of monoarthritis in children is:
    A. Septic arthritis
    B. Tuberculous arthritis
    C. Osteoarthritis
    D. Rheumatoid arthritis
    E. Any of the above

55. Tuberculous arthritis in advanced cases lead to:
    A. Bony ankylosis
    B. Fibrous ankylosis
    C. Loose joints
    D. Charcot's joints

56. Hong Kong procedure is useful for treating:

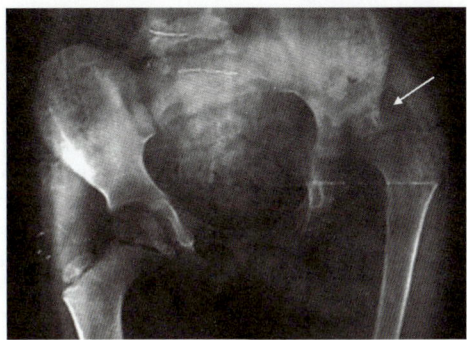

    A. Tuberculosis of cervical spine
    B. Gout
    C. AVN of hip
    D. Caffey's disease patients

57. Wandering acetabulum is seen in
    A. Fracture acetabulum
    B. CDH
    C. Dislocation of femur
    D. TB hip

58. Triple deformity of knee is classically seen in
    A. Fracture patella   B. TB knee
    C. RA   D. Rickets

59. The first neurological sign in a patient with TB spine is
    A. Sensory loss
    B. Spastic weakness
    C. Bladder involvement
    D. Ankle clonus

60. Patient with D7-D8 koch spine with paraplegia, treatment of choice:
    A. ATT
    B. Anterior decompression + ATT
    C. Laminectomy
    D. Posterior decompression

61. What causes both destruction of bone and reduction of joint space?
    A. Tuberculosis   B. Metastasis
    C. Multiple myeloma   D. Lymphoma

62. TB Sicca involves:
    A. Shoulder   B. Elbow
    C. Hip   D. Knee

63. Deformity of hip joint in case of tubercular synovitis of hip joint is:
    A. Flexion abduction external rotation
    B. Flexion adduction external rotation
    C. Flexion abduction internal rotation
    D. Flexion adduction internal rotation

64. Phemister's triad, true is A/E:
    A. Juxta-articular osteopenia
    B. Periarticular erosions
    C. Reduced joint space
    D. Joint swelling

ANSWERS

1. A. Spine
2. C. Increased deep tendon reflexes
3. A. Most common in thoracic spine; B. Long standing paraplegia carries poor prognosis; C. Has hematogenous spread; D. Middle path regime is used for treatment in our country.
4. A. Thoracic vertebrae T6–T8 is most commonly affected site (lower thoracic ic most common T9–T12) and D. Posterior part of vertebrae is more affected than anterior part
5. C. Narrowing of intervertebral disc space
6. A. Treatment for deformity correction
   In ancient times this maneuver was done for deformity correction in Pott's spine
7. D. MRI
8. A. Anterolateral decompression
9. B. Shoulder
10. C. Healed disease
11. C. Exaggerated lumbar lordosis
12. B. Always heals by chemotherapy
13. A. Spina ventosa
14. A. Spine
15. C. Dorosolumbar
16. A. Spinal tuberculosis
17. A. Poncet's disease
18. C. Meningitis
19. A. Tuberculosis
20. D. CT guided biopsy
21. A. Paucibacillary and hematogenous
22. D. Tuberculosis
23. A. Acute onset of paraplegia; B. Sudden progression of paraplegia; D. Long-standing paraplegia
24. C. Pain
25. B. Bony ankylosis
26. C. Lamina spinous process
27. B. Pott's spine
28. B. Spinal artery compression
29. A. Narrowing of intervertebral space. The earliest feature is loss of curvature due to paravertebral spasm
   The next radiological feature of spinal tuberculosis is reduction of intervertebral disk space and osteoporosis of two adjacent vertebrae sometime with fuzziness of the endplates.
30. A. TB spine
31. A. Vertebral body
32. D. Paradiscal
33. A. T12/L1
34. B. Tuberculosis
35. C. TB
36. B. Anterior decompression and bone grafting
37. D. Cold abscess pressing on the cord
38. A. Progressive loss of function in spite of medical treatment and B. No improvement in motor power in spite of 3 months of treatment.
39. B. Tuberculosis
40. A. Painless, no movement
41. D. ATT and decompression as bladder symptoms are present.
   Indications of surgery in any disease of spine.
   • Deterioration in neural or clinical status on treatment.
   • No improvement in neural or
42. C. ALD laminectomy is always a part
43. 90–90 traction
   90–90 traction to correct triple deformity of knee.
44. D. TB of hip
45. A. 1
46. C. Chronic hip infection.
47. C. Mortar and pestle acetabulum
48. B. TB hip
49. A. Posterior subluxation of tibia
50. A. Fibrous ankylosis
51. D. ATT + Replacement: Treatment of triple deformity is replacement/ arthrodesis.
52. B. Tuberculosis
53. A. Hip + spine
54. B. Tuberculous arthritis
55. B. Fibrous ankylosis.
56. A. Tuberculosis of cervical spine
57. D. TB hip
58. B. TB knee
59. D. Ankle clonus
60. B. Anterior decompression + ATT
   Since patient has paraplegia with dorsal Koch's, decompression will be performed.
61. A. Tuberculosis
62. A. Shoulder
63. A. Flexion abduction external rotation
64. D. Joint swelling

Pediatric Orthopedic Deformities

SPECIAL FEATURES OF PEDIATRIC BONE

- **Plastic deformation**—immature (pediatric) bone may undergo plastic deformation before fracture and is most commonly seen in ulna. Severe angulation (>20°) require reduction and immobilisation (Fig. 14.1A).
- **Torus/buckle fracture**—buckling of cortex classically occurring at metaphysio-diaphyseal junction. Most commonly occurs at distal radius and treatment involves splintage only (Fig. 14.1B).
- **Greenstick fracture**—one cortex breaks and other cortex remains intact because of stronger/thicker periosteum resisting the deforming force. It is the most common fracture pattern seen in children and most commonly occurs in forearm bones.
- Pediatric bone has thicker periosteum, soft bones, increased resiliency to stress, increase potential to remodel (metaphysis > diaphysis, angulation > rotation), shorter healing time, and presence of physis. In children bony injury occurs more easily than ligamentous injury, while in adults opposite is true.

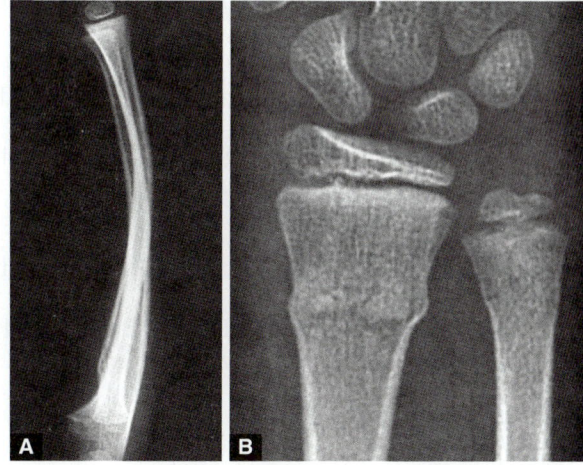

Fig. 14.1: (A) Plastic deformation, (B) Torus/buckle fracture

- In children whenever in doubt, it is always better to get X-ray of bilateral side for comparison.
- Most common fracture—distal both bone forearm (for adults is clavicle).
- Most common dislocation—elbow (for adults is shoulder).

PHYSEAL INJURIES

Pediatric periosteum, adjacent ligaments and joint capsule are stronger compared to adults and physis is the weakest part of bone, fractures mostly occurring in the hypertrophic zone of physis. Phalanx are the most common site of physeal injury followed by distal radius. Physeal injury may not be diagnosed initially on X-ray (as its cartilaginous) and present later with deformity.

Physeal injuries are classified by "Salter and Harris classification" (Fig. 14.2)

- Type I: Slip, i.e. fracture line separates epiphysis from metaphysis. Best prognosis.
- Type II: This is the most common type. Epiphysis separates from metaphysis carrying with it a chip of metaphyseal bone. Metaphyseal fragment is known as "Thurstan Holland fragment".
- Type III: Fracture line travels through the epiphysis, fracturing it.
- Type IV: Fractured epiphysis carries with it a part of metaphysis.
- Type V: Rammed/crushed physis by an axial force. It is rarest and has worst prognosis (diagnosis is generally made retrospectively when deformity/growth arrest is encountered).
- Rang's Type VI: Perichondrial ring injury.
- Ogden added a few more types.

The salter-Harris classification of growth plate injuries

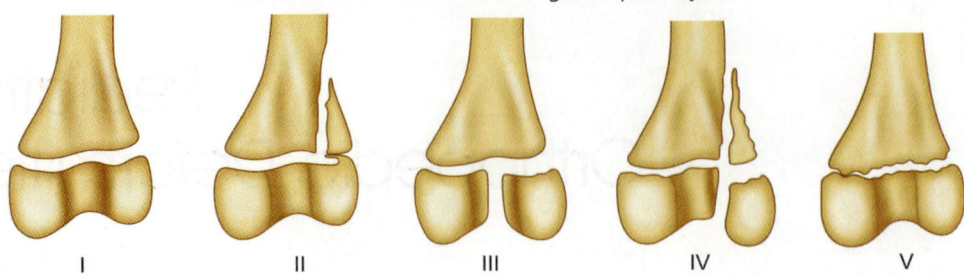

Fig. 14.2: Salter-Harris classification of physeal injuries. The metaphyseal fragment in type II injury is known as **Thurstan Holland** fragment

Treatment: Types I and II do not involve joint surface (epiphysis) and can be managed by closed reduction. Types III and IV pass through epiphysis and hence involve articular surface, thus accurate reduction is necessary which is achieved best by open reduction. Type V is generally a retrospective diagnosis when child presents with a growth arrest. Treatment here is mostly directed to resultant deformity.

Xtra edge
- Epiphyseal enlargement—juvenile rheumatoid arthritis, hyperthyroidism, rickets, spondylo-epiphyseal dysplasia.
- Epiphyseal dysgenesis/fragmented or punctate epiphysis—hypothyroidism.

PEDIATRIC HIP PROBLEMS

Limping Child

It means walking with difficulty due to causes in hip or any other parts of lower limb.
- **Painless limp**
  - 1–3 years: DDH, cerebral palsy, muscular dystrophy, infantile coxa vara
  - >3 years: Polio, limb length discrepancy, Perthes (classically painless)
- **Painful limp**
  - SCFE (10–14 years).
  - Osteochondritis dissecans.
  - Arthritis (septic/aseptic), osteomyelitis, synovitis.
  - Perthes (6–10 years) (may be painful at later stage).

Coxa Vara

Neck shaft angle at birth is 140° and femoral anteversion is 40°. When the child starts walking (i.e. bearing weight) neck shaft angle decreases to adult value of 125°+/–5° and anteversion to 15–20°, this happens till 8 years of age, after which there are no changes. When neck shaft angle is <120°, it is known as coxa vara and coxa valga when neck shaft angle >130°. Caused by growth anomaly at femoral epiphysis (congenital) or other acquired hip pathologies—SCFE, Perthes, Rickets, AVN, fractures of proximal femur.

Congenital coxa vara: Due to cartilaginous growth defect in inferomedial part of neck, cartilaginous area known as "Fairbank's triangle"(Fig. 14.3A). Complains of painless limp (characteristic), limitation of abduction and internal rotation, Trendelenburg gait in a child at an age, when he starts walking.

X-ray: Neck shaft angle <120°, vertical epiphysis, Fairbank's triangle.

Differential diagnosis: DDH (telescopy positive in DDH), Perthes' (age 6–10 years).

Treatment depends on HE (Hilgenreiner's epiphyseal) angle (Fig. 14.3B). It is angle between Hilgenreiner's line (horizontal line through triradiate cartilage) and line parallel to physis.
- Normal—0–25°
- <45°—observation
- >60°—surgery

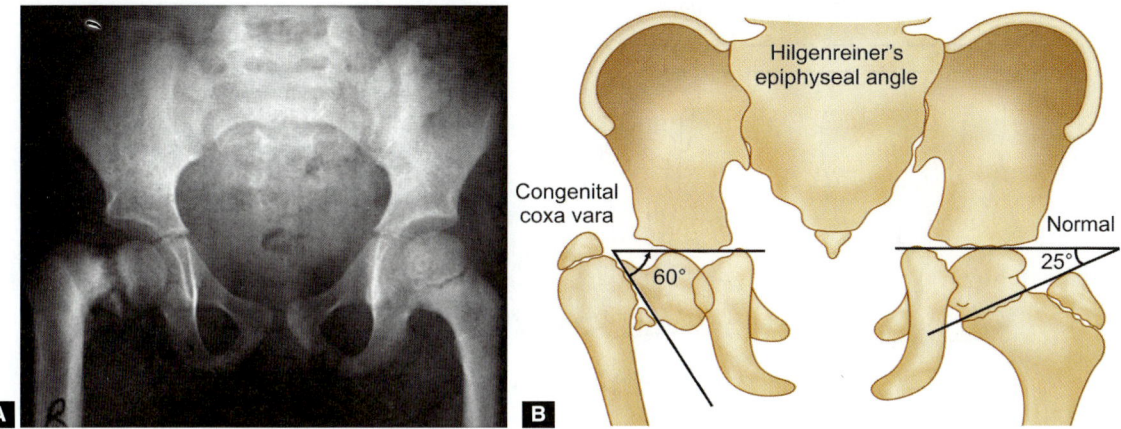

Fig. 14.3: (A) Note Fairbank's triangle in R side, (B) HE angle

- 45–60°—if progressive symptoms then surgery
- Surgery—subtrochanteric valgus osteotomy

Xtra edge
Fairbank's triangle: Differentials include—congenital coxa vara, non-union fracture neck of femur, Perthes' disease.

Developmental Dysplasia of Hip (DDH)
Spontaneous dislocation of hip due to dysplastic hip (head or acetabulum). Most common deformity however is shallow acetabulum and child may acquire compensatory genu valgum.

Sex: Females >> male.

Side involved: Left side most commonly involved, bilateral in 1/3rd cases.

Risk factors: 1st born female child, positive family history and intrauterine crowding—oligohydramnios, breech delivery. Diseases that are associated with intrauterine crowding—DDH, torticollis and metatarsus adductus (note: Twin pregnancy and CTEV is not a risk factor).

Clinical features
- Limited abduction/asymmetry in abduction of two limbs (especially in flexion), limb shortening, telescopy present and increased internal/external rotation of the dislocated hip.
- Vascular sign of Narath (absent femoral pulsations but present distal pulses) positive, prominent greater trochanter.
- Trendelenburg gait (U/L case) and waddling/duck/scissor gait (B/L cases), with increased lumbar lordosis (B/L > U/L).
- Asymmetrical thigh/buttock folds, and in B/L cases there is widened perineum with short stature.
- Galeazzi's sign/Allis sign (to assess limb shortening in U/L cases) is positive. In B/L cases there is no leg length discrepancy thus Galeazzi's sign is negative. In B/L cases, limb shortening is assessed by Klisic test. In Galeazzi's test, child is supine with both hips and knee flexed, affected limb will appear lower compared to unaffected side (Fig. 14.4A).
- In neonates/<3 months age, clinically screening can be done by:
  - Barlow's test (preferred)—we try to dislocate the hip, thus not positive in already dislocated hip. Child is placed supine with both hips and knee flexed, 1st part—limb adducted and pushed leading to dislocation and in 2nd part—limb abducted and pulled causing a clunk, indicating reduction (BARLOW = BAHARLO, i.e. dislocate).
  - Ortolani's test—it is similar to 2nd part of Barlow's test and here we try to reduce the already dislocated hip (Fig. 14.4B).

Screening: Clinical examination is enough to screen majority cases. If investigations are required, then USG is considered the screening tool for DDH in neonatal age group as it allows evaluation of cartilaginous femoral head prior to appearance of ossific nucleus, subluxation, dislocation,

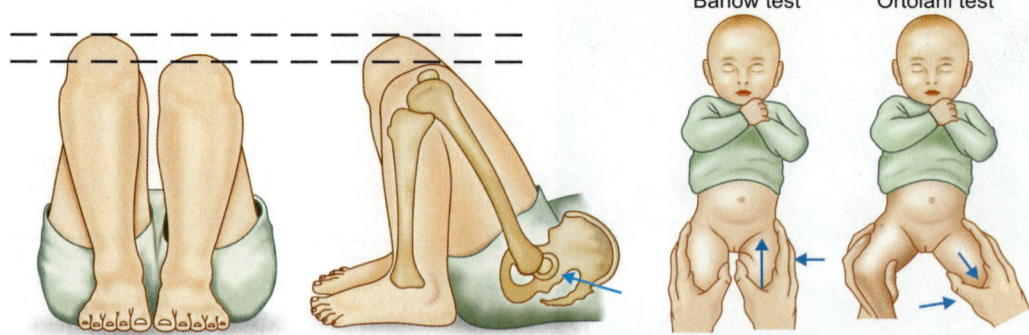

Fig. 14.4: (A) Galeazzi's sign, (B) Barlow's and Ortolani's test

pulvinar or inverted labrum, hypoplastic ossific nucleus, acetabular dysplasia and ossification. However, MRI allows assessment of complete disease spectrum, management and complications of DDH and is considered the best investigation. T1W image displays exact position of the cartilage and T2W images are useful for complications like ischemic necrosis (AVN) and effusions which are not demonstrated with USG/X-ray. USG measures alpha and beta angle for DDH, with increasing disease severity alpha angle decreases and beta angle increases.

IOC for DDH depends on the type of que:
- **In first 6 months of life:** USG is the IOC—as femoral head is primarily cartilagenous, so USG picks up well and getting MRI is un-necessary and challenging in this age group.
- **After 6 months of life:** MRI is the IOC as femoral head starts ossifying, USG cannot pick up bone. X-ray can still diagnose after 6 months but MRI is the IOC to evaluate complete disease process.
- **If que is asked simply IOC for DDH:** MRI.

X-ray indices (assessed on Von Rosen view)
- Perkin's line (vertical line from outer edge of acetabulum) and Hilgenreiner's line (line connecting the two triradiate cartilages) divide hip into four quadrants with the head lying in the lower and inner quadrant normally. When the head lies in lower and outer quadrant it is subluxed, and when lies in upper and outer quadrant it is dislocated. Center edge angle of Wiberg decreases in DDH.
- Acetabular index (angle between Hilgenreiner's line and line from triradiate cartilage to outer lip of acetabulum) calculated for acetabular dysplasia. Normal the angle is <30° and greater values will imply a dysplastic acetabulum (vertical and shallow).
- Broken Shenton's line, dysplastic acetabulum with delayed appearance of femoral head ossification center/retarded development of femur head.

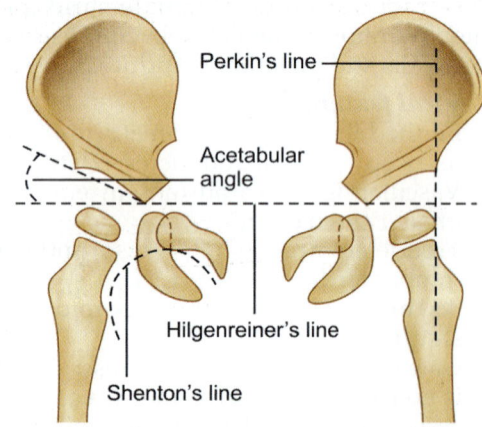

Fig. 14.5: Normal hip lines/angles seen in Von Rosen view

Treatment
- **Till 6 months**—closed reduction, forceful closed reduction (abduction and internal rotation) may lead to AVN of head > femoral nerve palsy. After closed reduction hip is immobilised in hip abduction splint–Pavlik harness (most common), Ilfeld-Craig splint, Von Rosen splint, Frejka pillow, etc. Reduction is assessed by USG/arthrography (rose thorn appearance). If the hip is unstable, i.e. dislocates again, hip is maintained in cast (Spica cast/bachelor's cast).
- 6–18 months—closed reduction and maintain reduction in hip spica cast/bachelor's cast.
- 18–36 months—closed reduction is difficult because of contracted hip capsule (capsule assumes hour glass shape); hypertrophied ligamentum teres, transverse acetabular ligament, pulvinar

fat, inverted acetabular labrum; interposition by iliopsoas tendon. **Attempts at closed reduction may end up in AVN.** Hence, open reduction + femoral rotational osteotomy and shortening (pelvic osteotomy may also be required in some cases) remains standard approach.
- >3 years—pelvis osteotomy is always required with femur shortening and rotational osteotomy.
- >10 years no treatment is given as child adapts to the situation, but if painful osteoarthritis is present, then total hip replacement may be done once bony maturity is attained.

Legg Claive Perthes Disease

Perthes disease also known as coxa plana/osteochondritis deformans juvenilis is AVN of proximal femoral epiphysis in a growing child.

Age/sex: 4–8 years (most susceptible age group because of femoral head blood supply), male > female.

Clinical features: Limp is the most common symptom that is aggravated by work/play and relieved by rest. Limp (most common symptom) is painless to start with and later becomes painful (2nd most common symptom). Limited abduction and internal rotation and when hip is flexed it goes into external rotation (Catterall sign). Trendelenburg gait is seen. All coagulopathies are risk factors for the development of disease.

Prognosis: It depends on age at presentation > duration of disease. **Head at risk signs** (poor prognostic sign) on X-ray include:
- Lateral subluxation of head.
- Horizontal growth plate.
- Metaphyseal cysts.
- Gage sign (radiolucent V sign).
- Calcification lateral to the capital epiphysis.
- Sagging rope sign—metaphyseal sclerotic band.

Classification: Salter Thompson, Catterall, Herring lateral pillar, Stulberg.

Investigations: MRI is the IOC, X-ray shows (Fig. 14.6)—fragmentation of epiphysis, subarticular fracture, flattening of head (coxa plana).

Treatment: Principle is to abduct the limb, so that head remains contained in the acetabular cavity. For abduction treatment may be done conservatively by applying abduction braces or by surgery.
- Abduction brace—broomstick/Petrie's cast.
- Surgery—femoral varus derotation osteotomy (most important) for containment of head. Chielectomy is removing osteophytes from head.

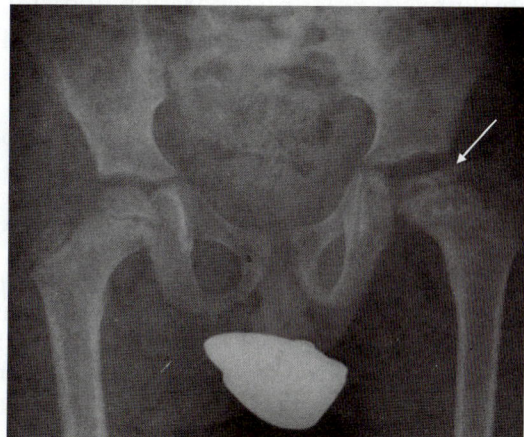

Fig. 14.6: Perthes' disease. Note the fragmented and flattened head

Slipped Capital Femoral Epiphysis (SCFE)

The term is a misnomer, as it is the neck which displaces, while capital epiphysis (i.e. head) remains in its position. Displacement occurs through hypertrophic zone of physis (Salter-Harris Type I injury) and neck is displaced anteriorly and superiorly relative to the epiphysis. It occurs in the age of growth spurt (12–15 years, male > female) due to shearing forces acting on the physeal plate.

Syndromes associated with SCFE: Endocrinopathies like hypothyroidism (most common), growth hormone excess, chronic renal failure (hyperparathyroidism), Turner's syndrome, etc.

Clinical features: The child is usually short and overweight boy (may be thin and tall), sexually immature, with endocrine disturbance, with complain of painful limp, antalgic gait, limitation of abduction and internal rotation with increased external rotation is characteristic. Hip is externally rotated when flexed. The slip may be acute or acute on chronic or chronic (most common). It may be B/L and chances increase when associated with endocrinopathy, thus opposite hip should also be evaluated.

Investigations
- X-ray—frog lateral view is ideal and best to detect minimal slip. Earliest finding is wide and irregular physis. When a line is drawn on superior border of neck on AP view (Klein's line), it will intersect a small portion of capital epiphysis laterally. When there is a slip, it will intersect a very small amount of epiphysis and in large slip there would not be any intersection, known as **Trethowan's sign**.
- Other X-ray signs—metaphyseal sign of steel, where there is a crescentic shaped area of increased density due to overlapping of head and neck due to slippage.
- MRI provides earliest diagnosis in pre-slip stage as it can study physeal cartilage.
- Bone scan—increased uptake in head, in AVN decreased uptake.

Treatment is always surgical. Aim is to prevent further slip and minimal or no attempt is made at reducing the slip, as it may be harmful and lead to AVN. Reduction is never done in chronic cases but in acute cases a gentle single attempt at reduction can be done. *In situ* fixation (screws or pins) is the treatment of choice.

Complications
- AVN
- Chondrolysis—presents with acute pain and global restriction of movement and on bone scan increased uptake in both sides of joint (acetabulum and head).

PEDIATRIC KNEE PROBLEMS

Traumatic Dislocation of Distal Femoral Epiphysis
Most (70–80%) of the femur length is gained by distal femur physis and that of tibia by proximal tibial physis. Fracture separation of distal femur epiphysis may occur and lead to growth abnormality. Distal femur epiphysis is displaced laterally in valgus force and anteriorly in hyperextension injury.

Congenital Dislocation of Knee
- It is a packing problem of intrauterine period, due to abnormal fetal position knee joint is locked in hyperextension. The disease spectrum ranges from hyperextension to dislocation, genu recurvatum/congenital hyperextension being the most common.
- Tibia is displaced anteriorly and laterally. Quadriceps and TFL is contracted/fibrosed, ACL is absent with hypoplastic patella.
- Since it is a intrauterine overcrowding problem, it may be associated with CTEV, DDH (ipsilateral), Metarsus adductus and Torticollis. It may also be associated with hyperlaxity syndromes like Ehlers-Danlos syndrome, Larsen's syndrome, etc.
- Treatment—if reduction can be done, then managed conservatively by serial casting till 90° flexion and if reduction is not possible, then surgery.

Angular Deformities of Knee
At birth, there is a varus alignment of knee which decreases to attain neutral alignment at about 2 years of age. After that, it increases towards valgus and attains max valgus at 4 years age then reduces to attain adult value of 6° valgus by 5–6 years age. For angular deformities, scannogram (full length X-ray of lower limb) is done.

Genu Valgum (Knock Knees)
It is abnormal valgus (i.e. greater than physiological valgus of 6°) of knees, presenting clinically as abnormal approximation of knees with divergent ankles, defined clinically as intermalleolar distance >8 cm in a standing child with knees approximated and patella facing forwards.

Causes
- Most common cause is idiopathic (physiological valgus persisting into adult life)
- Renal osteodystrophy
- Rickets
- Rheumatoid arthritis (OA causes varus deformity)
- OA of lateral compartment of knee joint
- Post-traumatic—fracture of lateral condyle of femur/tibia leading to growth arrest of lateral side.

Clinical features: Symptoms are due to overloading of lateral compartment of knee. Recurrent dislocation of patella is a common association.

Treatment is done only in symptomatic cases after the age of physiological valgus, in hope of spontaneous correction. Valgus deformity is generally due to femur and varus deformity due to tibia.
- If significant growth remaining—boys <12 and girls <10 years, are managed by growth modulation. Medial side physis growth is arrested temporarily by staples till deformity gets corrected and process is known as reversible "hemiepiphysiodesis".
- If child presents near or after skeletal maturity—corrective varus osteotomy in distal femur (closed wedge).

Genu Varum (Bow Legs)
When child is standing with the ankles approximated, if the distance between the medial joint line of knees is >6 cm, then genu varum is said to be present. Normal physiological varus persists till 2 years age and varus after that is pathological. Deformity may be in distal femur/knee or proximal tibia (most common).

Causes
- *Toddler*: Most common cause is physiological varus.
- *Pathological*:
  - Most common is rickets (India) and Blount's disease (worldwide)
  - Physeal injury of medial side (trauma, infection)
  - Osteoarthritis (most common cause in older adults)
  - Epiphyseal dysplasia.

Rickets: There is a gentle curve/bowing involving distal thigh and proximal legs, B/L deformity, child is short statured, stigmata of rickets present. X-ray shows signs of rickets—cupping, fraying, etc.

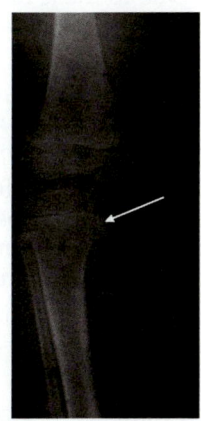

Fig. 14.7: Tibia vara (note beaking of metaphysis)

Tibia vara/Blount's disease: Osteochondrosis/disturbed growth of the medial proximal tibial physis leads to progressive varus and limb shortening. There is abrupt varus angulation below the knee and it is associated with internal tibial torsion (intoeing gait) and genu recurvatum. Siffert-katz sign may be present, i.e. medial femoral condyle may be subluxating posteromedially in the depressed medial tibial plateau. It may be U/L or B/L. X-ray—beaking of the proximal tibial metaphysis (Fig. 14.7). Infantile form (age at onset, 3 years) is most common and severe.

Treatment: Reassurance and observation till 2 years of age. Treatment is aimed at correcting the underlying cause, especially rickets. With correction of rickets deformity may resolve. Full time orthosis (HKAFO—hip knee ankle foot orthosis), medial upright elastic brace may be given to prevent deformity from increasing. If deformity not corrected/cause not known and child presents when significant growth remaining (boys <12 years and girls <10 years) hemi-epiphysiodesis (by staples) is done on lateral side. After correction staples are removed. After skeletal maturity lateral closing wedge osteotomy is done. Surgical treatment should be done before 4 years age.

Chondromalacia Patellae
It is softening of deeper layers of cartilage due to decrease in sulphated mucopolysaccharides affecting mostly young females and causing deep boring pain in knee anteriorly. Most important risk factor is malalignment in the extensor mechanism of lower limb leading to stress in patella. Skyline view X-ray is done for diagnosis.

PEDIATRIC LEG/FOOT PROBLEMS
Rocker Bottom Foot
It is a foot deformity either congenital or acquired where plantar surface of foot is convex, apex of convexity is at talar head.

Causes
- Congenital vertical/oblique talus—talus is vertical forming the most prominent part of sole. Syndromes associated are myelomeningocele, arthrogryposis, prune-belly syndrome, etc.

- Faulty/overcorrection of CTEV—forceful correction of equinus before adduction and varus are fully corrected, may cause equinus correction at mid-tarsal joint (ankle joint) leading to convex plantar surface.

Treatment: For congenital vertical talus—Grice-Green procedure (extra-articular arthrodesis of subtalar joint).

Congenital Talipes Equinovarus (CTEV) /Club Foot

It is the most common congenital orthopedic deformity in India (DDH worldwide). Males > females, B/L in 50% cases.

CTEV involves foot, ankle and leg and the deformities are:
- **C**avus at intertarsal joint (prominent medial longitudinal arch)
- **A**dduction of forefoot at tarsometatarsal joint
- **V**arus/inversion at subtalar joint   } CAVE
- **E**quinus at ankle joint, and
- Medial rotation of distal tibia.

    Due to these deformities, patient bears weight on the lateral border of foot and if untreated callosity and bursa may develop laterally.

Etiology
- Idiopathic (most common and present at birth)
- Secondary/atypical/acquired—neural tube defects (myelomeningocele), spina bifida, Friedreich's ataxia, etc. Acquired cases are not present at birth and develop CTEV later.

Pathogenesis: Deformities gets fixed by posteromedial soft tissue contracture and calf muscle contracture/fibrosis (decreased calf circumference). Talus is most severely affected and talo-navicular joint complex/dislocation is the cornerstone of the deformity. Syndromic clubfoot/acquired clubfoot is more severe and resistant to treatment.

Screening test: Dorsiflexion test—in newborn child foot can be dorsiflexed till its dorsum touches anterior surface of leg, this is normal. In CTEV this is not possible.

Scoring systems:
- Pirani score: 6 components, each graded on scale of (0–.5–1) in increasing severity and total possible score is 6.
    - Hindfoot—posterior heel crease, rigidity of equinus and empty heel.
    - Midfoot—medial crease, curvature of lateral border of foot and lateral head of talus.
- Dimeglio score.

X-ray: Diagnosis of CTEV is clinical, X-rays may be done in relapsed/recurrent cases.
- Talocalcaneal angle (Kite's angle): Normal is 20–40 and decreased in CTEV.
- Meary's angle.

Management: Treatment can be started as early as possible after birth, and serial manipulation with casting (above knee) is the treatment of choice. Order of correction is CAVE and is done by Ponseti technique. First cast is applied in supination to correct supination and from next cast, adduction and varus are corrected simultaneously and equinus is corrected at last. Equinus is most resistant to correction and Achilles tendon tenotomy is often required to correct equinus. Last cast is applied in dorsiflexion and abduction for 3 weeks. Earlier it was corrected by Kite's technique, where one deformity was addressed at a time adduction–varus–equinus (Table 14.1).

Table 14.1		
	Kite's method	*Ponseti technique*
At birth	Manipulation by mother	Manipulation and cast by doctor
Intervals between cast	Every 2 weeks	Every week (total 5–7 cast)
Order	A > V > E (cavus not addressed)	C > AV > E
Fulcrum while reducing	Calcaneocuboid joint (Kite's error)	Head of talus
Treatment duration	6–9 months	6–8 weeks

Once the deformity gets corrected it is maintained in foot abdution orthosis (Dennis Browne splint—Fig. 14.8) in dorsiflexion and foot abduction/external rotation. Till 1 year it is worn full time and after that CTEV shoes (designed by Thomas) in daytime and Dennis Browne splint at night till 7 years of age. As recurrence occurs till 7 years of age.

Surgery: Ponseti technique alone is not sufficient after 1–2 years age, soft tissues are not that pliable and these also get contracted/fibrosed. Thus, after 1–2 years, surgical procedures are required.

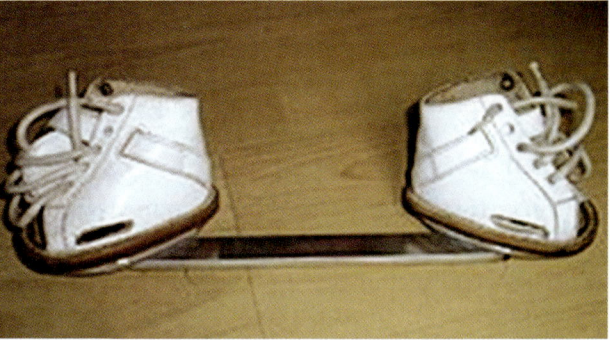

Fig. 14.8: Dennis Browne splint

- Posteromedial soft tissue release (1–3 years age): Tibialis posterior, FHL, FDL and TA lengthening. Turco's or McKay incision is used.
- After 3–5 years, bony procedures are added to PMSTR, mostly lateral column shortening procedures.
  - Dillwyn Evans procedure—ideal procedure for <8 years age group. Resection and fusion of calcaneocuboid joint.
  - Dwyer's osteotomy—in calcaneus to correct varus.
  - Lichtblau—shortening of calcaneal neck, i.e. extra-articular procedure.
- 8–10 years—wedge tarsectomy of lateral column.
- >10 years—triple arthrodesis for recurrent/resistant/persistent CTEV ideally done after 10 years age (as bones are ossified and fusion is possible). It involves fusion of 3 joints—talonavicular, calcaneocuboid and talocalcaneal. Pseudoarthrosis is the most common complication and occurs at talonavicular joint.
- JESS/Illizarov external fixator can also be used to correct deformity in skeletally matured children.

Congenital Pseudoarthrosis

Pseudoarthrosis is a false (pseudo) joint that may develop after non-union of a fracture. If too much motion exists at the nonunion site, fracture callus undergoes cystic degeneration, creating a false joint lined by synovial cells and fluid filled cavity. It may be also be seen after fracture or failed arthrodesis. The proximal fragment is cupped and distal end is pointing making shape of a joint (Fig. 14.9B).

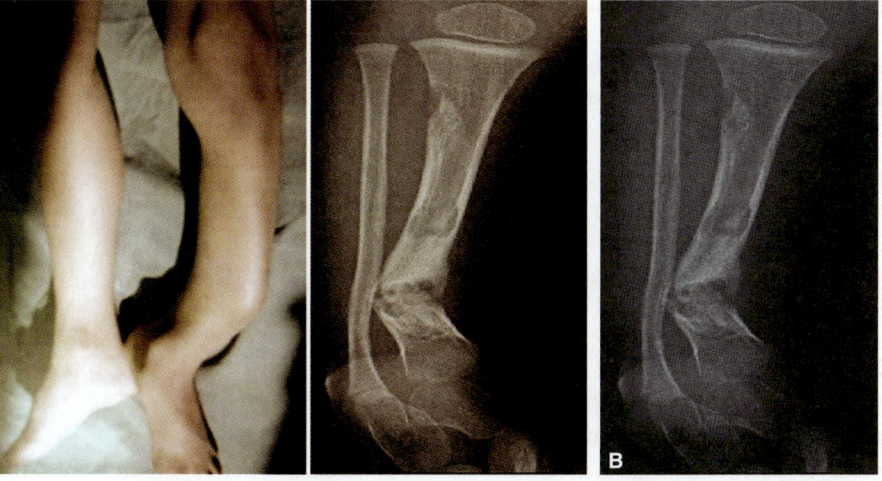

Fig. 14.9: (A) Congenital pseudoarthrosis of tibia (note the anterolateral bowing), (B) X-ray showing the pseudoarthrosis site resembling a joint

In *congenital pseudoarthrosis of tibia*, there is dysplasia (most commonly of tibia) of the distal third tibia and it is bowed **anterolaterally** (Fig. 14.9 A). It has high tendency for fracture and they often fail to unite leading to pseudoarthrosis. It is always unilateral and most common cause is idiopathic. Neurofibromatosis-I is associated in >50% cases. Classified by Boyd's classification; type II (hour glass constriction) is having highest risk, most commonly leads to pseudoarthrosis and associated with NF-I.

Differential diagnosis: Fibula hemimelia is a close D/D presenting with **anteromedial** bowing.

Treatment: Resection of pseudoarthrosis site, shortening, intramedullary nailing and bone grafting. Shortening may be addressed later by Illizarov technique. Vascularised fibula grafting after multiple failed attempts at union.

PEDIATRIC UPPER LIMB PROBLEMS

Radial Club Hand
There is congenital deficiency of radial side of upper extremity, with absence of radius that is either partial or complete (most common), thumb may be hypoplastic or absent. Forearm is short and radially deviated (Manus valgus).

Syndromes associated
- Holt-Oram syndrome (cardiac defect with absent radius)
- Fanconi's syndrome
- TAR syndrome (thrombocytopenia absent radius)
- VACTERL.

Investigations: Thorough investigations should always be done to rule out any associated syndromes. Echocardiography > platelet.

Treatment
- Centralisation of ulna.
- Pollicization of index finger, i.e. reconstruction of thumb by index finger.

Madelung Deformity
Madelung deformity is due to premature closure or defective development of the ulnar third of the distal epiphysis of the radius. This deformity results in a radial shaft that is bowed with increased interosseous space and dorsal subluxation of the distal radioulnar joint.

Congenital Radioulnar Synostosis
It is due to absence of longitudinal separation of radius and ulna, leading to osseous fusion of these two bones, proximal third being the most common. Forearm is most commonly fixed in pronation and supination/pronation movements are restricted. Surgery (osteotomy) is reserved for B/L cases.

Congenital Absence of Pectoral Muscle
Pectoral major and pectoral minor are the most common congenitally absent muscles. Diagnosis is made by USG.

Poland syndrome: Flattened chest wall, hypoplastic ribs, higher nipple and U/L increased radiolucency of lung on X-ray.

PEDIATRIC SPINE

Congenital (Infantile) Muscular Torticollis (Wry Neck)
- *Torticollis is of two types:* Congenital and secondary.
- Congenital/infantile torticollis is commonest type (due to fibrosis of sternocleidomastoid due to ischemia) and is associated with breech delivery, shoulder dystocia, birth injury (traumatic delivery) and SCM ischemia/tumor.

- Head is tilted towards affected side and chin to contralateral side producing "**Cock robin**" appearance (Fig. 14.10).
- SCM of affected side may be felt like hard fibrotic cord/a mass in body of SCM muscle (SCM tumor) in first 3 months of life and can resolve spontaneously over time.
- In long run there may be asymmetrical development of face (asymmetry flattening of skull—**plagiocephaly**).
- It is a type of packaging disorder and often associated with other packaging disorders like (DDH (5–20%) and metatarsus adductus).
- Can also be associated with atlanto-occipital abnormalities.
- *Treatment*: Passive stretching of affected SCM muscle/unipolar or bipolar release of SCM (optimum age—1 to 4 years).

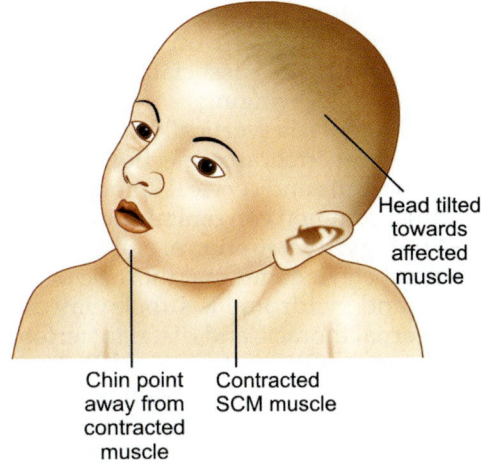

Head tilted towards affected muscle

Chin point away from contracted muscle

Contracted SCM muscle

Fig. 14.10: Deformities in congenital torticollis

Klippel-Feil Syndrome

Defined as multiple abnormal segments of cervical spine (i.e. defect of segmentation) and congenital fusion of 2 or more cervical vertebrae presenting with classic triad (seen in fewer than 50%).

- Low posterior hair line
- Short webbed neck
- Limited neck movements

Cervical fusion may be craniocervical (occiput to C2) or subaxial (i.e. below C2) or both (Fig. 14.11 A and B). If the features of triad are present without any apparent SCM contracture (i.e. torticollis is ruled out), then X-ray should be done to evaluate cervical spine to make the diagnosis of this syndrome.

Associated disorders

- Sprengel's shoulder
- Scoliosis
- Torticollis
- Neurological involvement due to trauma/scoliosis

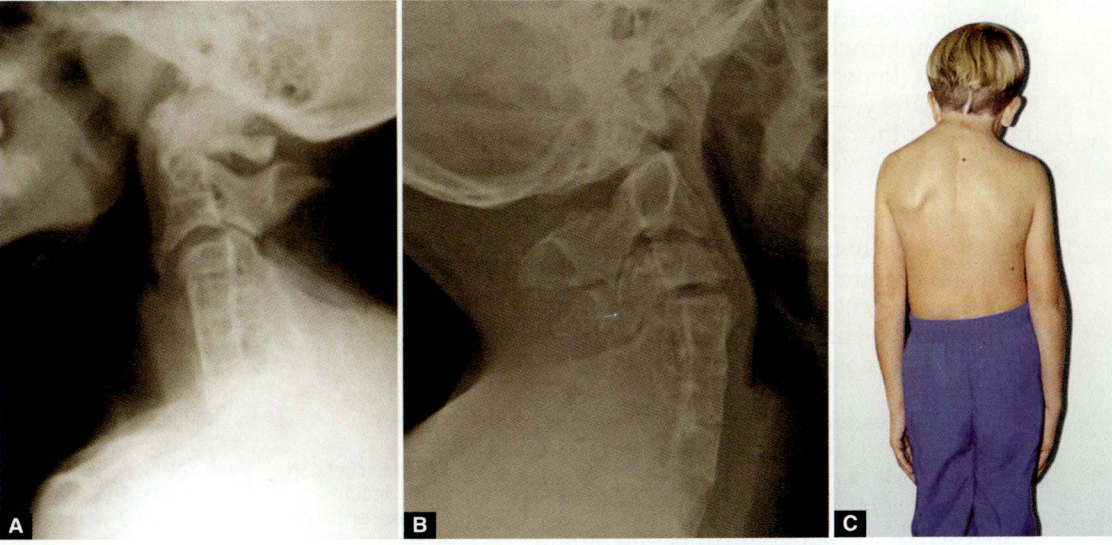

Fig. 14.11: (A) Preaxial fusion, (B) Subaxial fusion, (C) Clinical picture

Sprengel Shoulder

- Congenital condition with a small and undescended scapula (Fig. 14.12) often associated with
  - scapular winging
  - hypoplasia (vertically small and broad)
  - omo-vertebral connection (bar) between superior medial angle of scapula and cervical spine (30–50%)
- Most common congenital shoulder anomaly in children
- **Etiology:** Interruption of embryonic subclavian blood supply at level of subclavian, internal thoracic or suprascapular artery in contrast, Poland syndrome is subclavian artery interruption proximal to internal thoracic and distal to vertebral artery
- **Associated diseases:** Klippel-Feil (approximately 1/3 have Sprengel deformity), congenital scoliosis, kidney diseases.

Vertebra Plana

Vertebra plana (a.k.a. **pancake/silver dollar/coin-on-edge vertebra**) is the term given when a vertebral body has lost almost its entire height anteriorly and posteriorly, representing a very advanced compression fracture (Fig. 14.13). Disc spaces are fairly maintained.

Causes of vertebra plana—**ILLEGAL**
- **I**nfection (TB/pyogenic spondylitis)
- **L**eukaemia
- **L**ymphoma
- **E**wing's sarcoma
- **G**aucher's disease
- **A**neurysmal bone cyst
- **L**CH (eosinophilic granuloma–commonest cause).

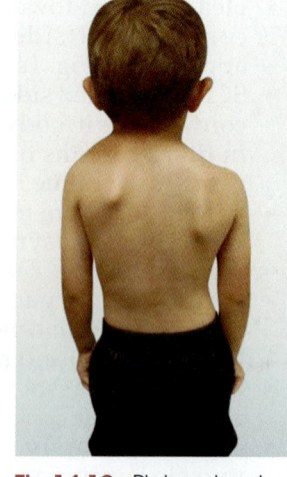

Fig.14.12: Picture showing elevated scapula on left side

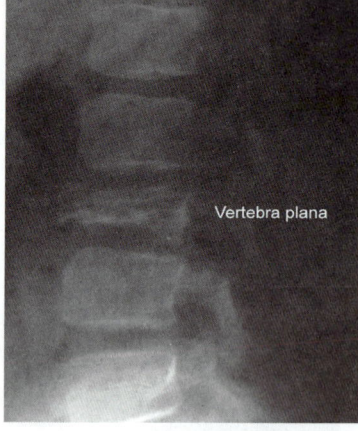

Vertebra plana

Fig. 14.13: X-ray of vertebra plana

Scoliosis

- Scoliosis (lateral curvature of spine) is a 3-dimensional deformity of spine as there is also rotational deformity of spine along with lateral deviation.
- It may be structural (permanent and fixed) or non-structural (temporary). Types under temporary:
  - **Postural**—most common type of non-structural scoliosis, where on forward bending the scoliotic curve disappears, whereas in structural variety, the curve becomes more prominent (known as Adam's test).
  - **Compensatory**—it is due to some deformity outside/below the spine in pelvis, hip or lower limb and spine compensates to the deformity by making a scoliotic curvature. On sitting, the effect of lower limb deformity on spine nullifies and thus scoliotic curvature also disappears.
- *Classification of structural scoliosis* (Fig. 14.14A)
  1. **Cause** is mostly unknown and **idiopathic** scoliosis is the most common form.
  2. **Congenital** scoliosis is present at birth and is due to some vertebral anomalies (Fig. 14.14B), mostly affects girls.
     Prognosis
     - *Unilateral unsegmented bar with contralateral hemivertebra*: Carries worst prognosis with greatest risk of progression.
     - *Block vertebra*: Have best prognosis and lowest risk of progression (most stable and least progression).

Idiopathic scoliosis classification	
Approximately 80% of patients with scoliosis have idiopathic scoliosis	
– Old classification	
• Infantile	Onset <3 years age
• Juvenile	Onset 3–10 years age
• Adolescent	Onset > years age
– New classification	
• Early onset	Onset < 8 years age
• Late onset	Onset > 8 years age

Fig. 14.14A: Classification of scoliosis

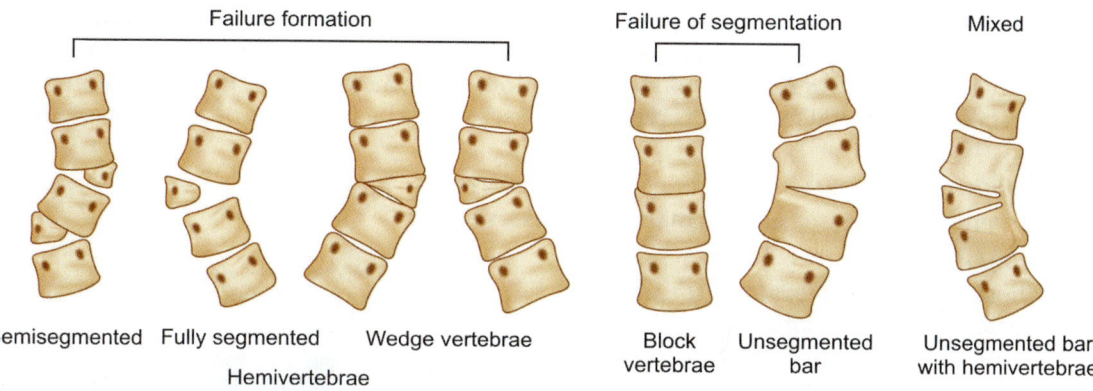

Fig. 14.14B: Congenital anomalies in vertebral formation leading to congenital scoliosis

3. **Neuromuscular scoliosis** caused by polio, cerebral palsy, spina bifida, muscular dystrophy, neurofibromatosis.

Associated conditions

May occur in isolation or with associated conditions
- Cardiac defects
- Genitourinary defects
- Spinal cord malformations
- VACTERL syndrome
- Klippel-Feil syndrome

Evaluation

- **Cobb's angle:** It measures severity of scoliosis (from upper and lower border of vertebrae) and thus guides in management of scoliosis (Fig. 14.15A).

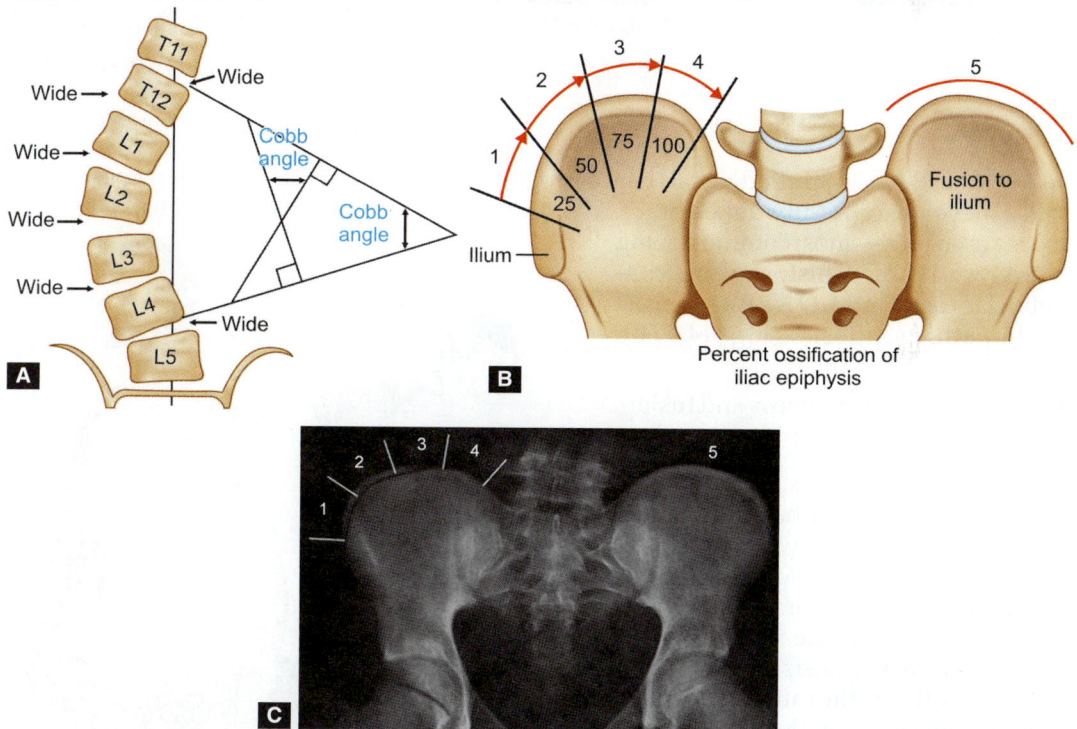

Fig. 14.15: (A) Cobb's angle, (B) Grading of Risser's sign, (C) X-ray showing grade 5 in left and grade 3 in right side

- **Risser sign:** The **Risser sign** is an indirect measure of skeletal maturity, whereby the ossification stage of the iliac apophysis is used to judge the ossification of the spinal vertebrae. On a scale of 5, it gives a measure of progression of ossification; grade 5 means that 100% of iliac apophysis is ossified (i.e. skeletal maturity is reached). Risser sign is based on the observation of an X-ray image (Fig. 14.15B).

Management of scoliosis

Non-structural scoliosis is always managed conservatively.

Structural scoliosis

- Scoliosis due to vertebral malformation/neurological disorders are high risk for rapid progression and thus mostly managed surgically.
- In idiopathic variety (Fig. 14.16 and Table 14.2), it depends on curve severity (Cobb's angle) and amount of growth remaining (Risser's grade/triradiate cartilage open or fused). If curve is more and significant growth remaining (i.e. Risser's grade lower), then it has high risk of curve progression and thus managed surgically. Curves <25° is managed conservatively and >45° is managed surgically. Between 25 and 45°, depends on curve progression and symptoms.

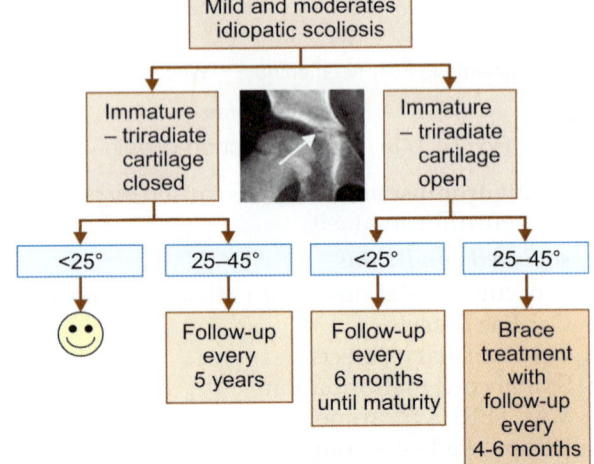

Fig. 14.16: Management of Idiopathic scoliosis

Curve magnitude (degrees)	Risser's grade 0/premenarchal	Risser's grade 1/2	Risser's grade 3,4,5
<25	Observation	Observation	Observation
25–45	Brace	Brace	Observation
>45	Surgery	Surgery	Surgery (>50°)

Table 14.2: Management of idiopathic scoliosis

Conservative: Brace is applied to halt curve progression and is useful only when apex of curve is below T7 level (except Milwaukee brace which was used for higher apex curves). DLSO/TLSO brace are used now—most common being Boston brace. Braces of historical braces—Turnbuckle cast (Fig. 14.17A), Risser's cast (for idiopathic scoliosis) (Fig. 14.17B), Minerva cast.

Surgery: Corrective osteotomy and fusion, (Harrington rod was used in past).

Scheuermann's Kyphosis

A rigid thoracic hyperkyphosis defined by > 45° caused by anterior wedging of >5° across three consecutive vertebrae and is differentiated from postural kyphosis by rigidity of curve. It is the most common type of structural kyphosis in adolescents located usually in thoracic spine (less common form occurs in thoracolumbar/lumbar region).

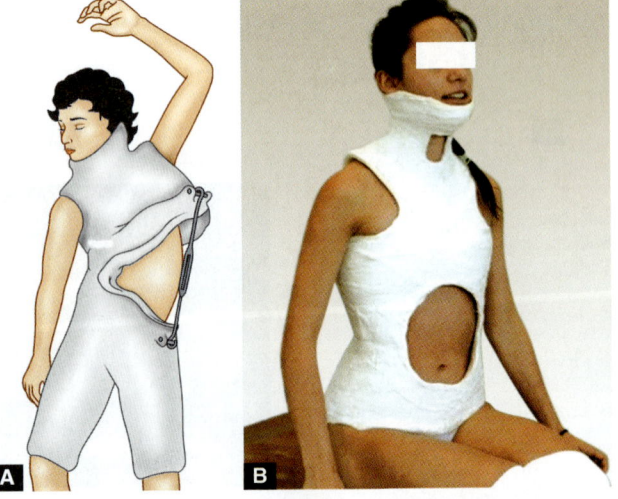

Fig. 14.17: (A) Turnbuckle cast, (B) Risser's cast

MISCELLANEOUS

Battered Baby Syndrome

Characteristic orthopedic findings:

- Subtle fractures like—subepiphyseal microfractures (detected on MRI).
- Due to abuse/rough handling of the child, a chip fracture of long bone results where a corner of long bone metaphysis is torn off with damage to epiphysis and periosteum (**characteristic**).
- Metaphyseal bucket handle fractures (**characteristic**).
- Fractures are most often spiral and involve proximal portion of limbs, i.e. femur > humerus > tibia.

MULTIPLE CHOICE QUESTIONS

1. A 4-year-old child is brought to emergency with complain of severe pain in arm after a fall, immediate X-ray done shows fracture distal radius and ulna. Which of the following term best describes the fracture?

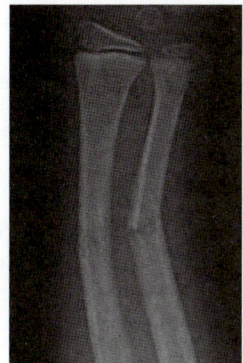

   A. Torus   B. Greenstick
   C. Barton's   D. Colles

2. A 4-year-old child presented to the clinic with a history of fall on outstretched hand. Radiographs revealed a broken anterior cortex with an intact posterior cortex of the radius with an exaggerated bowing of the radius. The fracture sustained is known as:
   A. Torus fracture
   B. Greenstick fracture
   C. Galeazzi fracture
   D. Monteggia fracture dislocation

3. Greenstick fractures are seen in:
   A. Children
   B. Elderly
   C. Young adults
   D. Common in all age group

4. Which of the following is true about fracture in children?
   A. Brittle bone
   B. Angulation and rotation not tolerated
   C. Immobilization leads to fixity of adjacent joints
   D. Complete fracture is more common than greenstick

5. What type of fracture is shown on X-ray?

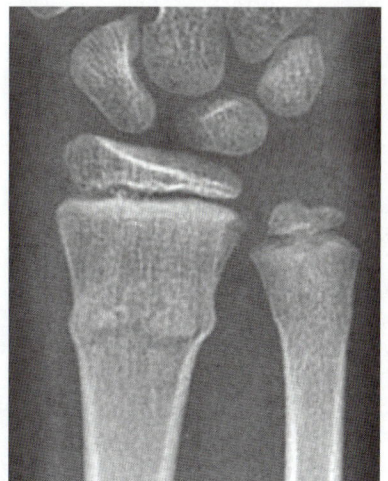

   A. Plastic deformation
   B. Greenstick fracture
   C. Torus fracture
   D. Epiphyseal injury

6. Most common bone to be fractured in children is:
   A. Distal radius   B. Clavicle
   C. Supracondylar   D. Radius/ulna

7. Greenstick fracture is:
   A. Fracture in adults   B. Complete fracture
   C. Incomplete fracture D. Fracture spine

8. A 6-year-old child falls in right-sided forearm region and develops fracture in dorsal surface of mid region of radius. The best treatment is:
   A. Antibiotics and sedative
   B. Bone plating and external fixation
   C. Slab with wait for bone imperfect
   D. Break the cortex other side and immobilization by POP

9. In children, all are true *except*:
   A. Dislocations are rare
   B. Comminuted fractures are common
   C. Thick periosteum
   D. Soft bones

10. **What type of fracture is shown on X-ray?**

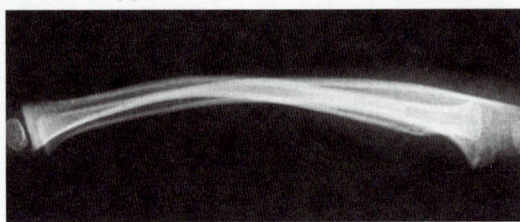

   A. Plastic deformation
   B. Greenstick fracture
   C. Torus fracture
   D. Epiphyseal injury

11. **Which statements pertaining to greenstick fracture is correct?**
   A. Any fracture in child
   B. Is generally incomplete
   C. Fracture only in rickets children
   D. All of the above

12. **In children, best remodeling is seen in fracture with:**
   A. Angulation in diaphysis
   B. Angulation in metaphysis
   C. Rotation in diaphysis
   D. Rotation in metaphysis

13. **Which is the commonest fracture in children?**
   A. Fracture clavicle
   B. Supracondylar fracture
   C. Greenstick fracture of lower end of radius
   D. All of the above

14. **Salter-Harris classification is used for:**
   A. Supracondylar humerus fractures in children
   B. Estimation of growth of the physes
   C. Physeal injuries
   D. Severity of degloving injuries to the limb

15. **A 4-year-old child suffered from a fall on outstretched band. X-rays revealed a fracture with the fracture line at the physes with a small metaphyseal fragment. There was no epiphyseal fracture. What type of injury by Salter-Harris classification is this?**
   A. I   B. II
   C. III   D. IV

16. **Metaphyseal fracture touching physis but not crossing it, comes under which type of Salter-Harris physeal injury?**
   A. I   B. II
   C. III   D. IV

17. **Thurston Holland sign is seen in:**
   A. Type I   B. Type II
   C. Types III   D. Type IV

18. **Salter-Harris classification is for:**
   A. Fracture supracondylar humerus
   B. Fracture epiphysis in children
   C. Fracture lateral condyle humerus
   D. Fracture shaft femur

19. **Perichondrial ring is:**
   A. Seen around foramen magnum
   B. Seen around epiphyseal plate
   C. More prominent in adults
   D. Shear strength increases with age

20. **Type VI Rang's injury includes:**
   A. Transverse fracture of metaphysic with longitudinal extension into physis
   B. Open injury with loss of physis
   C. Thurston Holland's sign
   D. Perichondrial ring injury

21. **An 8-year-old boy with a history of fall from 10 feet height complains of pain in the right ankle. X-ray taken at that time are normal without any fracture line. But after 2 years, he developed a calcaneovalgus deformity. The diagnosis is:**
   A. Undiagnosed malunited fracture
   B. Avascular nercrosis of talus
   C. Tibial epiphyseal injury
   D. Ligamentous injury of ankle joint

22. **Epiphyseal enlargement occurs in:**
   A. Paget's disease
   B. Sheurmann's disease
   C. Epiphyseal dysplasia
   D. Juvenile rheumatoid arthritis

23. **Epiphyseal dysgenesis is a feature of:**
   A. Hyperparathyroidism
   B. Hypoparathyroidism
   C. Hypothyroidism
   D. Hyperthyroidism

24. **All the following are causes of a painful limp** *except*:
   A. Slipped femoral epiphysis
   B. TB of the hip
   C. Perthes' disease
   D. Infantile coxa vara

25. **Causes of a painless limp in infancy includes:**
   A. Congenital dislocation of hip
   B. Infantile coxa vara
   C. Poliomyelitis
   D. All of the above

26. **Cause of coxa vara:**
   A. Congenital   B. Perthes' disease
   C. SCFE   D. All of the above

27. **Fairbank's triangle is seen in:**
   A. CTEV   B. DDH
   C. SCFE   D. Coxa vara

28. **Congenital coxa vara is treated by:**
   A. Fixation by SP nail B. Osteotomy
   C. Bone grafting   D. Traction

29. **Coxa vara is found in:**
   A. Perthes' disease   B. SCFE
   C. Rickets   D. All of the above

30. Name the test performed:

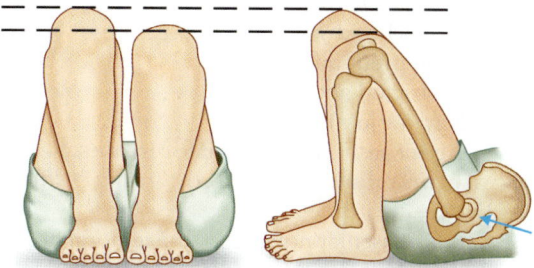

   A. Galeazzi's sign   B. Barlow's test
   C. Ortolani's test   D. Trendelenburg test

31. All of the following are true regarding congenital dislocation of hip *except*:
   A. Asymmetric thigh folds may be seen
   B. Galeazzi sign and Ortolani test may be positive
   C. It may be bilateral
   D. Polyhydramnios is a known risk

32. The following pelvic X-ray was seen in a patient. All the following signs will be present *except*:

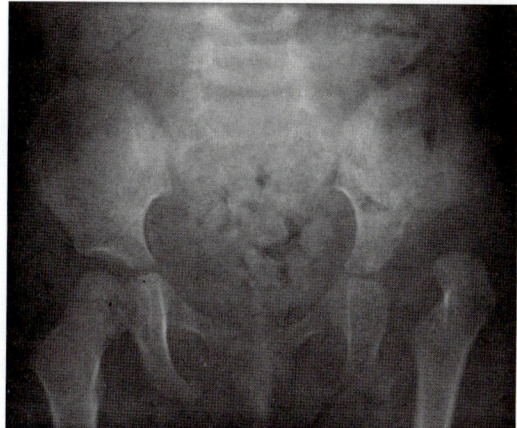

   A. Ortolani   B. Barlow
   C. Narath   D. Gaenslen's test

33. A 4-month-child diagnosed with DDH, cast used after closed reduction is:
   A. Hip spica   B. Pavlik harness
   C. Minnerva cast   D. Risser's cast

34. Pavlik harness is used to treat:
   A. Developmental dysplasia of hip
   B. Perthes' disease
   C. Slipped capital femoral epiphysis
   D. Congenital coxa vara

35. Irregular thigh folds are seen in:
   A. Developmental dysplasia of hip
   B. Perthes' disease
   C. Slipped capital femoral epiphysis
   D. Congenital coxa vara

36. Which of the following is not seen in a child with DDH?
   A. Wadding gait
   B. Feeling of femoral artery pulsation is difficult
   C. Decreased growth hormone
   D. Ortolani test is positive

37. Ortolani's test is used to diagnose:
   A. Congenital coxa vara
   B. Slipped capital femoral epiphysis
   C. Developmental dysplasia of the hip
   D. Perthes' disease

38. Positive Galeazzi sign is seen in:
   A. Unilateral DDH
   B. Bilateral DDH
   C. Distal radioulnar dislocation
   D. Distal radius fracture

39. Perkin's line on X-ray is used for diagnosis of:
   A. Perthes' disease   B. CDH
   C. CTEV   D. AVN hip

40. Ortolani test is positive when the examiner hears the:
   A. Clunk of entry on abduction and flexion of hip
   B. Clunk of entry on extension and adduction of hip
   C. Click of exit on abduction and flexion of hip
   D. Click of exit on extension and adduction of hip

41. Which of the following is NOT a feature of DDH?
   A. Smaller epiphysis of femoral head
   B. Inclination of acetabular roof is increased
   C. Shenton's line disrupted
   D. Femoral head is anteverted

42. Salter's pelvic osteotomy is done for treatment of:
   A. CTEV   B. SCFE
   C. DDH   D. None

43. Von Rosen's sign is positive in:
   A. Perthes' disease   B. SCFE
   C. DDH   D. CTEV

44. Bachelors' cast is used in:
   A. Fracture radius   B. Club foot
   C. DDH   D. Fracture calcaneum

45. Provocative test for detecting CDH:
   A. Peterson test   B. Barlow test
   C. Perkin's test   D. Von Rosen tests

46. Dysplastic hip in a child, investigation of choice:
   A. X-ray   B. MRI
   C. USG   D. CT scan

47. Primary pathology in CDH:
   A. Large head of femur
   B. Shallow acetabulum
   C. Excessive retroversion
   D. Everted limbus

48. Alpha angle in DDH:
A. Decreases   B. Increases
C. Constant   D. Variable

49. True about bilateral DDH:
A. Exaggerated lordosis
B. B/L genu valgum
C. Wadding gait
D. Shenton's line broken
E. Short stature
F. All of the above

50. All of the following statements are true about development dysplasia (DDH) of the hip, except:
A. It is more common in females
B. Oligohydramnios is associated with a higher risk of DDH
C. The hourglass appearance of the capsule may prevent a successful closed reduction
D. Twin pregnancy is a known risk factor

51. Beta angle in DDH:
A. Decreases   B. Increases
C. Constant   D. Variable

52. Barlow's test is done for testing:
A. CDH in child
B. DDH in infancy
C. Femoral neck fracture
D. Slipped femoral epiphysis

53. In a newborn child, abduction and internal rotation produces a click sound. It is:
A. Ortolani's sign   B. Telescoping sign
C. Lachman's sign   D. McMurray's sign

54. Commonest deformity in congenital dislocation of hip:
A. Small head of femur
B. Angle of torsion
C. Decreased neck shaft angle
D. Shallow acetabulum

55. What is the diagnosis in a boy of 8 years old presenting with the following X-ray:

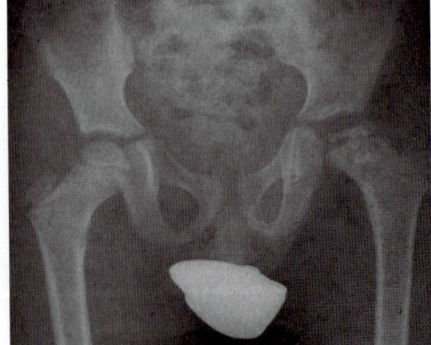

A. Perthes' disease
B. SCFE
C. Nonunion fracture neck of femur
D. Coxa vara

56. Regarding Legg-Calvé-Perthes' disease all are correct except (PGI type):
A. Osteochondritis
B. Male predominance
C. Restricted abduction
D. Narrow joint space
E. Age of onset is not related to disease severity

57. All of the following are true regarding Perthes' disease except:
A. It is avascular necrosis of the femoral head
B. Commonly affects children in the first decade
C. Limp and restricted rotations of the hip are common clinical features
D. MRI is not a good confirmatory investigation

58. Which of the following are true about Perthes' disease?
A. Self-limiting condition
B. Bilateral in 20% cases
C. Painful condition
D. Femoral head is displaced laterally
E. More common in females

59. Which of the following movements is restricted in Perthes' disease?
A. Adduction and external rotation
B. Abduction and external rotation
C. Adduction and internal rotation
D. Abduction and internal rotation

60. True about perthes' disease is:
A. Avascular necrosis of femoral head
B. Onset before 10 years of age
C. Osteotomy is used for treatment
D. Limb shortening
E. Joint space obliterated

61. Which one of the following is the IOC for evaluation of suspected Perthes' disease?
A. Plain X-ray
B. Ultrasonography (US)
C. Computed tomography (CT)
D. Magnetic resonance imaging (MRI)

62. The commonest cause of limp in a child of seven years is:
A. TB hip
B. CDH
C. Perthes' disease
D. Slipped upper femoral epiphysis

63. An 8-year-old male with painless limp on examination and restricted abduction and internal rotation left hip, probable diagnosis is:
A. Septic arthritis of hip
B. Tuberculosis arthritis of hip
C. Cong dislocation of hip
D. Perthes' disease

64. **Perthes' disease is treated by:**
    A. High dose of calcium with steroids
    B. Total hip replacement
    C. Supervised containment of femoral head in acetabulum
    D. Relieving weight bearing

65. **Steels metaphyseal sign is seen in:**
    A. Perthes' disease   B. SCFE
    C. DDH   D. Coxa vara

66. **All are true about slipped capital femoral epiphysis *except*:**
    A. Usually occur after 10 years of age
    B. Obesity is a risk factor
    C. Frog-leg lateral view is helpful
    D. More common in girls

67. **SCFE is most commonly seen in age:**
    A. 1–5 years   B. 6–10 years
    C. 10–15 years   D. 15–20 years

68. **Slipped capital femoral epiphysis is seen most commonly in which age group?**
    A. Infants   B. Adolescents
    C. Old age   D. Childhood

69. **Slipped capital femoral epiphyses slips in which direction?**
    A. No slip
    B. Posteromedial
    C. Anterolateral
    D. Medical

70. **An 11-year-old 70 kg child presents with limitation of abduction and internal rotation. There is tenderness in scarpas triangle. On flexing the hip the limb is externally rotated. The diagnosis is:**
    A. Perthes' disease
    B. Slipped capital femoral epiphyses
    C. Observation hip
    D. Tuberculosis hip

71. **A 14-year-old boy with 78 kg weight and hypothyroidism developed sudden onset of severe pain and tenderness on left hip as a result of minor fall. Most diagnosis is:**
    A. Fracture neck femur
    B. SCFE
    C. Perthes
    D. Hip dislocation

72. **Trethowan's sign is seen in:**
    A. Perthes' disease
    B. CDH
    C. SCFE
    D. Fracture neck femur

73. **Treatment of SCFE is:**
    A. Conservative
    B. Surgery by osteotomy
    C. Reduction and pinning
    D. *In situ* pinning

74. **Traumatic dislocation of epiphysial plate of distal femur occurs:**
    A. Medially   B. Laterally
    C. Posteriorly   D. Rotationally
    E. Anteriorly

75. **Commonest presentation of congenital dislocation of knee is:**
    A. Varus   B. Valgus
    C. Flexion   D. Hyperextension

76. **A 7-year-old young boy, had fracture of lateral condyle of femur. He developed malunion as the fracture was not reduced anatomically. Malunion will produce:**
    A. Genu valgum   B. Genu varum
    C. Genu recurvatum   D. Dislocation of knee

77. **Most common cause of genu valgum in children is:**
    A. Osteoarthritis
    B. Rickets
    C. Paget's disease
    D. Rheumatoid arthritis

78. **A child with 4 years age and angular deformity in knee with the following X-ray, diagnosis is:**

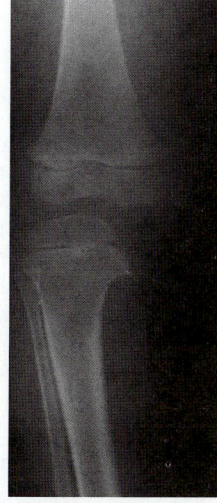

    A. Blount's disease   B. Rickets
    C. Genu valgum   D. Genu recurvatum

79. **Blount's disease results in a bowleg deformity due to:**
    A. Defect in posteromedial part of upper tibial epiphysis
    B. Endocrinopathy
    C. Recovery stage of rickets
    D. Deformity in proximal tibia

80. **Varus is:**
    A. Distal part towards midline
    B. Distal part away from the midline
    C. Proximal part towards midline
    D. Proximal part away from midline

81. **Which of the following is not a treatment option in this deformity?**

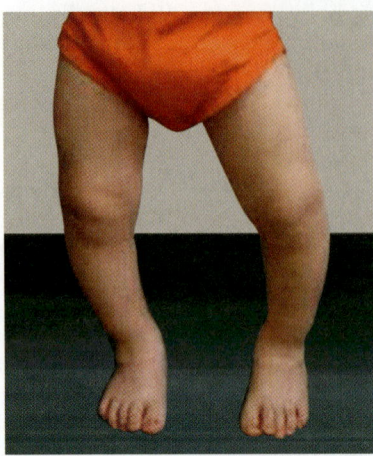

    A. Medial closing wedge osteotomy
    B. Lateral closing wedge osteotomy
    C. Full time orthosis
    D. Correction of metabolic disorder

82. **Charlie Chaplin gait is seen in:**
    A. CDH
    B. Congenital coxa vara
    C. Genu valgum
    D. External tibial torsion

83. **Blount's disease is:**
    A. Genu valgus   B. Tibia vara
    C. Flat foot   D. Genu recurvatum

84. **Which statement is true regarding bowleg?**
    A. In infants, it may be considered normal
    B. Occurs due to epiphyseal dysplasia
    C. Seldom associated with tibial angulation
    D. Affects only tibia but never femur

85. **Critical age of osteotomy for genu varum is:**
    A. 4 years   B. 6 years
    C. 8 years   D. 10 years

86. **True regarding genu varum is:**
    A. Orthosis is a must only during weight bearing
    B. Orthosis is recommended during daytime
    C. Orthosis is recommended during nighttime
    D. Orthosis is recommended full time

87. **Rocker bottom foot is due to:**
    A. Overtreatment of CTEV
    B. Malunited fracture calcaneum
    C. Horizontal talus
    D. Neural tube defect

88. **Rocker bottom foot is seen in:**
    A. Congenital vertical talus
    B. Arthrogryposis
    C. Holding club foot in too long corrected position
    D. All of the above

89. **In nail patella syndrome the patella is:**
    A. Small of absent   B. Larger
    C. Triangular   D. Square

90. **Pirani scoring includes all *except* (PGI type):**
    A. Medical crease
    B. Protrusion of cuboid bone
    C. Lateral crease
    D. Curvature of lateral border
    E. Concavity of sole

91. **Who devised correction of CTEV by serial casting?**
    A. Ignacio Ponseti   B. Gerhard Kuntscher
    C. Gavriil Ilizarov   D. Hugh Owen Thomas

92. **Club foot clinically presents as:**
    A. Calcaneovalgus   B. Equinovarus
    C. Equinocavovarus   D. Calcaneovarus

93. **Overcorrection of CTEV may lead to which of the following deformity:**
    A. Rocker bottom foot
    B. Calcaneovalgus
    C. Metatarsus adductus
    D. Hammer toe

94. **All of the following are described procedures for CTEV *except*:**
    A. Dwyer's osteotomy
    B. Posteromedial soft tissue release
    C. Triple arthrodesis
    D. Salter's osteotomy

95. **All of the following are done for management of clubfoot at birth *except*:**
    A. Manipulation
    B. Serial casting
    C. Recording the deformity to see improvements serially
    D. Posteromedial soft tissue release

96. **The last deformity to be corrected by Ponseti method for CTEV is:**
    A. Heel varus   B. Equinus
    C. Foot adduction   D. Cavus

97. **The typical deformity in CTEV is:**
    A. Ankle equinus
    B. Subtalar inversion
    C. Forefoot adduction
    D. All of the above

98. **Not true about atypical CTEV:**
    A. Foot is flexed downward
    B. Sole creases are not found
    C. Difficult to treat than typical variety
    D. May be associated with meningomyelocele

99. **What is the best management of CTEV in newborn?**
    A. Manipulation alone
    B. Manipulation and corrective splint
    C. Corrective surgery
    D. Wait and watch

100. **In correction of CTEV, which one of the following deformities resists?**
 A. Equinus
 B. Varus
 C. Adduction
 D. Cavus

101. **True about clubfoot:**
 A. Abduction of forefoot
 B. Associated with breech presentation
 C. Dennis-Brown splint used
 D. Adduction of forefoot
 E. Associated with spina bifida

102. **These shoes are used in:**

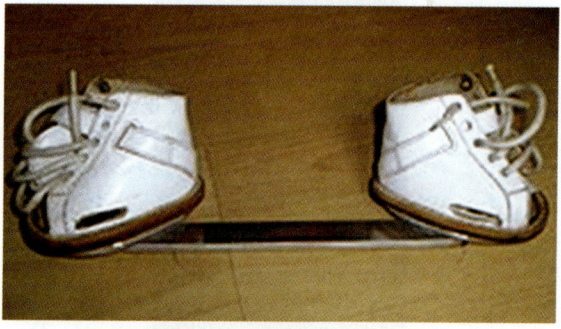

 A. CTEV
 B. Congenital vertical talus
 C. Rocker bottom foot
 D. Metatarsus adductus

103. **Causes of secondary clubfoot at birth are all *except*:**
 A. Idiopathic
 B. Arthrogryposis multiplex congenita
 C. Poliomyelitis
 D. Spina bifida

104. **Splint used in CTEV after correction:**
 A. Bohler-Brown splint
 B. Thomas splint
 C. Dennis-Brown splint
 D. None of the above

105. **In neglected cases of CTEV, joint fused are:**
 A. Calcaneocuboid, talonavicular and talo-calcaneal
 B. Tibiotalar, calcaneocuboid and talonavicular
 C. Ankle joint, calcaneocuboid and talonavicular
 D. None of the above

106. **Most common cause of CTEV:**
 A. Arthrogryposis multiplex congenita
 B. Spina bifida
 C. Idiopathic
 D. Neural tube defect

107. **Most common congenital anamoly in India:**
 A. CTEV
 B. DDH
 C. Genu valgum
 D. Hallux valgus

108. **Single step posteromedial release is:**
 A. Ponseti
 B. Kite's
 C. Turcos
 D. Cincinnati

109. **CTEV shoe was designed by:**
 A. Kite's
 B. Ponseti
 C. Turcos
 D. Thomas

110. **CTEV surgery at 2 years of age:**
 A. No surgery
 B. Soft tissue release
 C. Arthrodesis
 D. Bone osteotomy

111. **A newborn child presents with inverted foot and the dorsum of the foot cannot touch the anterior tibia. The most probable diagnosis:**
 A. Congenital vertical talus
 B. Arthrogryposis
 C. Congenital talipes equinovarus
 D. PES planus

112. **The ideal treatment of bilateral idiopathic clubfoot in a newborn is:**
 A. Manipulation by mother
 B. Manipulation and Dennis Brown splint
 C. Manipulation and casts
 D. Surgical release

113. **Triple arthrodesis involves:**
 A. Calcaneocuboid, talonavicular and talo-calcaneal
 B. Tibiotalar, calcaneocuboid and talonavicular
 C. Ankle joint, calcaneocuboid and talonavicular
 D. None of the above

114. **CTEV is caused by:**
 A. Neurological disorder
 B. Idiopathic
 C. Spina fibida
 D. Cubitus varus
 E. Arthrogryposis multiplex

115. **The clubfoot characteristically involves:**
 A. Foot and ankle
 B. Foot, ankle and leg
 C. Foot only
 D. Foot, ankle, leg and knee joint

116. **Most important pathology in clubfoot is:**
 A. Congenital talonavicular dislocation
 B. Tightening of tendoachilles
 C. Calcaneal fracture
 D. Lateral derangement

117. **A child 3 years of age is treated for CTEV by:**
 A. Triple arthrodesis
 B. Posteromedial soft tissue release
 C. Lateral wedge resection
 D. Tendo-Achilles lengthening and posterior capsulatomy

118. **Treatment for chronic cases of clubfoot is:**
 A. Triple arthrodesis
 B. Dorsomedial release
 C. Amputation
 D. None

119. In correction of clubfoot by manipulation which deformity should be corrected first?
A. Forefoot adduction   B. Varus
C. Upper end tibia   D. Calcaneum

120. Triple arthrodesis is NOT done before skeletal maturation because of:
A. Shortening of foot
B. Recurrence of deformity
C. Inadequate fusion
D. Complete correction not possible

121. The most common congenital anomaly among the following is encountered in our country:
A. Congenital pseudoartosis of tibia
B. Congenital dislocation of hip
C. Congenital talipes equinovarus
D. Multiple congenital contractures

122. 'Pseudoarthrosis' in triple fusion is seen at the joint of:
A. Calcaneocuboid   B. Calcaneonavicular
C. Naviculocuboid   D. Talonavicular

123. Pollicization is:
A. Amputation of thumb
B. Equalization of fingers
C. Toe to thumb transplantation
D. Reconstruction of thumb

124. Madelung's deformity involves:
A. Humerus   B. Proximal ulna
C. Distal radius   D. Carpals

125. The following deformity is seen in a child. What is the likely cause?

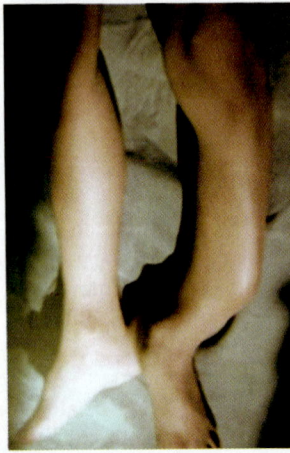

A. Tibial hemimelia
B. Fibula hemimelia
C. Congenital pseudoarthrosis of tibia
D. Congenital posteromedial angulation of tibia

126. In some old fractures, cartilaginous tissue forms over the fractured bone ends with a cavity in between containing clear fluid. This condition is called:
A. Delayed union   B. Slow union
C. Nonunion   D. Pseudoarthrosis

127. Pseudoarthrosis may be seen in all of the following conditions *except*:
A. Fracture   B. Idiopathic
C. Neurofibromatosis   D. Osteomyelitis

128. A child presenting with anterolateral bowing of leg with the following X-ray, diagnosis is:

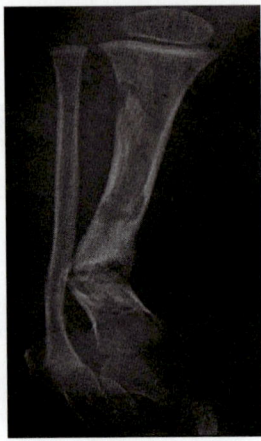

A. Fibula hemimelia
B. Congenital pseudoarthrosis of tibia
C. Infected nonunion
D. Tibia hemimelia

129. Pseudoarthrosis can be due to all *except*:
A. Congenital   B. Post-inflammatory
C. Trauma   D. None of the above

130. Pseudoarthrosis of tibia is best treated by:
A. Internal fixation
B. Internal fixation and bone grafting
C. Above knee POP cast
D. Below knee POP cast

131. Cause of congenital pseudoarthrosis is:
A. Intrauterine fracture
B. Neurofibromatosis
C. Fibrous dysplasia
D. Unknown

132. Congenital pseudoarthrosis is seen in the following:
A. Hip joint   B. Femur
C. Radius ulna   D. Tibia

133. The characteristic triad of Klippel-Feil syndrome includes all the following, *except*:
A. Short neck
B. Low hair line
C. Limited neck movements
D. Elevated scapula

134. In Klippel-Feil syndrome, the patient has all of the following clinical features *except*:
A. Low hair line
B. Bilateral neck webbing
C. Bilateral shortness of sternomastoid muscles
D. Gross limitations of neck movements

135. Sprengel's shoulder is due to deformity of:
    A. Scapula   B. Humerus
    C. Clavicle   D. Vertebra

136. The muscle affected in congenital torticollis is:
    A. Trapezius
    B. Rhomboideus major
    C. Rhomboideus minor
    D. Sternocleidomastoid

137. Which of the following is not true in case of congenital torticollis?
    A. Seen only in cases of breech vaginal delivery
    B. It can disappear spontaneously
    C. It is also known as sternomastoid tumour
    D. Untreated, neglected cases can result in plagiocephaly

138. Name of the deformity:

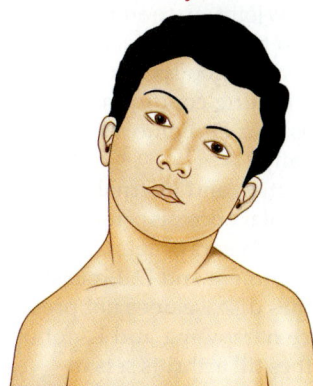

    A. Torticollis
    B. Fracture clavicle
    C. Sprengel deformity
    D. Absent pectoralis major muscle

139. All the following are true in infantile torticollis, *except*:
    A. It arises before birth
    B. There is facial asymmetry
    C. Commonest form of wryneck
    D. Infarction of sterno-cleidomastoid muscle

140. Vertebra plana is seen in all *except*:
    A. Histiocytosis X
    B. Leukemia
    C. Excessive use of systemic steroids
    D. Scheuermann's disease

141. Vertebra plana is not seen in:
    A. Trauma disease   B. Paget's disease
    C. Malignancy   D. Ewing's sarcoma

142. Idiopathic scoliosis can be treated by:
    A. Minerva cast   B. Milwaukee brace
    C. Crutchfield traction D. PTB cast

143. Cobb's angle is used to measure the degree:
    A. Kyphoscoliosis
    B. Angular deformity of the knee
    C. Extent of depression in calcaneal fracture
    D. Extent of spondylolisthesis

144. Vertebral rotation in scoliosis is checked in:
    A. Forward bending   B. Backward bending
    C. Sideways   D. Without bending

145. Turnbuckle cast is used for:
    A. Fracture shaft humerus
    B. Fracture shaft femur
    C. Scoliosis
    D. Cervical spine injury

146. In scoliosis degree of deformity is calculated by:
    A. Cobb's method   B. Hamburger method
    C. Haldane method   D. Milwaukee method

147. Angle measured for measurement of scoliosis:
    A. Cobb's   B. Bohler's
    C. Kite's   D. Baumann's

148. Risser's sign is for:
    A. Kyphosis   B. Scoliosis
    C. Shortening   D. Lengthening

149. Progression of congenital scoliosis is least likely in which of the following vertebra anomalies?
    A. Fully segmented hemivertebra
    B. Wedge vertebra
    C. Block vertebra
    D. Unilateral unsegmented bar with hemi-vertebra

150. Risser localiser cast is used in the management of:
    A. Kyphosis   B. Spondylolysthesis
    C. Idiopathic scoliosis D. Lordosis

151. Child abuse all the following are X-ray feature *except*:
    A. Metaphyseal corner fracture
    B. Metaphyseal bucket handle fracture
    C. Metaphyseal fragment displacement
    D. Subepiphyseal microfractures

152. An 8-year-old child is brought by parents to the casualty with a spiral fracture of femur and varying degree of ecchymosis all over body. The etiology is:
    A. Hit and run accident
    B. Battered baby syndrome
    C. Hockey stick injury
    D. Osteogenesis imperfect

153. All are true regarding pes planus *except*:
    A. There is collapse of medial longitudinal arch
    B. The heel becomes valgus and foot pronates at the subtalarmid complex joint
    C. Jack's test differentiates between flexible and rigid deformity
    D. One of the common type of tarsal coalition is calcaneonavicular
    E. Tarsal coalition is inherited as X-linked recessive condition

154. Pes planus is seen in:
    A. Perthes' disease
    B. Congenital vertical talus
    C. CTEV
    D. RA
    E. Infection

ANSWERS

1. B. Greenstick
2. B. Greenstick fracture
3. A. Children
4. B. Angulation and rotation not tolerated
5. C. Torus fracture
6. D. Radius/ulna
7. C. Incomplete fracture
8. D. Break the cortex other side and immobilization by POP
9. B. Comminuted fractures are common
10. A. Plastic deformation
11. B. Is generally incomplete
12. B. Angulation in metaphysis
13. C. Greenstick fracture of lower end of radius
14. C. Physeal injuries
15. B. II
16. B. II
17. B. Type II
18. B. Fracture epiphysis in children
19. B. Seen around epiphyseal plate
20. D. Perichondrial ring injury
21. C. Tibial epiphyseal injury
    - It is a case of epiphyseal injury, and may not be diagnosed on X-ray at the time of injury. Later the patient may present with deformity if not diagnosed initially.
22. D. Juvenile rheumatoid arthritis
23. C. Hypothyroidism
24. D. Infantile coxa vara
    Perthes' disease causes painless limp initially, but later may become painful, while infantile (congenital) coxa vara is characteristically painless
25. D. All of the above
26. D. All of the above
27. D. Coxa vara
28. B. Osteotomy
29. D. All of the above
30. A. Galeazzi's sign
31. D. Polyhydramnios is a known risk
32. D. Gaenslen's test
33. A. Hip spica
34. A. Developmental dysplasia of hip
35. A. Developmental dysplasia of hip
36. C. Decreased growth hormone
37. C. Developmental dysplasia of the hip
38. A. Unilateral DDH
39. B. CDH
40. A. Clunk of entry on abduction and flexion of hip
41. D. Femoral head is anteverted
    When head remains dislocated, growth of head is hampered resulting in small head and acetabulum undergoes dysplasia resulting in vertical (i.e. increased inclination) orientation

42. C. DDH
43. C. DDH
44. C. DDH
45. B. Barlow test
46. B. MRI
47. B. Shallow acetabulum
48. A. Decreases
49. F. All of the above
50. D. Twin pregnancy is a known risk factor
51. B. Increases
52. B. DDH in infancy
53. A. Ortolani's sign
54. D. Shallow acetabulum
55. A. Perthes' disease
56. D. Narrow joint space and, E. Age of onset is not related to disease severity
57. D. MRI is not a good confirmatory investigation
58. A. Self-limiting condition, B. Bilateral in 20% cases and D. Femoral head is displaced laterally
59. D. Abduction and internal rotation
60. A. Avascular necrosis of femoral head; B. Onset before 10 years of age; C. Osteotomy is used for treatment and D. Limb shortening
    Perthes disease does not present with joint space narrowing and is not obliterated in perthes till arthritis sets in
61. D. Magnetic resonance imaging (MRI)
62. C. Perthes' disease
63. D. Perthes' disease
64. C. Supervised containment of femoral head in acetabulum
65. B. SCFE
66. D. More common in girls
67. C. 10–15 years
68. B. Adolescents
69. A. No slip
70. B. Slipped capital femoral epiphyses
71. B. SCFE
72. C. SCFE
73. D. *In situ* pinning
74. B. Laterally; E. Anteriorly
75. D. Hyperextension
76. A. Genu valgum
    - 7-year-old boy means growth plate is intact. Now when injury occurs laterally, medial side will grow uninterrupted and will produce valgus deformity, similarly medial injury will produce varus deformity.
77. B. Rickets
78. A. Blount's disease
    - Note the metaphyseal beaking, characteristic of Blount's disease.

79. A. Defect in posteromedial part of upper tibial epiphysis
80. A. Distal part towards midline
81. A. Medial closing wedge osteotomy
82. D. External tibial torsion
83. B > D. Tibia vara > Genu recurvatum
84. A. In infants, it may be considered normal; B. Occurs due to epiphyseal dysplasia and C. Seldom associated with tibial angulation
85. A. 4 years
86. D. Orthosis is recommended full time
87. A. Overtreatment of CTEV
88. D. All of the above
89. A. Small or absent
90. B. Protrusion of cuboid bone, C. Lateral crease, E. Concavity of sole
91. A. Ignacio Ponseti
92. C. Equinocavovarus
93. A. Rocker bottom foot
94. D. Salter's osteotomy
95. D. Posteromedial soft tissue release
96. B. Equinus
97. D. All of the above
98. B. Sole creases are not found
99. B. Manipulation and corrective splint
100. A. Equinus
101. C. Dennis-Brown splint used, D. Adduction of forefoot and E. Associated with spina bifida
102. A. CTEV
103. C. Poliomyelitis
    Poliomyelitis does not cause clubfoot at birth.
104. C. Dennis-Brown splint
105. A. Calcaneocuboid, talonavicular and talo-calcaneal
    • These three joints are fused and is know as "triple arthrodesis"
106. C. Idiopathic
107. A. CTEV
108. C. Turcos
    Turcos incision is used in PMSTR
109. D. Thomas
110. B. Soft tissue release
111. C. Congenital talipes equinovarus
    The test mentioned is dorsiflexion test which can be used as a screening test in newborn children for CTEV.
112. C. Manipulation and casts
113. A. Calcaneocuboid, talonavicular and talo-calcaneal

114. A. Neurological disorder; B. Idiopathic; C. Spina fibida and E. Arthrogryposis multiplex
115. B. Foot, ankle and leg
116. A. Congenital talonavicular dislocation
117. B. Posteromedial soft tissue release
118. A. Triple arthrodesis
119. A. Forefoot adduction
120. C. Inadequate fusion
121. C. Congenital talipes equinovarus
122. D. Talonavicular
123. D. Reconstruction of thumb
124. C. Distal radius
125. C. Congenital pseudoarthrosis of tibia
126. D. Pseudoarthrosis
127. D. Osteomyelitis
128. B. Congenital pseudoarthrosis of tibia
129. B. Post-inflammatory
130. B. Internal fixation and bone grafting
131. D. Unknown
    Neurofibromatosis is an association, it is not a cause
132. D. Tibia
133. D. Elevated scapula
    Triad of Klippel-Feil syndrome: Short neck, low hair line and restriction of neck motion. Sprengel shoulder has a common association with Klippel-Feil syndrome, but its not a part of the triad.
134. C. Bilateral shortness of sternomastoid muscles
135. A. Scapula
136. D. Sternocleidomastoid
137. A. Seen only in cases of breech vaginal delivery
138. A. Torticollis
139. A. It arises before birth
140. D. Scheuermann's disease
141. B. Paget's disease
142. B. Milwaukee brace
143. A. Kyphoscoliosis
144. A. Forward bending
145. C. Scoliosis
146. A. Cobb's method
147. A. Cobb's
148. B. Scoliosis
149. C. Block vertebra
150. C. Idiopathic scoliosis
151. D. Subepiphyseal microfractures
152. B. Battered baby syndrome
153. E. Tarsal coalition is inherited as X-linked recessive condition
154. B. Congenital vertical talus; D. RA and E. Infection

Bone Tumors

GENERAL FACTS

Orthopedic oncology is a vast subject in itself, for better learning/memory/diagnosis, readers should be acquainted with the following classifications and should always consider osteomyelitis as an important differential, especially in metaphyseal tumors.

A. Location of Tumor

Most important tumors locationwise; mnemonic is "EOG" for Dia/meta/epiphysis [E = Ewing's sarcoma, O = Osteosarcoma, G = Giant cell tumor].

- *Epiphysis*
    - Osteoclastoma/GCT (after physeal closure in adults), most commonly an epiphyseal tumor.
    - Chondroblastoma (before physeal closure)—it is purely epiphyseal
    - Articular osteochondroma (rare)
    - Clear cell type of chondrosarcoma

- *Metaphysis*
    - Bone cyst (SBC/ABC)
    - Osteosarcoma
    - Enchondroma
    - Chondrosarcoma (except clear cell variety)
    - Osteochondroma aka exostosis (except articular)
    - Osteoclastoma/GCT (before physeal closure, i.e. in children)

- *Diaphysis*
    - Ewing's sarcoma—important differential for osteomyelitis.
    - Multiple myeloma
    - Admantinoma
    - Lymphoma
    - Osteoid osteoma
    - Osteoblastoma
    - Fibrous lesions:
        - Fibrous dysplasia
        - Fibrous cortical defect
        - Nonossifying fibroma

they all make important D/Ds of diaphyseal lesion

B. Cell of Origin

WHO classification		
Cell/tissue	*Benign*	*Malignant*
Osteoblast	Osteoid osteoma Osteoblastoma	Osteosarcoma
Chondroblast	Osteochondroma Chondroblastoma Chondromyxoid fibroma	Chondrosarcoma
Fibrous	Fibrous dysplasia Fibrous cortical defect Nonossifying fibroma	Fibrosarcoma
Histiocytic	Fibrous histiocytoma	Malignant fibrous histiocytoma
Osteoclast	GCT (highly aggressive) Admantinoma ABC	Malignant GCT
Notochord remnant		Chordoma
Vascular	Hemangioma	Hemangioma endothelioma Hemangioma pericytoma
Hematopoietic		Multiple myeloma NHL, Hodgkin's lymphoma Ewing's sarcoma (round cell)
Neurogenic	Neurilemmoma	
Lipogenic	Lipoma	Liposarcoma

C. Age

Most primary bone tumors arise in <20 years age group, while secondary/metastatic bone tumors arise in elderly population.

- Ewing's sarcoma: 5–15 years age group.
- Osteosarcoma: bimodal: 1°: 10–20 years
  2°: 40–60 years } any age group is possible
- Osteoclastoma: 20–40 years
- Enchondroma: 20–40 years
- Chondrosarcoma/hemangioma: 40–60 years
- Multiple myeloma: >50 years
- SBC: 1st decade
- ABC: 2nd decade

Xtra Edge
- Location of GCT is epimetaphyseal > epiphysis > diaphysis (before skeletal maturity—rare).
- Ewing's sarcoma is the most common tumor in 1st decade, but most common age group of Ewing's is 2nd decade.
- Other tumors of 1st decade—retinoblastoma, metastasis from neuroblastoma.

D. Most Common Site of Bone Tumors

- Fibrous dysplasia: Neck of femur (commonest for monostotic and overall) and craniofacial bones (polyostotic)
- Enchondroma: Hand bones (metaphysis of small bones of hand and feet, especially phalanges, commonest in little finger)
- ABC: Proximal femur > tibia
- Simple bone cyst: Proximal humerus

- Chordoma: Sacrum > spheno-occipital region (clivus)> anteriorvertebral body (i.e. only axial bones)
- Ivory osteoma: Frontal sinus
- Chondrosarcoma: Pelvis (ilium)> proximal femur > scapula
- Osteochondroma: Distal femur > Proximal tibia
- Osteoid osteoma: Femur > Tibia (diaphysis)
- Osteoblastoma: Vertebra (posterior elements) > Femur diaphysis
- Ameloblastoma (also referred as Adamantinoma): Mandible adamantinoma of long bones is separate entity and its most common site is Tibia
- Chondroblastoma: Distal femur
- Chondromyxoid fibroma: Proximal tibial metaphysis
- Osteosarcoma: Distal femur
- Ewing's sarcoma: Femur diaphysis > Flat bones
- Hemangioma: Spine (T4-L4 region) > Skull
- Giant cell tumor: Distal femur > proximal tibia > distal radius
- Eosinophilic granuloma: Skull
- Pigmented villonodular synovitis (PVNS): Knee
- Multiple myeloma: Spine
- Glomus tumor: Subungual area of fingers
- Synovial cell sarcoma: Knee
- Solitary plasmacytoma: Spine
- Metastasis/secondaries: Dorsal vertebrae.

E. Some 'Most Common (M/C)' Facts about Bone Tumors (tm)

- M/C bone tm—metastasis/secondaries
- M/C malignant bone tm—metastasis/secondaries
- M/C primary benign bone tm—osteochondroma/exostosis (not a true benign tm).
- M/C true primary benign bone tm—osteoid osteoma
- M/C benign bone lesion—fibrous cortical defect.
- M/C primary malignant bone tm—multiple myeloma (if bone marrow included)
- M/C primary malignant bone tm/2nd M/C primary malignant bone tm—osteosarcoma
- 3rd M/C primary malignant bone tm—chondrosarcoma
- M/C malignant bone tm of hand—chondrosarcoma 2° to enchondroma, otherwise most common malignant tumor of hand—squamous cell carcinoma
- M/C primary malignant bone tm on flat bones—chondrosarcoma
- M/C primary malignant bone tm—osteosarcoma
- M/C bone tm in pediatric age group—osteosarcoma
- 2nd M/C bone tm in pediatrics—Ewing's sarcoma
- M/C bone tm <10 years old—Ewing's sarcoma
- M/C bone tm in adult—osteosarcoma
- M/C bone tm in elderly—metastasis/secondaries.
- M/C tm of hand bone and M/C intra-osseous cartilage tm—enchondroma
- M/C bone tm with multicentric origin—Ewing's sarcoma
- Most common radiation induced tumor—osteosarcoma > fibrosarcoma
- Most radiosensitive and chemosensitive bone tumor—Ewing's sarcoma
- M/C tumor of jaw is squamous cell carcinoma of oral mucosa, while most common bone tumor of mandible is ameloblastoma
- M/C malignant bone tumor of chest wall—chondrosarcoma
- Tumor with history night pains showing diagnostic response to aspirin/NSAIDs—osteoid osteoma
- M/C site of primary in female is breast and in male is prostate
- Bone metastasis is mostly lytic (kidney, thyroid) > blastic (breast, prostate). Breast metastases are both lytic and blastic.

F. Grading—Enneking's System (Table 15.1)

Xtra Edge
- Edmonton system—used for grading cancer pain.
- Mirel's criteria is used for measuring risk of pathological fracture in bone metastasis. A score of more than or equal to 8 warrants prophylactic fixation of the lesion to avoid an impending pathological fracture.

Investigations

1. **X-ray**
   - Type of margin and pattern of bone destruction, dictate about the nature of tumor (benign/malignant) to some extent.
     - Benign—margin is well defined/zone of reactive sclerosis with geographic pattern of bone destruction, i.e. narrow zone of transition.
     - Benign aggressive—margins may have multiple scattered lytic areas, i.e. motheaten type of appearance.
     - Malignant—margins are ill-defined with permeative type of lesion, i.e. wide zone of transition.
   - Some classical X-ray signs (Table 15.2).
2. CT scan is helpful to study tumor calcification, cortex, nidus of osteoid osteoma (thin slice CT is IOC), and in detecting lung metastasis.

Table 15.1: Grading—Enneking's system

Benign

1. Latent—low biologial activity; well marginated; often incidental findings (i.e. nonossifying fibroma).
2. Active—symptomatic; limited bone destruction; may present with pathological fracture (i.e. aneurysmal bone cyst).
3. Aggressive—aggressive; bone destruction/soft tissue extension; do not respect natural barriers (i.e. giant cell tumor).

Malignant

Stage	Grade	Site	Metastases
IA	Low	Intracompartmental	None
IB	Low	Extracompartmental	None
IIB	High	Extracompartmental	None
III	Any	Any	Regional or distant metastases

Table 15.2: X-ray sign

Periosteal reaction	Solid-osteoid osteoma
	Lamellated-Ewing's (onion)
	Complex (sunburst)—osteosarcoma
Sunray/Codman's triangle	Osteosarcoma
Onion peel	Ewing's, osteomyelitis
Ground glass/Shepherd crook	Fibrous dysplasia
Soap bubble	GCT
Fallen leaf appearance	SBC>ABC
Trap door	
Winking owl sign	One pedicle destroyed due to vertebral metastasis
Blind bat sign	Both pedicles destroyed
Hemangioma	Corduroy (polka dot in MRI/CT)
Popcorn calcification	Chondrosarcoma
Punched out appearance of spine	Multiple myeloma

3. MRI is the IOC, identify extent of marrow involvement, soft tissue extension of the tumor and involvement of neurovascular structures.
   - T2 halo sign—sign of active lesion
   - T1 halo sign—sign of good response to therapy
4. Technetium (Tc) bone scan helps to identify multiple bone metastasis and its activity level. It accumulates in the area of increased activity and thus mostly positive in malignant/osteoblastic lesions. However, it appears cold in pure osteolytic lesions, e.g. multiple myeloma. False positive (any area of high bone turnover), e.g. trauma, infection, arthropathy, Paget's disease, osteoid osteoma, osteoblastoma, fibrous dysplasia, arthritis, etc.
5. PET scan is helpful in assessing response to treatment.
6. Biopsy is the gold standard investigation and all non-invasive investigation must be completed before doing biopsy. All samples (infective/neoplasm) should be cultured and biopsied.
   - Chinese letter pattern—fibrous dysplasia
   - Herringbone pattern—fibrosarcoma
   - Biphasic pattern—synovial cell sarcoma
   - Chicken wire pattern—chondroblastoma.

Differential diagnosis
- Infection is always the most important differential and it mimics Ewing's sarcoma > osteosarcoma.
- Fibrous dysplasia mimics GCT
- Bone infarct mimics enchondroma
- Myositis ossificans mimics osteosarcoma
- Bone islands mimics osteoid osteoma
- Brown tumor
- Stress fracture
- Vertebra plana (*Mnemonic:* **ILLEGAL**)
  - Infection (TB/pyogenic spondylitis)
  - Leukemia
  - Lymphoma
  - Ewing's sarcoma
  - Gaucher's disease
  - ABC
  - LCH (eosinophilic granuloma is the commonest cause)
- Multicentric bone lesions (*Mnemonic:* Steamed **BEEF MOMO**)
  - **S**yndrome—Goltz (GCT)
  - **B**one infarct
  - **E**nchondroma
  - **E**wing's sarcoma
  - **F**ibrous dysplasia
  - **M**ultiple myeloma
  - **O**steomyelitis
  - **M**etastasis
  - **O**steochondroma
    - Pulsatile bone tumors: Secondaries from renal cell carcinoma > secondaries from follicular carcinoma thyroid > ABC > GCT > telengiectatic osteosarcoma.

METASTASIS
- After 40 years of age, every bone tumor must be considered metastatic unless proven otherwise.
- Periosteum/perichondrium constitutes the most effective barrier to tumor extension.
- Blastic: Prostate, medullary carcinoma of thyroid.
  - Lytic: Kidney, lung, thyroid
  - Mixed: Breast, ovary, cervix, testis (genitals)

- Most common site of primary in secondary bone tumors:
  - Male: Prostate > lung
  - Female: Breast > lung
  - Children: Neuroblastoma
  - If primary unknown: Most common is lung > kidney
  - Overall most common: Breast > prostate > lung > kidney > thyroid
  - Most common area of metastasis from bone is lung
- Most common site of primary is spine (thoracic > thoralumbar) and metastasis distal to knee/elbow (acral) are rare and most commonly due to lung > kidney. Commonest site of acral metastasis is tibia.
- Bone to bone metastasis (*Mnemonic*: **ONE**): **O**steosarcoma, **N**euroblastoma, **E**wing's.
- Proximal humerus and proximal femur are the commonest site of metastasis among long bones and femoral neck accounts for most common site of pathological fracture.
- Microscopic appearance of a metastatic lesion is similar to primary lesion.
- Pathological fracture is not an emergency and always managed after proper evaluation of primary.
- Pulmonary metastasis when present rules out multiple myeloma.
- Renal cell carcinoma—mostly the secondary deposits are found as a single focus.
- Thyroid carcinoma—the metastatic growth appears at epiphysis and along suture lines.
- Bone graft is avoided in pathological fracture, as radiation therapy may prevent incorporation of the graft.
- The IOC for detecting occult osteoblastic metastasis is Tc scan and for lytic metastasis is PET scan.
- Sarcomas metastasizing through lymphatic channels are (*Mnemonic:* **CLEAR—MS**)
  - **C**lear cell sarcoma
  - **L**ymphosarcoma
  - **E**pithelial sarcoma
  - **A**ngiosarcoma
  - **R**habdomyosarcoma
  - **M**alignant fibrous histiocytoma
  - **S**ynovial cell sarcoma.

Treatment

- **Radiotherapy:** Most primary and secondary bone malignancies are radioresistant. Exception to primary includes—multiple myeloma, lymphoma and Ewing's and tumors secondary to renal cell carcinoma. Most common acute side effect is skin irritation and most severe side effect is radiation induced carcinoma, commonest being osteosarcoma.
- **Chemotherapy** has a well-defined role in high-grade malignancy of bone but not in low-grade ones and in cartilaginous lesions. It is also useful for high grade soft tissue malignancy of childhood but not for adult soft tissue malignancy.
- **Surgery** involves excision of tumor and/or curettage.
  Terms used in tumor excision:
  - *Intralesional:* The plane of dissection lies within the tumor tissue.
  - *Marginal excision:* Plane of excision is through the pseudocapsule/reactive zone around tumor.
  - *Wide excision:* Plane of excision includes a cuff on normal tissue (usually about 3 cm).
  - *Radical excision:* Involves removing the entire compartment containing the tumor.
  Curettage: It is scooping out the contents, done mostly for benign slow growing tumors (e.g. SBC). If curettage is followed by additional chemical (phenol, liquid nitrogen, bone cement) treatment, then it is called extended curettage. It is done to reduce the rate of recurrence (best agent is liquid nitrogen) in aggressive lesions like GCT, ABC, enchondroma, etc.
  After the tumor is excised/curetted out, the cavity may be filled with bone graft or cement. Cement provides immediate stability/rapid mobilization after surgery but detecting recurrences is difficult in comparison to bone graft.

SIMPLE (UNICARMEL) BONE CYST (SBC)

It is the true cystic bony lesion. The cyst wall is lined by a thin fibrous membrane and it contains serous straw/yellow fluid (unlike ABC that has hemorrhagic fluid).

Age/Sex: 1st two decades of life; M:F = 2:1.

Site: Metaphysis of the long bones (proximal humerus > distal femur > proximal tibia). The lesions are most active during periods of skeletal growth and heals spontaneously after skeletal maturity. Although it starts at metaphysis, active lesions are those which are closer to physis (within 1 cm) and latent grow towards diaphysis.

Clinical features: Patients are mostly asymptomatic and diagnosed incidentally when a pathological fracture has occurred.

X-ray features: Single (aseptate) metaphyseal cyst, centrally located, symmetrically expansile with a well-defined margin. Its width never exceeds the width of the neighboring growth plate. Fallen leaf/trap door appearance are diagnostic (since SBC is aseptate) (Fig. 15.1 A).

Treatment
- Small/asymptomatic/upper limb → observation.
- Large/symptomatic/lowerlimb → 1st line is aspiration and injection (steroids>bone marrow aspirate > demineralised bone matrix > sclerosant). Curettage and bone graft +/– fixation is reserved as last line/lower limb which are at high risk of fracture. Pathological fracture in upper limb cases may be managed conservatively (as it may initiate healing of lesion), while in lower limb needs fixation.

ANEURYSMAL BONE CYST (ABC)

It is a benign, locally aggressive blood-filled tumor of bone.

Age/Sex: <20 years age, with female dominance.

Site: Most common in metaphysis of proximal femur > tibia > proximal humerus. It also involves post elements of spine (important D/D osteoblastoma—they are nonexpansile and partly ossified). The cyst may arise primary or secondarily due to osteoclastoma (most common), osteoblastoma, SBC, fibrous dysplasia, chondroblastoma, etc.

X-ray: Eccentric metaphyseal asymmetric expansile lesion, that may elevate periosteum or expand cortex (i.e. ballooned out) and has septations (Figs 15.1B and C). Margins may be well defined/permeative. MRI shows double density fluid level and intralesional septations (diagnostic).

Treatment: Extended curettage and bone grafting.

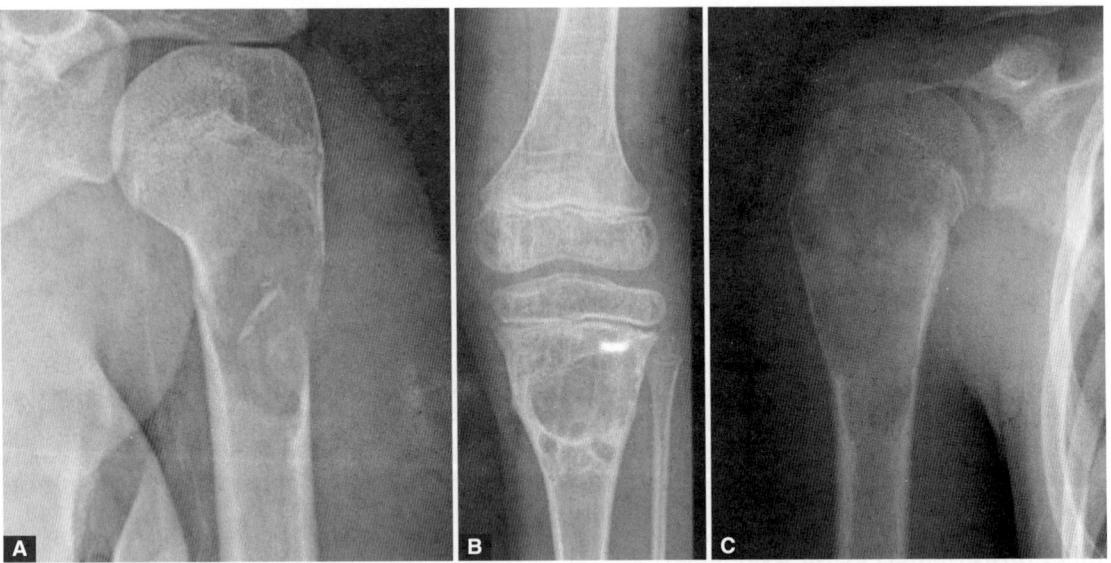

Fig. 15.1: (A) SBC showing trap door appearance (fallen leaf will be at the bottom); (B) and (C) ABC with visible multiple septations

GIANT CELL TUMOR (OSTEOCLASTOMA)

It is benign but locally aggressive with uncertain origin (likely cell of origin in monoclonal).

Age/Sex: 20–40 years age group (after physeal closure), F > M.

Site: It is an epiphyseal, more specifically epi-metaphyseal lesion in adults and metaphyseal in children (i.e. before closure of physis). The commonest site is distal femur > proximal tibia (2nd) > distal radius (3rd). The commonest site in spine is the sacrum followed by lumbar vertebrae.

Clinical presentation: Mostly it is asymptomatic. Commonest symptom is pain >> pathological fracture. Egg shell crackling felt on palpation is characteristic.

Metastasis: Although benign, pulmonary metastasis can occur rarely.

Primary malignant transformation of GCT is rare, it is mostly secondary due to radiation. Multiple giant cell like bone tumor called **GOLTZ** syndrome.

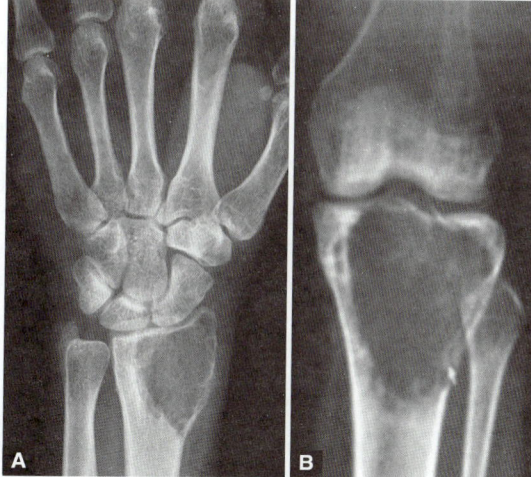

Fig. 15.2: (A) GCT distal radius (distal radius lytic lesion X-ray, diagnosis is mostly GCT for MCQ purpose. (B) GCT proximal tibia. GCT is differentiated from ABC by its proximity to epiphysis and skeletal maturity (ABC arises in skeletally immature patient)

X-ray: Eccentric expansile lytic lesion, just below subchondral bone (soap bubble appearance). Intra-articular extension is rare, but cortical break and soft tissue extension is possible (locally aggressive). Matrix is never calcified (Fig. 15.2). Campanacci grading is based on X-ray. MRI findings include T1- dark, on T2-bright image.

Biopsy: Multinucleated giant cells (non-neoplastic, benign and reactive) in a background of mononuclear stromal cell (neoplastic component of the tumor). The nuclei of both cell types are identical which is differentiating point with other giant cell containing tumors (giant cell variants).

Giant cell variants (*Mnemonic:* **FAN OUCH**)
- **F**ibrous dysplasia
- **A**BC
- **N**onossifying fibroma
- **O**steitis fibrosa cystica
- **U**nicameral bone cyst
- **C**hondromyxoid fibroma, chondroblastoma
- **H**yperparathyroidism

Treatment
- Extended curettage (TxOC). Sandwich technique (a type of extended curettage) where < 1 cm of subchondral bone is preserved.
- Excision is TxOC for distal end ulna/upper end of fibula.
- Distal end radius—excision followed by reconstruction with upper end fibula.
- Treatment of recurrent lesions is same as primary.
- Radiotherapy is opted only for unresectable spinal GCT (as it may turn GCT malignant).
- Recent advances—bisphosphonates/Denozumab may hold disease progression.

OSTEOCHONDROMA (EXOSTOSIS)

It is a developmental malformation (aberration of growth plate), not a true neoplasm. Growth parallel patient's skeletal growth and ceases after skeletal maturity is reached.

Site: Metaphyseal lesion and growth occurs in a direction opposite to the physis with a stalk (Fig. 15.3). Metaphyseal area of any bone developed by endochondral ossification may be involved. Most common bones involved are distal femur > proximal tibia > proximal humerus.

X-ray: Pedunculated (M/C) or broad based/sessile lesions.

The lesion has both cortical and cancellous part with an intramedullary cavity which all are continuous with the parent bone. It also has a cartilaginous cap which is only a few mm thick. Lesions are always larger than they appear on X-ray, because cartilaginous cap is not visible on X-ray. X-ray is sufficient to make a diagnosis (Fig. 15.3 A).

Clinical features: Mostly asymptomatic and diagnosed incidentally on X-ray. May cause pressure symptoms like bursitis (presents with pain),tendinitis, neurovascular complications, fracture, etc.

Malignant transformation (chondrosarcoma): It is suspected in a rapidly growing tumor, which was previously silent, grows after skeletal maturity, has cartilage cap >2 cm thick (seen on MRI). Incidence of malignant transformation is, however, rare (1% with exostosis and 5% with HME).

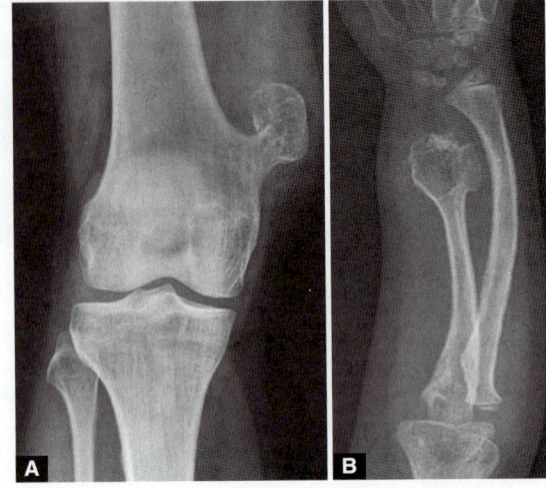

Fig. 15.3: (A) Classical pedunculated osteo-chondroma, which is growing away from physis. (B) Forearm deformity in HME (osteo-chondroma is in distal ulna with radial bowing)

Hereditary multiple exostosis (HME) or diaphyseal aclasis is an AD inheritance (chromosome 8,11,19) disorder. Genes involved are EXT 1 (Chr 8) and EXT2 (Chr 11). Growth abnormalities like bowing of long bones (radius bowing, ulna shortening) have been described by MASADA (Fig. 15.3B).

Differential diagnosis: Trevor's disease (osteochondroma on only half side of growth plate, in only one side of the body).

Treatment: It is most observation unless symptomatic where an extraperiosteal resection is done.

ENCHONDROMA

Chondroma (chordoma is different) is a benign neoplasm of hyaline cartilage and mostly they arise inside medullary canal, hence the name "enchondroma" (eccentric chondroma is called osteochondroma).

Site: Any bone formed of cartilage can be involved, commonest being small bones of hand (especially phalanges with middle phalanx of little finger being commonest) and foot.

Clinical features: Generally, they are asymptomatic but pain may be present due to pathological fracture.

X-ray: Expansile radiolucent lesion with stippled intra-lesional calcification (Fig. 15.4).

Differentials: Bone infarct, spina ventosa, ABC.

Malignant transformation: Maffucci syndrome (almost all cases) > Ollier's disease > Solitary enchondroma (rare)
- *Ollier's disease:* Multiple enchondromatosis.
- *Maffucci's syndrome:* Multiple enchondroma, sub-cutaneous hemangioma and phleboliths.

Treatment: It is reserved for symptomatic cases where excisional curettage and bone grafting are done.

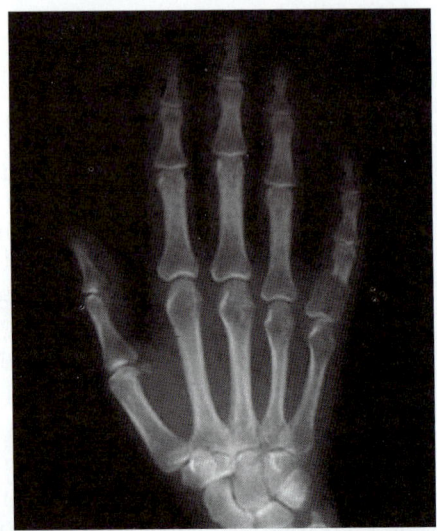

Fig. 15.4: Enchondroma

CHONDROBLASTOMA (CODMAN'S TUMOR)

Rare benign cartilaginous tumor.

Site: Epiphysis (D/D is GCT) of distal femur.

Clinical features: Since epiphyseal tumor it may cause joint symptoms like chronic synovitis and arthritis.

X-ray: Well-defined epiphyseal lesion with surrounding reactive bone/sclerosis (absent in GCT) with matrix calcification (absent in GCT) (Fig. 15.5).

Biopsy: Chicken wire calcification.

Treatment: Extended curettage.

CHONDROMYXOID FIBROMA

Rare benign cartilaginous metaphyseal tumor, which unlike other cartilaginous tumors, does not show matrix calcification.

Site: Most common site is proximal tibial metaphysis.

X-ray: Bubbly lesion with sclerotic margins.

Differentials: Nonossifying fibroma (closest D/D).

Treatment: Extended curettage.

Xtra Edge

In MCQs, if matrix calcification is mentioned, answer is cartilaginous tumor >> osteogenic.

FIBROUS CORTICAL DEFECT (FCD)/NONOSSIFYING FIBROMA (NOF)

FCD is the commonest benign bone lesion (i.e. not a true neoplasm) characterised by fibrous proliferation in the metaphysis of long bones. It is a developmental disorder, usually asymptomatic and diagnosed incidentally, and has a natural tendency to involute and ossify in adulthood (i.e. with skeletal maturity). When FCD persists and increase in size with medullary invasion, then it is called nonossifying fibroma.

Age/sex: 1st–2nd decades of life.

Site: Commonest site is lower femur metaphysis.

X-ray: Well defined, lytic lesion with sclerotic margins, placed eccentrically in the metaphyseal region, oval in shape with long axis parallel to axis of bone. FCD is confined to the cortex and measures < 2 cm in diameter while NOF is > 2 cm in diameter.

Biopsy: Foam cells and giant cells are almost always present (commonest GCT variant).

Treatment: Curettage in symptomatic cases.

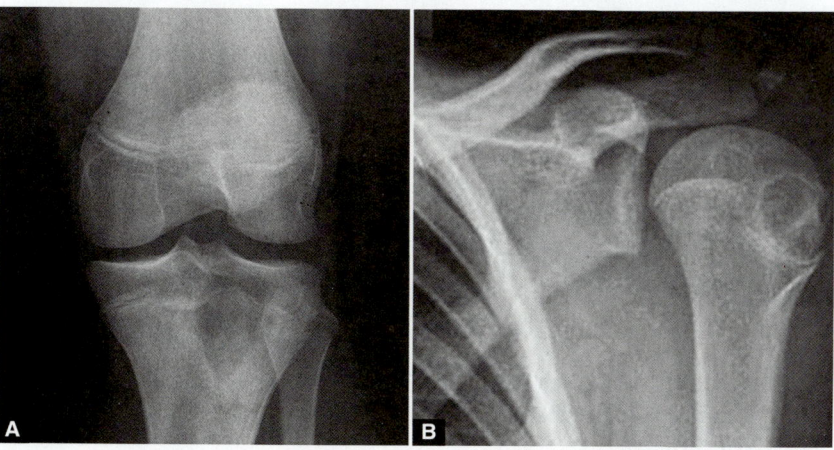

Fig. 15.5: Lytic lesion with marginal sclerosis in epiphysis of skeletally immature patient is chondroblastoma

FIBROUS DYSPLASIA

It is a developmental anomaly of bone with replacement of normal bone/marrow with fibrous tissue and small woven spicules of bone giving it, its characteristic radiological ground glass appearance. The basic defect is the inability to produce mature lamellar bone and the process of bone maturation is arrested at woven bone formation. It can exist in epiphysis, metaphysis and diaphysis and can be of two types:

- Monostotic: Most common form, single bone affected, 20–30 years age group, proximal femur is commonest site; most cases do not progress with age.
- Polyostotic: <10 years age group, zygomatic-maxillary area (craniofacial) is commonest site; may progress with after skeletal maturity.
- Overall commonest site is proximal femur.

Syndromes associated with polyostotic forms:

- McCune-Albright syndrome: Polyostotic fibrous dysplasia + cutaneous café-au-lait spots + endocrine dysfunction (e.g. precocious puberty). The skin lesions (café-au) have irregular borders and located ipsilateral to the bony lesions, females > males. Café-au-lait spots of neurofibromatosis have smooth borders called "coast of California".
- Mazabraud's syndrome: Soft tissue myxoma + polyostotic fibrous dysplasia.
- Cherubism: Symmetric involvement of maxilla and mandible. Lesions become static at skeletal maturity.

Clinical features: Pain is the commonest symptom. Deformities result due to microfractures, commonest in proximal femur. Deformity called "Shepherd crook deformity" is caused by varus, antalgic gait and limb shortening. Symptoms may exacerbate during pregnancy.

X-ray features: Well-defined lesion k/a ground glass appearance/smoky milky appearance (due to loss of trabecular pattern), with a sclerotic rim called "rind sign".

Biopsy: Chinese letter like pattern.

Treatment: Excisional curettage with bone grafting.

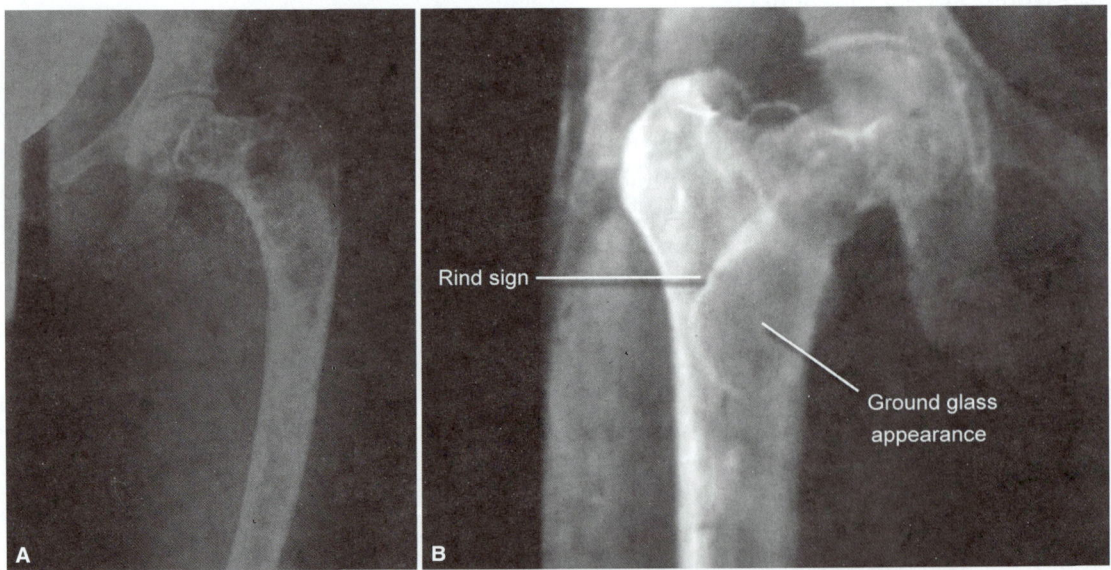

Fig. 15.6: (A) Shepherd crook deformity, (B) Ground glass appearance with rind sign

OSTEOFIBROUS DYSPLASIA/CAMPANACCI DISEASE/OSSIFYING FIBROMA

- Middle third of tibia > fibula is most common affected site
- Occurs in 1st two decades of life
- Presents with anterolateral bowing of long bones

- *X-ray:* Eccentric intracortical osteolysis with cortical expansion
- *Treatment:* Observation, as most regress spontaneously. If symptomatic resection is the TxOC.

NEUROFIBROMATOSIS (NF)
It is a hereditary hamartomatous disorder affecting central/peripheral nervous system, skeletal, skin and soft tissue.

NF1/Peripheral NF/von Recklinghausen Disease
- Commonest single gene disorder affecting nervous system.
- AD with 100% penetrance.
- Defect in chromosome 17.

Clinical features: Café-au-lait spots/coast of California (most common feature), axillary and inguinal freckling (2nd commonest), skeletal abnormalities (scoliosis; most common, pseudo-arthrosis of tibia), intraspinal NF-hour glass/dumb-shaped tumor of nerve root, neurological deficit may occur due to enlarging tumor but paraplegia never develops, cognitive deficit.

Diagnostic criteria (2/7):
- 6 or more café-au-lait spots, each with a minimum diameter of 15 mm in adults and 5 mm in children.
- A positive family history (1st degree relative) of NF.
- 2 or more NF of any type or one plexiform NF.
- Characteristic bony lesion (scoliosis, pseudoarthrosis of tibia, hemihypertrophy, sphenoid dysplasia).
- Freckling in the axilla.
- Optic glioma.
- 2 or more Lisch nodules (iris hamartoma).

NF 2/Central NF
- Less common type
- AD inheritance
- Defect in chromosome no. 22

Clinical features: B/L acoustic neuroma is a characteristic feature (absent in NF1) and visual defect due to posterior subcapsular lenticular opacity. Musculoskeletal abnormality characteristic of NF 1 is absent in NF 2. Cranial nerve (e.g. facial nerve) and brain/spinal cord tumors (e.g. meningioma) are also common. NF especially the deep-seated ones may undergo sarcomatous degeneration and metastasize by hematogenous route.

Diagnostic criteria (either of the following):
- B/L acoustic neuroma
- 1st degree relative with NF 2 and
  - either a unilateral acoustic neuroma or
  - any 2 of the following
    - Meningioma, glioma, neurofibroma, schwannoma
    - Posterior subcapsular lenticular opacity

Biopsy: Stained by Rio-Hortega stain which identify specific cells called lemmocytes.

Treatment: Kyphoscoliosis warrants early correction and fusion as they progress invariably in all patient. Complete excision is the only treatment of the tumor.

Xtra Edge
Kyphoscoliosis with single and sharp lower thoracic curve involving less than 5 vertebrae is the commonest skeletal lesion. In cervical kyphosis, single vertebra is involved.

HEMANGIOMA
- It is a hamartoma in bone composed of vascular channels.
- It is the commonest benign neoplasm of spine.

Commonest site: Spine (dorsal and lumbar regions) >> skull.

Clinical features: Mostly it is asymptomatic diagnosed incidentally on CT/MRI done for other reasons. Due to classical radiological image, biopsy is almost never required.

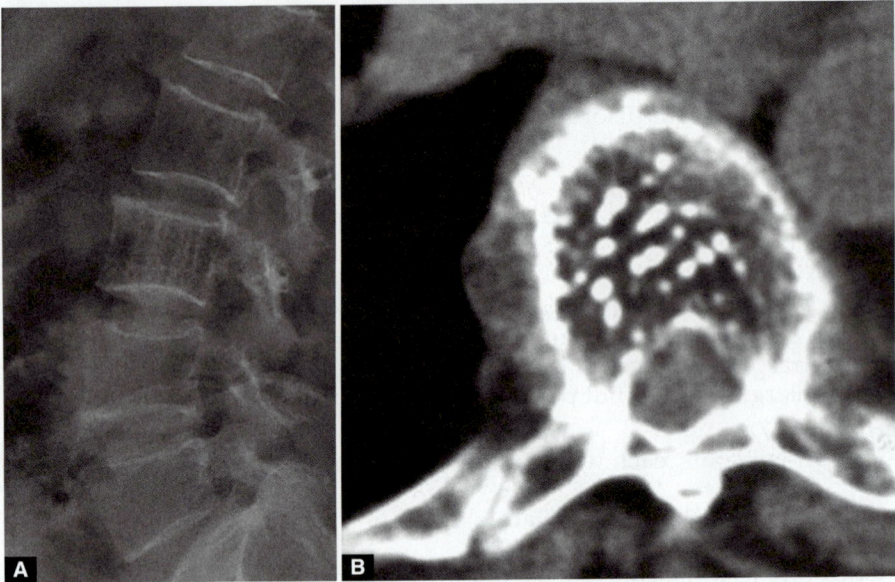

Fig. 15.7: (A) X-ray LS spine showing hemangioma in L3 vertebra with corduroy appearance, (B) CT scan showing Polka dot pattern

Imaging: X-ray of vertebrae shows vertically oriented trabeculae (Fig. 15.7A) showing classical "Jailhouse/corduroy appearance". CT scan shows "Polka dot appearance" on cross-sectional images (Fig. 15.7B).

Treatment: Symptomatic cases are managed by angio-embolization/vertebroplasty (injection of bone cement into vertebral body) +/– radiotherapy.

OSTEOID OSTEOMA

This slow growing benign tumor of osteoblasts is the commonest true benign bone tumor.

Commonest site: Diaphyseal and cortical in location affecting femur > tibia. It is also common in posterior elements of spine.

Clinical features: Typical presentation is pain that worsens at night and is dramatically relieved by aspirin. Pain may be due to elevated levels of PGs and COX and thus relieved by aspirin.

Imaging: X-ray (Fig. 15.8A) shows a radiolucent nidus (made of fibrovascular stoma) surrounded by thick sclerotic bone (it contains both osteoblastic and clastic cells). Thin slice CT is the IOC to diagnose and identify the nidus. Size of the nidus is generally <1.5 cm. Tc scan shows increased uptake in nidus (double density sign).

Treatment
- Conservative with NSAIDs.
- Surgery: "Burr down technique" for removal of entire nidus is advised in patients with persistent symptoms despite conservative treatment. Recent advance CT-guided radio-frequency ablation.

OSTEOBLASTOMA

It is a vascular, benign, bone forming skeletal neoplasm resembling osteoid osteoma, but usually lacks reactive sclerosis (Fig. 15.8B). Lesions are more aggressive and bigger in size (nidus more than 1.5 cm in diameter) as compared to osteoid osteoma.

Site: Commonest site is posterior elements of spine > diaphysis of femur.

Clinical features: Pain is the most common symptom, but unlike osteoid osteoma, it is not nocturnal or relieved by NSAIDs.

Treatment: Extended curettage with bone grafting.

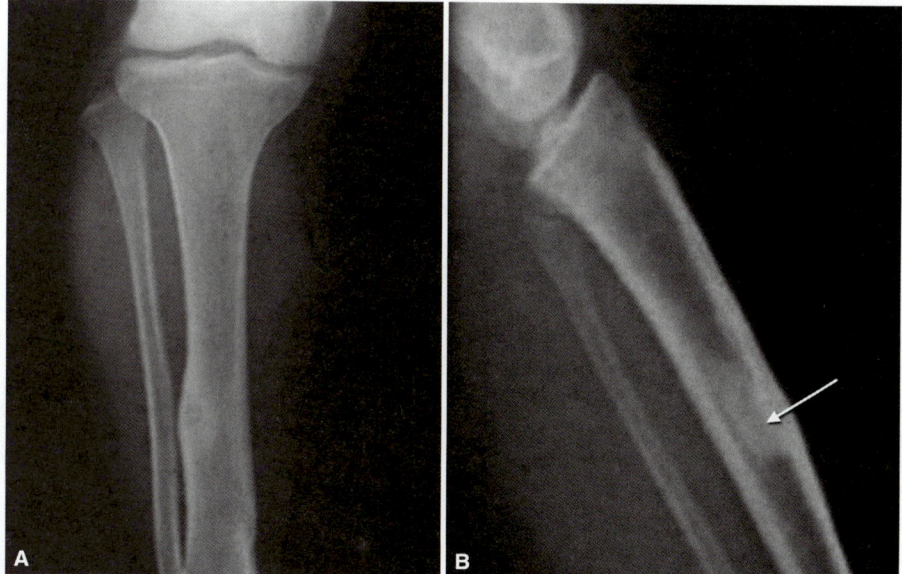

Fig. 15.8: (A) Osteoid osteoma showing nidus with sclerotic rim. (B) Osteoblastoma in tibial diaphysis (arrow)

OSTEOMA

Benign slow growing osteogenic lesions, involving almost exclusively head and neck area. Paranasal sinuses (frontal and ethmoid) are the commonest location.

Malignant Tumors

ADAMANTINOMA

It is a low grade malignant tumor that arises from tissues similar to 'ameloblasts' located over bones in subcutaneous location.

Age: 2nd–3rd decades of life

Site: Commonest in tibial diaphysis followed by fibula

Clinical features: Pain is the commonest symptom. Since it is a slow growing tumor, metastasis occurs late to inguinal lymph nodes and lungs.

X-ray: Multiple sharply demarcated radiolucent lesions (soap bubble appearance), similar to Campanacci disease.

Biopsy: It may reveal islands of epithelial cells in fibrous stroma (hallmark).

Treatment: Wide resection with adequate margins. Recurrence, if any, occurs quite late (since slow growing) and may require amputation.

Xtra Edge

Ameloblastoma: It is a separate entity (benign) from adamantinoma (malignant) arising from ameloblasts (enamel forming cells in mandible). It is the commonest 'bone' tumor of the jaw (overall commonest tumor of jaw is squamous cell carcinoma of the oral mucosa). The commonest site of occurrence is posterior mandible in the area of molar teeth.

X-ray: Soap bubble appearance.

Treatment: Wide local excision.

OSTEOSARCOMA

It is the commonest non-hematological malignancy of bone or 2nd most common primary malignancy of bone (1st is multiple myeloma).

It is highly malignant metaphyseal tumor (tm) where malignant mesenchymal cells produce osteoid (immature bone).

Tumor can be:
- Osteosclerotic ⎫
- Osteolytic   ⎬ or
- Mixed (M/C) ⎭

Osteoblastic ⎫
Chondroblastic ⎬ as the tumor cells are pleuripotent
Fibroblastic ⎭

Age: Bimodal age distribution   1°: 10–20 years ⎫
                                    2°: 40–60 years ⎭ any age group is possible

Site: Area of rapid growth—distal femur > proximal tibia > proximal humerus.

Syndromes associated: Retinoblastoma, Li-Fraumeni syndrome, Rothmund-Thomson syndrome.

Premalignant lesions associated with 2° osteosarcoma: Paget's disease (pelvis most common site), post-radiation, fibrous dysplasia, bone infarct, multiple osteochondromatosis. Osteosarcoma is the commonest radiation induced tumor and occurs at unusual sites like skull, clavicle, spine, ribs, etc. It has been reported to occur even 10–15 years after radiation exposure.

Clinical feature: Progressive persistent pain is the most common symptom (due to micro-infarcts) and 25% of patients have characteristic nocturnal pain. Later tender, warm and swollen limb/mass with dilated veins.

Imaging features: X-ray features (Fig. 15.9A and B): Permeative bone forming lesion with ill-defined borders. Periosteal reactions—Codman's triangle (subperiosteal new bone at tumor host cortex junction) or sunray appearance (due to calcification along the Sharpey's fibers). In late cases, tumor extends to soft tissue.

MRI: To detect marrow extension/soft tissue extension of tumor and its proximity to neurovascular structures.

Bone scan: To detect skip lesions/skeletal metastasis and to detect lung metastasis (most common site) CT is the IOC.

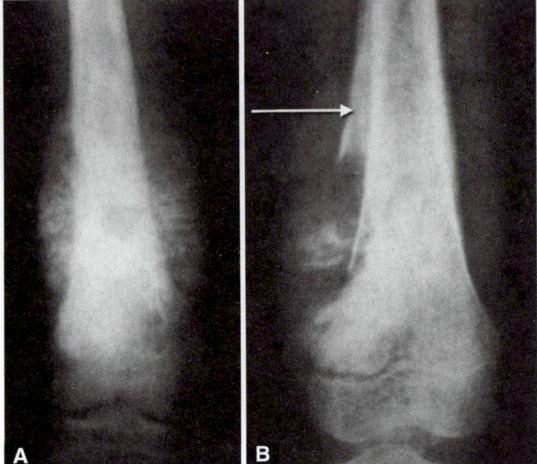

Fig. 15.9: (A) Sunray appearance, (B) Codman's triangle

Biopsy: Characterised by osteoid production, is taken from softer peripheral location and marrow examination has no role.

Blood investigations: Increased ALP, LDH, used for follow-up of lesion/detecting tumor recurrence. Osteocalcin A and anti-sarcoma antibodies are also raised.

Treatment: Neoadjuvant chemotherapy followed by limb salvage surgery/wide resection (whichever is appropriate) followed by chemotherapy. Chemotherapy regimen is T10 regimen, given for 4–6 weeks pre-operatively, containing the following drugs:
- High dose MTx (HDMTx) with citrovorum factor rescue.
- BCD—Bleomycin, Cyclophosphamide, Dactinomycin.
- Doxorubicin.

    After surgery, histological examination of the specimen is done, and response to chemotherapy is graded by Huvos grading. If the response is good, same regimen is followed postoperatively. But if response is not good, HDMTX is omitted and cisplatin is added with BCD and either of vincristine/doxorubicin*.

Prognostic factors: Osteosarcoma is the commonest tumor to metastasize and hence carries the worst prognosis. Most common route of metastasis is hematogenous; lymphatic is rare and most common site is lung. The most important prognostic factor is tumor stage (extent of disease). Pulmonary metastasis has poor prognosis but non-pulmonary metastasis has even worse prognosis. Skip metastasis (metastasis within same bone or across joint), osteosarcomas secondary to Paget's disease and radiation have equally bad prognosis. The next important prognostic feature is grade of the lesion, however, age/sex has no role in prognosis.

---

*(question asked—etoposide is not a component of T10 regimen).

Variants of osteosarcoma
- Parosteal osteosarcoma—low grade tumor with a favorable prognosis arising directly to external surface of a bone, commonest site is posterior aspect of distal femur. Lies directly on cortical surface (juxtacortical) with eventual destruction of cortex with medullary cavity invasion. Treatment—surgical en block excision without chemotherapy.
- Periosteal osteosarcoma—low grade osteosarcoma arising from diaphyseal cortex/periosteum (most commonly femur > tibia).
- Telangiectatic osteosarcoma—purely lytic variant of osteosarcoma, with invasive/ballooned appearance of the lesion similar to ABC.

Differentials: Myositis ossificans—differentiated by MRI. The mature cells/ossification in osteosarcoma is seen at the center, whereas in myositis ossificans, mature ossified cells are more abundant in the periphery.

Xtra Edge
- Radiation induced sarcoma—osteosarcoma (most common), fibrosarcoma, malignant fibrous histiocytoma.
- Recently extracorporeal radiation/immunotherapy has found some role in the treatment of osteosarcoma.
- FBI virus has been found to be associated with the pathogenesis of osteosarcoma.

EWING'S SARCOMA
It is a small round blue cell tumor with PNET (primitive neuroectodermal tumors) like features arising from endothelial cells in the bone marrow (mesenchymal origin). Trl (11;22) occurs in 90% of these mesenchymal cells that impart it the PNET biopsy features.

Age: Classically affects 5–15 years old; commonest bone tumor in <10 years old. However, per se the incidence is maximum in 2nd decade of life.

Site: Diaphysis of long bones (most commonly femur) >>Pelvis. 1/3rd cases occur in flat bones. Occasionally it might have a multicentric origin.

Clinical features: Pain is the commonest symptom, and systemic/local features are florid mimicking osteomyelitis (fever, increased counts). A needle aspirate of the tumor may grossly resemble pus making osteomyelitis the most important differential (thus all specimen should be cultured and biopsied).

X-ray: Permeative lytic bony lesion in diaphysis with onion peel periosteal reaction (lamellated periosteal reaction), extending to soft tissue (Fig. 15.10).

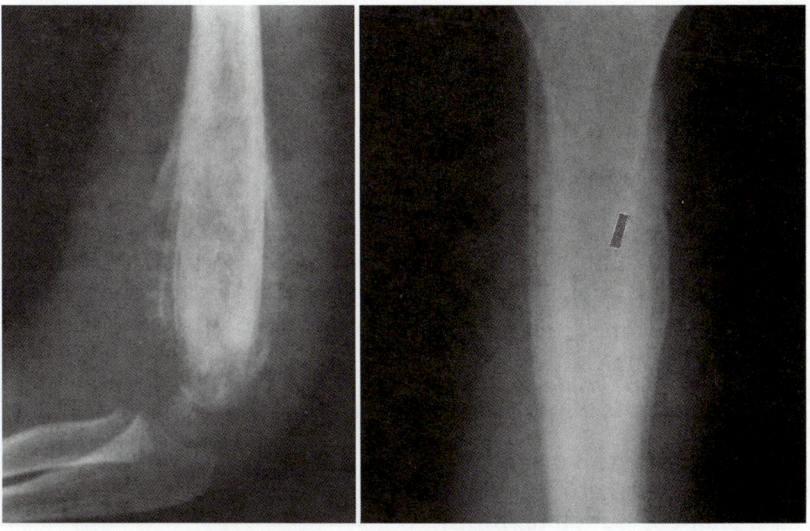

Fig. 15.10: Ewing's sarcoma of distal humerus and tibia showing onion peel appearance

MRI: To know the complete extent of the disease, as the complete bone may be involved and may not be apparent on X-ray and to see soft tissue extension.

CT scan for lung metastasis (most common site).

Bone scan: To see bone metastasis (2nd most common site). It is the commonest tumor showing bone to bone metastasis.

Bone marrow aspirate which is rarely used in other tumors, is a regular investigation in Ewing's sarcoma to rule out diffuse systemic disease.

Biopsy: Reveals pseudorosette formation typical of PNET, Homer Wright rosettes, perithelioma, neural elements on electron microscopy and stains positive for S-100 and neuron-specific enolase.

Tumor markers: CD99 positivity, MIC-2 gene positivity and PAS positivity but reticulin negative (lymphoma are CD45, reticulin positive but PAS negative).

Genetics: Tumors are part of PNET group and share a common MIC-2 gene (CD99) and trl (11; 22) (detected by RT-PCR). It is poorly differentiated, whereas PNET shows definite neural differentiation (N-Myc positive). Trl (11;22) > trl (21;22) > trl (7;22) are of diagnostic significance.

Treatment: It is the most radiosensitive and chemosensitive tumor. Neoadjuvant-adjuvant chemotherapy is always given to treat distant metastasis that may not be apparent initially. VDCA regimen is used (vincristine, doxorubicin, cyclophosphamide and actinomycin D). Chemotherapy is followed by wide resection. For unresectable tumors, radiotherapy becomes the mainstay (tumor melts on radiotherapy).

Prognosis: The tumor is most chemosensitive and radiosensitive and has best prognosis amongst the malignant lesions. The worst prognostic factor is the presence of distant metastasis. Systemic features, i.e. increased counts, old age and male sex are also associated with poor prognosis. However, histological grade is of no prognostic value, as all Ewing's sarcomas are considered to be of high grade.

Xtra Edge
- Ewing's sarcoma: PAS (+), reticulin (–).
- Lymphoma: PAS (–), reticulin (+).
- Embryonal rhabdomyosarcoma: Desmin, myoglobin, MSA(+).
- Hemangiopericytoma: Factor VIII (+).
- Melanoma: Cytokeratin (+).

CHONDROSARCOMA
It is the malignant tumor of cartilage producing cells. It is third most common primary malignant bone tumor (2nd most common primary non-hematological malignancy).

Types
- Primary/central/conventional: Most common type, seen in older age, in flat bones (pelvis most common) and in proximal bones—proximal femur and proximal humerus.
- Secondary/peripheral arises in pre-existing benign cartilage tumor, e.g. enchondroma, multiple exostosis. Develop somewhat earlier than primary chondrosarcoma.
- Although chondrosarcoma rarely occurs in hand, they are the commonest malignant bone tumors of hand, and also the most common malignant chest wall tumors.

  Pain is the commonest symptom in the absence of pathological fracture (differentiating point from enchondroma).

X-ray: Expansion of the medullary portion of bone, cortical thickening and matrix calcification (popcorn/comma shaped/punctate/mottled) (Fig. 15.11).

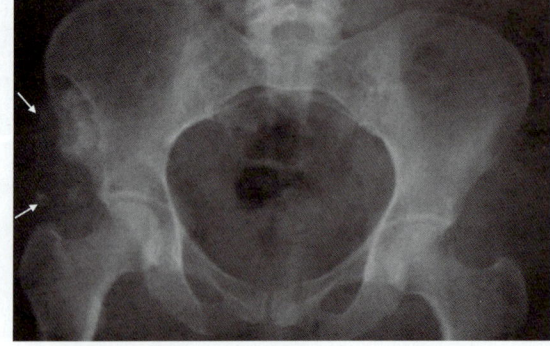
Fig. 15.11: Chondrosarcoma of ilium

Biopsy: Malignant cells full of cartilaginous matrix without any osteoid tissue. If any osteoid tissue is present, then the diagnosis is of 'chondroblastic osteosarcoma'.

Treatment: Wide local excision/radical excision.

Xtra Edge
- Since cartilage is relatively avascular, the cells survive transplantation easily and rate of local recurrence after intra-operative tumor contamination is high.
- Chondrosarcoma can produce hyperglycemia.

CHORDOMA
It is a rare, low grade malignant bone tumor of cranium and spine arising from notochordal remnants. In fact it is the 2nd most common primary malignancy in the spine (after multiple myeloma) and the commonest primary malignancy of sacrum.

Site: More than 50% arise in the sacrococcygeal area (below S3 level) and 30% at the base of skull.

Clinical features: Pain is the commonest symptom and is located in lower back in rectal/anal area.

Imaging features: They are often missed on X-ray/MRI because most arise below the S3 level. X-ray (in AP view findings are obstructed by bowel gas shadow) lateral view of sacrum should be done and in MRI LS spine sacrococcygeal area should be included in suspected cases.

Biopsy: Physaliferous cells (pathognomic).

Treatment: Wide surgical resection (effort should be made to protect S2, S3 nerve roots to preserve bowel/bladder function). Radiotherapy may be useful in unresectable tumor but chemotherapy has no role. Proton beam therapy has been the recent addition to the list of treatment options.

MULTIPLE MYELOMA/KAHLER'S DISEASE
- Neoplastic proliferation of single clone of plasma cells in the bone marrow producing excess of monoclonal immunoglobulins. While the multisystem disorder is called multiple myeloma (MM), isolated bony lesion is called plasmacytoma.
- Multiple myeloma is the most common primary malignancy of bone.
- It is diagnosed (Table 15.3) in adults over 40 years of age (median age at diagnosis 65 years). Multiple myeloma and metastatic carcinoma are always considered in patients >40 years age with new bone tumor.
- Radiation exposure, pesticide (dioxin) exposure and infection with HHV-8 and HIV have been found to be causative.
- The most common presentation of MM is generalized bone pain in an elderly patient.
- Features indicating end organ damage may include **anemia** (due to replacement of marrow by abnormal plasma cells) or **hypercalcemia** and **uremia** due to renal failure. **Hyperviscosity** may lead to neural ischemia manifesting as paraesthesias and areas of sensory loss. **Amyloidosis** may develop in some patients causing macroglossia, skin lesions and peripalpebral purpuras.
- **Punched out lesions without a reactive zone/sclerotic zone** with a sharp zone of transition to normal bone, are found throughout the skeleton.

Table 15.3: Diagnostic criteria for multiple myeloma
Major criteria
1. Biopsy confirmation of plasmacytoma
2. >30% plasma cells on bone marrow biopsy
3. Serum IgG> 3.5 g/dL, IgA > 2 g/dL
4. Urine IgA > 1g/24 hr or presence of Bence Jones proteins
Minor criteria
• 10–30% plasma cells on bone marrow biopsy
• Serum or urine protein levels below those listed for major criteria
• Multiple lytic bone lesions
• Decreased serum IgG levels

- Common sites of involvement (in order of frequency) are spine (commonest), pelvis, ribs, upper extremities, face, skull, femur and sternum.
- Bone scan is usually negative (cold spot) because of lack of osteoblastic overactivity.
- Screening tool of choice is a skeletal survey.
- *Blood tests*:
  - Screening tests include: Paraproteins in serum and Bence Jones protein in urine.
  - Low hemoglobin, raised serum calcium (due to marked osteolytic action of myeloma cells), increased uric acid (due to increased cell breakdown), elevated urea (in patients in renal failure), markedly increased ESR and a high total protein value but with reversal of A: G (albumin: globulin) ratio (due to increase in globulin fraction of proteins).
  - Serum electrophoresis shows an increase in gamma fraction of globulin called the M-spike detectable in both blood and urine.
  - Serum β_2-microglobulin is a tumor marker, increase of which is a poor prognostic sign.
- On urine examination one can also detect the presence of Bence Jones proteins by the heating method or by immuno-electrophoresis (more sensitive method).
- *On histological examination*:
  - The tumor cells have an eccentric nucleus with clumped nuclear chromatin arranged in a clock face pattern (cartwheel appearance) and stain positive for **CD56** and **CD38** (while normal plasma cells do not).
  - Hoffa's clear zone (clear zone near nucleus representing golgi apparatus) is characteristic in these cells.

Treatment
- Chemotherapy is the mainstay of treatment. Drugs used are melphalan in combination with prednisolone. Other agents which may be used are cyclophosphamide, doxorubicin and thalidomide. Bisphosphonates are used to decrease bone pain and control hypercalcemia.
- Autologous stem cell transplantation, although not curative (i.e. does not cause remission) improves overall survival by 2–3 years. It is an option in relatively young (<65 years) patients without comorbidities.
- Impending (Mirel's score > 8) or actual pathological fractures may require long bone stabilization with intramedullary implants (to splint the entire length of bone).

Xtra Edge
1. The commonest site for an extramedullary myeloma is skin and subcutaneous tissues > liver. Over 80% of these arise in the region of head and neck, especially the upper respiratory tract.
2. The most common site for a solitary plasmacytoma is spine.
3. Multiple myeloma is one tumor which can have dural deposits without bone lesions.
4. The levels of alkaline phosphatase are not raised in multiple myeloma.
5. The commonest site for an extramedullary myeloma is skin and subcutaneous tissues > liver.
6. Over 80% of these arise in the region of head and neck, especially the upper respiratory tract.
7. The most common site for a solitary plasmacytoma is spine.

EOSINOPHILIC GRANULOMA OF BONE
Eosinophilic granuloma (EG) is a part of spectrum of disease Langerhans' cell histiocytosis (formerly called histiocytosis X).
- *Letterer-Siwe disease*: A fulminant systemic disease, in <3 years old.
- *Hand-Schüller-Christian disease*: Triad of lytic skull lesions, exopthalmos, diabetes insipidus.
- *Eosinophilic granuloma*: It may occur in the bone as either a solitary lesion of bone destruction (more common) or as multiple lesions in the skeleton. Common sites include the skull (most common site), mandible, spine, ribs and the long bones.

Age: Usually children presenting with localized pain, tenderness, swelling, fever, elevated ESR and leukocytosis.

X-ray features
- The skull may have a lesion with sharp, punched out borders that are uneven across the inner and outer table causing a **"bevelled edge"** that gives them the characteristic **double contour**.
- In long bones, EG is found in the diaphysis or metaphysis mostly in the center of the medullary cavity. Good periosteal reaction and may expand to cause endosteal scalloping.

Biopsy: The gold standard for confirmation.
- Electron microscope demonstrates racket-shaped cytoplasmic inclusion bodies called **Birbeck's granules** and the cells stain positive for S-100, CD1a and Neuron specific enolase.

Treatment: Treatment is mostly not required. Regress spontaneously in about 6 months to 2 years. They are **highly radiosensitive** and excision and curettage is done for resistant cases. Chemotherapy is limited to systemic form of the disease. Overall, prognosis is very good.

Xtra edge
- Punched out lesions in skull
  - Eosinophilic granuloma
  - Multiple myeloma
  - LCH
  - Hyperparathyroidism
  - Metastasis
  - TB

Most important differential is eosinophilic granuloma/multiple myeloma. They can be differentiated by the fact that in EG, the lesions have a double contour (due to bevelled edge) as there is uneven destruction of the inner and outer table of the skull.

SYNOVIAL CELL SARCOMA
This is a mesenchymal malignant tumor (no synovial origin despite its name).

Site: They arise from soft tissue in the vicinity of tendon, bursae, joint capsule and mostly they are extra-articular. The tumor is most commonly located around the knee and also the most common soft tissue sarcoma of foot.

Clinical features: It is a slow growing tumor with an indolent course with the chief complaint of deep seated mass/swelling.

Biopsy: "Biphasic tumor" (epithelial and mesenchymal differentiations).

Genetics: **trl (X; 18)** leading to SYT-SSX gene fusion.

Treatment: Wide excision is the treatment of choice and radiotherapy is also effective.

PIGMENTED VILLONODULAR SYNOVITIS (PVNS)
It is a rare benign disease of the synovial membrane which is characterized by hypervascular neoplastic proliferation of the synovium with deposition of hemosiderin.

Sites: Knee > hip > shoulder.

Clinical features: Slowly progressive mild pain, decreased range of movement and episodes of catching/joint locking.

On knee aspiration, the finding of blood-tinged synovial fluid is highly suggestive, although not pathognomonic of PVNS. On arthroscopy typical brownish pigmentation of synovium is seen due to deposition of hemosiderin pigment.

Treatment: Low dose external beam radiotherapy and arthroscopic/open synovectomy have been tried with varying success for the treatment. Malignant transformation has been reported, but very rare.

BONE ISLAND
Bone island is an unossified piece of cartilage in the bone. At times a person may have multiple bone islands scattered in whole body, a condition called "osteopoikilosis".

SOFT TISSUE SARCOMAS
- Rhabdomyosarcoma is the most common soft tissue tumor in children.
- Liposarcoma is the commonest soft tissue tumor in adult.
- Sarcomas of soft tissue origin do not frequently involve bone, except the following:
  - Synovial cell sarcoma
  - Angiosarcoma
  - Rhabdomyosarcoma
  - Liposarcoma.

MULTIPLE CHOICE QUESTIONS

1. **A 55 years old male having bony pains for last two years, presents with the image shown below. Most probable diagnosis is:**

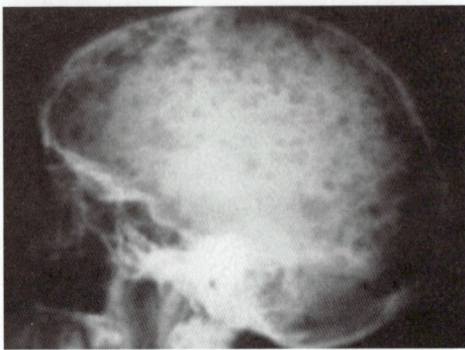

   A. Multiple myeloma
   B. Paget's disease
   C. Hyperparathyroidism
   D. Eosinophilic granuloma

2. **Fallen fragment sign is characteristic of:**
   A. ABC
   B. SBC
   C. GCT
   D. Hyperparathyroidism

3. **After radical resection of chordoma, which radiation therapy is best?**
   A. Photons   B. Neutrons
   C. Protons   D. Electrons

4. **In which of the following multiple lesions are not seen?**
   A. Enchondroma   B. Osteoid osteoma
   C. Fibrous dysplasia D. GCT

5. **Background lesions simulating bone tumors are all *except*:**
   A. Fibrous dysplasia B. Bone island
   C. Hurler's syndrome D. Bone infarct

6. **Epiphysis involved in which bone tumor:**
   A. Osteosarcoma   B. Multiple myeloma
   C. Giant cell tumor   D. Ewing's sarcoma

7. **Epiphyseal tumor before fusion of epiphysis:**
   A. Chondroblastoma   B. Chondrosarcoma
   C. Ewing's sarcoma   D. Giant cell tumor

8. **Which is not a metaphyseal tumor?**
   A. Osteosarcoma
   B. Chondrosarcoma
   C. Giant cell tumor
   D. Aneurysmal bone cyst

9. **Tumor in diaphysis:**
   A. Osteogenic sarcoma
   B. Ewing's sarcoma
   C. Osteoclastoma
   D. Osteochondroma

10. **GCT is:**
    A. Epiphyseal
    B. Epiphyseometaphyseal
    C. Metaphyseal
    D. Metaphyseodiaphyseal

11. **Most common tumor of hand:**
    A. Enchondroma
    B. Squamous cell carcinoma
    C. Chondroblastoma
    D. Melanoma

12. **Solitary bone cyst is most common in the:**
    A. Upper end of humerus
    B. Lower end of humerus
    C. Upper end of fibula
    D. Lower end of femur

13. **The following lesions are classically seen in metaphysis:**
    A. Osteomyelitis   B. Osteosarcoma
    C. Osteochondroma   D. Osteoclastoma
    E. Ewing's sarcoma

14. **Most common site of osteogenic sarcoma is:**
    A. Femur, upper end B. Femur lower end
    C. Tibia upper   D. Tibia lower end

15. **Chondroblastoma is tumor of:**
    A. Epiphysis   B. Metaphysis
    C. Diaphysis   D. Flat bone

16. **Bone tumors seen in diaphysis:**
    A. Chondrosarcoma   B. Ewing's tumor
    C. Osteoclastoma   D. Chondroblastoma
    E. Osteoid osteoma

17. **Chordoma can occur over all the following sites *except*:**
    A. Rib   B. Clivus
    C. Sacrum   D. Vertebral body

18. **Not a common tumor of 1st decade of life:**
    A. Ameloblastoma   B. Neuroblastoma
    C. Retinoblastoma   D. Rhabdomyosarcoma

19. **True about bone tumor is:**
    A. Multiple myeloma is seen in more than 55 years age and above
    B. Osteogenic sarcoma fourth decade
    C. Chondrosarcoma first decade
    D. Osteoclastoma fifth decade

20. **A 10-year-old boy, LEAST common cause of proximal lytic lesion head of femur is:**
    A. Plasmacytoma   B. Metastasis
    C. Histiocytosis   D. Bone tumor

21. **Which of the following is wrongly matched?**
    A. Osteosarcoma: Sunray appearance
    B. Chondroblastoma: Soap bubble appearance
    C. Ewing's sarcoma: Onion peel appearance
    D. Secondaries of spine: Winking owl sign

22. **Which of the following childhood tumors most frequently metastasizes of bone?**
    A. Neuroblastoma   B. Ganglioneuroma
    C. Wilms' tumor   D. Ewing's sarcoma
23. **Radioresistant bone tumor among the following:**
    A. Ewing's sarcoma   B. Osteosarcoma
    C. Multiple myeloma D. Chondrosarcoma
    E. Lymphoma
24. **Soap bubble appearance in X-ray suggests:**
    A. Osteogenic sarcoma
    B. Ewing's sarcoma
    C. Osteoclastoma
    D. Chondrosarcoma
25. **Active benign tumor (Enneking) all are true** *except*:
    A. Intracapsular
    B. Well defined
    C. Wide area of activity (>5 cm)
    D. Treated by extended curettage
26. **Classification system of bone tumor is:**
    A. Enneking   B. Manchester
    C. Edward   D. TNM
27. **All of the following tumor are benign tumor** *except*:
    A. Chondroma   B. Chordoma
    C. Osteochondroma   D. Enchondroma
28. **According to a newer hypothesis Ewing's sarcoma arises from:**
    A. Epiphysis   B. Diaphysis
    C. Medullary cavity D. Cortex
29. **X-ray upper end humerus, diagnosis is:**

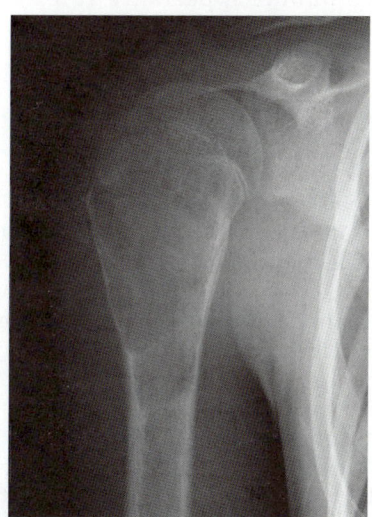

    A. Giant cell tumor
    B. Simple bone cyst
    C. Aneurysmal bone cyst
    D. Osteosarcoma

30. **All are true about aneurysmal bone cyst** *except*:
    A. Eccentric
    B. Expansile and lytic
    C. Treated by simple curettage
    D. Metaphysis of long bones
31. **Fallen fragment sign is a feature of:**
    A. Simple bone cyst
    B. Aneurysmal bone cyst
    C. Giant cell tumor
    D. Fibrous dysplasia
32. **Pediatric patient with upper humerus lytic lesion with cortical thinning which is not a treatment modality?**
    A. Sclerosant
    B. Radiotherapy
    C. Curettage and bone grafting
    D. Steroids
33. **True about simple bone cyst is A/E:**
    A. Seen in children
    B. Present as well demarcated radiolucent lesions
    C. Pathological fracture seen
    D. Commonest site is diaphysis
34. **A classical expansile lytic lesion in the transverse process of a vertebra is seen in:**
    A. Osteosarcoma
    B. Aneurysmal bone cyst
    C. Osteoblastoma
    D. Metastasis
35. **A 8 years male has expansile lytic cavity in upper end of humerus. Cavity in center has a cortical fragment. What is the diagnosis?**
    A. UBC   B. ABC
    C. GCT   D. Enchondroma
36. **Secondary aneurysmal bone cyst arises in:**
    A. Osteoclastoma   B. Chondroblastoma
    C. Fibrous dysplasia D. GCT
    E. All of the above
37. **Regarding GCT of bone true is:**
    A. Common in 20–40 years age group
    B. Proximal femur involvement may be seen
    C. Best managed by extended curettage followed by bone grafting
    D. Closest differential is ABC
    E. 3% cases have metastasis to lungs
38. **About giant cell tumor, all are true** *except*:
    A. Commonly presents in the 20–40 years age group
    B. Matrix consists of proliferating mono-nuclear cells
    C. Osteoclast gaint cells constitute the proliferative component of the tumor
    D. It is a benign tumor which may have lung metastasis

39. A 30-year-old male presented with hip pain for last 6 months. Hip X-ray is shown below. What is the likely diagnosis?

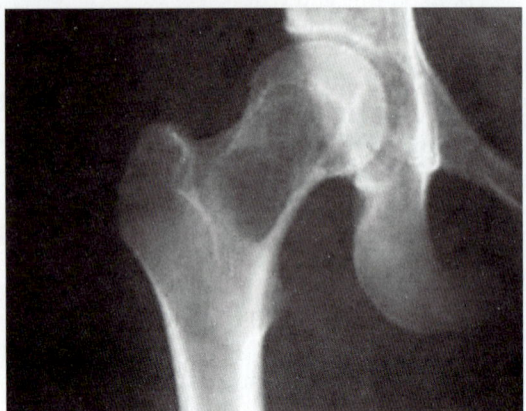

A. Giant cell tumor   B. Simple bone cyst
C. Adamantinoma   D. Ewing's sarcoma

40. True statement regarding GCT is:
A. Malignant tumor
B. Most commonly seen around knee
C. Local radiation is the treatment
D. Seen before puberty

41. The most likely diagnosis for the tumor at upper end of tibia is:

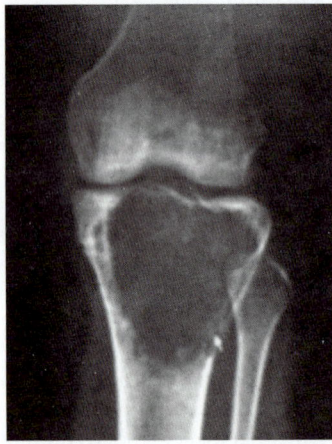

A. GCT   B. UBC
C. ABC   D. CB

42. Soap bubble appearance on X-ray is seen in which bone tumor?
A. Osteogenic sarcoma B. Giant cell tumor
C. Multiple myeloma   D. Chondroblastoma

43. Which of the following is epiphyseal tumor?
A. Giant cell tumor   B. Osteogenic sarcoma
C. Ewing's sarcoma   D. Osteoid sarcoma

44. GCT malignant component is:
A. Giant cells   B. Mononuclear cells
C. Both   D. None

45. Which of the following is variant of giant cell tumor?
A. Ossifying fibroma
B. Non-ossifying fibroma
C. Osteogenic sarcoma
D. Chondroblastoma

46. What is the most likely diagnosis of the X-ray depicted below?

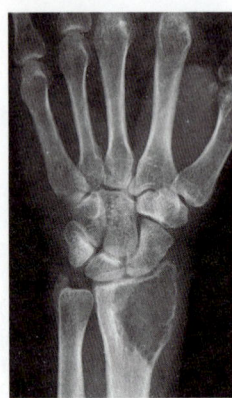

A. Chondrosarcoma   B. Osteoclastoma
C. Osteogenic sarcoma D. Osteoid sarcoma

47. The differential diagnosis of lesion, histologically resembling giant cell tumor in the small bones of the hands or feet, includes all of the following *except*:
A. Aneurysmal bone cyst
B. Fibrosarcoma
C. Osteosarcoma
D. Hyperparathyroidism

48. Soap bubble appearance at lower end of radius, the treatment of choice is:
A. Local excision
B. Excision and bone grafting
C. Amputation
D. Radiotherapy

49. Osteoclastoma is treated with:
A. Joint replacement   B. Excision
C. Curettage   D. Arthrodesis
E. Chemotherapy

50. Most common benign tumor of the bone is:
A. Giant cell tumor   B. Simple bone cyst
C. Osteochondroma   D. Enchondroma

51. Factors indicating malignant degeneration in osteochondroma:
A. Size   B. Pain
C. Weight loss   D. Thickness of cartilage

52. All of the following are the causes of sudden increase in pain in osteochondroma, *except*:
A. Sarcomatous changes
B. Fracture
C. Bursitis
D. Degenerative changes

53. **All the statements are true about exostosis,** *except*:
   A. It occurs at the growing end of bone
   B. Growth continues after skeletal maturity
   C. It is covered by cartilaginous cap
   D. Malignant transformation may occur

54. **Diaphyseal aclasia is etiologically:**
   A. Congenital   B. Developmental
   C. Metabolic   D. Inflammatory

55. **Which of the following statement is false about osteochondromatosis?**
   A. Usually affects long bones, but can also occur in skull and pelvis
   B. Usual site is metaphyseal region
   C. Also known as multiple exostoses, diaphyseal aclasia
   D. It does not interfere with general body stature
   E. Autosomal dominant in inheritance

56. **Maffucci syndrome:**
   A. Multiple enchondromatosis with hemangiomas
   B. Multiple osteochondromatosis with hemangiomas
   C. Multiple osteochondromas
   D. Multiple giant cell tumor

57. **Development of chondrosarcomas is related with:**
   A. Maffucci syndrome B. Felty syndrome
   C. Oliver's disease   D. None of the above

58. **Most common tumor in bones of hand:**
   A. Exostosis   B. Giant cell tumor
   C. Enchondroma   D. Synovial sarcoma

59. **Maffucci syndrome is:**
   A. Multiple osteochondromas
   B. Multiple enchondromas
   C. Multiple enchondromas with soft tissue malignancies
   D. Multiple hemangiomas

60. **Identify the lesion in the X-ray:**

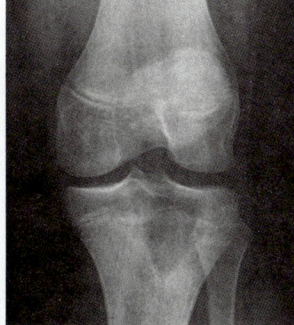

   A. Chondroblastoma
   B. Osteoclastoma
   C. ABC
   D. Eosinophilic granuloma

61. **Which one of the following bone tumors typically affects the epiphysis of a long bone?**
   A. Osteosarcoma
   B. Ewing's sarcoma
   C. Chondroblastoma
   D. Chondromyxoid fibroma

62. **Dense calcification is found in:**
   A. Osteosarcoma
   B. Chondroblastoma
   C. Synovial sarcoma
   D. Osteoblastoma

63. **A 15-year-old boy presented with painful swelling over the left shoulder. Radiograph of the shoulder showed an osteolytic area with stippled calcification over the proximal humeral epiphysis. Biopsy of the lesion revealed an immature fibrous matrix with scattered giant cells. Which of the following is the most likely diagnosis?**
   A. Giant cell tumor
   B. Chondroblastoma
   C. Osteosarcoma
   D. Chondromyxoid fibroma

64. **Not true about non-ossifying fibroma of bone:**
   A. Present until 3rd and 4th decades
   B. Eccentric
   C. Sclerotic margin
   D. Histologically giant cell with foam cell
   E. Metaphyseal lesion

65. **McCune-Albright syndrome features are A/E:**
   A. High calcium
   B. Presents around puberty
   C. Cysts in long bones
   D. Precocious puberty
   E. High ACTH levels

66. **Mandible most common tumor:**
   A. Ameloblastoma
   B. Squamous cell carcinoma
   C. Osteoid osteoma
   D. Metastasis

67. **Characteristic radiological feature of fibrous dysplasia is:**
   A. Cortical thickening
   B. Cortical calcification
   C. Ground glass appearance
   D. Bone enlargement

68. **True about ameloblastoma:**
   A. Cystic lesion
   B. Rapidly growing
   C. Malignant disease
   D. MC site is tibia

69. A 33-year-old man presented with a slowly progressive swelling in the middle 1/3rd of his right tibia. X-ray examination revealed multiple sharply demarcated radiolucent lesions separated by areas of dense and sclerotic bone. Microscopic examination of a biopsy specimen revealed island of epithial cells in a fibrous stroma. Which of the following is the most probable diagnosis?
   A. Adamantinoma
   B. Osteofibrous dysplasia
   C. Osteosarcoma
   D. Fibrous cortical defect

70. Fibrous dysplasia, true is:
   A. X-ray shows increase bone density
   B. More common in females as compared to males
   C. Rare in <40 years age
   D. Monostotic fibrous is seen in McCune-Albright syndrome

71. X-ray proximal femur in a patient with pain hip. The deformity shown is:

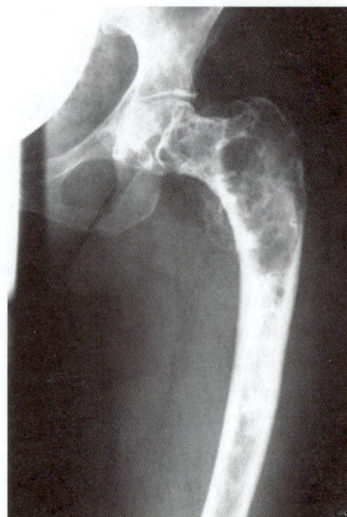

   A. Blade of grass deformity
   B. Shepherd crook deformity
   C. Chicken wire appearance
   D. Corduroy appearance

72. Most common site of admantinoma of the long bones is:
   A. Femur   B. Ulna
   C. Tibia   D. Fibula

73. Most common site of origin of ameloblastoma is:
   A. Mandible near molar tooth
   B. Middle alveolar margins
   C. Hard palate
   D. Mandible near symphysis menti

74. Neurofibromatosis inheritance:
   A. Autosomal dominant
   B. Autosomal recessive
   C. X-linked dominant
   D. X-linked recessive

75. Musculoskeletal abnormalities in neurofibromatosis is:
   A. Hypertrophy of limb
   B. Scoliosis
   C. Pseudoarthrosis
   D. All of the above

76. The common features of neurofibromatosis include all, *except*:
   A. Optic glioma
   B. Dumbbell neurofibroma
   C. Scoliosis
   D. Periventricular calcifications

77. Striated vertebra are seen in:
   A. Metastasis   B. Tuberculosis
   C. Hemangioma   D. Osteoblastoma

78. Which of the following statements is not true regarding hemangioma of the bone?
   A. Occurs commonly in skull bones
   B. Requires observation as it is premalignant
   C. Hamartomatous in origin
   D. Forms 10–12% of the bone tumors
   E. Local gigantism occurs when it occurs in an extremity

79. Osteoid osteoma consists of:
   A. Osteoblasts   B. Osteoclasts
   C. Both of the above   D. None of the above

80. Which is the commonest true benign bone tumor?
   A. Osteoid osteoma   B. Hemangioma
   C. Osteochondroma   D. Enchondroma

81. A 10-year-old child has a lesion in the diaphysis of bone in the cotex with central lysis and surrounding sclerosis
   A. Osteoid osteoma
   B. Eosinophilic granuloma
   C. Fibrous cortical defect
   D. Fibrous dysplasia

82. A patient presents with pain in the thigh, relieved by aspirin. X-ray shows a radiolucent mass surrounded by sclerosis. Diagnosis is:
   A. Osteoma   B. Osteoid osteoma
   C. Osteoblastoma   D. Osteoclastoma

83. Pain in osteoid osteoma is specifically relieved by:
   A. Salicylates   B. Narcotic analgesics
   C. Radiation   D. Splinting

84. Babu, a 19-year-old male, has a small circumscribed sclerotic swelling over diaphysis of femur, likely diagnosis is:
   A. Osteoclastoma   B. Osteosarcoma
   C. Ewing's sarcoma   D. Osteoid osteoma

85. **Nidus is seen in:**
    A. Chondroblastoma B. Osteosarcoma
    C. Osteoid osteoma D. Giant cell tumor
86. **Tumor with maximum bone matrix:**
    A. Osteoid osteoma   B. Chondrosarcoma
    C. Enchondroma   D. None
87. **Which of the following is true about osteosarcoma?**
    A. Sunburst appearance due to bony involvement
    B. Lung metastasis common
    C. Seen in epiphysis
    D. Secondarys osteosarcoma is seen in younger age group
88. **Calcification in osteosarcoma is due to presence of:**
    A. Osteoid matrix
    B. Osteoblasts
    C. High calcium levels in serum
    D. High calcitonin
89. **The following reaction is associated with which tumor?**

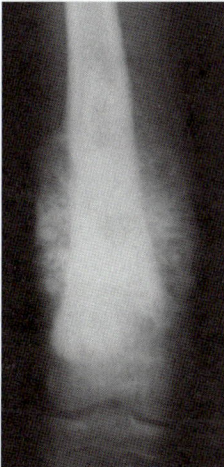

    A. Osteosarcoma   B. Chondroblastoma
    C. Ewing's sarcoma   D. Codman's tumor
90. **Osteosarcoma occurs in:**
    A. Osteoma   B. Osteoporosis
    C. Osteomalacia   D. Osteitis deformans
91. **In young person most common cancer among following is:**
    A. Giant cell   B. Osteosarcoma
    C. Chondrosarcoma   D. Ewing sarcoma
    E. Multiple myeloma
92. **In osteogenic sarcoma predominant histological finding is:**
    A. Giant cells
    B. Osteoid forming tumor cells
    C. Fibroblastic proliferation
    D. Chondroblasts

93. **Children with germline retinoblastoma are more likely to develop other primary malignancies in their later lifetime course. Which of the following can occur in such patients?**
    A. Osteosarcoma of lower limbs and soft tissue sarcoma
    B. Thyroid carcinoma
    C. Seminoma
    D. Squamous cell carcinoma
94. **Which of the following bone tumor presents with secondaries in lung with pneumothorax?**
    A. Osteosarcoma   B. Ewing's sarcoma
    C. Osteoclastoma   D. Chondroblastoma
95. **X-ray appearance of osteosarcoma are all *except*:**
    A. Periosteal reaction
    B. Codman's triangle
    C. Soap bubble appearance
    D. Sunray appearance
96. **Codman's triangle is most commonly seen in:**
    A. Chondroblastoma B. Osteosarcoma
    C. Multiple myeloma D. Hemangioma
97. **Characteristic histopathological feature of osteosarcoma is:**
    A. Codman's triangle
    B. Matrix new bone formation with Codman's triangle
    C. Malignant cell with osteoid formation
    D. Spindle cells
98. **True about osteosarcoma is A/E:**
    A. Primary osteosarcoma most commonly occurs in age group of less than 20 years
    B. Periosteal reaction is present
    C. Presented as elevated soft tissue mass
    D. Commonly associated with osteiod osteoma
    E. Formation of bone by the tumor cells is characteristic
99. **Codman's triangle and onion seen in:**
    A. Benign bone tumors
    B. Malignant bone tumors
    C. Traumatic conditions
    D. Paget's disease
100. **Osteosarcoma most commonly affects:**
    A. Femur   B. Humerus
    C. Tibia   D. Vertebrae
101. **Radiation induced tumor:**
    A. Osteosarcoma   B. Ewing's sarcoma
    C. Multiple myeloma D. Chondrosarcoma
102. **Which of the following malignant tumors is radioresistant?**
    A. Ewing's sarcoma   B. Retinoblastoma
    C. Osteosarcoma   D. Neuroblastoma
103. **Which of the following is a pulsatile tumor?**
    A. Osteosarcoma   B. Chondrosarcoma
    C. Osteoclastoma   D. Ewing's sarcoma
104. **Matrix forming tumor is:**
    A. Osteosarcoma   B. Chondrosarcoma
    C. Fibrosarcoma   D. Ewing's sarcoma

105. **An 8-year-old boy with progressive swelling over upper end tibia with raised local temperature, variable in consistency and ill-defined margins:**
    A. Giant cell tumor
    B. Ewing's sarcoma
    C. Osteogenic sarcoma
    D. Secondary metastasis

106. **'T -10 protocol' for treatment of osteosarcoma includes all of the following, *except*:**
    A. High dose methotrexate
    B. Bleomycin, cyclophosphamide, doxorubicin (BCD)
    C. Vincristine
    D. Etoposide

107. **All of the following investigations are needed for the diagnosis of osteosarcoma, *except*:**
    A. MRI of femur   B. Bone marrow biopsy
    C. Bone scan   D. CT chest

108. **True about osteosarcoma:**
    A. Involves epiphysis of long bones
    B. Most commonly involve knee and distal femur
    C. Spread to lung through hematogenous route
    D. Exclusively found in adolescent and early adult life
    E. X-ray has sunray appearance

109. **Management plan for osteogenic sarcoma of the lower end of femur must include:**
    A. Radiotherapy, amputation, chemotherapy
    B. Surgery alone
    C. Chemotherapy + limb salvage surgery + chemotherapy
    D. Chemotherapy + Radiotherapy

110. **Characteristic translocation seen in Ewing's sarcoma:**
    A. t(2; 8)   B. t(11; 22)
    C. t(x; 18)   D. t (14; 18)

111. **Small round cell tumor among the following:**
    A. Ewing's sarcoma   B. Chandrosarcomas
    C. Metastasis   D. Rhabdomyosarcoma

112. **Ewing's sarcoma is characterized by all *except*:**
    A. Duaphysis in location
    B. Locally malignant
    C. Soap bubble appearance
    D. Onion peel appearance on X-ray

113. **A 7-year-old boy presents with swelling and pain over tibia. On X-ray there is periosteal reaction in diaphysis. Probable diagnosis is:**
    A. Osteomyelitis   B. Chondroblastoma
    C. Ewing's sarcoma   D. Osteosarcoma

114. **Most common site of Ewing's sarcoma:**
    A. Upper end of tibia B. Shaft of tibia
    C. Lower end of femur D. Shaft of femur

115. **A 5-year-old child with pain and swelling over tibia, X-ray done, most probable diagnosis based on periosteal reaction seen on X-ray:**

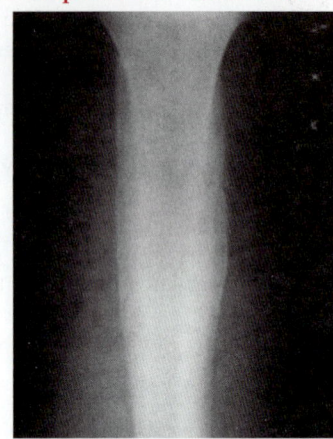

    A. Osteosarcoma   B. GCT
    C. Ewing's sarcoma   D. Chondrosarcoma

116. **Maximum incidence of Ewing's sarcoma occurs in:**
    A. 1st decade   B. 2nd decade
    C. 3rd decade   D. 4th decade

117. **Glycogen positive cells are seen in:**
    A. Ewing's sarcoma   B. Osteosarcoma
    C. Fibrosarcoma   D. Osteoid osteoma

118. **Mass in anterior aspect of thigh fixed to bone the procedure to be carried out:**
    A. Incisional biopsy B. Excisional biopsy
    C. FNAC   D. Radiotherapy

119. **Ewing's sarcoma most common age group:**
    A. 1st decade   B. 2nd decade
    C. 3rd decade   D. 4th decade

120. **PAS positive cells are seen in:**
    A. Ewing's sarcoma   B. Osteosarcoma
    C. Chondrosarcomas   D. Multiple myeloma

121. **Mic 2 positive cells are seen in:**
    A. Ewing's sarcoma   B. Osteosarcoma
    C. Chondrosarcomas   D. Multiple myeloma

122. **CD 99 is marker of:**
    A. Dematofibrosarcoma protuberans
    B. Ewing's sarcoma
    C. Osteosarcoma
    D. Metastasis

123. **Ewing's sarcoma is associated with which genetic defect:**
    A. 13q 14   B. c-myc
    C. Trisomy 8   D. T(22,11)

124. **Poor prognostic sign for Ewing's sarcoma is:**
    A. Fever   B. Age, 12 years
    C. Grade   D. Females

125. **1st decade most common bone tumor:**
    A. Ewing's sarcoma   B. Osteosarcoma
    C. Multiple myeloma   D. Metastasis

126. A 15-year-old boy is injured while playing cricket. X-rays of the leg rule out a possible fracture. The radiologist reports the boy has an evidence of aggressive bone tumor with both bone destruction and soft tissue mass. The bone biopsy reveals a bone cancer with neural differentiation. Which of the following is the most likely diagnosis?
   A. Chondroblastoma B. Ewing's sarcoma
   C. Neuroblastoma D. Osteosarcoma

127. Commonest site of occurrence of chondro-sarcoma is:
   A. Pelvis   B. Femur
   C. Ribs   D. Proximal tibia

128. Tumor with calcification is seen in:
   A. Unicameral bone cyst
   B. Chondroblastoma
   C. Osteoclastoma
   D. Chondrosarcoma

129. A 7-year-old boy with H/o trauma 2 months back, now presents with fever and acute pain over thigh. On X-ray femoral shaft shows lesions with multiple laminated periosteal reaction, next line of management:
   A. CRP measurement B. Core biopsy
   C. Tc99 MDP scan   D. MRI

130. Which of the following tumor is associated with hyperglycemia?
   A. Ewing's sarcoma   B. Osteosarcoma
   C. Multiple myeloma D. Chondrosarcoma

131. A 45 years male presented with an expansile lesion in the center of femoral metaphysic. The lesion shows endosteal scalloping and punc-tuate calcifications. Most likely diagnosis is:
   A. Osteosarcoma   B. Chondrosarcoma
   C. Simple bone cyst D. Fibrous dysplasia

132. Physaliferous cells are seen in:
   A. Phyllodes tumor   B. Chordoma
   C. Meningioma   D. Pheochromocytoma

133. Chordoma commonly involves:
   A. Dorsal spine   B. Clivus
   C. Lumbar spine   D. Sacrum

134. Which of the following is not a benign bone tumor?
   A. Osteoid osteoma   B. Chondroma
   C. Enchondroma   D. Chordoma

135. Most common primary bone tumor is:
   A. Multiple myeloma B. Osteosarcoma
   C. Chondrosarcoma   D. Metastasis

136. Lytic punched out lesions in the skull X-ray, most likely diagnosis:
   A. Osteosarcoma
   B. Multiple myeloma
   C. Metastasis
   D. Eosinophilic granuloma

137. A 70-year-old male complains of multiple bone pains, on evaluation he has high ESR, high calcium values, lytic lesion in multiple bone >20% plasma cells in peripheral smear. Most likely diagnosis is?
   A. Multiple myeloma
   B. Hairy cell leukemia
   C. Plasma cell leukemia
   D. Metastasis periosteal

138. True for multiple myeloma:
   A. Hypercalcemia
   B. Increased serum alkaline phosphatase
   C. Monoclonal M band
   D. Bone marrow plasma cells <5%

139. A patient with pain in back. Lab investigation shows elevated ESR. X-ray skull shows multiple punched out lytic lesions. Most important investigation to be done is:
   A. Serum acid phosphatase
   B. CT head with contrast
   C. Whole body sacn
   D. Serum electrophoresis

140. Most common malignancy that metastasizes to the spine is:
   A. Lung   B. Prostate
   C. Breast   D. Thyroid

141. Bone to bone metastasis is most commonly seen in:
   A. Osteosarcoma
   B. Ewing's sarcoma
   C. Chondrosarcoma
   D. Reticulum cell carcinoma

142. Night pains are characteristically seen with:
   A. Osteoid osteoma
   B. Osteosarcoma
   C. Ewing's sarcoma
   D. Fibrous cortical defect

143. Which of the following is a GCT variant?
   A. Chondroblastoma
   B. Aneurysmal bone cyst
   c. Osteosarcoma with giant cells
   d. Fibrous dysplasia

144. Increased LDH levels are a bad prognostic factor in which tumor?
   A. Osteosarcoma
   B. Osteoid osteoma
   C. Giant cell tumor
   D. Ewing's tumor

145. All of the following statements about synovial cell sarcoma are correct except:
   A. Occurs more often at extra-articular sites
   B. Originates from synovial lining
   C. Usually seen in people under 50 years age
   D. Knee is the most common site

146. **A 30-year-old lady presented with pain and tenderness in index finger just under the nail. She was unable to wash her hands with cold water. Patient did not reveal any history of trauma or injury. What could be probable finding noted in this case?**
    A. Sausage digits
    B. Ridging of nail, bluish discoloration and pinhead tenderness
    C. Stiffness of whole hand
    D. Hypersensitivity of finger

147. **Generally radiotherapy should not be used for treating benign conditions, the only possible exception being:**
    a. Chondromyxoid fibroma
    b. Extensive pigmented vilonodular synovitis
    c. Benign fibrous histiocytoma
    d. Desmoplastic fibroma so extensive that it cannot be surgically excised

148. **Vertebra plana is seen in all *except*:**
    A. Ewing's sarcoma   B. Paget's disease
    C. Trauma disease   D. Malignancy

149. **Which of the following is biphasic tumor?**
    A. Rhabdomyosarcoma
    B. Osteosarcoma
    C. Synovial sarcoma
    D. Osteoblastoma

150. **Pigmented villo-nodular synovitis most commonly occurs at:**
    A. Knee   B. Hip
    C. Shoulder   D. Elbow

151. **True about bone metastasis:**
    A. 5% bone metastasis are symptomatic
    B. MC secondary in females is breast
    C. High serum levels of alkaline phosphatase
    D. Prostate produces osteosclerotic lesion
    E. Commonly involves hand and feet bones

152. **Metastases are least common in:**
    A. Vertebra
    B. Pelvis
    C. Proximal parts of long bones of the upper limb
    D. Small bones of the hand

153. **Most common soft tissue tumor in a child:**
    A. Rhabdomyosarcoma
    B. Fibrosarcoma
    C. Histiocytoma
    D. Liposarcoma

154. **Expansile lytic osseous metastases are characteristics of primary malignancy of**
    A. Breast
    B. Prostate
    C. Bronchus
    D. Kidney

155. **A 60-year-old male has bone pain, vertebral collapse and pathological fracture in pelvis. The most probable diagnosis is:**
    A. Multiple myeloma
    B. TB
    C. Hemangioma of bone
    D. Secondaries

156. **When size of osteoclastoma exceeds the size of metaphysis (PGI type):**
    A. Tumor will be covered by cortex
    B. Tumor will be covered by fibrous capsule
    C. Tumor will be covered by a thin layer of bone
    D. It is limited to metaphysis
    E. It is covered by periosteum

157. **The following bone tumor may cause dural deposits without causing bony changes:**
    A. Hodgkin's lymphoma
    B. Multiple myeloma
    C. Secondaries
    D. Fibrous dysplasia

158. **Which is not a feature of malignant transformation in an ostechondroma?**
    A. Weight loss
    B. Pain
    C. Rapid increase in size
    D. Calcification on CT more than 2 cm

159. **The treatment of choice for Ewing's sarcoma is:**
    A. Radiotherapy
    B. Chemotherapy
    C. Wide surgical excision
    D. Amputation

ANSWERS

1. A. Multiple myeloma
2. B. SBC
3. C. Protons (*Ref*: Skull Base. 2011 May; 21(3): 201–206. Prepublished online 2011, Mar 25. doi: 10.1055/s-0031-1275636)
   A type of radiation called proton beam therapy is most often recommended for chordoma patients because it allows delivery of very high doses of radiation to the tumor while minimizing doses to tissues just

millimeters away. Another type of particle beam radiation called carbon ion therapy has similar properties to proton beam therapy, but is only available at a small number of centers.

4. B. Osteoid osteoma
5. C. Hurler's syndrome
6. C. Giant cell tumor
7. A. Chondroblastoma
8. C. Giant cell tumor

9. B. Ewing's sarcoma
10. B. Epiphyseometaphyseal
    • Epiphyseometaphyseal > epiphyseal
11. B. Squamous cell carcinoma
12. A. Upper end of humerus
13. A. Osteomyelitis; B. Osteosarcoma; and
    C. Osteochondroma
14. B. Femur lower end
15. A. Epiphysis
16. B. Ewing's tumor; E. Osteoid osteoma
17. A. Rib
18. A. Ameloblastoma
19. A. Multiple myeloma is seen in more than
    55 years age and above
20. A. Plasmacytoma
21. Chondroblastoma: Soap bubble appearance
22. A. Neuroblastoma
23. B. Osteosarcoma and D. Chondrosarcoma
24. C. Osteoclastoma
25. C. Wide area of activity (>5 cm)
26. A. Enneking
27. B. Chordoma
28. C. Medullary cavity
29. C. Aneurysmal bone cyst
30. C. Treated by simple curettage
31. A. Simple bone cyst
32. B. Radiotherapy
33. D. Commonest site is diaphysis
34. B. Aneurysmal bone cyst
    • Posterior element of vertebrae:
      – Expansile and purely lytic: ABC
      – Non-expansile and ossified: Osteo-
        blastoma
    • Body of vertebrae: GCT
35. A. UBC
    Lytic lesion in upper end of humerus—
    favorite answer is always SBC and cortical
    fragment points towards "fallen fragment
    sign".
36. E. All of the above
37. All
38. C. Osteoclast gaint cells constitute the
    proliferative component of the tumor
39. A. Giant cell tumor
40. B. Most commonly seen around knee
41. A. GCT
42. B. Giant cell tumor
43. A. Giant cell tumor
44. B. Mononuclear cells
45. B. Non-ossifying fibroma
    • Non-ossifying fibroma is a relatively
      better answer here, as GCT has no matrix
      calcification, while all other options present
      with matrix calcification.

46. B. Osteoclastoma
    Lytic, expansile and eccentric lesion in distal
    radius, always think of GCT first.
47. C. Osteosarcoma
    • Osteosarcoma is extremely rare in small
      bones of hand and feet and does not
      contain giant cells.
48. B. Excision and bone grafting
49. A. Joint replacement; B. Excision; C. Curettage
    and D. Arthrodesis.
50. C. Osteochondroma
51. D. Thickness of cartilage
52. D. Degenerative changes
53. B. Growth continues after skeletal maturity
54. B. Developmental
55. D. It does not interfere with general body
    stature
    Osteochondromatosis means multiple
    osteochondromas/diaphyseal aclasia and
    osteochondromas are known to cause
    growth disturbances.
56. A. Multiple enchondromatosis with heman-
    giomas
57. A. Maffucci syndrome
58. C. Enchondroma
59. C. Multiple enchondromas with soft tissue
    malignancies
60. A. Chondroblastoma
    • Epiphyseal lytic lesion before fusion of
      epiphysis is chondroblastoma
61. C. Chondroblastoma
62. B. Chondroblastoma
    • Cartilageneous lesion presents with
      stippled calcification and among the given
      options only chondroblastoma is such
      tumor.
63. B. Chondroblastoma
64. A. Present until 3rd and 4th decade
65. A. High calcium and E. High ACTH levels
66. B. Squamous cell carcinoma
67. C. Ground glass appearance
68. A. Cystic lesion
69. A. Adamantinoma
70. B. More common in females as compared to
    males
71. B. Shepherd crook deformity
72. C. Tibia
73. A. Mandible near molar tooth
74. A. Autosomal dominant
75. D. All of the above
76. D. Periventricular calcifications
77. C. Hemangioma
78. B. Requires observation as it is premalignant
    and D. Forms 10–12% of the bone tumors

79. C. Both of the above
80. A. Osteoid osteoma
81. A. Osteoid osteoma
82. A. Osteoid osteoma
83. A. Salicylates
84. D. Osteoid osteoma
85. C. Osteoid osteoma
86. A. Osteoid osteoma
    Osteosarcoma has maximum bone matrix followed by osteoid osteoma.
87. B. Lung metastasis common
88. A. Osteoid matrix
89. A. Osteosarcoma
90. D. Osteitis deformans
91. B. Osteosarcoma
92. B. Osteoid forming tumor cells
93. A. Osteosarcoma of lower limbs and soft tissue sarcoma
94. A. Osteosarcoma
    Although both osteosarcoma and Ewings sarcoma can have lung metastasis, but osteosarcoma is more common with much more incidence of lung metastasis, as compared to Ewing's sarcoma. Moreover, pneumothorax is more commonly seen in osteosarcoma.
95. C. Soap bubble appearance
96. B. Osteosarcoma
97. C. Malignant cell with osteoid formation
98. D. Commonly associated with osteiod osteoma
99. B. Malignant bone tumors
100. A. Femur
101. A. Osteosarcoma
102. C. Osteosarcoma
103. A. Osteosarcoma
104. A. Osteosarcoma
105. C. Osteogenic sarcoma
106. D. Etoposide
107. B. Bone marrow biopsy
    • Biopsy always remains the gold standard investigation for neoplasic lesions, in osteosarcoma biopsy is taken from the leading edge of the lesion, not from marrow.
108. B. Most commonly involve knee and distal femur; C. Spread to lung through hematogenous route and E. X-ray has sunray appearance.
109. C. Chemotherapy + limb salvage surgery + chemotherapy
110. B. t(11; 22)
111. A. Ewing's sarcoma
112. C. Soap bubble appearance

113. C. Ewing's sarcoma
    • Both osteomyelitis and Ewing's sarcoma seem to be answer here, osteomyelitis starts in metaphysis and very rarely/lately involve diaphysis, while Ewing's sarcoma site of origin is diaphysis.
114. D. Shaft of femur.
    • Tricky question, as we are in a habit of 'lower end femur', but Ewing's sarcoma involves diaphysis of femur and thus the answer is shaft of femur.
115. C. Ewing's sarcoma
116. B. 2nd decade
117. A. Ewing's sarcoma
118. B. Excisional biopsy
119. B. 2nd decade
120. A. Ewing's sarcoma
121. A. Ewing's sarcoma
122. B. Ewing's sarcoma
123. C. Trisomy 8
124. A. Fever
125. A. Ewing's sarcoma
126. B. Ewing's sarcoma
    • Peripheral neurectodermal tumors (PNET) that share a common t(11:22) and round cells, differing only in their degree of neural differentiation, Ewing's sarcoma is poorly differentiated, whereas PNET exhibits definite neural differentiation.
127. A. Pelvis
128. D. Chondrosarcoma
    • Cartilaginous tumors are preferred answer in matrix calcification and malignant > benin tumor shows matrix calcification .
129. D. MRI
    • Diagnosis here is "Ewing's sarcoma" and next best investigation is MRI. Biopsy remains the gold standard, but before biopsy all noninvasive investigation should be done.
130. D. Chondrosarcoma
131. B. Chondrosarcoma
132. B. Chordoma
133. A. Dorsal spine; D. Sacrum
134. D. Chordoma
135. A. Multiple myeloma
136. B. Multiple myeloma
137. C. Plasma cell leukemia
138. A. Hypercalcemia and C. Monoclonal M band
    • ALP is generally normal in multiple myeloma, but may be increased when fracture occurs.
    • Bone marrow plasma cells are > 10% in multiple myeloma
    • More than 20% plasma cells in peripheral smear is 'plasma cell leukemia'.

139. D. Serum electrophoresis

140. C. Breast

141. B. Ewing's sarcoma

142. A. Osteoid osteoma

143. B. Aneurysmal bone cyst

144. D. Ewing's tumor

145. B. Originates from synovial lining

146. B. Ridging of nail, bluish discoloration and pin-head tenderness

147. B. Extensive pigmented vilonodular synovitis

148. B. Paget's disease

149. C. Synovial sarcoma

150. A. Knee

151. B. MC secondary in females is breast, C. High serum levels of alkaline phosphatase, D. Prostate produces osteosclerotic lesion

152. D. Small bones of the hand

153. A. Rhabdomyosarcoma

154. D. Kidney

155. D. Secondaries

- It could be metastasis, more likely than multiple myeloma, considering the site, the age and the incidence

156. A. Tumor will be covered by cortex, B. Tumor will be covered by fibrous capsule, C. Tumor will be covered by a thin layer of bone, E. It is covered by periosteum

157. B. Multiple myeloma

158. A. Weight loss

159. B. Chemotherapy

Neuromuscular and Genetic Disorders

SKELETAL DYSPLASIAS

Skeletal dysplasias are a heterogenous group of developmental disorder of bone with a wide spectrum of manifestations ranging from early onset of osteoarthritis with normal survival to death *in utero* or in early infancy.

Osteogenesis imperfecta is the most common skeletal dysplasia (Box 16.1) while thanatophoric dysplasia is the most common lethal skeletal dysplasia.

Most skeletal dysplasias are associated with short stature. Achondroplasia is the commonest variety associated with abnormally short stature (dwarfism).

> **Box 16.1:** Common skeletal dysplasias
>
> - Osteogenesis imperfecta—most common
> - Multiple epiphyseal dysplasia (MED)
> - Spondyloepiphyseal dysplasia (SED)
> - Achondroplasia
> - Pseudochondroplasia
> - Metaphyseal chondrodysplasia

Some common terms

- *Amelia*—complete absence of limb.
- *Amelia totalis*—complete absence of all four limbs.
- *Phocomelia* (meaning seal-like limbs) is a birth defect wherein the proximal bones of the limbs are shortened, such that the hands and the feet are located very close to the trunk. It was the prime concern in children whose mothers had been on antiemetic drug thalidomide, which led to the stoppage of the drug.
- *Rhizomelia* indicates shortening of the proximal portion of a limb due to shortening of femur or humerus.
- *Mesomelia* indicates shortening of the middle portion of a limb due to shortening of leg or forearm bones.
- *Acromelia* is due to the shortening of foot and hand bones.
- *Dysostosis*: It is isolated dysplasia of a bone or a group of bones, i.e. craniofacial dysostosis, polydactyly, syndactyly, etc.

Achondroplasia

It is a primary defect in endochondral bone formation due to point mutation in FGFR-3 gene. It has AD transmission but most cases are sporadic (due to spontaneous point mutation).

- Paternal age >36 years is linked with new mutation.
- Endochondral ossification (responsible for longitudinal growth) is abnormal resulting in dwarfism.
- Intramembranous ossification is normal, hence normal clavicle and skull.

Clinical features

- Rhizomelic micromelia, i.e. arms and thighs are most severely shortened, i.e. disproportionate dwarfism. Trunk height tends to be normal, but arm span and standing height are diminished. Short stature is apparent at birth.
- It is the commonest cause of disproportionate dwarfism.
- Hands are short and broad. All fingers are approximately of the same length (**starfish** hand) with wide separation between the middle and ring finger (**trident** hand).
- There may be protuberant belly and obesity and child walks with waddling gait.

- Achondroplasia has large head with prominent mandibles, small maxillae and depressed nasal bridge.
- However, these children have normal intelligence (**circus dwarf**).

X-ray features
- Long bones are short with increase in diameter and density.
- Posteriorly scalloped vertebrae, short pedicles and short inter-pedicular distance. Vertebrae are flat and have beak.
- **Bullet-shaped** vertebrae are seen in infants.
- Pelvis is broad and flat (**champagne glass pelvis**, i.e. width is greater than depth) with squared iliac wings, horizontal acetabular roofs and narrow sciatic notches.
- Epiphyses of bones are, however, normal.

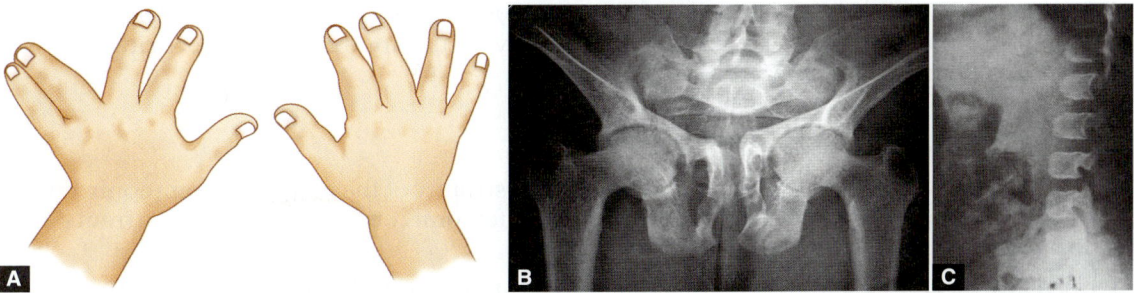

Fig. 16.1: (A) Trident and star fish hand, (B) champagne glass pelvis, (C) bullet shaped vertebrae

Cleidocranial Dysostosis

Autosomal dominant, mutation in CBFA gene on chromosome 6 leading to defective intramembranous ossification, so that clavicle, skull and pelvis are abnormal.
- Child is short statured and skull involvement has typical **Elfin facies, i.e. skull is wider than normal and the face appears small and flat looking (hypoplastic).**
- Skull X-ray shows wide suture lines, hypoplastic facial bones and multiple wormian bones.
- The eyes are widely set and deciduous teeth erupt normally but permanent teeth are delayed and maldeveloped.
- Clavicles may be underdeveloped or absent. Most common defect is loss of lateral 1/3rd clavicle > loss of middle third clavicle. Due to absence of clavicle shoulders look droopy, chest appears narrow and when bilateral loss is there, both shoulders can touch each other in front of the chest.
- X-ray pelvis shows a wide symphysis pubis, wide sacroiliac joint, small iliac wings and thin rami.
- Lengthening of 2nd metacarpal bone, coxa vara.

Xtra edge
Wormian bones, also known as intra-sutural bones (most common in lambdoid suture), are extra bone pieces that occur within a suture (joint) in the cranium (Fig. 16.2). To be significant they should be >10 in number, measure at least 6 mm × 4 mm and be arranged in general mosaic pattern.

Causes of wormian bones → **CHORD (mnemonic)**
- Cleidocranial dysostosis.
- Hypothyroidism/hypophosphatasia.
- Osteogenesis imperfecta.
- Rickets.
- Down's syndrome.

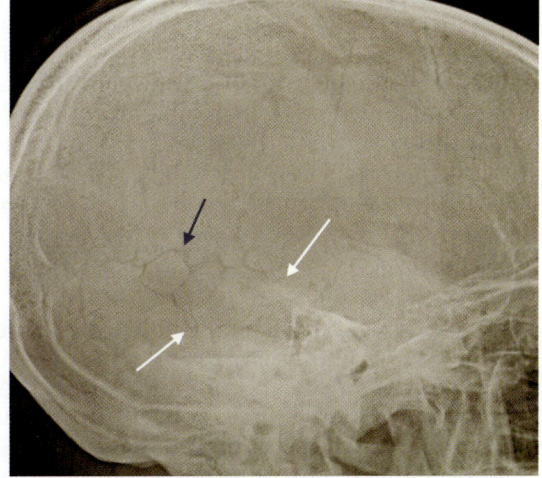

Fig. 16.2: X-ray showing intra-sutural bone, i.e. wormian bones

Large 2nd metacarpal—achondroplasia

   Short metacarpals $\longrightarrow$ **IITP**atna (mnemonic)

- **I**diopathic
- **P**ost-Infarction.
- **T**urner's syndrome
- **P**seudohypoparathyroidism

Dysplasia epiphysealis hemimelica (Trevor's disease/Fairbank's disease): Involvement of only one and a half of epiphysis on only one side of body leading to asymmetrical limb deformity. Knee is the commonest site.

Osteopoikilosis (spotted bones): It is characterized by presence of multiple bone islands (cartilage remnants) across the skeleton.

Melorheostosis/Leri's disease (candle bone disease): X-ray picture is characteristic (Fig. 14.8) showing asymmetrical, irregular cortical sclerosis giving the appearance of wax dripping down the side of a candle appearance.

Pyle's disease: Metaphyseal dysplasia.

Camurati-Engelmann disease: Diaphyseal dysplasia.

Nail-patella syndrome (onycho-osteodysplasia): Dystrophy of the nail (most commonly thumb) and hypoplastic or absent patella, hypoplastic lateral femoral condyle leading to recurrent patella dislocation.

X-ray features: Hypoplastic or absent patella, bilateral posterior iliac horns (Fong's prongs), and prominent anterior iliac spine are characteristic features.

OSTEOGENESIS IMPERFECTA (OI)

OI (Lobstein-Vrolik's disease/brittle bone disease/fragilitas ossium) is a connective tissue disorder-cum-skeletal dysplasia characterized by imperfect formation of type I collagen. So, there is defective osteoid formation and there is alteration in the structural integrity of skin, ligaments, tendon, bone, sclera and teeth.

It is transmitted in AD form, may also occur as sporadic/spontaneous mutation or rarely AR transmission.

Pathogenesis

Type I collagen is composed of three strands of collagen protein: Two α_1 strands and one α_2 strand, encoded by two separate genes—**COL1A1** (chromosome 17) for pro-α_1 and **COL1A2** for pro-α_2. These combine to form type 1 pro-collagen molecules.

The defect may be **quantitative**—when there is no formation of type 1 collagen molecule (due to stop codon) or **qualitative** when there is substitution/deletion in the glycine peptide residue, leading to abnormal and ineffective collagen molecule. If the substitution occurs at the carboxy terminal end of the chain, it can lead to severe consequences, since the cross-linking of the triple helix is initiated at the carboxy terminal position.

Clinical Features
Orthopedic manifestations

- There is marked osteopenia that leads to frequent/recurrent fractures after trivial trauma (Fig. 16.3). Fractures can even occur *in utero* or at the time of birth with severe forms presenting as stillbirths. Any fracture pattern may be present.
- Lower limb fractures are more common than upper limb. Femur is commonest bone fractured followed by tibia.

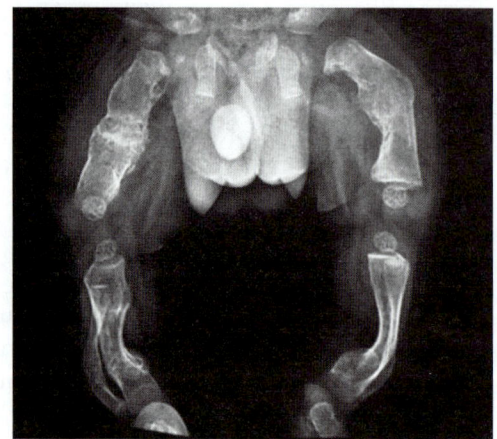

Fig. 16.3: Osteogenesis imperfecta—see multiple fractures in various stages of healing, callus formation and bony deformities

- Frequency of fractures usually declines after puberty but in women rises again after menopause.
- Bone remodeling is defective; fracture healing, however is normal, but fractures tend to heal with abundant callus, although the callus is of poor quality.
- Hyperlaxity of ligaments with hypermobility of the joints is also present. **Wormian** bones (Fig. 16.2) are characteristically found in the skull.
- Kyphosis, scoliosis, bowing of legs, basilar invagination, protrusio acetabuli are other features.

Ocular involvement: As a consequence of the thin collagen layer in the sclera, sclera appears blue owing to the hue of underlying uveal vessels. Following features may be present in addition:

- *Saturn's ring*: White sclera immediately surrounding the cornea.
- *Arcus juvenilis:* White opacity concentric to limbus in the periphery of cornea.
- Hypermetropia and retinal detachment.

Auditory involvement: Onset is in adolescence or adulthood. It is mainly conductive deafness, due to otosclerosis (abnormal bone material grows around stapes due to defective remodeling) and sensorineural deafness can also coexist due to pressure on the auditory nerve as it emerges through the skull.

Dental involvement: Dentinogenesis imperfecta (dentin dysplasia) is characteristic. Yellowish brown/bluish gray discoloration of teeth is seen. Enamel, which is ectodermal in origin, is normal. Deciduous and permanent teeth both are involved, they break easily and are prone to carries. Lower incisors are particularly more severely affected.

Skin and muscle involvement: The skin is thin and translucent and is prone to subcutaneous hemorrhages. Muscles are hypotonic due to multiple fractures and deformities. Hernias are common.

Metabolic features: A hypermetabolic state exists, resulting in excessive sweating and heat intolerance. The patient is susceptible to hyperthermia during general anesthesia.

Diagnosis

Prenatal: PCR can be conducted on chorionic villi biopsy at 8–12 weeks.

Postnatal: Skeletal survey (radiographs) shows multiple fractures in various stages of healing, abundant callus formation and bony deformities (Fig.16.3). Bone cortices are thin with generalized osteopenia. The skull has a mushroom appearance with a very thin calvarium. Wormian bones (Fig. 16.2), may be seen in the skull X-ray.

Most definite: A molecular defect in type I procollagen is detected by incubating the skin fibroblasts with radioactive amino acids and analyzing the pro-alpha chains by **polyacrylamide gel electrophoresis**.

Treatment

Bisphosphonates are the preferred drugs, given to reduce fracture rate and pain and to increase cortical thickness by inhibiting osteoclast function. They do not prevent development of scoliosis. patients who receive cyclical bisphosphonate therapy may show Zebra strip sign (Fig. 16.4) on X-rays. Zebra lines appear after 8–10 weeks of therapy and progressively migrate toward diaphysis and disappear after physeal closure.

Surgery: For children above the age of 2 years, fracture fixation with special implants like **Bailey-Dubow rods** (telescoping rods that can telescope and increase in size with growth) is preferred. Bowing deformities of long bones are treated with multiple realignment osteotomies with rod fixation (**Sofield-Miller procedure/seek-kebab treatment**).

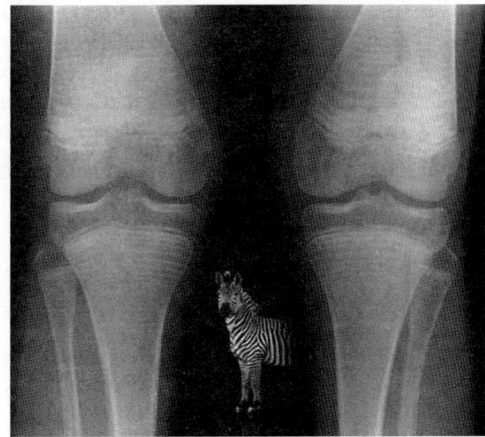

Fig. 16.4: Zebra strip sign following bisphosphonate therapy in osteogenesis imperfecta

CAFFEY'S DISEASE

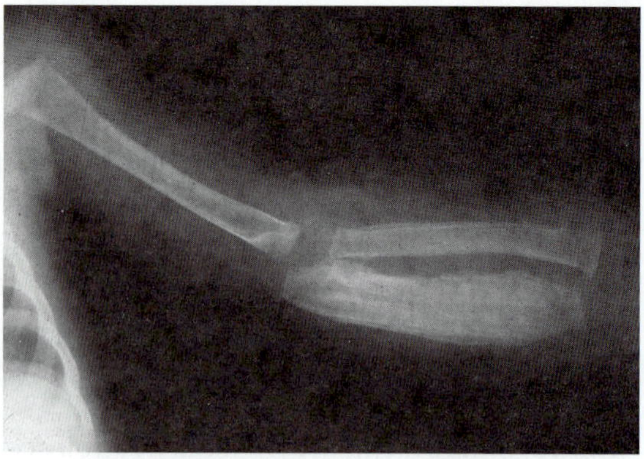

- It is a self-limiting inflammatory disease of unknown etiology, characterized by intense **diaphyseal** periostitis (Fig. 16.5) and hyperostosis (thickening of cortex of bone often leading to doubling of width of bone), occurrence of soft tissue nodules and growth abnormalities.
- *Types*: Familial and sporadic (most common).
- Seen mainly in infants < 6 months old.
- The characteristic triad includes—cortical bone thickening, painful soft tissue swellings and systemic symptoms (irritability and fever). It mimics osteomyelitis.
- Most common site of involvement is mandible and its presentation in mandible often mimics

Fig. 16.5: Cortical hyperostosis due to Caffey's disease

  jaw tumors. In familial form tibia and ulna are most commonly involved bones. Hands and feet are spared.
- *Treatment*: NSAIDs (indomethacin). Antibiotics have no role.
- *Caffey's sign*: It is seen in Perthes' disease and has no relation with this condition.

OSTEOPETROSIS

Osteopetrosis (marble bone disease, Albers-Schonberg disease) is characterized by defective osteoclastic bone resorption due to defects in their carbonic anhydrase type II proton pump, as evidenced by absence of ruffled borders and inability to respond to PTH. Defective bone resorption interferes with normal bone remodeling leading to thickened, radiologically dense (white) bones and hence the term, marble bone disease.

Types
- *Malignant form (AR)*: Congenital.
- *Benign form (AD)*: Adult/adolescent type. Symptom-free and diagnosed incidentally.

Clinical features
- Malignant form presents at birth and infancy with pancytopenia due to obliteration of marrow cavity by bony overgrowth (abnormal bleeding, anemia, infections and failure to thrive).
- Bone pain and pathological fractures (fragile brittle bone) are common and mostly involve vertebrae and base of skull.
- Due to pancytopenia, there is extramedullary hematopoiesis (hepatosplenomegaly).
- It is associated with renal tubular acidosis due to carbonic anhydrase II deficiency. (In CRF there is osteosclerosis not petrosis).
- Healing of fractures is normal, but internal fixation is difficult in these patients.
- Osteomyelitis (most commonly in mandible) is common due to decreased immunity.
- Cranial nerve palsy is due to bony overgrowth of cranial foramen—2nd, 7th and 8th.

Blood investigations: Decreased bone resorption leads to low serum calcium and high alkaline phosphatase → high PTH → low phosphate levels.

X-ray features
- Thickened, sclerotic (white) bones (due to loss of distinction between cortical and cancellous bone) are characteristic features (Fig. 16.6B).
- **Endobones** (Fig. 16.6A) or bone within a bone appearance (radio-dense tissues inside the cortices of long bones) is pathognomonic for osteopetrosis.
- Defective bone remodeling around the knee joint causes typical **Erlenmeyer flask** deformity (Fig. 16.6C).
- Rugger jersey spine may also be present.

Treatment: Bone marrow transplantation.

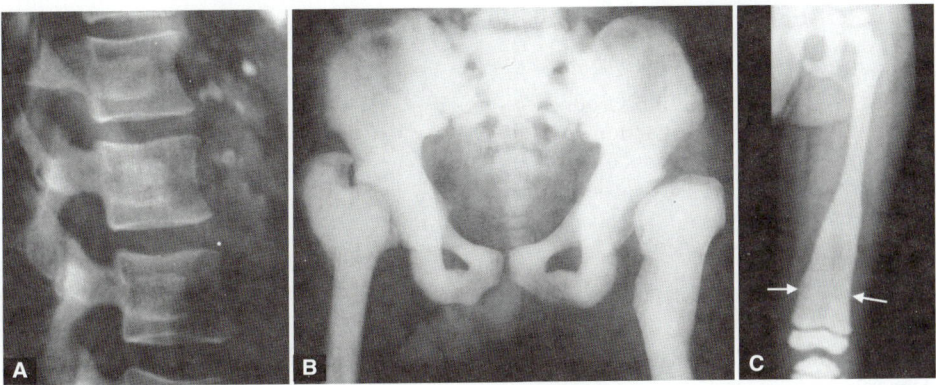

Fig. 16.6: (A) Endobones, (B) white out appearance of osteopetrosis, (C) Erlenmeyer flask deformity

Xtra edge
Bone within a bone appearance → **SLOPE** (mnemonic)
- **S**ickle cell disease
- **L**ead poisoning
- **O**steopetrosis
- **P**aget's disease
- Acrom**E**galy

Erlenmeyer flask deformity → **GOLT** (mnemonic)
- **G**aucher's disease
- **O**steopetrosis
- **L**ead poisoning
- **T**halassemia.

Sclerosing bone (white bone) disorders → osteopetrosis, osteopoikilosis, osteomyelitis, osteopathia striata, melorheostosis, Caffey's disease and pycnodysostosis.

MULTIPLE CHOICE QUESTIONS

1. **Bone dysplasia is due to:**
   A. Faulty nutrition   B. Faulty development
   C. Trauma   D. Parathyroid tumor
2. **Musculoskeletal abnormalities seen in neuro-fibromatosis:**
   A. Pseudoarthrosis   B. Hypertrophy of limb
   C. Scoliosis   D. All of the above
3. **The following is false about achondroplasia:**
   A. Due to gene mutation
   B. Mental retardation
   C. AD
   D. Shortening of limbs present
4. **A 9-year-old child has high arched palate with shoulders meeting in front of his chest. Diagnosis is:**
   A. Cleidocranial dysostosis
   B. Erb's palsy
   C. Chondro-osteodystrophy
   D. Cortical hyperostosis
5. **Phocomelia is characterized by:**
   A. Absence of short bones
   B. Complete absence of extremities

   C. Defects of long bones of limb
   D. Partial absence of extremities
6. **Nail-patella syndrome is characterized by:**
   A. Iliac horn   B. Sacral horn
   C. Knee deformity   D. Dislocation of patella
7. **"Trident hand" is seen in:**
   A. Achondroplasia
   B. Mucopolysaccharoidosis
   C. Diphyseal achalasia
   D. Cleidocranial dysostosis
8. **The features of achondroplasia include all *except*:**
   A. Defective head
   B. No mental retardation
   C. Autosomal recessive
   D. Familial
9. **The characteristics of Morquio's disease include all *except*:**
   A. Spinal kyphosis
   B. Subnormal intelligence
   C. Excessive excretion of keratan sulfate in urine
   D. Dwarfism

10. **The characteristic mutation seen in achondroplasia:**
   A. Fibrilin -1   B. FGFR-3
   C. NOTCH1 gene   D. COL5A1 gene

11. **The following is false about achondroplasia:**
   A. Autosomal dominant
   B. Mental retardation
   C. Due to gene mutation
   D. Shortening of limbs present

12. **A short statured patient brought to orthopedics OPD with an X-ray showing flattened vertebra with beak. The probable diagnosis is:**
   A. Achondroplasia
   B. Ochronosis
   C. Eosinophilic granuloma
   D. Calve's disease

13. **Absent lateral 1/3 rd of clavicle is seen in:**
   A. Hyperparathyroidism
   B. Turner's syndrome
   C. Fibrous dysplasia
   D. Cleidocranial dysostosis

14. **Cleidocranial dysostosis may show:**
   A. Wide foramen magnum
   B. Absence of clavicles
   C. Coxa vara
   D. All of the above

15. **Osteogenesis imperfecta, true is:**
   A. Marble bone disease is another name of it
   B. Hyperlaxity of ligaments with hypermobile joints
   C. Cranial nerve compression may occur
   D. Treatment involves bone marrow transplantation

16. **Which of the below is a feature of osteogenesis imperfecta?**
   A. Blue sclera   B. Cataract
   C. Anterior uveitis   D. Retinal detachment

17. **Osteogenesis imperfecta has abnormality in which type of collagen?**
   A. Collagen 3   B. Collagen 2
   C. Collagen 4   D. Collagen 1

18. **A child presented with hip pain:**
   A. Osteogenesis imperfecta
   B. Osteoporosis
   C. Osteopetrosis
   D. Osteopoikilocytosis

19. **Ring-shaped epiphyses are seen in:**
   A. Osteogenesis imperfecta
   B. Morquio's syndrome
   C. Zellweger syndrome
   D. Multiple epiphyseal dysplasia

20. **Brittle bone disease is:**
   A. Osteogenesis imperfecta
   B. Osteopertrosis
   C. Paget's disease
   D. Osteoporosis

21. **Prenatal determination of osteogenesis imperfecta is done by:**
   A. Acid phosphatase
   B. Alkaline phosphatase
   C. Abnormal pro-α chain
   D. FGF3 mutation

22. **All are features of osteogenesis imperfecta** *except*:
   A. Blue sclera   B. Multiple fractures
   C. Cataract   D. Hearing loss

23. **Not true about osteogenesis imperfecta:**
   A. Impaired healing of fracture
   B. Deafness
   C. Laxity of joint
   D. Fragile fracture

24. **In which of the following conditions bilateral symmetrical fractures occur?**
   A. Rickets
   B. Osteopetrosis
   C. Osteogenesis imperfecta
   D. Fluorosis

25. **All are commonly seen in osteogensis imperfecta** *except*:
   A. Blue sclera
   B. Bilateral hip dislocation
   C. Lax ligament
   D. Osteoporosis

26. **Osteogenesis imperfecta is due to the following:**
   A. Excessive osteoblastic activity
   B. Defective osteoid function
   C. Defective osteoclast function
   D. Defective mineralization of bone

27. **Wormian bones are seen in:**
   A. Osteogenesis imperfecta
   B. Scheuermann's disease
   C. Paget's disease
   D. Osteoclastoma

28. **Osteogenesis imperfecta:**
   A. Autosomal dominant (AD)
   B. Autosomal recessive (AR)
   C. Both AD and AR
   D. Sex-linked dominant
   E. None of the above

29. **Brittle bones disease is:**
   A. Osteoprosis
   B. Osteoetrosis
   C. Osteogenesis imperfecta
   D. Osteomalacia

30. **Osteopetrosis, false is:**
   A. Low levels of serum calcium
   B. Raised levels of alkaline phosphatase
   C. Low levels of PTH
   D. Low levels of serum phosphate

31. **Marble bone disease is:**
    A. Paget's disease
    B. Ankylosing spondylitis
    C. Osteopetrosis
    D. Melorheostosis
32. **Albers-Schönberg disease is also known as:**
    A. Osteoprosis   B. Osteopetrosis
    C. OI   D. Paget's disease
33. **A 3-year-old male presented with progressive anemia, hepatosplenomegaly and osteomyelitis of jaw with pathological fracture. X-ray shows chalky white deposits in bone. Probable diagnosis is:**
    A. Alkaptonuria
    B. Osteopetrosis
    C. Myositis ossificans progerssiva
    D. Osteopoikilosis
34. **Regarding osteopetrosis all the following statement are true *except*:**
    A. Pancytopenia
    B. Delayed fracture healing
    C. Cranial nerve compression
    D. Osteomyelitis of mandible
35. **Raju, a 10-year-old boy, presents with predisposition to fractures, anemia, hepatosplenomegaly and a diffusely increased radiographic density of bones. The most likely diagnosis is:**
    A. Osteopetrosis
    B. Osteoporosis
    C. Myelofibrosis
    D. Osteopetrosis
36. **Dripping candle wax appearance on X-ray of spine is seen in:**
    A. Osteopetrosis
    B. Metastasis
    C. TB spine
    D. Melorheostosis
37. **Albers-Schönberg disease is:**
    A. Osteopetrosis   B. Osteoporosi
    C. Osteochondritis   D. Osteomalacia

38. **Not seen in osteopetrosis:**
    A. Compression of cranial nerves
    B. Osteomyelitis of mandible
    C. Pancytopenia
    D. Delayed healing of bone
39. **Generalized osteosclerosis is seen in:**
    A. Osteoporosis
    B. Osteochondritis
    C. Osteogenesis imperfecta
    D. Osteopetrosis
    E. Osteomalacia
40. **Dripping candle wax lesion in spine:**
    A. Meyastasis   B. TB spine
    C. Osteopetrosis   D. Melorheostosis
41. **Increased bone density in X-ray seen in:**
    A. Collapse cancellous bone
    B. Periosteal reaction
    C. Paget's disease
    D. AVN
    E. Osteomyelitis
42. **Increased bone density in X-ray seen in:**
    A. Increased thickening of trabeculae
    B. Fracture and collapse of cancellous bone
    C. Defective mineralization
    D. Myositis ossificans
    E. Relative disuse atrophy and surrounding bone response
43. **Caffey's disease is:**
    A. Renal osteodystrophy
    B. Infantile cortical hyperostosis
    C. Osteomyelitis of jaw in children
    D. Chronic osteomyelitis in children
44. **Caffey's disease occurs in:**
    A. Infants below 6 months
    B. Above 5 years
    C. Above 10–20 years
    D. 20–40 years
45. **Jaw swelling is seen in:**
    A. Osteoporosis   B. Osteomalacia
    C. Osteopetrosis   D. Caffey's disease

ANSWERS

1. B. Faulty development
2. D. All of the above
3. B. Mental retardation (Fundamentals of Orthopaedics, 2nd ed., pg. 394)
4. A. Cleidocranial dysostosis
5. C. Defects of long bones of limb
6. A. Iliac horn
   - Nail-patella syndrome (onycho-osteo-dysplasia)—dystrophy of the nail (M/C thumb) and hypoplastic or absent patella, hypoplastic lateral femoral condyle l/t recurrent patella dislocation.

- X-ray features: Hypoplastic or absent patella, bilateral posterior iliac horns (Fong's prongs) and prominent anterior iliac spine are characteristic features.
7. A. Achondroplasia
8. C. Autosomal recessive
9. B. Subnormal intelligence (Fundamentals of Orthopaedics, 2nd ed., pg. 399)
   - Achondroplasia has large head with prominent mandibles, small maxillae and depressed nasal bridge. However, these children have normal intelligence (circus dwarf).

10. B. FGFR-3
11. B. Mental retardation
12. A. Achondroplasia
13. D. Cleidocranial dysostosis
14. D. All of the above
15. B. Hyperlaxity of ligaments with hypermobile joints
16. A. Blue sclera
17. D. Collagen 1
18. A. Osteogenesis imperfecta
19. A. Osteogenesis imperfecta
20. A. Osteogenesis imperfecta
21. C. Abnormal Pro-α chain
22. C. Cataract
23. A. Impaired healing of fracture
24. C. Osteogenesis imperfecta
25. B. Bilateral hip dislocation
26. B. Defective osteoid formation
27. A. Osteogenesis imperfecta
28. C. Both AD and AR
29. C. Osteogensis imperfecta
30. C. Low levels of PTH
31. C. Osteopetrosis

32. B. Osteopetrosis
33. B. Osteopetrosis
34. B. Delayed fracture healing
35. A. Osteopetrosis
36. D. Melorheostosis
    - Melorheostosis/Leri's disease (candle bone disease)—ray picture is characteristic showing asymmetrical, irregular cortical sclerosis giving the appearance of wax dripping down the side of a candle appearance.
37. A. Osteopetrosis
38. D. Delayed healing of bone
39. D. Osteopetrosis
40. D. Melorheostosis
41. 'All' Collapse cancellous bone; B. Periosteal reaction; C. Paget's disease; D. AVN and E. Osteomyelitis
42. A. and B. Increased thickning of trabeculae and fracture and collapse of cancellous bone
43. B. Infantile cortical hyperostosis
44. A. Infants below 6 months
45. D. Caffey's disease

17

Metabolic Bone Diseases

OSTEOPOROSIS

Osteoporosis (the commonest metabolic bone disease) is a quantitative reduction in bone density without changes in bone quality (i.e. chemical composition). It results when the rate of bone resorption exceeds the rate of bone formation. It is commonly associated with ageing process (senile osteoporosis) where bone formation generally proceeds at a normal rate, but bone removal occurs at an increased rate. The loss of bone in cancellous bone is rapid compared to cortical bone.

Classification
- **Primary:**
  - *Type I*: *Postmenopausal*. The loss is mainly from trabecular bone rather than cortical bone. It predisposes the patient to vertebral fracture and distal radius fracture.
  - *Type II*: *Senile*. Bone loss is gradual involving both trabecular and cortical bone, predisposing patient to hip and vertebral fracture.
- **Secondary** due to external factors.

Risk Factors
- Corticosteroids when given at a dose greater than 7.5 mg/day for a long duration, causes osteoporosis largely from trabecular bone, more so in the first 6 months of therapy.
- Heparin can cause **reversible** osteoporosis by a hypocalcemia induced increase in PTH activity that leads to the condition.
- Diuretics like furosemide cause calciuria and lead to osteoporosis, while thiazides decrease urinary calcium excretion and are considered to be protective and may be used as a therapy in recalcitrant cases of steroid-induced osteoporosis

Clinical Features
- Mostly asymptomatic, but back pain and pathological fractures are other m/c symptoms.
- Distal radius is the commonest site of fracture in <70 years, while in patients >70 years DL spine becomes the most common site. Overall vertebral fractures are the most common site.
- Loss of vertebral height, kyphotic dorsal spine, stooped habitus and shortened stature are classical features.

Investigations
- Serum calcium, phosphorous, alkaline phosphatase and serum vitamin D levels are usually normal.
- **X-ray features** (Fig. 17.1)
  - At least 30% of the bone mass must be lost for osteoporosis to be apparent on the radiographs.
  - Transverse trabeculation disappears, vertical trabeculae of vertebrae are thinned.

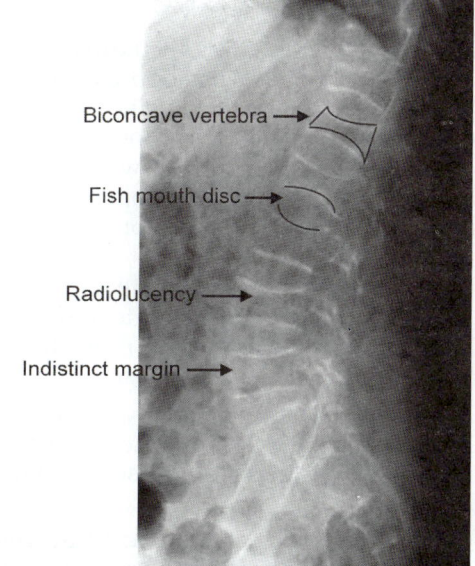

Biconcave vertebra ➞

Fish mouth disc ➞

Radiolucency ➞

Indistinct margin ➞

Fig. 17.1: LS spine X-ray depicting classical X-ray features of osteoporosis

Table 17.1: WHO diagnostic criteria for osteoporosis	
	BMD T-score
Normal	<1 SD below normal
Osteopenia	1–2.5 SD below normal
Osteoporosis	≥2.5 SD below normal with no history of fractures
Severe osteoporosis	≥2.5 SD below normal with history of non-violent fractures

- – Compression fractures, reduced vertebral height, wedge-shaped dorsal vertebra, biconcave lumbar bodies and lumbar discs (cod fish mouthed vertebrae) are noted.
- – Singh's index can be used for grading on X-ray (type I—severe osteoporosis and type VI—normal).
- **Gold standard** is biopsy from iliac crest (Beck and Nordin scale).
- **Bone mineral density (BMD):** BMD is measured best by DEXA (dual energy X-ray absorptiometry) scan. Three site DEXA (hip, distal radius, lumbar spine) provides fair estimate of the severity. For patients on treatment, repeat DEXA is done every 2 years. BMD in a hemiplegic patient is reduced maximum in humerus.
  - – *T-score*: It measures BMD and compares to the reference value (30 years old of the same sex, ethnicity). WHO definition of osteoporosis is based on T score (Table 17.1).
  - – *Z-score*: It compares BMD with a subject of the same age and sex.
- FRAX tool can be used to estimate the probability of an individual sustaining an osteoporotic fracture over next 10 years.

Management

Medical Management

- Drugs that stimulate formation—calcium, calcitriol, fluorides, teriparatide (rPTH analogue).
- Drugs that inhibit resorption—bisphosphonate, denosumab, calcitonin, estrogen, SERMs, gallium nitrate.
- Both action—strontium ranelate.
  - – Drugs that stimulate bone formation can increase BMD throughout the period of treatment, while drugs inhibiting bone resorption reaches a plateau in 2–3 years because bone formation also decreases.

Dietary fibres, iron therapy and tetracyclines inhibit calcium absorption. A gap of two hours must be maintained between the two drugs.

Bisphosphonates: These are the drugs of choice for both senile and postmenopausal osteoporosis. They are not metabolised and are excreted intact in urine. Their cessation of treatment does not lead to rapid bone loss.

1st generation: Etidronate was the first bisphosphonate to be introduced but not for osteoporosis. Etidronate inhibits both bone formation and resorption, and thus has a role in Paget's disease.

2nd generation: Alendronate and risedronate.

3rd generation: Ibandronate and zolendronic acid; these inhibit bone resorption much more than inhibiting formation, thus have a role in osteoporosis.

Precautions: The patient is advised to take the medicine empty stomach with one glass of water and not to lie down for at least half an hour as these can cause esophageal complications.

Complications

- Long term use can cause an atypical fracture of sub-trochanteric femur. These are generally transverse insufficiency fractures with thickening of the lateral femoral cortex and are associated with slow healing (Fig. 17.2).

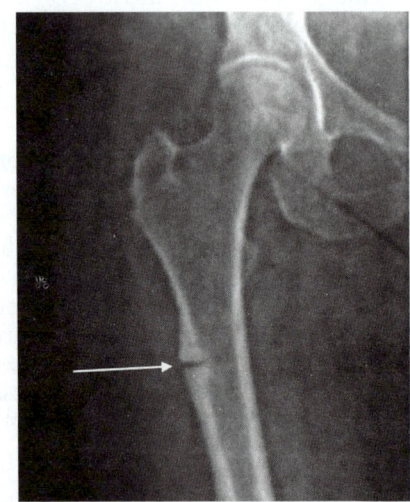

Fig. 17.2: Bisphosphonate induced subtrochanteric insufficiency fracture (arrow)

- Another peculiar side effect of the bisphosphonate therapy is **osteonecrosis of the jaw (ONJ).** It is caused by both oral and IV bisphosphonates and may be related to the inhibition of osteoclast-mediated resorption of bone. Denosumab and antiangiogenic medications can cause similar effects.

Calcitonin: Calcitonin selectively reduces the risk of vertebral fractures only, with no effect on incidence of peripheral fractures. The drug acts by the following four mechanisms:
1. Inhibits calcium absorption by the intestine
2. Inhibits osteoclast activity in the bones
3. Stimulates osteoblastic activity in the bones
4. Inhibits renal reabsorption of Ca.

Dose: 50 IU I/M or S/C every day; 200 IU nasal spray in alt. nostril every day.

Indications
- Hypercalcaemia of malignancy
- Paget's disease (pain relief)
- Prevention of acute bone loss from sudden immobilisation
- Treatment of osteoporosis (not used prophylactically). Use for shortest possible duration and dose.

Side effects: Rhinitis is the most common reported side effect.

Hormone replacement therapy (HRT): Used mainly in treatment of postmenopausal osteoporosis. Daily dose of 0.625 mg of conjugated estrogen in combination with progestin is indicated. Progestin are indicated to reduce the side effect of estrogen. Women receiving combination therapy can get withdrawal bleeding. Due to these side effects HRT is not used primarily to **prevent** osteoporosis.

Selective estrogen receptor modulators (SERMs): They act as estrogen antagonist in breast tissue and as an agonist in bone (Table 17.2).
- Raloxifene selectively stimulates estrogen receptor in bone and is used in treatment of osteoporosis. It reduces the risk of breast cancer also. However, raloxifene reduces the risk of vertebral fractures only.
- Tamoxifene is used in breast cancer not in osteoporosis (Table 17.2).
- Newer SERMs like Lasofoxifene have been shown to reduce the risk of nonvertebral fractures as well.

Teriparatide: It is recombinant human PTH. On large doses it removes calcium from bone while in small pulses it can directly stimulate osteoblasts to form new bone.
- It decreases the risk of vertebral and nonvertebral fractures.
- It is the DOC in bisphosphonate resistant osteoporosis.
- The drug is contraindicated in Paget's disease due to the potential of developing sarcoma.
- It can rapidly increase bone mass, thus indicated pre-operatively in osteoporotic patient undergoing bone surgery.

Denosumab: It is a fully human monoclonal IgG2 antibody against RANKL. Like osteoprotegerin, it inhibits binding of RANKL to RANK receptors (Fig. 17.3), thereby inhibiting osteoclast function. It is contraindicated in severe hypocalcemia.

Table 17.2: Commonly used selective estrogen receptor modulators

- **Tamoxifen**
  - *Agonist*: Bone, lipoprotein system, uterus (increased thromboembolic events and endometrial cancer are side effects)
  - *Antagonist*: Breast (used in breast cancer)
- **Raloxifene**
  - *Agonist*: Bone, lipids
  - *Antagonist*: Breast, endometrium

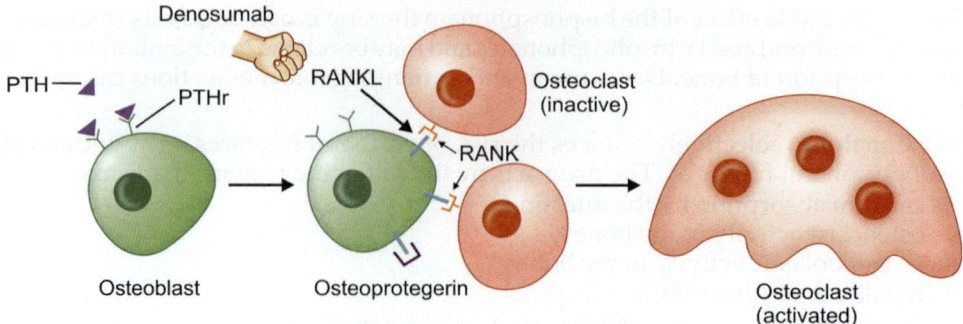

Fig. 17.3: Mechanism of action of denosumab

Operative Management

Vertebroplasty: Injecting bone cement (PMMA) into compressed vertebrae via a *trans*-pedicular route.

Kyphoplasty: Initially the height of vertebra is restored by inflating a balloon and then injecting the cement.

Xtra Edge
- Disuse osteoporosis: In hemiplegics maximum drop in bone mineral density occurs in non-weight bearing bones of upper limb (maximum in humerus) on the side of hemiplegia.
- Bisphosphonates are drugs of choice for both senile and postmenopausal osteoporosis. In bisphosphonate resistant osteoporosis teriparatide is the DOC.
- Etidronate may prevent bone loss secondary to heparin therapy.
- Vitamin K deficiency decreases bone mineral density and increases the risk of fractures. Vitamin K along with vitamin D is increasingly being given to prevent and treat osteoporosis.
- Only two drugs which act on osteoblast: Teriparatide and strontium ranelate.
- Vertebroplasty is also used in the treatment of vertebral hemangiomas.

RICKETS
Rickets is a disorder of defective mineralization of the growing skeleton (before epiphyseal closure), the pediatric counterpart of osteomalacia, that occurs due to deficiency of vitamin D in children.

Pathophysiology
The prime pathology in rickets is inadequate mineralization or calcification of physis (growth plates) in growing bones due to deficiency of vitamin D, but osteoid matrix is secreted at a normal rate leading to increased osteoid maturation (i.e. mineralisation) time. The zone of provisional calcification is inadequately mineralized and bony trabeculae become weak. Osteoid is laid irregularly with widened osteoid seams, osteoid islands may even persist down into the diaphysis. Under increasing stresses of body weight, the physis gets deformed (broadened and cupped), leading to defective growth and bony deformities.

Signs and Symptoms
- Generalized features include failure to thrive, muscle weakness, listlessness, delayed milestone and lethargy.
- The child may present with tetany (positive trousseau or Chvostek sign) or convulsions because of hypocalcemia.
- Pathological fractures may result due to weak bones. Once the patient starts walking, bony deformities may develop.
- Frontal bossing (thickening of frontal bone) is usually evident after the age of 6 months.
- Delayed closure of fontanel and delayed dentition are noted.
- Craniotabes is usually the **first** manifestation and refers to soft skull bones that can be pressed like a ping-pong ball.
- Enlarged costochondral junctions (called Rickets rosary, R = Rounded; c/f Scorbutic rosary— S = sharp) result due to subluxation of the physis (Fig. 17.4A).

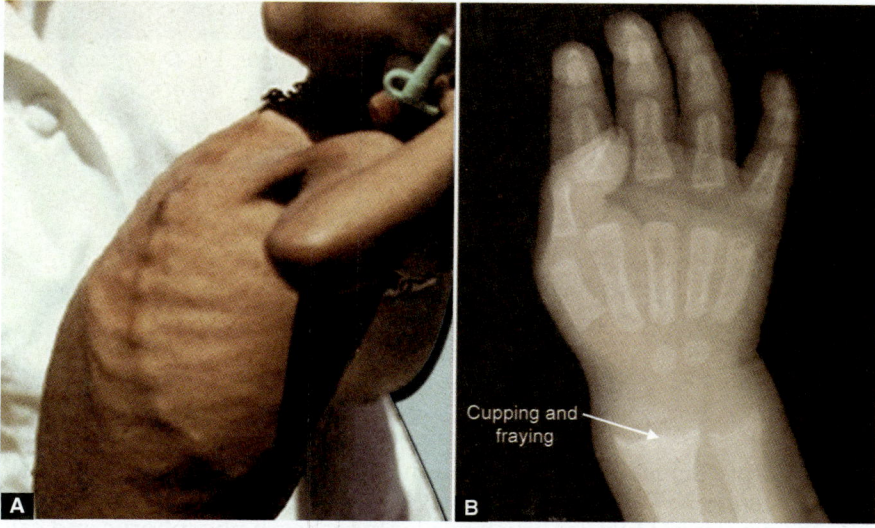

Fig. 17.4: (A) Rachitic rosary, (B) X-ray of rickets

- Indentation over the lower chest at attachment of diaphragm (Harrison's sulcus).
- Due to abdominal muscle hypotonia patients develop 'Pot belly'.
- Pigeon chest (pectus carinatum) refers to a protruding sternum.
- Bow legs (genu varum; more common) and knock knees (genu valgum; in older children), both may be seen. Windswept deformity of the legs (varum at one knee and valgum at the other) may be seen as well.
- Broadening of ankle, wrist and knee joints occurs due to deformed physis.
- Double malleoli sign may be seen due to metaphyseal widening.
- Kyphosis/scoliosis.
- Hypocalcemia induced hyperparathyroidism.

X-ray Features (Fig. 17.4B)
- Delayed appearance of epiphysis
- Thickening and widening of physis
- Loss of provisional zone of calcification
- Metaphysis—cup shaped, splayed and frayed
- Generalised osteopenia and thin cortices
- Deformity of bone in later stage

Viamin D Deficiency

25-Hydroxy Vitamin D Levels
Sufficiency: >30 ng/ml
Insufficiency: 21–29 ng/ml
Deficiency: <20 ng/ml

Types of Rickets (Table 17.3)
1. Nutritional rickets: Due to dietary deficiency of vitamin D, so active vitamin D $(1,25\text{-}OH_2)$ levels are low.
2. Vitamin D dependent rickets (VDDR): Dietary intake is normal, but there is a problem in its metabolism.
   a. VDDR type I—deficiency of 1-alpha-hydroxylase renal enzyme.
   b. VDDR type II—Vitamin D receptor insensitivity due to mutation of VDR gene. End organs are insensitive to vitamin D $(1, 25\text{-}OH_2)$. Alopecia is present in addition to rachitic features.
3. Vitamin D resistant rickets/renal tubular rickets/familial hypophosphatemic rickets: Inability of renal tubules to retain phosphates leading to hypophosphatemia. Calcium is normal thus PTH not stimulated.

Table 17.3: Diagnosis of different rickets

	Nutritional rickets	Vit. D-dependent rickets I hydroxylation problem	Vit. D-dependent rickets II end organ insensitivity	Vit. D-resistant rickets renal tubular rickets	Renal osteodystrophy
S. calcium	N – ↓	↓	↓	N	N – ↓
S. phosphorus	↓ – N	↓	↓	↓↓	↑
Alkaline phosphatase	↑	↑	↑	↑	↑
PTH	↑	↑	↑	N	↑↑↑
25 (OH) vitamin D	↓↓	↑↑	↑↑	N	N
1,25 $(OH)_2$ vitamin D	↓	↓↓	↑↑↑	N	↓↓
Urine Ca	↓	X	X	↓	↓
Urine phosphorus	↓			↑↑	↓

4. **X-linked hypophosphatemic rickets:** Mutations in the phosphate regulating gene (PHEX gene) present on chromosome X. This leads to excessive urinary excretion of phosphate by restricting the ability of proximal renal tubular brush border to reabsorb phosphorus and calcium.

5. **Renal osteodystrophy:** This is seen in children who have a chronic renal disease that leads to renal failure. The problem begins with a damaged renal glomerulus inability to excrete phosphorus leading to **hyperphosphatemia**. Because of kidney failure, less of 1,25 $(OH)_2$ vitamin D is produced which eventually leads to hypocalcemia. This stimulates PTH and causes secondary hyperparathyroidism. Increased PTH resorbes calcium from bone in heavy amount, leading to **osteitis fibrosa cystica** (multiple cysts in the bone). Spine radiograph may show alternate bands of sclerosis and lysis referred to as the **rugger jersey spine**. Ectopic calcification can occur due to high phosphate levels. Prolonged stimulation of parathyroid hormone secretion leads to hyperplasia of the parathyroid glands. Parathyroid gland becomes autonomous and insensitive to changes in calcium, phosphate and vitamin D. This causes hypercalcemia and known as tertiary hyperparathyroidism. High serum phosphate level, markedly raised PTH levels and decreased active vitamin D levels with low urinary calcium and phosphorus, in the presence of other features of renal failure are enough to establish the diagnosis.

In almost all types of rickets there is inability to absorb calcium and phosphorus. PTH is elevated in response to hypocalcemia, corrects the serum calcium, so calcium levels are normal to low while phosphate levels may be low to normal. Alkaline phosphatase (ALP) is elevated.

ALP is a marker of osteoblastic activity

- *Increased*: Paget's disease, hyper PTH, osteomalacia, rickets, lytic bony neoplasm/metastasis.
- *Normal*: Osteoporosis, osteopetrosis, fibrous dysplasia, multiple myeloma and hypoparathyroidism.
- *Decreased*: Achondroplasia, hypophosphatasia, and cretinism.

Treatment

1. Nutritional rickets: Stoss therapy (3 lac–6 lac IU I/M or oral stat).
2. Hypophosphatemic rickets: Oral phosphorus (Ph) (Joules solution) and vitamin D supplements.
3. VDDR I: Calcitriol, Ca and Ph.
4. VDDR II: Large doses of calcitriol, Ca and Ph (treatment not satisfactory).
5. CRF: Calcitriol, Ca supplementation and Ph restriction.
6. RTA: Bicarbonate supplementation (Shohl's solution) and Ph supplementation.

Treating rickets with a deformity (e.g. Genu valgum/clubfoot): Resolution of skeletal deformities occurs completely with treatment with vitamin D and calcium. If the deformity persists even after radiological healing (the best way to predict healing) in rickets, surgery (i.e. corrective osteotomy) to correct that deformity can be done. However, surgery should be done only after the levels of ALP are brought to normal as when ALP is raised, bone is soft and not in a state to hold the fixation implant.

Xtra Edge
- Vitamin D content of human milk is low, so breastfed infants if not exposed to adequate sunlight tend to develop rickets.
- Mother's supplementation of vitamin D and mother's sunlight exposure if increased also increases the vitamin D content of breast milk.
- The clinical evidence of florid Rickets may not be evident in children with severe protein–energy malnutrition, since ricket is a disease of growing bones and growth is retarded in severe malnutrition.
- Magnesium deficiency also causes rickets (magnesium dependent vitamin D resistant rickets) which does not respond to high dose vitamin D therapy. In these patients excellent response is seen with oral magnesium chloride supplementation. Therefore serum magnesium levels should be assessed in all cases of vitamin D resistant rickets.
- In renal osteodystrophy (tertiary hyperparathyroidism) metaphyseal changes resembling rickets are seen in children. Together with cortical erosions this gives a "**rotting fence-post**" appearance specially at the femoral neck.
- *Hypervitaminosis*: Vitamin D has an anti-proliferative effect on cells like keratinocytes, breast cancer cells and prostate cancer cells. It l/t alopecia and Ca mobilisation from bones and metastatic calcification.

HYPOPHOSPHATASIA
It is a different entity from hypophosphatemia. There is a genetic error in synthesis of ALP and thus serum level of ALP is low. Serum Ca and Ph levels are normal. Diagnosis is made by phosphoethanolamine in urine/serum.

OSTEOMALACIA
Osteomalacia is basically a disorder of inadequate mineralization of bone that occurs 'in adults' due to deficiency of vitamin D in the body. The osteoid production however is unaffected, but inadequately mineralized osteoid leads to soft and weak bones and hence the term osteo-malacia.

Signs and Symptoms
Diffuse bone pains, backache, muscular weaknesss leading to waddling gait.

X-ray Features
Characteristic X-ray finding: Looser's zones, also known as cortical infarctions, Milkman's fractures, increment fractures, umbauzones or pseudofractures (Fig. 17.5A): They occur due to incomplete healing of stress fractures by a calcium-deficient callus. They appear as thin transverse lucencies, running at right angles to the involved cortex since the indentations are caused by vascular crossings/muscular pull pressing on a soft bone. The margins may be irregular and sclerotic. Often, they are multiple, bilateral and symmetrical. Common sites include pubic and ischial rami (most common site), medial proximal femur, axillary edge of scapula immediately below the glenoid, lumbar vertebrae, ribs and clavicle.

Other X-ray findings
- Biconcave cod fish vertebrae.
- Trefoil or Champagne glass pelvis (Fig. 17.5B).
- Protrusioacetabuli (bilateral is called Otto pelvis).
- Coxa vara (atraumatic).

Conditions with Looser's zones
- Osteomalacia (characteristic)
- Renal osteodystrophy
- Fibrous dysplasia
- Hyperthyroidism
- Paget's disease of bone
- X-linked hypophosphatemia
- Osteogenesis imperfect

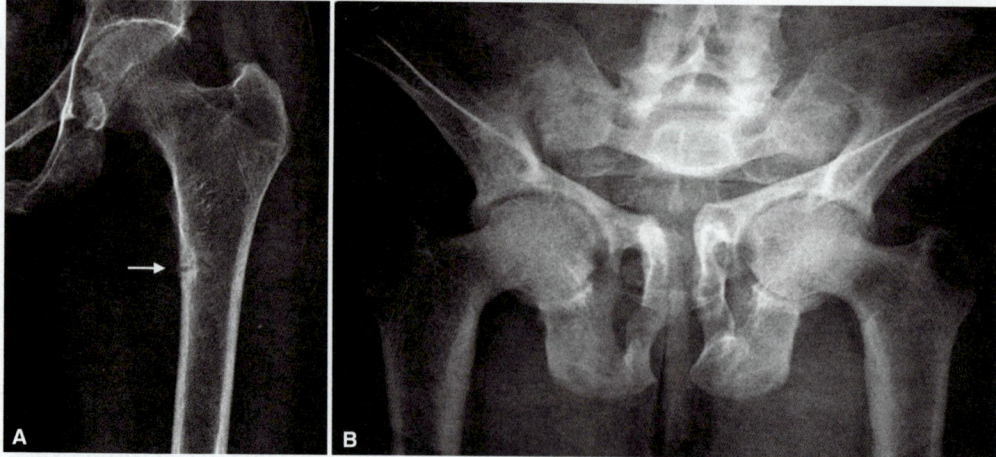

Fig. 17.5: (A) Looser zone, (B) Champagne glass pelvis

Xtra Edge
- Most common cause of osteomalacia (vitamin D deficiency) is lack of adequate exposure to sunlight.
- Sunscreen lotions reduce vitamin D synthesis in the skin.
- Darker skin people require longer exposure to make the same amount of vitamin D as a person with a white skin tone.
- Obesity is associated with vitamin D deficiency.
- Most common cause of (nontraumatic) protrusio acetabuli in India is osteomalacia and in the world is rheumatoid arthritis.
- Hypovitaminosis associated proximal myopathy (osteomalacic proximal myopathy).

HYPERPARATHYROIDISM
Hyperparathyroidism is a condition due to excessive secretion of PTH, either by the parathyroid glands or by an ectopic focus. Osteoclasts have RANK receptors on their surface while osteoblasts have the complimentary RANKL on their surface (Fig. 17.3), that remains covered by special proteins called osteoprotegrins. PTH attaches to osteoblasts via its receptor (PTHr) and makes the osteoprotegrins dissociate exposing the RANKL. This enables osteoclasts to attach to osteoblast via their RANK receptors, thereby activating them and leading to bone resorption.

Types
- 1° hyperparathyroidism—due to adenoma (most common) or hyperplasia.
- 2° hyperparathyroidism—due to persistent hypocalcemia.
- 3° hyperparathyroidism—when 2° hyperplasia leads to autonomous activity.

Clinical Features
- Abdominal pain, depression, muscle fatigue (not tetany) and urinary stones.
- Generalized osteopenia secondary to diffuse bone resorption.
- Generalized bone pains (tender to palpation).
- Pathological fractures: Generally involve the DL spine, neck and shaft of femur and pubic rami.
- *Brown tumors*: In regions where bone loss is particularly rapid, hemorrhage, reparative granulation tissue, and vascular, fibrous tissue replace the normal marrow, resulting in a brown tumor. Since hemosiderin is present in the area, it gives the characteristic brown color on histology. The lesion has a collection of osteoclasts and giant cells.

X-ray Features
- Generalized osteopenia.
- *Brown tumors*: Appear as expansile cystic lytic lesions seen mostly in mandible, maxilla, ribs, clavicle and pelvis. Multiple lesions are referred to as **osteitis fibrosa cystica/ von Recklinghausen disease** of bone (Fig.17.6A).

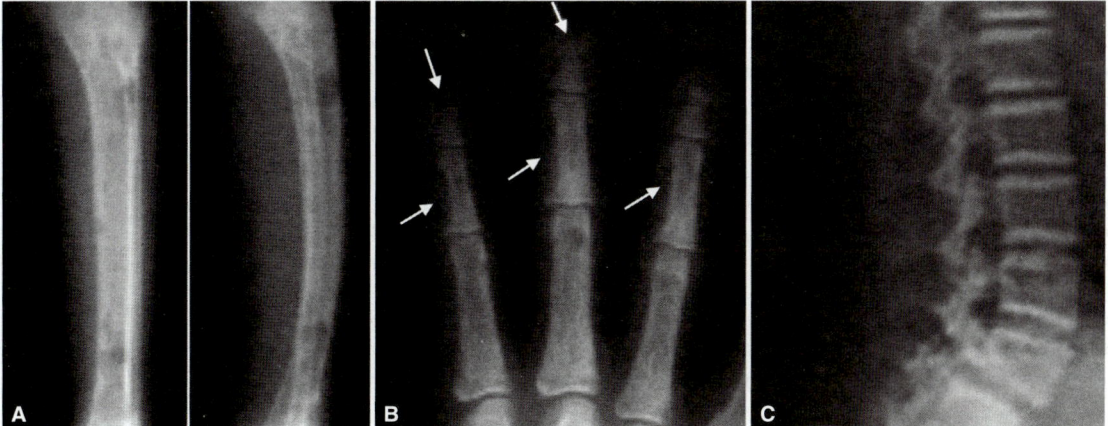

Fig. 17.6: (A) Osteitis fibrosa cystic, (B) Subperiosteal resorption, (C) Rugger jersey spine (appearance resembles that of a football player's jersey/ dress)

- Subperiosteal resorption of the phalanges is **diagnostic** (commonly seen on radial sides of middle phalanges) (Fig. 17.6B).
- Resorption of the lateral ends of the clavicle.
- Loss of lamina dura of the teeth.
- Diffuse stippling may be seen in the skull called the salt and pepper appearance.
- *Rugger jersey spine*: It refers to appearance of horizontal striped vertebrae seen as a result of alternate bands of bone loss and osteosclerosis in patients with **renal osteodystrophy**. The changes are also commonly seen at the base of skull apart from vertebrae (Fig. 17.6 C).

Investigations (Table 17.4)

Table 17.4: Differentiating primary from secondary hyperparathyroidism		
	1° adenoma	*2° hyperparathyroidism*
Clinical features	More	Less
Ca	High	Less/N
Ph	Low	variable
PTH	High	High
ALP	High	High

Treatment

- Supportive and includes adequate hydration and decreased calcium intake.
- Parathyroidectomy in severe case of unresolved long standing hypercalcemia, recurrent kidney stones and severe osteoporosis.

Xtra Edge

- *Hungry bone syndrome*: Postoperative complication of parathyroidectomy. It refers to rapid, profound and prolonged hypocalcemia associated with hypophosphatemia, and hypomagnesemia that result because of suppressed PTH levels, which follows parathyroidectomy.
- Hyperparathyroidism can be part of MEN 1, 2A and 2B.
- In hyperparathyroidism due to malignancy, the serum levels of PTH are low. Instead, one can detect high levels of PTH related peptide.
- Rugger jersey spine is seen in renal osteodystrophy and osteopetrosis (marble bone disease).

SCURVY

It is a nutritional disorder caused by deficiency of vitamin C leading to defective osteoid formation. Its main effect is on the cells/tissues of mesodermal origin.

Pathology

Deficient vitamin C impairs hydroxylation of lysine and proline which are essential for collagen formation. Consequently, capillary hemorrhages occur beneath mucous membrane and other locations of abundant capillary accumulations. The most vascular skeletal sites are beneath the periosteum, marrow in the metaphysis and actively growing epiphysis (mainly knee and shoulder).

Clinical Features

- The deficiency develops after 6–12 months of deprivation, so neonates generally get spared.
- *Generalized features*: Infant is restless, pale, febrile, lethargic, having malaise.
- The joints are swollen, painful, tender and extremities are held immobile, a condition called pseudoparalysis.
- The gums are bluish, spongy especially the upper central incisors.
- Subperiosteal hemorrhages mostly occurring beneath the periosteum of the metaphyseal growing ends of long bones of the lower extremity. They are painful and contribute to pseudo-paralysis.
- Other features of hemorrhage—hematuria, hematemesis.
- Pathological fractures may be reported but more commonly there occur epiphyseal separations. Sites for epiphyseal separation and subperiosteal hemorrhages include lower end femur, upper end tibia and upper humerus.
- Costochondral separations lead to **S**corbutic rosary, **S**harp and painful (**R**achitic = **R**ound/non-tender).

X-ray Features (Fig. 17.7)

- Ground glass appearance (osteopenia–1st sign) and Pencil thin cortex
- Subperiosteal hemorrhages: Lower end of the femur and tibia are most commonly involved. It is visualized in the healing phase of scurvy.
- White line of Frankel
- *Wimberger ring*: Circular, opaque, dense band around the epiphysis of a long bone.
- *Pelkan spur*: Metaphyseal spur at outward projection of zone of provisional calcification and periosteal reaction.
- *Trummerfeld zone*: Lucent metaphyseal band underlying the Frankel's line.
- *Corner/angle sign*: Peripheral metaphyseal cleft.

Treatment

- Vitamin C supplementation forms the mainstay.
- Joint pain disappears in 48 hours and symptoms of scurvy are completely cured in 7–10 days.

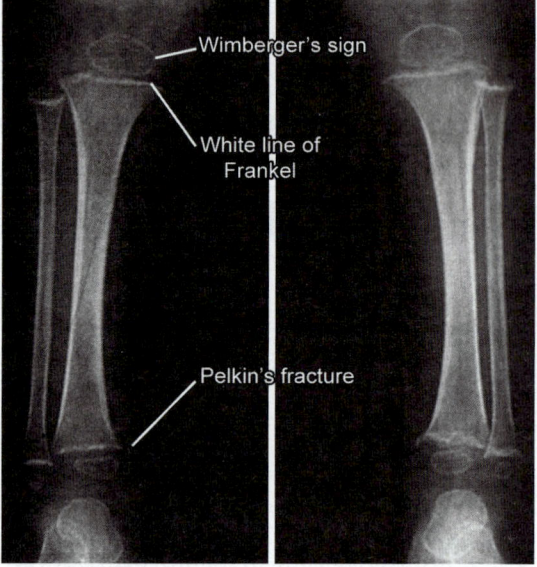

Fig. 17.7: X-ray showing signs of scurvy

Xtra Edge

- Vitamin C is destroyed by heat.
- *Barton's disease*: It includes features of both rickets and scurvy.
- *Barlow's disease*: Infantile scurvy with pseudoparalysis.
- Causes of White line of Frankel:
    - Scurvy
    - Healing rickets
    - Lead poisoning
    - Acute leukemia
    - Growth arrest lines due to chronic diseases like bronchial asthma, cystic fibrosis
    - Methotrexate therapy
    - Healing in renal osteodystrophy
- *Ring epiphysis*: Rickets, scurvy, osteogenesis imperfecta, hypothyroidism and osteopetrosis.

FLUOROSIS

Fluorine in very low concentration (1 ppm) is essential for formation of dental enamel and mineralisation of bone. Inadequate ingestion leads to dental caries and overingestion is characterised by fluorosis.

Fluorosis is seen in parts of India (Punjab, Andhra Pradesh and Tamil Nadu) and Africa where the fluorine content of drinking water is high (2–4 ppm).

- Fluorine stimulates osteoblastic activity; fluorapatite crystals are laid down in bone and these are usually resistant to osteoclastic resorption.
- It leads to subperiosteal new bone accretion and osteosclerosis most marked in axial bone and forearm/leg bones.
- Bony attachment of tendons, ligaments and fascia are also thickened due to new bone formation (hyperostosis).
- In the human body, almost 95% of fluoride is contained in the bones and teeth. Thus, the symptoms of this disorder primarily span over these two systems.
- Bone disease in fluorosis is more severe in those with concurrent calcium deficiency.

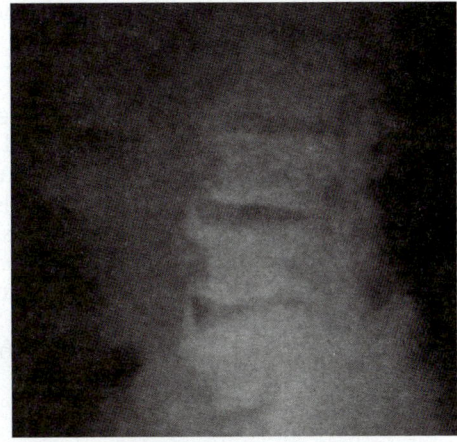

Fig. 17.8: X-ray showing ossification of spinal ligaments

- **Dental fluorosis:** Teeth lose their shiny appearance followed by chalky white and later yellowish resulting in mottling of teeth, most commonly 1st incisors of the upper jaw, and occurs only in permanent teeth when they are erupting. It is not seen after they are completely formed.
- **Skeletal fluorosis:** Backache, joint pain and stiffness are common clinical features. The bone becomes weak and pathological fracture may occur and later on bones may deform and bowed (**genu valgum**). Calcification of the posterior longitudinal ligament occurs in the spine and leads to narrowing the spinal canal. In advanced stages, this may lead to compression of the cord leading to **spastic** paralysis.

X-ray Features

- Osteosclerosis
- Hyperostosis of tendons/ligaments (Fig. 17.8)
- Calcification of the interosseous membrane of the forearm (Fig. 17.9) and leg is characteristic.

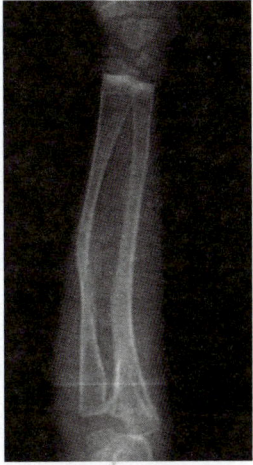

Fig. 17.9: X-ray showing interosseous membrane calcification

Differential Diagnosis

Osteosclerotic conditions: Paget's disease, DISH, osteopetrosis, renal osteodystrophy, secondaries from prostate and Engelmann's disease.

PAGET'S DISEASE

Paget's disease (osteitis deformans) is a disease of abnormal bone turnover characterised by excessive osteoclastic activity initially followed by disorganised excessive new bone formation. It may be one bone (monostotic) or multiple bone involvement (polyostotic).

Etiopathogenesis

Exact etiology is unknown although paramyxovirus and respiratory syncytial virus has been implicated.

- **1st phase:** Extensive osteoclastic destruction accompanied by increased vascularity (radiologically seen as advancing lytic wedge or blade of grass) and fibrosis. Trabeculae are thinned and haversian canals are enlarged.

- **2nd phase** (phase of bone formation): The resorbed bone is replaced by structurally weak bone that is brittle and breaks easily. Repair and destruction are taking place at the same time. Fracture are most common in 2nd stage.
- **3rd phase** (sclerotic/burnout phase): Bone resorption declines progressively resulting in hard, dense, avascular pagetic/mosaic bone. When fracture occurs in 3rd stage, union is delayed.

Clinical Features
- **Mostly asymptomatic** and involves males >females.
- Pelvis is most common site affected and pain is the most common symptom.
- Bones are weak and bend/deform and fracture easily. Limb looks bent and warm due to high vascularity and thus the condition is called osteitis deformans.
- Cranial nerve—2nd, 5th, 7th, 8th palsy is seen.
- Nerve compression and spinal stenosis is seen.
- Deafness is due to nerve compression > osteosclerosis (loss of BMD in cochlear capsule).
- High output cardiac failure.
- Steal syndrome—blood is diverted from internal organs to skeletal system l/t cerebral ischemia and spinal claudication.
- Osteoarthritis and osteosarcoma (1% cases) may develop.

X-ray Features
- Ivory vertebrae (diffusely sclerotic vertebrae)
- Picture frame vertebrae (thickening at superior and inferior end plates, Fig. 17.10)
- Osteoporosis circumscripta (osteoporotic patch) initially that later leads to cotton wool spots (Fig. 17.11 A and B) in the skull.
- *Brim sign*: Sclerotic iliopectineal line in pelvis.
- *Blade of grass appearance*: It is "V"-shaped radiolucency seen in the diaphysis of long bones.
- A banana fracture or incremental fracture refers to a complete, horizontally oriented pathological fracture seen in deformed bones affected by Paget disease.

Other Investigations
- Serum Ca and Ph levels are usually normal.
- Markers of bone formation and resorption are increased (Table 17.5).
- Biopsy of bone characteristically shows the mosaic pattern, but is rarely indicated.

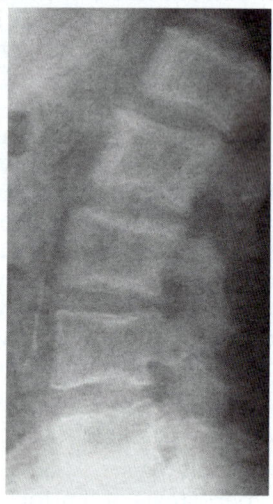

Fig. 17.10: Picture frame vertebrae

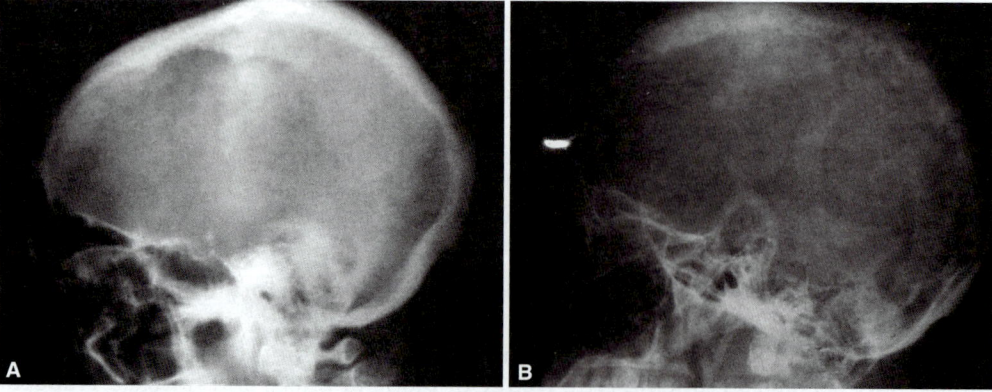

Fig. 17.11: (A) Osteoporosis circumscripta, (B) Cotton wool skull

Table 17.5: Markers of bone formation and resorption

Markers of bone resorption
- Urine and serum cross-linked N telopeptides
- Urine and serum cross-linked C telopeptides
- Urine hydroxyproline
- Urine deoxypyridinoline
- Urine hydroxylysine glycosides
- Serum TRAP (tartarate resistant acid phosphatase)—Serum bone sialoprotein

Markers of bone formation
- Serum bone specific alkaline phosphatase—Serum osteocalcin
- Serum carboxy terminal extension peptide of pro-collagen-1
- Serum type I collagen extension peptide

Table 17.6: Differentiating various metabolic bone disorders

Disease	Ca	Ph	ALP	PTH
Osteoporosis	N	N	N	N
Rickets/osteomalacia	N/↓	↓	↑	↑
Primary hyperparathyroidism	↑	↓	↑	↑
Paget's disease	N	N	↑	N

Treatment
- Mithramycin (plicamycin), an anti-neoplastic agent (toxic to osteoclast) was the first drug used for Paget's disease.
- DOC now are Bisphosphonates. Etidronate was used first; Risedronate is preferred now.
- Calcitonin is used for acute relief of pain (temporary effect).

Xtra Edge
- Weight bearing bones (lower limb/vertebrae) show active reparative process, while repair in skull bone (subjected to less stress and strain) lags behind in the early stages and resorption predominates.
- There is no attempt at repair of haversian system.
- In Paget's disease, the bones of hand and feet are seldom affected (differential point from polyostotic fibrous dysplasia).
- Differentiating feature of various metabolic disorders have been tabulated in Table 17.6.

MULTIPLE CHOICE QUESTIONS

1. **All of these drugs inhibit resorption of bone except:**
   A. Teriparatide B. Raloxifene
   C. Risedronate D. Strontium ranelate

2. **Which of the following statement is incorrect regarding osteoporosis?**
   A. I/V parathormone is useful in severe osteoporosis
   B. T-score is less than 2.5
   C. Bisphosphonates are the mainstay of treatment
   D. Calcitonin is useful in acute pain

3. **Which bisphosphonate is approved for the treatment of osteoporosis and is given on yearly basis?**
   A. Alendronate B. Zolendronate
   C. Risedronate D. Ibandronate

4. **A 60-year-old female with long term steroid intake, presents with backache. X-ray spine done as shown below, next investigation to be done is:**

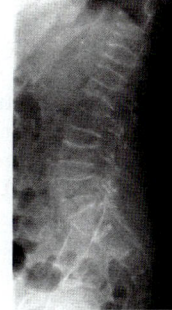

   A. DEXA B. PTH
   C. Calcium D. Calcitriol

5. **Most common site for the osteoporotic vertebral fracture is:**
   A. Dorsolumbar spine B. Cervical spine
   C. Lumbosacral spine D. Dorsal spine
6. **Z score measures the bone mineral density compared to:**
   A. Age, race and sex matched individuals
   B. Race and sex matched individuals
   C. Sex matched individuals
   D. None of the above
7. **Osteoporosis is characterized by all the following *except*:**
   A. Decreased bone mineral density
   B. Decreased serum calcium, phosphorus and alkaline phosphatase are seen
   C. Glucocorticoids can cause osteoporosis
   D. Dorsolumbar spine is the most common site of osteoporotic fracture
8. **The bodies of spine are biconcave and are called "cod fish spine" most commonly seen in:**
   A. Scurvy
   B. Osteomalacia
   C. Fluorosis
   D. Hyperparathyroidism
9. **Osteoporosis which of the following is false?**
   A. Osteoporosis is defined, if t score is less than 1.5
   B. Severe osteoporosis PTH is used for treatment
   C. Calcitonin decreases the bone pain
   D. Bisphosphonates are cornerstone of treatment
10. **Osteoporotic female on prolonged bisphosphonates has hip pain, next investigation is:**
    A. X-ray   B. Vitamin D
    C. ALP   D. DEXA
11. **Osteoporosis is caused by all *except*:**
    A. Fluorosis
    B. Hypogonadism
    C. Hyperthyroidism
    D. Hyperparathyroidism
12. **Gold standard for diagnosis of osteoporosis:**
    A. DEXA
    B. Single beam densitometry
    C. Quantitative computed tomography
    D. Bone histomorphometry
13. **In osteoporosis, bone formation is increased by which drug?**
    A. Bisphosphonates   B. Estrogen
    C. Calcitonin   D. Teriparatide
14. **A 70-year-old female present to OPD after a trivial trauma, MRI shows L1 collapse. Next best management is:**
    A. Vitamin D therapy
    B. CT
    C. Bisphosphonates
    D. Screw fixation
    E. Aggressive physiotherapy

15. **Most common site of osteoporosis:**
    A. Humerus   B. Vertebrae
    C. Scapula   D. Flat bones
16. **Decreased osteoid content is a feature of:**
    A. Osteoporosis   B. Osteopetrosis
    C. Osteomalacia   D. Paget's disease
17. **In osteoporosis which of these is seen?**
    A. Normal calcium, decreased ALP
    B. Decreased calcium, increased ALP
    C. Normal calcium, normal ALP
    D. Decreased calcium, normal ALP
18. **Most common area affected in osteoporotic fracture is:**
    A. Vertebra   B. Pelvis
    C. Radius   D. Hip
19. **Which of the following is not a treatment option for osteoporosis?**
    A. Denosumab   B. Alendronate
    C. Vertebroplasty   D. Corticosteroids
20. **Rickets in infancy is characterised by all of the following *except*:**
    A. Wide open fontanelle
    B. Bow legs
    C. Rachitic rosary
    D. Craniotabes
21. **Denosumab—a monoclonal antibody against RANKL receptor is used in the treatment of:**
    A. Osteoarthritis   B. RA
    C. SLE   D. Osteoporosis
22. **Cod fish vertebrae are seen in:**
    A. Osteomalacia   B. Osteoporosis
    C. Spinal ALP   D. Fractures
23. **Osteoporosis treatment in 60 years female is:**
    A. Estrogen   B. Tamoxifen
    C. Alendronate   D. Calcitonin
24. **Senile osteoporosis patient is on bisphosphonates for 7 years and has pain in left hip, next investigation is:**
    A. BMD by DEXA   B. X-ray
    C. Serum ALP   D. USG
25. **MC fracture in postmenopausal women:**
    A. Spine   B. Hip
    C. Radius   D. Tibia
26. **Steroids have the following effect on bone:**
    A. Osteomalacia   B. Osteoporosis
    C. Calcific deposits D. Myositis ossificans
27. **Which of the following is used in osteoporosis for decreasing bone resorption and increasing bone formation?**
    A. Teriparatide   B. Calcitonin
    C. Strontium ranelate D. Bisphosphonate
28. **Most common cause of kyphotic deformity:**
    A. Trauma
    B. Osteoporosis
    C. Ankylosing spondylitis
    D. Rickets

29. Osteoporosis is seen in:
   A. Thyrotoxicosis   B. Cushing's disease
   C. Menopause   D. All of the above

30. A bald child with swollen abdomen, hyperosseous bones have?
   A. Hypervitaminosis C
   B. Hypervitaminosis D
   C. Down's syndrome
   D. Tuberous sclerosis

31. Hypervitaminosis of which of the following will cause bony abnormalities?
   A. Vitamin A   B. Vitamin D
   C. Vitamin C   D. Vitamin E

32. Oncogenic rickets not seen in:
   A. Osteosarcoma
   B. Nonossifying fibroma
   C. Chondroblastoma
   D. Angiosarcoma

33. Treatment of postmenopausal osteoprosis:
   A. Tamoxifen   B. Progesterone
   C. Estrogen   D. Alendronate
   E. Calcitonin

34. Denosumab—a monoclonal antibody against RANKL receptor is used in treatment of:
   A. Rheumatoid arthritis
   B. Osteoporosis
   C. Osteoarthritis
   D. SLE

35. Osteoporosis is characterized by:
   A. Increased serum alkaline phosphatase
   B. Decreased bone density
   C. Wasting of muscles
   D. Looser's zone seen

36. Which of the following is not a recognized risk factor for osteoporosis?
   A. Early menarche
   B. Sedentary life style
   C. Smoking
   D. Low dietary calcium intake

37. Treatment of postmenopausal osteoporosis:
   A. Calcitonin   B. Alendronate
   C. Progesterone   D. Tamoxifen

38. Which of the following is seen in osteoporosis?
   A. Low Ca, high PO_4, high alkaline phosphatase
   B. Low Ca, low PO_4, low alkaline phosphatase
   C. Normal Ca, normal PO_4, normal alkaline phosphatase
   D. Low Ca, low PO_4, normal alkaline phosphatase

39. The most common manifestation of osteoporosis is:
   A. Compression fracture of the spine
   B. Asymptomatic, detected incidentally by low serum calcium
   C. Bowing of legs
   D. Loss of weight

40. A patient of osteoporosis on medication, complained of hip pain. X-ray was done. What drug was she taking?

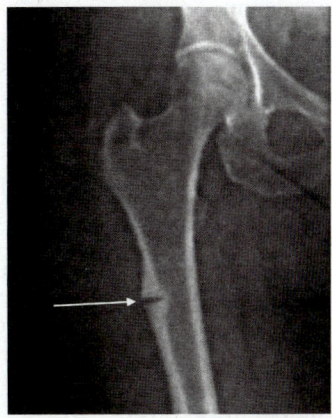

   A. Bisphosphonates   B. Strontium ranelate
   C. Calcium   D. Teriparatide

41. Drug of choice for senile osteoporosis is:
   A. Estrogens   B. Androgens
   C. Calcitonin   D. Etidronate

42. The maximum change in bone mineral density in hemiplegic patients after 1 year is seen in:
   A. Lumbar spine
   B. Proximal femur of the paralysed side
   C. Distal radius of the paralysed side
   D. Humerus of the paralysed side

43. Blade of grass lesion is seen in:
   A. Thalassemia
   B. Osteoporosis
   C. Carcinoma prostate
   D. Paget's disease

44. An elderly female is on treatment for osteoporosis with alendronate for 7 years. She now presents with complaints of hip pain. The next investigation for her should be:
   A. X-ray   B. DEXA scan
   C. Vitamin D levels   D. ALP levels

45. As per current recommendations which vitamin is required with vitamin D for treatment of osteoporosis?
   A. Vitamin A   B. Vitamin B
   C. Vitamin C   D. Vitamin K

46. All the following are used in osteoporosis except:
   A. Denosumab   B. Strontium
   C. PTH   D. Milnacipran

47. Child diagnosed with hypophosphatemic rickets; choose the correct statement:
   A. Serum calcium levels are mostly normal
   B. Raised levels of alkaline phosphate seen
   C. Has XLD inheritance
   D. PTH is markedly raised
   E. Pigeon chest is one of the characteristics of skeletal deformity

48. **Biochemical abnormality in rickets:**
    A. High calcium   B. High PO_4
    C. Low ALP   D. ALP is high
    E. Low calcium

49. **Wrist X- ray:**
    A. Rickets   B. Colles' fracture
    C. Scaphoid fracture   D. Osteoporosis

50. **X- ray hand, most probable diagnosis:**
    A. Scurvy   B. Rickets
    C. Hyper PTH   D. Achondroplasia

51. **Which of the features are seen in pediatric vitamin D deficiency?**
    A. Rachitic rosary   B. Harrison's sulcus
    C. Wimberger sign   D. Pigeon chest

52. **A 2-year-old child with rickets is on calcium supplements and has a foot deformity. The child will be referred to a surgeon for the correction of the deformity when:**
    A. Serum calcium levels are normal
    B. Serum vitamin D levels are normal
    C. Growth plate healing becomes normal
    D. Serum ALP becomes normal

53. **Hypervitaminosis of which of the following vitamins can cause bony abnormalities?**
    [*PGI type*]
    A. Vitamin A   B. Vitamin C
    C. Vitamin D   D. Vitamin K
    E. Vitamin E

54. **Osteomalacia is due to:**
    A. Vitamin C deficiency
    B. Vitamin D deficiency
    C. Vitamin E deficiency
    D. None

55. **In Rickets all are seen *except*:**
    A. Bowing of legs   B. Rachitic rosary
    C. Bleeding   D. Craniotabes

56. **A 30 years female has low serum calcium and phosphate with elevated parathormone. Diagnosis is:**
    A. Vitamin D deficiency
    B. Primary hyperparathyroidism
    C. Osteoporosis
    D. Paget's disease

57. **Pectus carinatum is seen in:**
    A. Scurvy
    B. Rickets
    C. Hemophilia
    D. Orthogenesis imperfect

58. **Rickets osteotomy is carried out once:**
    A. Calcium is normal
    B. ALP is normal
    C. Healing of growth plate takes place
    D. Knee movement is normally carried out

59. **Test for vitamin D deficiency:**
    A. Vitamin D levels   B. ALP levels
    C. Calcium levels   D. Phosphate level

60. **Hypophosphatemic rickets mode of inheritance is:**
    A. Autosomal dominant
    B. Autosomal recessive
    C. X-linked dominant
    D. X-linked recessive

61. **Which of the drugs cause osteomalacia?**
    A. Phenytoin   B. Valproate
    C. Carbamazepine   D. Aspirin

62. **Looser zone is fracture of:**
    A. Osteoporosis   B. Osteomalacia
    C. Metastasis   D. Scurvy

63. **Osteomalacia is associated with:**
    A. Decrease in osteoid volume
    B. Decrease in osteoid surface
    C. Increase in osteoid maturation time
    D. Increase in mineral apposition rate

64. **Rickets in infancy is characterized by the following *excepts*:**
    A. Craniotabes
    B. Rachitic rosary
    C. Wide open fontanelles
    D. Bow legs

65. **Decreased mineralization of epiphyseal plate in a growing child is seen in:**
    A. Rickets   B. Osteomalacia
    C. Scurvy   D. Osteoporosis

66. **Osteomalacia/rickets may be seen in A/E:**
    A. Neurofibroma
    B. Osteoblastoma
    C. Hemangiopericytoma
    D. Ewing's sarcoma

67. **Basic pathological defect in rickets is:**
    A. Decreased osteoblastic activity
    B. Nonfunctional osteoclast
    C. Defective osteoclastic resorption of uncalcified osteoid and cartilage
    D. Defective proliferation of physis

68. **A patients with raised serum alkaline phosphatase and raised parathormone level along with low calcium and low phosphate level is likely to have?**
    A. Primary hyperparathyroidism
    B. Paget's disease
    C. Osteoporosis
    D. Vitamin D deficiency

69. **Action of vitamin D is that it:**
    A. Stimulates bone marrow
    B. Increases calcium loss
    C. Stimulates absorption of calcium
    D. Stimulates osteoclasts

70. **Primary hyperparathyroidism is associated with:**
    A. Increased serum PTH and hypercalcemia
    B. Decreased serum PTH and hypercalcemia
    C. Increased serum PTH and hypocalcemia
    D. Decreased serum PTH and hypocalcemia

71. **A 70-year-old male, known case of chronic renal failure, suffers from a pathological fracture of right femur, the diagnosis is:**
    A. Primary hyperparathyroidism
    B. Secondary hyperparathyroidism
    C. Scurvy
    D. Vitamin D resistant rickets

72. **A middle aged female has resorption of 2nd and 3rd metacarpal and multiple lytic lesions in pelvis femur ribs clavicle:**
    A. Hyperthyroidism
    B. Hyperparathyroidism
    C. Osteomalacia
    D. Renal osteodystrophy

73. **Osteitis fibrosa is seen in:**
    A. Hyperparathyroidism
    B. Hypoparathyroidism
    C. Hypothyroidism
    D. Hyperthyroidism

74. **This X-ray skull is a feature of:**

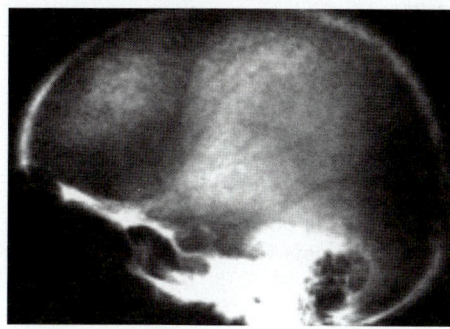

    A. Paget's syndrome
    B. Eosinophilic granuloma
    C. Primary hypoparathyroidism
    D. Multiple myeloma

75. **Hypoparathyroidism causes:**
    A. Multiple bone cysts
    B. Subperiosteal bone resorption
    C. Brown's tumor
    D. All of the above

76. **This X-ray is a feature of:**

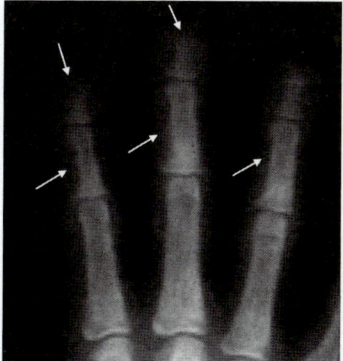

    A. Hyperthyroidism
    B. Hypothyroidism
    C. Hypoparathyroidism
    D. Hyperparathyroidism

77. **Hyperparathyroidism is characterized by:**
    A. Hypocalcemia
    B. Osteoprotegerin
    C. Hyperphosphatemia
    D. Multiple bone cyst

78. **Brown tumor is seen in:**
    A. Hyperparathyroidism
    B. Hypoparathyroidism
    C. Hypothyroidism
    D. Hyperparathyroidism

79. **A 50-year-old man presented with multiple pathological fracture. His serum calcium was 11.5 mg/dl and phosphate was 2.5 mg/dl. Alkaline phosphatase was 940 1.U/dl. The most probable diagnosis is:**
    A. Osteoporosis
    B. Osteomalacia
    C. Multiple myeloma
    D. Hyperparathyroidism

80. **Soft tissue calcification with hypercalcemia is observed in:**
    A. Hyperparathyroidism
    B. Alkaptonuria
    C. Gout
    D. Cushing's disease

81. **Absence of lamina dura in the alveolus occurs in:**
    A. Rickets
    B. Osteomalacia
    C. Deficiency of vitamin
    D. Hyperparathyroidism

82. **Looser's zone is seen in which of the following conditions?**
    A. Osteoprosis
    B. Osteomalacia
    C. Rickets
    D. Scurvy

83. **Looser zone/pseudofracture are commonly seen in the following areas *except*:**
    A. Scapula   B. Ribs
    C. Pelvis   D. Radius

84. **Looser's zones are seen in:**
    A. Osteomalacia
    B. Paget's disease
    C. Renal osteodystrophy
    D. All of the above

85. **Short 4th metacarpal is a fracture of:**
    A. Hyperparathyroidism
    B. Hypoparathyroidism
    C. Pseudohypoparathyroidism
    D. Scleroderma

86. **Milkman's frature is:**
    A. Pseudofracture in adults
    B. Fracture of clavicle in children
    C. Fracture humerus
    D. Fracture first metacarpal

87. **"Rugger jersey spine" is seen in:**
    A. Fluorosis
    B. Achondroplasia
    C. Renal osteodystrophy
    D. Marfan's syndrome

88. **Rugger jersey spine in CRF is due to:**
    A. Osteomalacia
    B. Trauma
    C. Hyperparathyroidism
    D. Aluminium osteodystrophy

89. **A female eating only junk food, pinpoint ecchymoses around follicle. Bleeding into joints and subperiosteal hemorrhages, swollen tongue and gingivitis. What are the defects?**
    A. Hydroxylation of lysine and proline
    B. Carboxylation of clothing factors
    C. Deficiency factor Vlll
    D. Deficiency factor IX

90. **Wimberger's ring sign is seen in:**
    A. Scurvy
    B. Syphilis
    C. Paget's
    D. Hemophilia

91. **Barton's disease is:**
    A. Scurvy and rickets
    B. Scurvy and fracture
    C. Rickets and fracture
    D. Scurvy and syphilis

92. **Vitamin C deficiency leads to:**
    A. Defective mineralisation
    B. Defective osteoid formation
    C. Normal collagen and bone matrix
    D. X-ray shows normal evidence

93. **A young patient presents with enlargement of costochondral junction and with the white line of Frankel at the metaphysis. The diagnosis is:**
    A. Scurvy
    B. Rickets
    C. Hyperparathyroidism
    D. Osteomalacia

94. **Vitamin required for collagen is:**
    A. Vitamin A
    B. Vitamin C
    C. Vitamin D
    D. Vitamin E

95. **Metaphyseal fracture is commonly seen in:**
    A. Osteogenesis imperfecta
    B. Scurvy
    C. Rickets
    D. None

96. **Increase bone density with hyperostosis seen in skeletal fluorosis is likely to occur when fluorine concentration in drinking H_2O is above:**
    A. 6 ppm
    B. 10 ppm
    C. 15 ppm
    D. 20 ppm

97. **Increased bone density occurs in:**
    A. Cushing syndrome
    B. Hypoparathyroidism
    C. Fluorosis
    D. Hyperthyroidism

98. **What is the diagnostic radiological finding in skeletal fluorosis?**
    A. Sclerosis of sacroiliac joint
    B. Interosseous membrane ossification
    C. Osteosclerosis of vertebral body
    D. Ossification of ligaments of knee joint

99. **Increased density in skull vault is seen in:**
    A. Hyperparathyroidism
    B. Multiple myeloma
    C. Fluorosis
    D. Renal osteodystrophy

100. **Manifestations of fluorosis include:**
    A. Stiffness of back ligaments
    B. Caries teeth
    C. Genu valgum
    D. Dental changes
    E. Stiffness of bones and tendons

101. **Osteosclerosis is a feature of which of the following?**
    A. Rickets
    B. Hyperparathyroidism
    C. Paget's disease
    D. Orthogenesis imperfect

102. **All of the following are true regarding Paget's disease *except*:**
    A. Pelvis is the most common site
    B. Cranial nerve involvement may be seen
    C. High output cardiac failure is one of the complications
    D. It may progress to secondary chondro-sarcoma

103. **Paget's disease commonly develops in which age group?**
    A. 1st decade
    B. 3rd decade
    C. 5th decade
    D. 7th decade

104. **Blades of grass lesion is found in:**
    A. Paget's disease
    B. Thalassemia
    C. Osteoporosis
    D. Carcinoma prostate

105. **Picture frame vertebra is seen in:**
    A. Paget's disease
    B. Osteopetrosis
    C. Osteoporosis
    D. Ankylosing spondylitis

106. **Increased alkaline phosphatase in seen in:**
   A. Osteoporosis   B. Multiple myeloma
   C. Paget's disease D. Osteolytic metastasis
107. **All are features of Paget's disease *except*:**
   A. Defect in osteoclasts
   B. Common in female
   C. Can cause deafness
   D. Can cause osteosarcoma
108. **Paget's disease after 10 years develops into:**
   A. Osteosarcoma
   B. Fibrous cortical defect
   C. Osteoid osteoma
   D. Ankylosing spondylitis
109. **Paget's disease is associated with which bone cancer?**
   A. Osteosarcoma   B. Chondrosarcoma
   C. Fibrosarcoma   D. Ewing's sarcoma
110. **Pain in Paget's disease is relieved best by:**
   A. Simple analgesics B. Narcotic analgesics
   C. Radiation   D. Calcitonin
111. **All of the following statements regarding Paget's disease are correct *except*:**
   A. Females are affected more than males
   B. It can lead to osteogenic sarcoma
   C. Serum alkaline phosphates level is increased
   D. Called osteitis deformans
112. **A 60- year-old male with bony abnormality at upper tibia associated with sensorineural hearing loss. On laboratory examination serum alkaline phosphatase levels are (440 mU/I) elevated and serum Ca^{++} and PO are normal. Skeletal survey shows ivory vertebrae and cotton wool spots in X-ray skull. Diagnosis is:**
   A. Fibrous dysplasia
   B. Paget's disease
   C. Osteosclerotic matastasis
   D. Osteoporosis
113. **Paget's disease of bone commonly affects:**
   A. Skull   B. Vertebra
   C. Pelvis   D. Femur
   E. Humerus

114. **Treatment of choice for Paget's disease of the bone is:**
   A. Vitamin D
   B. Immobilization of the limb
   C. Surgical treatment
   D. Calcitonin
115. **Which of the following is a primary defect in Paget's disease?**
   A. Osteoblast   B. Osteoclast
   C. Osteocyte   D. Fibroblast
116. **A 67-year-old man on biochemical analysis found to have threefold rise of level of serum alkaline phosphatase that of upper limit of normal value during a routine checkup but serum calcium and phosphorous concentration and liver function test results are normal. He is asymptomatic. The probable cause is:**
   A. Multiple myeloma
   B. Paget's disease of bone
   C. Primary hyperparathyroidism
   D. Osteomalcia
117. **Deafness in cases of Paget's disease is due to:**
   A. Thickened cranium
   B. Narrowing of foramina of skull
   C. Brain compression
   D. Otosclerosis
118. **The histopathologic feature of Paget's disease includes:**
   A. Simultaneous osteoblastic activity at places
   B. Osteoclastic resorption
   C. Replacement of bone marrow by fibrovascular tissue
   D. All of the above
119. **Vitamin D deficiency rickets is confirmed by demonstration of:**
   A. Epiphyseal changes in X-ray
   B. Hypocalcemia and hypophosphatemia
   C. Raised serum alkaline phosphatase
   D. Healing with physiologic doses of vitamin D$_3$
120. **Drug of choice for bisphosphonate resistant osteoporosis:**
   A. Teriparatide   B. Denosumab
   C. Anakinra   D. Calcitonin

ANSWERS

1. A. Teriparatide
   It is recombinant human PTH. On large doses it removes Ca from bone while in small pulses it can directly stimulate osteoblast to form new bone. The bone formation effect of teriparatide is far more than its minimal bone resorption effect.
2. A. I/V parathormone is useful in severe osteoporosis
   • It is given subcutaneously, not I/V

3. B. Zolendronate
4. A. DEXA
5. A. Dorsolumbar spine
6. A. Age, race and sex matched individuals
7. B. Decreased serum calcium, phosphorus and alkaline phosphatase are seen
8. B. Osteomalacia
9. A. Osteoporosis is defined, if t score is less than 1.5
10. A. X-ray

11. A. Fluorosis
12. A. DEXA
13. D. Teriparatide
14. A. Vitamin D therapy and C. Bisphosphonates
15. B. Vertebrae
16. A. Osteoporosis
17. C. Normal calcium, normal ALP
18. A. Vertebra
19. D. Corticosteroids
    • Steroids is not used in the treatment of osteoporosis, infact it is a risk factor for developing osteoporosis.
20. B. Bow legs
    • Leg deformities develop only after the child starts walking, i.e after the age of 1 year
21. D. Osteoporosis
22. B. Osteoporosis
23. A. Estrogen
24. B. X-ray
25. A. Spine
26. A. Osteomalacia
27. C. Strontium ranelate
28. B. Osteoporosis
29. D. All of the above
30. B. Hypervitaminosis D
31. A. Vitamin A and B. Vitamin D
32. D. Angiosarcoma
33. C. Estrogen, D. Alendronate, E. Calcitonin
34. B. Osteoporosis
35. B. Decreased bone density
36. A. Early menarche
37. A. Calcitonin, B. Alendronate
38. C. Normal Ca, normal PO_4, normal alkaline phosphatase
39. A. Compression fracture of the spine
    • MC presentation is asymptomatic, but out of the given options 'A' is best suited.
40. A. Bisphosphonates
41. A. Estrogens
42. D. Humerus of the paralysed side
43. D. Paget's disease
44. A. X-ray
45. D. Vitamin K
46. D. Milnacipran
47. A. Serum calcium levels are mostly normal, B. Raised levels of alkaline phosphate seen, C. Has XLD inheritance, E. Pigeon chest is one of the characteristics of skeletal deformity.
48. D. ALP is high; E. Low calcium
49. A. Rickets
50. B. Rickets
51. A. Rachitic rosary
52. D. Serum ALP becomes normal
53. A. Vitamin A, C. Vitamin D
54. B. Vitamin D deficiency

55. C. Bleeding
56. A. Vitamin D deficiency
57. B. Rickets
58. C. Healing of growth plate takes place
59. A. Vitamin D levels
60. C. X-linked dominant
61. A. Phenytoin
62. A. Osteoporosis
63. C. Increase in osteoid maturation time
64. D. Bow legs
    • Deformities of leg develops only after child starts walking, i.e. after the age of one year.
65. A. Rickets
66. D. Ewing's sarcoma
67. C. Defective osteoclastic resorption of uncalcified osteoid and cartilage
68. D. Vitamin D deficiency
    • In osteoporosis all these blood parameters generally remains normal.
69. C. Stimulates absorption of calcium; D. Stimulates osteoclasts
70. A. Increased serum PTH and hypercalcemia
71. B. Secondary hyperparathyroidism
72. B. Hyperparathyroidism
73. A. Hyperparathyroidism
74. C. Primary hypoparathyroidism
75. D. All of the above
76. D. Hyperparathyroidism
    • Subperiosteal bone resorption
77. D. Multiple bone cyst
78. A. Hyperparathyroidism
79. D. Hyperparathyroidism
80. A. Hyperparathyroidism
81. D. Hyperparathyroidism
82. B. Osteomalacia
83. D. Radius
84. D. All of the above
85. C. Pseudohypoparathyroidism
86. A. Pseudofracture in adults
87. C. Renal osteodystrophy
88. C. Hyperparathyroidism
89. A. Hydroxylation of lysine and proline
90. A. Scurvy
91. A. Scurvy and rickets
92. B. Defective osteoid formation
93. A. Scurvy
94. B. Vitamin C
95. B. Scurvy
96. B. 10 ppm
97. C. Fluorosis
98. B. Interosseous membrane ossification
99. C. Fluorosis
100. A. Stiffness of back ligaments; D. Dental changes—fluorosis causes mottling of teeth

101. C. Paget's disease
102. D. It may progress to secondary chondro-sarcoma
103. D. 7 th decade
104. A. Paget's disease
105. A. Paget's disease
106. C. Paget's disease
107. B. Common in female
108. A. Osteosarcoma
109. A. Osteosarcoma
110. D. Calcitonin
111. A. Females are affected more than males
112. B. Paget's disease
113. A. Skull; B. Vertebra; C. Pelvis; D. Femur
114. D. Calcitonin
115. B. Osteoclast

116. B. Paget's disease of bone
   - Many a times Paget's disease can have asymptomatic presentation with high ALP, normal calcium and phosphate, whereas multiple myeloma does not have increased ALP
   - Osteomalacia and hyperparathyroidism will have abnormality in calcium and phosphorus levels
117. B. Narrowing of foramina of skull
118. D. All of the above
119. D. Healing with physiologic doses of vitamin D_3
   - Healing with Vit D administration is the best way to diagnose rickets due to vitamin D deficiency
120. A. Teriparatide

Joint Diseases

JOINT ANATOMY

In a normal synovial joint, the ends of each bone are covered by hyaline cartilage referred to as articular cartilage. The joint is lined circumferentially by synovial membrane. The synovial membrane (made of Type I and III collagen) contains specialized cells called synovial cells that secrete a viscous yellowish fluid called synovial fluid that lubricates the joint cavity.

The synovial cells are of two types: Type A (macrophage like cells) is primarily involved in phagocytosis while Type B (fibroblast-like cells) possess a rich network of endoplasmic reticulum and secrete hyaluronic acid, proteins and prostaglandins present in synovial fluid.

Synovial Fluid

This specialized fluid is basically an ultradialysate of blood plasma to which hyaluronic acid has been added by the synovial cells. An absence of basement membrane in the synovium allows an easy passage of fluid from capillaries into the joint cavity.

Normal amount: 0–4 mL (varies from joint to joint).

Composition: Water content is around 95% and pH 7.3–7.6. Hyaluronic acid is the most important component that gives its thixotrophic properties (its viscosity decreases with increased rate of shear) and thereby allows it to follow non-newtonian kinetics (viscosity is shear rate-dependent).

Synovial fluid does not clot on standing as there is no fibrinogen. However, fluid in specific infections (e.g. TB) and rheumatoid arthritis coagulates and forms large clots because they contain fibrinogen.

Viscosity of synovial fluid may be estimated by allowing the fluid to drip from the end of a small syringe. Normally, the viscous fluid falls drop by drop. The thin, nonviscous fluid of inflammation flows freely and uninterruptedly.

- Normal—traumatic arthritis/degenerative arthritis (OA)/PVNS.
- Normal/decreased—SLE.
- Decreased—Rh. fever/RA/gout/pyogenic arthritis/TB arthritis.

Synovial Fluid Analysis (Table 18.1)

Inflammatory fluid has reduced hyaluronate and thus reduced viscosity and the fluid is turbid yellow.

Table 18.1: Synovial fluid analysis

Parameters	Normal	Degenerative Osteoarthritis	Inflammatory Gout	Inflammatory Rheumatoid arthritis	Infectious Pyogenic arthritis	Infectious Tuberculous arthritis
Appearance	Straw or clear yellow	Clear yellow	Yellow to turbid milky	Yellow, cloudy	Purulent	Yellow, turbid
Viscosity	Normal	Normal	Decreased	Decreased	Decreased	Decreased
Total WBC count	≤200	≤2,000	2,000–50,000	2,000–50,000	>50,000	10,000–20,000
Polymorphonuclear leukocytes	<20%	<20%	60–70%	50–60%	90%	60%
Crystals	Negative	Negative	Urate crystals	Negative	Negative	Negative
Glucose level	A bit lower than plasma level	↓	↓	↓	↓↓	↓↓

Cartilage and its Structure

Normal cartilage is smooth, glistening and bluish white with an average thickness of 1.5–3 mm. Chondrocytes constitute <10% of the total volume of cartilage; consequently, the functional properties of cartilage, including stiffness, durability and distribution of load rely primarily on the extracellular matrix. However, the synthesis and maintenance of the extracellular matrix depends on the chondrocytes.

The main constituents of ECM are Type II collagen (60%) and proteoglycans (30%).

Proteoglycans → Core protein → Negatively charged chondroitin sulphate
→ Aggrecan ⇌ Positively charged hyaluronic acid side chain.

The articular cartilage is divided into four zones from the articular surface to subchondral bone.

Superficial zone (Zone 1)
- It is the thinnest and forms the gliding surface of the joint
- It protects deeper layers from shear stress
- Chondrocytes and collagen fibrils have their axis parallel to the joint surface
- It has progenitor cells (for articular cartilage)
- There is high density of chondrocytes
- There is high water content.

Transitional zone (Zone 2)
- It indicates a transition whereby the collagen and proteoglycan content increases (least in superficial zone) while the water content goes down and chondrocytes are low in density.
- In this layer, collagen fiber orientation and chondrocytes arrangement transitions from parallel to columnar (arranged in columns).
- It provides 1st resistance to compressive forces.

Middle/deep/radial zone (Zone 3)
- Largest of all zones.
- The chondrocytes are spheroidal in shape with their major axis perpendicular to joint surface.
- The cells here are synthetically most active.
- Furthermore, the largest collagen fibrils of articular cartilage and the highest content of proteoglycans are also contained here.
- As the number of proteoglycans increases, the amount of water decreases from the superficial to the deep zone.
- Provides greatest resistance to compressive forces.

Tidemark
Tidemark forms the boundary between calcified and uncalcified cartilage. It is considered to be a part of Zone 4, i.e. calcified zone only.

Calcified zone (Zone 4)
- These chondrocytes contain very little cytoplasm and almost no endoplasmic reticulum (metabolically least active) but connect the articular cartilage to the underlying bone.
- Cell number is decreased and chondrocytes are hypertrophic.

    Age related changes in the articular cartilage include: Decreased number of chondrocytes, decreased water content, decreased proteoglycan content due to decreased synthesis (not increased enzymatic degradation, which is seen in OA), decreased chondroitin sulphate 4/6 ratio and increased keratan sulphate and hyaluronate.

Cartilage property	Aging	Osteoarthritis
Hydration	decreased	Increased (in late OA it is also decreased
Proteolytic enzymes	Normal	Increased
Proteoglycan content	Decreased (due to decreased synthesis)	Decreased (due to increased destruction)

Xtra Edge
- Articular cartilage has no nerve supply, so there is no pain in the initial stages of arthritis. When subchondral bone is exposed, nude nerve ends causes pain.
- Capsule is the most pain sensitive structure in the joint and joint effusion causes pain due to capsular stretching.

ARTHRITIS

- Inflammatory
  - Cardinal signs of inflammation are present.
  - Systemic symptoms (morning stiffness >1 hour, fatigue, fever, weight loss) present.
  - Increased ESR, CRP.
  - X-ray—osteoporotic/destructive features are present.
  - For example—infectious, crystal deposition, RA, seronegative arthritis, etc.
- Non-inflammatory
  - Cardinal signs of inflammation are absent.
  - Systemic symptoms (morning stiffness >1 hour, fatigue, fever, weight loss) absent.
  - ESR , CRP—normal.
  - X-ray—osteosclerosis/new bone formation/osteophytes.
  - For example—osteoarthritis, traumatic arthritis, PVNS.

Based upon the number of joints involved (Table 18.2) arthritis can be classified as monoarthritis (single joint involved), oligoarthritis (2–4 joints involved) and polyarthritis (5 or >5 joints involved).

Most common joints involved in various types of arthritis are given in Table 18.3.

OSTEOARTHRITIS

There is imbalance between normal cartilage repair mechanisms and its degradation which leads to net loss of cartilage. The cartilage loss is "asymmetric", greater where the stress on the joint is the greatest (in knee medial compartment, hip superolateral aspect of the head).

Types

- Primary—its idiopathic.
- Secondary—may be due to risk factors like previous trauma, congenital/developmental disorder, endocrinological disorder, metabolic disorder, obesity, smoking, etc.

Joints involved

Knee, hip, 1st MTP (D/D—gout), facet joints of cervical spine and LS spine.

Hand joints: Osteoarthritis involves DIP (Heberden's node/H = High), PIP (Bouchard's node/B = Below), 1st CMC joint (base of thumb), with sparing of MCP joint, all other CMC joint and wrist joint.

Pattern of involvement

- Monoarticular/pauciarticular—knee > hip (weight bearing joints)
- The most common bone involved in knee is patella
- Polyarticular—DIP
- Overall DIP is commonest.

Table 18.2: Classifying arthritis on the number of joints involved	
Monoarthritis	Gout, infective and trauma
Oligoarthritis	Gout, seronegative, spondyloarthritis, reactive arthritis
Polyarthritis	RA, SLE and psoriatic arthritis

Clinical Features

Table 18.3			
Septic	Knee	Senile osteoporosis	Vertebrae
Syphilitic	Knee	Paget's	Pelvic bone>femur>skull
Gonococcal	Knee	Actinomycosis	Mandible
Rheumatoid	MCP joint	Hemophilic	Knee (quadriceps bleeding)
Ankylosing spondylitis	SI joint> lumbar spine	Acute osteomyelitis	Lower end of femur
Gout	MTP joint of great toe	Brodie's abscess	Upper end tibia
Pseudo gout	Knee	Charcot's arthropathy	Most commonly mid-tarsal
Reactive arthritis	Knee		
Psoriatic arthritis	DIP, PIP and any joint		

- Middle/old age, weight bearing joints.
- Pain is the commonest symptom (waxing and waning).
- Pain aggravated by exertion and relieved on rest (unlike inflammatory arthritis).
- Crepitus, deformity (genu varum in OA knee), swollen joints due to excess osteophyte formation or synovial swelling (Heberden's node/ Bouchard's node).
- Bony ankylosis is uncommon except IP joints of fingers where it may be the end result.

X-ray Features (Fig. 18.1)
- Decreased joint space (asymmetric, medial > lateral)
- Subchondral sclerosis
- Subchondral cysts
- Marginal osteophytes
- Loose bodies
- *In late stages*: Deformities of the joint and joint subluxations
- The combination of cartilage space loss, central subchondral erosions, and marginal osteophyte proliferation results in a *gull-wing* appearance (called "**seagull-wing sign**") (Fig. 18.2). It is seen classically in erosive osteoarthritis and may be also seen in RA/psoriatic arthritis.

Blood Investigations
Erythrocyte sedimentation rate, CRP and serum uric acid are usually normal. Elevated homocysteine levels have recently been documented and may have a role in pathogenesis.

Grading
Hip: Tonnis grading

Knee: Ahlbäck, Kellgren and Lawrence grading.

Treatment
- Clinical picture is more imp. than X-ray for deciding treatment.
- Initial treatment is always conservative
  - Lifestyle modification, rest, weight reduction.
  - Quadriceps strengthening (because quadriceps weakness is common in OA esp. vastus medialis).
  - Orthosis, NSAIDs, SSRI, glucosamine, intra-articular hyaluronic acid and steroids.

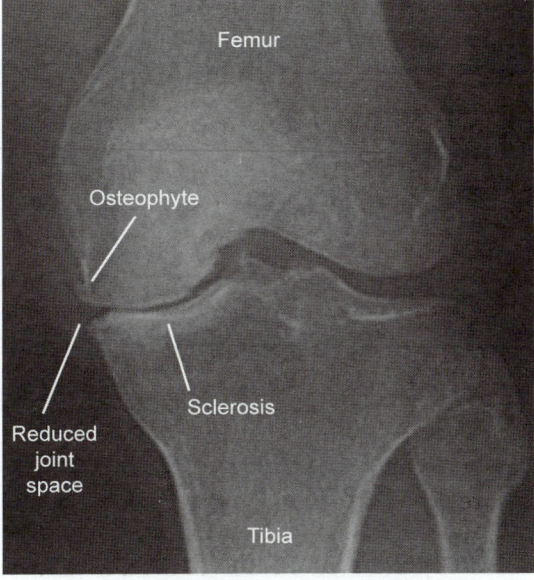

Fig. 18.1: OA knee

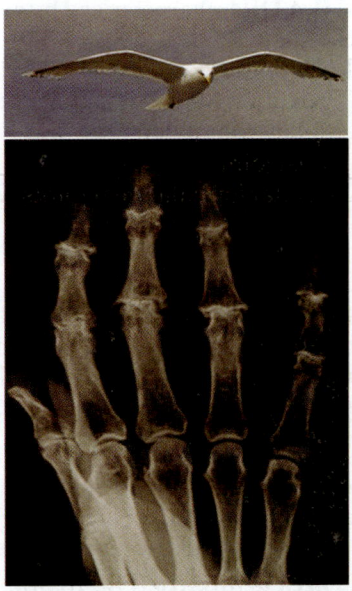

Fig. 18.2: Gull-wing sign in erosive arthritis

- In late stages
  - Arthroscopic debridement can provide temporary pain relief.
  - In adults with non-inflammatory arthritis with isolated medial compartment involvement, high tibial osteotomy (HTO) can be performed.
  - In tri-compartmental disease, old age, ligamentous instability—total knee replacement.

INFLAMMATORY ARTHRITIS

- *Seropositive*: Rheumatoid arthritis (RA factor +ve)
- *Seronegative*: Spondyloarthropathies (RA factor –ve)
  - Psoriatic arthritis
  - Enteropathy (IBD)
  - Ankylosing spondylitis } "PEARS"
  - Reactive arthritis
  - SAPHO syndrome

These diseases have common features like the involvement of the sacroiliac joints (sacroiliitis) and axial spine (spondylitis); oligoarthritis, inflammation at the attachment of tendon, fascia, and ligament insertion sites (enthesitis); association with HLA B-27 and extraskeletal features like eye involvement (uveitis), cardiac and other system involvement.

RHEUMATOID ARTHRITIS (RA)

It is a seropositive arthritis. It refers to presence of RF, an autoantibody (IgM) against the Fc portion of IgG.

Etiopathogenesis

- It is an erosive arthritis with pannus formation at the periphery of the joint,which denudes the articular cartilage off the subchondral bone. Adhesions between the opposing bone surface leading to fibrous and finally bony ankylosis.
- Joint swelling due to joint effusion and synovial hypertrophy.
- Ligaments/tendons are also involved/stretched and this may lead to joint subluxation/dislocation.
- Muscles may show polymyositis, vasculitis, subcutaneous nodules along the extensor surface of the limb, perineural fibrosis.

Clinical Features

It is a multisystem disorder of young and middle aged adults (female >> male), strongly associated with **HLA DR4**, characterised by **symmetric** polyarthritis that usually starts in the **small peripheral** joints.

The 14 specified joints (both sides) that are commonly involved in RA are:
1. Proximal interphalangeal joint
2. Metacarpophalangeal joint } sparing of DIP joint.
3. Wrist joint
4. Metatarsophalangeal joints (2nd only to hand involvement)
5. Elbow
6. Knee } involvement of large joints occurs later.
7. Ankle

Most common joints involved in RA: MCP > Wrist > PIP > Knee.
Less commonly involved joints: Hip, temporomandibular, subtalar, atlantoaxial joints.
Joints not involved include: Distal interphalangeal, lumbar spine, sacroiliac (SI) joints.
In RA most of the spine is spared except the C1–C2 articulation and facet joints.

Deformities

Hand

Boutonnière deformity (Fig. 18.3A): Flexion contracture of PIP joints and extension of DIP joint. It is due to rupture of the central extensor expansion of the fingers.

Swan neck deformity (Fig. 18.3B): Hyperextension of PIP joints with flexion of the DIP joint. It is due to rupture of the volar plate of the PIP joint.

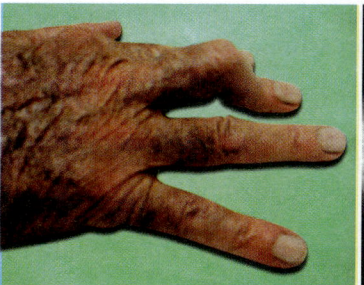 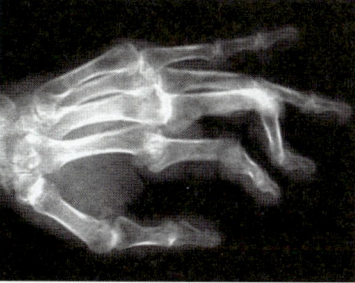 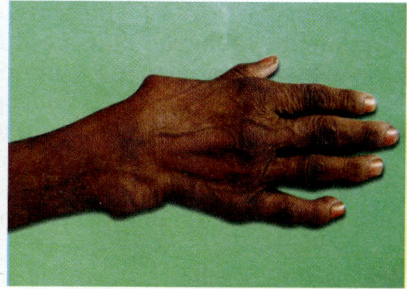

Fig. 18.3A: Boutonnière deformity of middle finger and X-ray of same patient showing advanced arthritic changes of PIP joint of middle finger

Fig. 18.3B: Ulnar deviation with swan neck deformity of little finger

Z-deformity (Fig. 18.4A and B): Radial deviation of the wrist with ulnar deviation of the digits.

Caput ulnae syndrome: It refers to the destructive process initiated by the synovitis of the distal radio-ulnar joint (DRUJ) which includes stretching of the tendon sheath of wrist extensors and volar subluxation of the carpal bones.

Hitchhiker thumb deformity: It refers to flexion of the MCP and extension of distal interphalangeal joint of the thumb.

Foot

Hallux valgus (most common), clawtoes, hammertoes, wind swept deformity of toes—valgus deformity of toes in one foot and varus in other.

Knee

Genu valgum is more commonly seen in rheumatoid knees (genu varum in OA).

Wind swept deformity: Genu varum at one knee and valgum at the other.

Extra-articular Manifestations

Besides the articular manifestations discussed above, the disorder also has some characteristic extra-articular manifestations that rarely may be the presenting mode. These extra-articular features may be seen in up to one-third of the patients and are as follows:
* *Systemic manifestations:* Generalized fatigue, low-grade fever, weight loss.
* Diffuse osteoporosis is almost always associated.

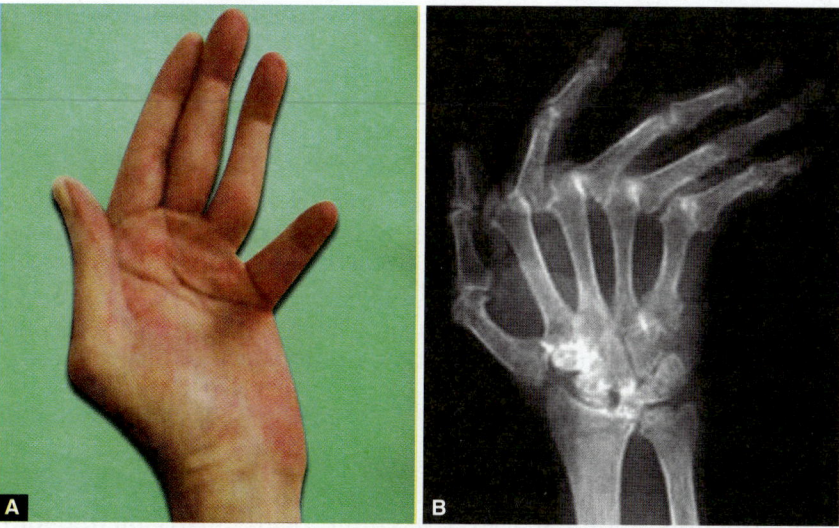

Fig. 18.4A and B: Z-deformity: Radial deviation of the wrist with ulnar deviation of the digits

- *Rheumatoid nodules*: These are the most pathognomic extra-articular feature and appear as nontender subcutaneous nodules. They present mainly over pressure areas or peri-articular extensor surfaces with olecranon being the commonest site.
- Rheumatoid vasculitis is widespread and can involve any organ. Vasculitis of vasa nervorum (the vessels supplying nerves) leads to mononeuritis multiplex, an asymmetric asynchronous painful motor-sensory peripheral neuropathy involving at least two separate nerves.
- Nerve entrapment syndromes may be there (like carpal tunnel syndrome, cubital tunnel syndrome, tarsal tunnel syndrome, etc.)
- *Eye changes*: Keratoconjunctivitis sicca (Sjögren's syndrome) (most common eye manifestation), episcleritis, scleritis (most severe eye manifestation) and secondary glaucoma.
- *Cardiac manifestations*: Pericarditis (most common cardiac manifestation), cardiomyopathy, arrhythmias, heart block.
- *Pulmonary manifestations*: Pleurisy, effusion, fibrosing alveolitis, pneumonitis and Caplan's syndrome.
- Pleural and pericardial effusions (with a very low glucose content).
- Anemia of chronic disorder, leukocytopenia, thrombocytosis, marrow hypoplasia, splenomegaly, generalized lymphadenopathy, pitting edema of foot and Felty's syndrome.

Blood Investigations

RA Factor
- It is not specific for RA and can be seen in other autoimmune disorders. 70–90% patients with RA have positive RA factor.
- Early in the course of the disease RA factor may be negative, thus a negative RA factor should never be the only reason to rule out RA. Thus low sensitivity and not used for screening purpose.
- Its presence is associated with worst prognosis (prognostic significance).
- It is associated with more severe articular disease.
- It is associated with all of the extra-articular features.
- The level of RA factor parallel the activity of the disease.

Anti-CCP
- Anti cyclic citrullinate peptide antibody (anti-CCP) is more specific/sensitive than RA factor for diagnosis of RA.
- It may be positive very early in the course of the disease.
- This test is particularly useful in case of chronic hepatitis infection, which is also associated with a positive RF but not with positive anti-CCP.

Other investigations: Normocytic normochromic anemia, thrombocytosis, increased ESR/CRP/haptoglobin. Their level parallel disease activity. WBC count may be elevated, normal or low in the case of Felty's syndrome.

Felty syndrome: This is triad of
- Chronic rheumatoid arthritis
- Splenomegaly
- Neutropenia

It is seen in patients with severe seropositive disease and may be accompanied by hepatomegaly, splenomegaly thrombocytopenia, lymphadenopathy and fever. Most of them do not require special treatment but treatment for severe rheumatoid involvement. If severe neutropenia exists with recurrent bacterial infection, splenectomy is indicated.

Caplan syndrome: This is rheumatoid arthritis associated with coal workers pneumoconiosis involving the upper lobes of the lung. The multiple pulmonary nodules in these patients show cavitation and specks of calcification.

X-ray Features
- Soft tissue swelling (earliest radiological feature)
- Juxta-articular osteopenia (an early feature)
- Symmetrical reduction of joint space (cf. asymmetrical; mostly medial joint collapse in degenerative arthritis)

- Subchondral erosions and cysts (cf. subchondral sclerosis in degenerative arthritis)
- Deformities of hands and foot joints
- Lack of hypertrophic bone changes (sclerosis or osteophyte).

Diagnosis

Is based on the presence of 4/7 of the following criteria:

1. Morning stiffness in and around joint that lasts for at least 1 hour and that has been present for at least 6 weeks.
2. Swelling/arthritis of 3 or more joints for at least 6 weeks.
3. Arthritis of hand joints—MCP, PIP, wrist for at least 6 weeks.
4. Swelling of the same joints on both sides of the body, i.e. symmetrical arthritis.
5. Changes in X-rays that are consistent with RA.
6. Rheumatoid nodules (pathognomic).
7. Serum RA factor.
   The 2010 revised ARA criteria for diagnosis of RA is given in Table 18.4.

Prognostic Factors

Factors that suggest poor prognosis in RA include:

- Males have better prognosis than young females.
- Positive family history
- High titres of RA and positive anti-CCP levels
- Elevated ESR and CRP levels
- X-ray showing bone erosions in early course of disease
- Synovitis persisting for a long time
- Presence of extra-articular manifestations
- Presence of HLA-DR4

Table 18.4: Diagnostic criteria (2010 ARA)

Revised American Rheumatism Association Criteria for Diagnosis of RA 2010

• Joint involvement*	
– 1 large joint	0
– 2–10 large joint	1
– 1–3 small joints (with or w/o large joint involvement)	2
– 4–10 small joints	3
– >10 joints (at least 1 small joint)	5
*Large joints: Shoulder, elbow, hips, knee, ankle	
*Small joints: MCP, PIP, 2nd-5th MTP, thumb, IP joints, wrists	
• Serology	
– Negative RF and negative anti-CCP	0
– Low positive RF or low positive anti-CCP	2
– High positive RF or high positive anti-CCP	3
• Acute phase reactants	
– Normal CRP and normal ESR	0
– Abnormal CRP and abnormal ESR	1
• Duration of symptoms*	
– <6 weeks	0
– ≥6 weeks	1
*With synovitis not better explained by another disease	

Result

Score ≤6 positive

Patients with score <6/10 are not classified as having RA; their status can be reassessed and the criteria may be fulfilled cumulatively over time.

Target population

Patients who have at least 1 joint with definite clinical synovitis (swelling)

Treatment

NSAIDs
Very effective in providing symptomatic relief but cannot halt the progression of disease.

Steroids
- Most potent anti-inflammatory drugs available.
- Not only provide symptomatic relief but also significantly decrease the radiographic progression of the disease.
- They are used to control the inflammation in RA, while the much slower acting DMARDs are starting to work.
- The paradigm is to shift toward DMARDs for long-term control and taper the steroids over a 2–3 months period.
- High-dose glucocorticoids are the mainstay in cases where extra-articular manifestations are present:
  - vasculitis (especially mono-neuritis multiplex),
  - scleritis,
  - pericarditis, or
  - endocarditis

Synthetic DMARDs
- Ability to halt/slow the progression of the disease in both early and advanced RA.
- Their main disadvantage is that they are slow acting and take 2–6 months for maximal effect.
- **Drugs**
  - *Methotrexate*: Methotrexate (MTX) is the most commonly used DMARD and is started as a single dose once a week (7.5–30 mg/week) tablet. It can be given as subcutaneous injection also. The dose is escalated from 7.5–15 mg per week to 20–30 mg per week if improvement is not seen in three months. Oral folic acid tablets are given at doses of 5–10 mg/week, 24–48 hours after MTX, to avoid toxicities secondary to inhibition of rapid cell turnover. The drug is contraindicated in pre-existing liver disease, hepatitis B or C infection, ongoing alcohol use, renal failure, bone marrow suppression and in women of childbearing potential who are not using contraception.
  - *Hydrochloroquine (HCQ)*: Least toxic but also least effective DMARD, so not used as mono-therapy. Retinal toxicity is a side effect.
  - Sulfasalazine.
  - Leflunomide.
  - Minocycline.
  - Gold (oldest DMARD)—less frequently used now.
  - Penicillamine.
- *Most commonly used DMARD combination*: Mtx + Sulfasalazine + HCQ.

Biological DMARDs
Their main advantage is rapid onset of action compared to synthetic DMARDs. Their main disadvantages are cost, risk of TB and demyelinating syndromes.
- Anti TNF-Alpha: Etanercept
  - Infliximab
  - Adalimumab
- Against IL-1: Anakinra
- Anti-CD-20: Rituximab
- IL-6 antagonist: Toclizumab

Xtra Edge
- Rheumatoid nodules are most common extra-articular feature. However, following diseases must be considered in patients with subcutaneous nodules and arthritis—gout, sarcoidosis, rheumatic fever, SLE and amyloidosis.
- *Sero-negative RA*: These are patients who have clinical picture of RA but have negative RF. They generally have better prognosis and fewer extra-articular manifestations.

- *RA and pregnancy*: The diseases improves during pregnancy although post partum it flares up. MTX, Leflunomide and biological DMARDs are contraindicated while HCQ and SSZ are allowed. Steroids may be given to control flares if required.
- *Ball Catcher's view (hands in ball catching position)* is a special X-ray view to detect early erosive changes in RA of hand.
- Rheumatoid arthritis tends to spare the central nervous system (CNS). Neuropathies are generally due to vasculitis.
- Although mononeuritis multiplex is a common extra-articular manifestation of RA, the most common cause of the same in India is leprosy.
- Juvenile idiopathic arthritis (JIA) is the commonest chronic rheumatic illness of childhood.

SERONEGATIVE SPONDYLOARTHROPATHIES (SSAS)

It is a group of autoimmune disorders with onset usually below the age of 40 years characterized by inflammatory arthritis of predominantly axial skeleton with or without large peripheral joints, with absence of RA factor in serum (hence seronegative).

Common features include:
- Involvement of the sacroiliac joints (sacroiliitis) and axial spine (spondylitis)
- Oligoarthritis
- Enthesitis (inflammation at the attachment of tendon, fascia and ligaments)
- Association with HLA B-27
- Extraskeletal manifestations (e.g. uveitis in eye, cardiac involvement, etc.)

Conditions included in the group (mnemonic: PEARS):
- Psoriatic arthritis
- Enteropathic arthritis (associated with ulcerative colitis/Crohn's disease)
- Ankylosing spondylitis
- Reiter's syndrome
- Reactive arthritis (Chlamydia/Shigella)
- Synovitis, acne, pustulosis, hyperostosis and osteitis (SAPHO) syndrome
  The mainstay of therapy in all seronegative arthritis is NSAIDs and indomethacin is the agent of choice.

ANKYLOSING SPONDYLITIS (AS)

Ankylosing spondylitis (Marie Strumpell disease/Bechtrew's disease) is a chronic progressive inflammatory seronegative spondyloarthropathy, involving mainly the axial skeleton (spine and the sacroilliac joints) with variable involvement of root joints (hip and shoulder). Patients are mainly young males (15–25 years old), rarely over the age of 40 years.

HLAB27
- Striking association of AS with HLAB27.
- This marker is present in 1–6% of the general population, but positive in almost 90% of the patients with AS.
- Antineutrophil cytoplasmic antibodies (ANCAs) are also associated with AS.
- Recently two genetic loci have been shown to be associated with AS:
  - Interleukin receptor IL-23R
  - Endoplasmic reticulum aminopeptidase (ERAP)-1.

Pathology
- The primary site of pathology in AS is the enthesitis.
- Autoimmune attack leads to enthesitis with edema in the adjacent bone that may result in erosive lesions in the affected joints.
- The joints involved undergo first fibrous and eventually bony ankylosis.
- Ossification also occurs in the ligaments that are ending up as enthesis, especially the ligaments of the spine that gradually get ossified, progressively leading to stiffness.

Clinical Features
- The symptoms are more prominent in the morning after getting from bed or after a period of inactivity and the pain is classically relieved by activity.

- Gradual onset of pain and stiffness of the lower back and patient often walks to the clinician with a straight stiff back
- Sacroiliac (SI) joint is the first joint to be involved (changes start first on the iliac side of the joint) followed by the lumbar spine. Eventually, the whole spine may be involved in severe cases (cervical spine is involved late).
- In late stages, the patient's spine adopts a "question mark" posture due to hyperkyphosis of thoracic spine and straightening of the lumbar spine, i.e. loss of lumbar lordosis (sniffing dog posture). Initially hips hyperextend and knee flexed to compensate the above, but later when hips are also involved, fixed flexion deformity develops and sagittal balance is decompensated.
- Chin on chest posture is classical of AS.
- Most serious complication of spinal disease is vertebral fracture even with minor trauma with high risk of cord damage. Most commonly fractures occur in lower cervical spine, especially C5–C6 and C6–C7 and the mechanism involved is hyperextension.
- The fractures involve all the three columns of spine, with secondary dislocation and neurological deficit.
- Peripheral arthritis seen in AS is mainly mono/oligoarticular involving mainly the lower limbs, hip joint being the commonest.
- Hip joint involvement is a sign of bad prognosis.
- Ethesitis leads to chest wall pain (costosternal joints), heel pain (TA insertion) and sole pain (plantar aponeurosis insertion).
- M/C extra-articular manifestation is acute anterior uveitis (iridocyclitis).
- Causes of sudden death in AS are conduction defects, SA node fibrosis.

Clinical Examination
- *Test for sacroiliitis*:
    - Gaenslen's test (Fig. 18.5A)
    - Pump handle test
    - Patrick/FABER test (Fig. 18.5 B)
    - Side-side compression test.
- *Lumbar spine*: Schober test/modified Schober test.
- *Thoracic spine*: Chest expansion less than 5 cm in full inspiration, at the level of nipples.
- *Cervical spine*: Fleche test (Fig. 18.5C).

X-ray Features
- **Sacroiliac joints** (Fig. 18.6)—B/L sacroiliitis is the hallmark of AS (never diagnose AS without sacroiliitis). Following features may be present:
    - Blurring of margins (changes starts in the lower third of the joint).
    - Juxta-articular erosions.

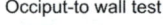

Occiput-to wall test

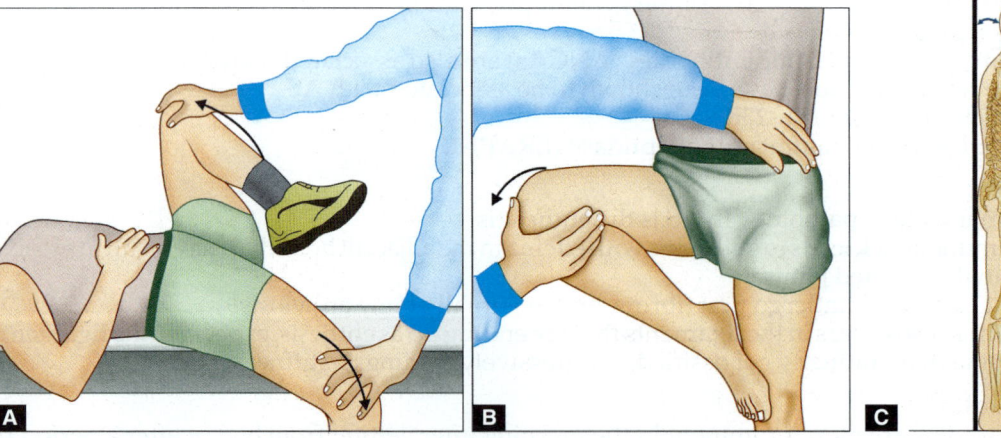

Fig. 18.5: (A) Gaenslen test, (B) FABER test, (C) Fleche test

- Pseudowidening due to erosions.
- Obliteration of joint and ankylosis (fibrous followed by bony).
- Destruction is first evident on iliac side of the joint.
- **Spine**
  - Loss of lumbar lordosis.
  - Inflammatory resorption of bone at the site of enthesitis—squaring of the corners of the vertebral body—subsequent ossification occurs at the annulus fibrosus.
  - Calcification of the anterior/posterior longitudinal ligaments l/t vertical/bridging syndesmophytes.
  - All these lead to classical "Bamboo spine appearance"(Fig. 18.7).
  - **Dagger sign** (Fig. 18.8)—refers to a

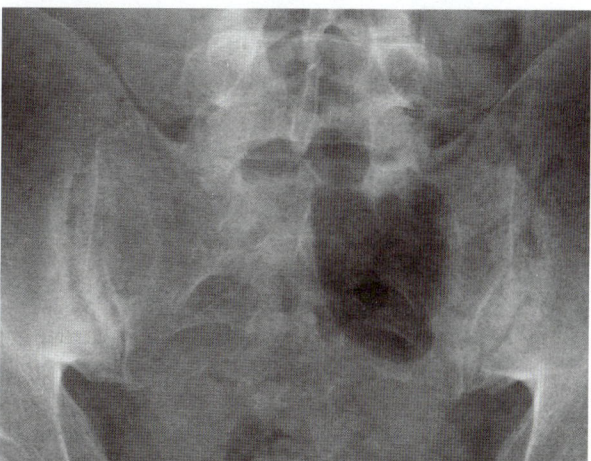

Fig. 18.6: X-ray showing sacroiliitis with marginal erosion

single central radiodense line in the AP radiographs of spine related to ossification of supraspinous and interspinous ligaments.

MRI Findings

MRI is considered best for earliest diagnosis. Following lesions may be seen:

- Romanus lesion—shiny corner sign (inflammatory erosion of edges of vertebral end plates)
- Anderson lesion—spinal pseudoarthrosis (inflammatory involvement of inter-vertebral disks).

Diagnosis

Diagnostic criteria for AS is given in Table 18.5. Before establishing the diagnosis especially in middle or elderly adults, a condition that needs to be excluded is diffuse idiopathic skeletal hyperostosis (Table 18.6).

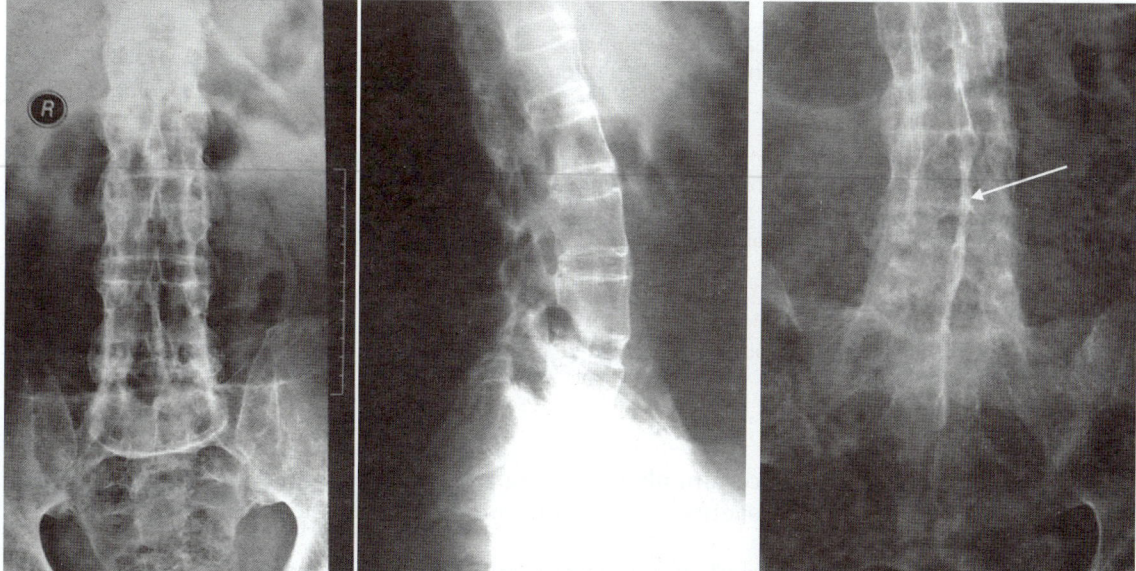

Fig. 18.7: AP and lateral view of spine showing bamboo spine appearance in AS

Fig. 18.8: Dagger sign

Table 18.5: Modified New York criteria (1984) for the diagnosis of AS

Clinical criteria
- Low back pain and stiffness for more than 3 months that improves with exercise but not with the rest.
- Limitation of lumbar spine mobility in both the sagittal and frontal planes.
- Limitation of chest expansion to 2.5 cm (1 inch) or less, measured at the level of the fourth intercostal space.

Radiologic criteria
- Unilateral sacroiliitis of grade 3–4 or
- Bilateral sacroiliitis of grade ≥2

Grading
Definite ankylosing spondylitis if: The radiological criterion is associated with at least one clinical criterion.
Probable ankylosing spondylitis if: Three clinical criteria are present or the radiologic criterion is present without any signs or symptoms satisfying the clinical criteria.

Difference with diffuse idiopathic skeletal hyperostosis is given in Table 18.6.
Taken from Fundamentals of Orthopedics by Mohindra and Jain (2nd Ed. Jaypee Publishers)

Table 18.6: Comparison of ankylosing spondylitis and diffuse idiopathic skeletal hyperostosis		
	Ankylosing spondylitis	*DISH(Forestier's disease)*
Sex/age	Common in males of 15–40 years of age	Common in males in 5th–6th decade
Etiology	It is chronic progressive inflammatory seronegative spondyloarthropathy	It is a form of degenerative arthritis
Pathogenesis	The primary site of pathology in ankylosing spondylitis is the enthesis (site of attachment of tendons and ligaments to bone). Ossification also occurs in the ligaments that are ending up as enthesis, especially the ligaments of the spine that gradually get ossified, progressively leading to stiffness	Characterized by ossification at sites of tendon, ligaments and joint capsule insertion (enthesitis) Anterior longitudinal ligament of the spine is most commonly involved
Distribution	SI joint, lumbar spine (eventually whole spine), the hip joints commonly involved	Marked predilection to the axial skeleton; mainly involves thoracic spine
Course	All patients invariably present early with pain and stiffness of back	It is usually asymptomatic and discovered incidentally
SI joint	Bilateral, symmetrical involvement (sacroiliitis) In late cases, erosion may cause pseudowidening of the SI joints	Not involved
ESR	Elevated	Normal
HLA B27	Positive in 90% cases	Negative
Disability	Marked disability of the spine and hip joints in advanced cases	Usually no disability
X-ray features	Bamboo spine, squaring of vertebrae, syndesmophytes	Candle wax appearance due to calcification along the anterior and lateral portion of the vertebral bodies (separated from vertebral bodies)
Treatment	NSAIDs, TNF inhibitors	Usually not required

Treatment
- NSAIDs
  - Indomethacin is the most commonly used drug.
  - Phenylbutazone is the most effective drug but causes aplastic anemia so reserved for non-responsive cases.
- Sulfasalazine and MTX (folic acid anatagonist) are used for peripheral joints.
- The anti-TNF agents currently approved are adalimumab, etanercept, infliximab and golimumab.

PSORIATIC ARTHRITIS

- It is characterised by seronegative polysynovitis with erosive arthritis. Joint symptoms are usually seen in 20–30% of adults with psoriasis.
- Almost any peripheral joint can be involved.
- Group-A streptococcal infection has been implicated as an initial trigger in inciting an immune response in guttate psoriasis.
- Destruction may sometimes be unusually severe (hence called arthritis mutilans).
- Genetic predisposition is often seen.
- The condition is associated with HLA-DR7, HLA-CW6.
- RA factor is almost always negative.
- 60% of those with spondylitis or sacroiliitis have HLAB27 positivity. In pure cutaneous lesions (i.e. without arthritis) HLA-B27 is absent.
- Eye involvement in form of uveitis, blepharitis, keratoconjuctivitis sicca may be seen.
- Psoriatic arthritis is capable of evolving into Reiter's syndrome and vice versa.

Clinical Features

The skin lesions mostly precede (10–12 years) arthritis, but about 20% patients may present with an initial arthritis.

- *Symmetrical polyarthritis* (most common form).
- *Asymmetrical oligoarthritis* (second most common form).
- *Distal arthritis* (DIP and PIP joints involved): Erosion of the terminal tufts (acro-osteolysis) occurs in association with nail changes. Dactylitis, or "sausage digit," is also a characteristic feature. It refers to the complete swelling of a single finger or more, commonly a toe.
- *Arthritis mutilans* (Fig. 18.9): In this rare subtype extreme destruction of the phalanges and MCP joints is seen, giving rise to shortened and subluxated digits that can be telescoped producing the classical "pencil in cup deformity" on X-rays.
- *Spondyloarthropathy* (SI joint, usually unilateral and spine involvement): This may be seen in up to one-third cases. The predominance of cervical spine involvement over thoracolumbar spine distinguishes it from AS.

Diagnosis

- *X-ray features*
  - Joint-space narrowing and erosions involving the DIP/PIP
  - DIP involvement with the classical "pencil in cup" deformity (Fig. 18.10)
  - Small joint ankylosis
  - Severe osteolysis of the phalanges and metacarpal bones (arthritis mutilans)
  - Periostitis and proliferative new bone at sites of enthesis
  - Periarticular osteopenia, which is seen in RA is usually absent in psoriatic arthritis. In contrast proliferative bony changes are seen along the shaft of the metacarpal and metatarsal bones adjacent to erosive changes, leading to fluffy periostitis. This is also known as "whiskering".

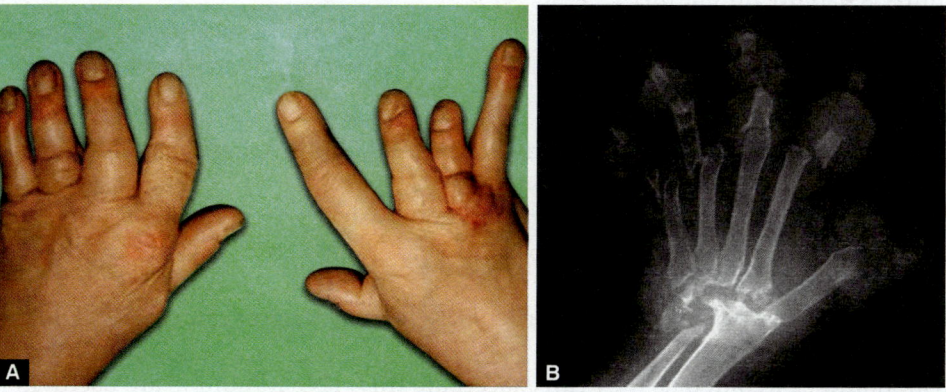

Fig. 18.9: Arthritis mutilans, clinical picture (A) and X-ray (B) showing telescoped digits

- CASPAR criteria
- Wright and Moll criteria
- *Acro-osteolysis*: This refers to bony erosions of terminal tufts of phalanges. Important causes include:
  - Primary acro-osteolysis (Hajdu-Cheney syndrome)
  - Psoriatic arthritis
  - Hyperparathyroidism
  - Polyvinyl chloride exposure
  - Ergot poisoning
  - Thermal injury
  - Extreme cold; frost bite
  - Leprosy
  - Juvenile chronic arthritis
  - Raynaud disease
  - Scleroderma

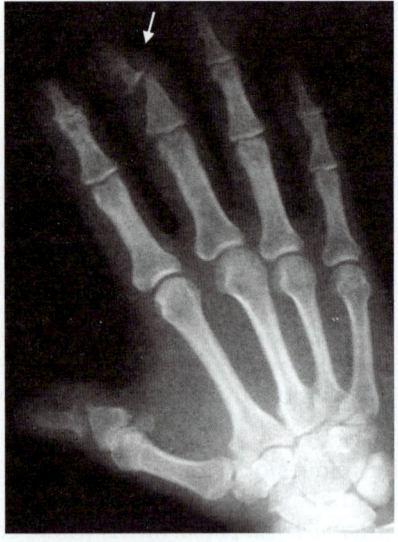

Fig. 18.10: Hand X-ray depicting the classical "Pencil in cup" deformity

Treatment
- Anti-psoriatic medicines form the mainstay of treatment
- MTX is the drug of choice
- Retinoids, psoralens, PUVA, sulfasalazine, cycloserine
- Anti TNF-alpha agents (etanercept and infliximab).

REACTIVE ARTHRITIS (REITER'S SYNDROME)

It is an inflammatory polyarthritis that occurs after **infection** (non-purulent) elsewhere in the body away from the affected joints.

Sexually transmitted (mostly in adults)
Chlamydia (commonest), mycoplasma, lymphogranuloma venerum

Dysentery(mostly in children)
Shigella (most common), salmonella, campylobacter

Overall commonest is chlamydia followed by shigella

- Strong association with HLAB27
- Reiter's triad
  - Nonerosive arthritis
  - Urethritis
  - Conjunctivitis.

  } occurs generally after 1–3 weeks of GI/genitourinary infection

- Extraskeletal features include ocular involvement (i.e. conjunctivitis, iritis, scleritis, episcleritis, and keratitis) and mucocutaneous lesions in the form of circinate balanitis (inflammatory lesion of the glans or shaft of the penis) and keratoderma blennorrhagicum (papular rash on the palm and soles).
- Sacroiliitis is usually unilateral.
- Antibiotics are of no benefit in treating the arthritis (c.f. antibiotics have a dramatic role in gonorheal arthritis).

ENTEROPATHIC ARTHRITIS
- It occurs in association with both ulcerative colitis and Crohn's disease and presents either as peripheral arthritis or sacroiliitis and spondylitis.
- The peripheral arthritis is often migratory and nonerosive.
- Often treatment of the underlying bowel disease leads to remission of the peripheral arthritis.
- DMARDs are useful in this condition, particularly sulfasalazine because of its additional effect on IBD.
- NSAIDs should be avoided as they can exacerbate IBD. TNF inhibitors are useful in resistant cases.

Xtra Edge
- Arthritis mutilans may be seen in
  - Psoriatic arthritis
  - RA
  - JIA
  - Diabetes
  - Leprosy
  - Neuropathic arthropathy
  - Reiter's syndrome
  - Differentiating features of various SSAs are given in Table 18.7.

GOUT

It is a hereditary disorder of disturbed purine metabolism that involves usually middle aged (30 years average) males, characterized by hyperuricemia (>6.8 mg/dl) that leads to deposition of monosodium urate crystals in joints and periarticular tissues and thereby precipitates recurrent attacks of acute synovitis that eventually lead to arthritis.

Risk Factors
- Obesity
- Male sex
- Alcoholism
- Dietary excess of purine-rich foods (meat, alcohol and fructose containing diet)
- Trauma or major surgery
- History of chronic inflammatory disease
- Presence of a hemolytic or myeloproliferative disorder
- Long-term use of drugs like aspirin, diuretics

Etiopathogenesis
- Due to increased total body urate levels there occurs precipitation of monosodium urate crystals (called tophi) into the joints.
- Serum urate level >6.8 mg/dl is defined as hyperuricemia because synovial fluids with urate concentration >7 are supersaturated with urate, and whenever there is fluctuation in its concentration (decrease >increase in concentration) the microtophi break apart and liberate the crystals into the synovial fluid, inviting macrophages that generate the acute attack of gout. Thus the level of uric acid at the time of acute attack may be normal.
- All patients with hyperuricemia does not develop gout (even a decade may elapse without symptoms) and asymptomatic hyperuricemia is not a disease.
- Occurrence of gout is directly related with the magnitude and duration of hyperuricemia.

Table 18.7: Differentiating features of various seronegative spondyloarthropathies (SSAs)				
Spondyloarthropathy	AS	Psoriatic arthritis	Enteropathic arthritis	Reactive arthritis
Male to female ratio	More common in men	1:1	1:1	More common in men
Joint involvement	Hip, shoulder, knee	DIP, PIP and knee	Knee, ankle	Knee, ankle
SI joint involvement	Bilateral	Unilateral	Bilateral	Unilateral
Dactylitis	Uncommon	Common	Uncommon	Common
Cutaneous changes	None	Nail pitting Onycholysis Rashes	Erythema nodosum, Pyoderma gangrenosum	Circinate balanitis, Keratoderma blennorrhagica

Taken from Fundamentals of Orthpedics by Mohindra and Jain (2nd Ed. Jaypee Publishers)

Hyperuricemia in gout patients may be due to:
- Under excretion of uric acid.
- Overproduction of uric acid—diseases of high cell turn over.
- Both underexcretion and over production (e.g. alcohol).

Tophi: These are pathognomic hallmark of gout and they evolve from repetitive precipitation of monosodium urate crystals (MSUC) during attacks. Tophi may deposit in connective tissue in and around joints —articular cartilage, synovium, bursae, tendons, ligaments, subcutaneous tissue, pinna of ear, kidney, etc. Tophi do not involve skin and muscle, but they may ulcerate through skin discharging white chalky material mimicking pus.

Clinical Features

The disease course is characterized by recurrent acute attacks that end up into the stage of chronic gouty arthropathy.
- **Acute attack:** Acute attack is preceded by a provocative factor and is sudden in onset occurring frequently at night. The joint is extremely painful and mimics features of cellulitis/septic arthritis. Most commonly involved joint is 1st MTP joint (great toe) followed by intertarsal joint. Other joints, viz. ankle, wrist, knee, elbow may also be involved. Patients are asymptomatic between attacks and intervals between attacks tends to become progressively shorter and more severe.
- **Chronic gout:** Recurrent acute attacks lead to chronic gouty arthropathy. Joint is eroded, painful, stiff and deformed. Tophi are deposited in and around joints which may vary in size from 1 mm to several centimetres in diameter. Tophi may ulcerate and discharge white chalky material mimicking pus.
  - Nerve tissue is resistant to invasion by tophi but may be compressed leading to sensory disturbance.
  - Secondary infection of gouty ulcer does not occur, suggesting that urate crystals possess bacteriostatic properties.
- **Chronic gout with renal complications**
  - Deposition of MSUC in medullary interstitium leads to gouty nephropathy (chronic urate nephropathy).
  - Nephrolithiasis: Amount of uric acid excreted in urine is a better predictor of nephrolithiasis than hyperuricemia is.
  - Calcium containing stones are more common in gout patients than general population.

Diagnosis

- Increased ESR, CRP levels.
- Increased uric acid levels (but may be normal in acute attack). Its baseline measurement is important for followup.
- 24 hours urinary uric acid excretion of greater than 800 mg/day indicates over production of uric acid. Its measurement is important before starting uricosuric drugs.
- **X-ray features:** Lesions are larger and slightly further from joint margin than typical RA erosions.
  - Soft tissue swelling (may be the only sign during acute attack)
  - Periarticular deep erosions
  - *G sign/Martel sign* (punched out lesion of bone with overhanging bony edges, Fig. 18.11)
  - Conspicuous absence of osteoporosis
  - Joint space narrowing (ultimately leading to secondary OA).
- **USG:** Double contour sign

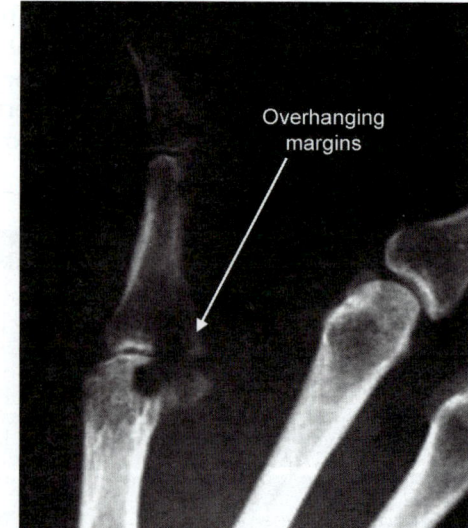

Overhanging margins

Fig. 18.11: Hand X-ray of a gout patient showing punched out lesions with overhanging bony margins

- Gold standard is joint aspiration and synovial fluid/tophi analysis with polarised light microscopy and identifying MSUC.
    - During attacks—crystals are intracellular (WBC) and needle shaped.
    - Between attacks—crystals are extracellular and rod/blunted shape.
    - Joint fluid is turbid/clowdy appearance and may be chalky.

Treatment

Acute attack
- Rest, ice, diet control.
- Analgesics—NSAIDs (indomethacin), colchicine (fastest acting but has side effects, so not used now), prednisolone.
- Urate lowering agents are contraindicated in acute gout.

Chronic gout (in between attacks): Urate lowering therapy is the mainstay.
- Uricosuric drugs (probenecid/sulfinpyrazone) in under excretors and if renal function is normal.
- Urate lowering drugs (given always under the cover of NSAIDs/colchicine as they may precipitate an acute attack)
    - Allopurinol (xanthine oxidase inhibitor): It is the most commonly used drug and the drug of choice if renal function is compromised
    - Febuxostat (non-purine xanthine oxidase inhibitor).

CALCIUM PYROPHOSPHATE DIHYDRATE (CPPD) ARTHROPATHY
It is characterised by deposition of CPPD crystals in articular tissue with aging (most important risk factor). It is spectrum includes three overlapping conditions:
1. ***Chondrocalcinosis:*** It is the asymptomatic appearance of calcific material in articular cartilage, intervertebral disks and knee menisci. A number of disorders are there where CPPD deposition is an associated finding—hemochromatosis, hyperparathyroidism, hypothyroidism (most common association), hypophosphatasia, hypomagnesemia, hepatolenticular degeneration (Wilson's disease) and alkaptonuria (ochronosis).
2. ***Pseudogout:*** This is acute synovitis due to CPPD crystals, typically affecting middle-aged **women**. Larger joints like **knee** (most common site) are commonly involved. Pain is lesser compared to gout. Confirmation comes with the demonstration of **positively** birefringent, **rhomboid**-shaped crystals in the synovial fluid on joint aspiration.
3. ***Chronic pyrophosphate arthropathy:*** It resembles osteoarthritis, but the X-ray features are distinctive.

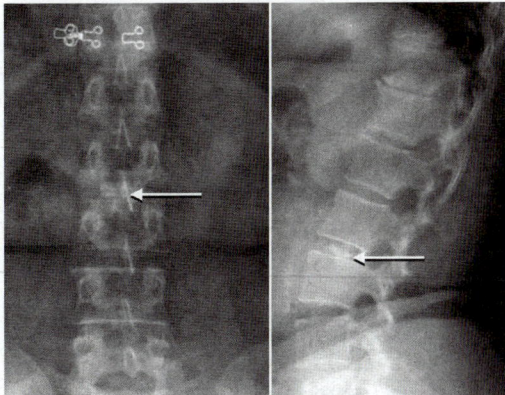

X-ray Features
The characteristic X-ray feature is chondro-calcinosis—calcification of articular cartilage in joints, the menisci in the knee, pubic symphysis, intervertebral disks (Fig. 18.12) and at times tendons and bursae around joints.

Fig.18.12: Disk calcification in chondro-calcinosis

HEMOPHILIC ARTHRITIS
- Hemophilia is an X-linked recessive disorder that manifests generally in males (females are carriers).
- It is characterized by the deficiency of clotting factors VIII (**hemophilia A**, 80% cases), IX (**hemophilia B**, Christmas factor) or XI (**hemophilia C**). The deficiency results in spontaneous hemorrhages into the joints that initiate a chronic synovitis that eventually culminates in progressive destructive arthritis.
- **von Willebrand's disease**—when both factor VIII and platelets are deficient.

- Bleeding incidence depends on level (% of normal) of clotting factors
  - >50%: Normal life
  - >5%: Hemorrhage after major injury or during an operative procedure
  - 1–5%: Hemorrhage after minor injury or unrecognized mild trauma
  - <1%: Spontaneous bleeding.

Orthopedic Manifestations

Joint bleeding (hemarthrosis)
- Most common orthopedic manifestation.
- Weight bearing joints are commonly involved (knee > elbow > shoulder > ankle > wrist > hip).
- Ankle is most commonly involved in children.
- Joints mimic features of infection and rest in position of ease.
- Joint aspiration is usually avoided unless distension is severe or there is suspicion of infection.

Intramuscular bleeding
- Although bleeding into muscles is relatively less common than joint bleeding, it can lead to muscle necrosis, fibrosis and development of contractures.
- Lower limb—quadriceps (most common overall) > triceps surae.
- Upper limb—deltoid.
- Abdomen—iliopsoas mimics appendicitis.
- Retroperitoneal bleeding mimics renal colic.

Pseudotumors
- Uncontrolled bleeding in a confined place of musculoskeletal system produces cystic swellings which can cause pressure changes of surrounding structures (bone/nerve).
- Most pseudotumor are caused by subperiosteal bleeding. Thigh is the most common site of pseudotumor formation followed by abdomen and pelvis. The quadriceps is the most common muscle to develop pseudotumor.
- Under appropriate factor replacement therapy, the iliacus pseudotumor recedes, the flexion deformity at hip subsides, and the femoral nerve deficit clears up gradually over a number of months.

Nerve palsy
- Bleeding into the peripheral nerve causes intense pain and sensory/motor symptoms.
- Hematomas may cause compression neuropathies/neuropraxia (generally transient).
- Femoral nerve followed by median nerve is the most common nerve involved.

Fractures
- Fractures in hemophilia may result from trauma or may occur pathologically after a trivial injury.
- They are most common in the lower limb, especially in patients with stiff knee, who sustain supracondylar fracture of the femur.

X-ray Features
- Soft tissue swelling
- Juxta-articular erosions/osteopenia (no sclerosis) and subchondral cysts
- Narrowing of the joint space
- Epiphyseal overgrowth
- Widening of the intercondylar notch and squaring of the patella in knee (Fig. 18.13A)
- Enlargement of the proximal radius and trochlear notch of ulna (Fig. 18.13B).

Treatment
- Factor replacement to 30–40% of normal.
- NSAIDs should be used cautiously.
- Aspiration/intra-articular injection/manipulation and massage is avoided.
- For disabling hemophilic arthropathy synovectomy, arthrodesis or arthroplasty may be required.
- Yttrium is most commonly used for radiosynovectomy (radiation synoviorthesis).

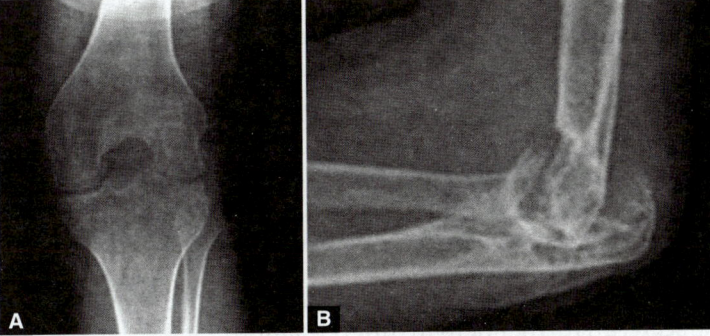

Fig. 18.13: (A) Widening of the intercondylar notch, (B) enlargement of the proximal radius and trochlear notch of ulna

Xtra Edge
Most commonly involved muscles:

Bennet's fracture	Reduction hindered by abductor pollicis
Compartment syndrome	Flexor digitorium profundus
Meyer's procedure	Bone muscle graft-quadriceps
OA	Quadriceps (V. medialis)
Most common site of intra-muscular bleeding in hemophilia	Quadriceps
de Quervain's disease	Abductor pollicis longus
	Extensor pollicis brevis
Tennis elbow	Extensor carpi radialis brevis
Stance phase of gait	Quadriceps/gluteus
Colles' fracture	Rupture of extensor pollicis longus tendon
Fracture distal end radius	Loss of function of extensor pollicis longus

NEUROPATHIC JOINT (CHARCOT'S JOINT)
- Neuropathic joint was first described by Charcot in tabes dorsalis. The condition is a progressive destructive (but painless) arthritis that arises as a result of loss of pain and proprioceptive joint sensations.
- Repetitive trauma leads to fragmentation and destruction of the joint cartilage, loose body formation and new bone formation (osteophytosis) in abnormal sites.
- The affected joint is markedly swollen, deformed, may be subluxated or have gross instability, but is classically minimally painful/nontender(diagnostic point).
- Crepitus may be felt about moving the joint owing to the presence of multiple loose bodies.
- The patient may exhibit features of underlying disease.
- Charcot's triad includes gross joint swelling, exaggerated movements and painless presentation.
- The commonest joints involved are the mid-tarsal joints of the foot. Table 18.8 gives the list of commonly involved areas as per the cause of arthropathy.

Table 18.8: Sites of Charcot's arthropathy	
• Diabetes	• Mid-tarsal joint
• Leprosy	• MTP (feet)/IP joint (hand)
• Syringomyelia	• Shoulder joint
• Tabes dorsalis	• Knee joint
• Myelomeningocoele	• Ankle/intertarsal joint
• Chronic alcoholism	• Foot
• Amylodosis	• Peroneal muscle atrophy
• Congenital insensitivity to pain	• Ankle and foot

X-ray Features (Fig. 18.14)
- Marked destructive changes with periarticular erosions
- Joint space narrowing
- Osteophyte formation
- Subchondral sclerosis
- Loose bodies.
  The changes simulate osteoarthritis, but the absence of pain is diagnostic.

It may be difficult to differentiate Charcot's arthropathy from osteomyelitis but joint margins in Charcot's arthropathy are distinct, while in osteomyelitis they are blurred. MRI/Bone scan can further help in differentiation but CT scan is not useful.

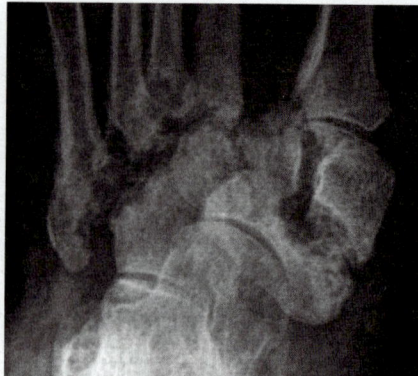

Fig. 18.14: X-ray showing marked destructive changes in Charcot's arthropathy

Treatment
- Minimizing the trauma by efficient bracing, weight-relieving calipers or leather corset.
- In troublesome cases, joint debridement (arthrocentesis) and arthrodesis may be necessary, although the results are often disappointing. Joint arthroplasty is relatively contraindicated in Charcot's disease.

ALKAPTONURIC ARTHRITIS (OCHRONOSIS)
- Joint symptoms occur, usually after the age of 40 years.
- The pigment deposit in articular cartilage, synovium, menisci and intervertebral disks causes periarticular, meniscal and intervertebral disk calcifications.
- Spine and shoulder joints are common sites of affection.
- Symptoms simulate osteoarthritis.
- *X-ray features*
  - Narrowing/calcification of intervertebral discs
  - Peripheral joints show chondrocalcinosis and severe OA.
- *Treatment*
  - Vitamin C supplementation.
  - Nitisinone is a newer disease modifying drug.
  - Arthroplasty in later stages.

Xtra Edge
- Differential diagnosis of intervertebral disc calcification
  - Alkaptonuria
  - CPPD deposition
  - Gout
  - AS
  - DISH
  - Hemochromatosis
  - Degenerative spondylosis.
- Clutton joints: The term is used in congenital syphilis to refer to the physical appearance of bilateral painless joint swellings that are usually there in the knees.

SYNOVIAL CHONDROMATOSIS
- In this condition, there occurs cartilaginous (hyaline) metaplasia in the intimal layers of synovium of the joint (most common), bursae or tendon sheath; leading to formation of multiple (may be even more than 50) loose bodies.
- The cartilage body may remain unchanged or may become calcified or ossified particularly at the centre by metaplasia or by endochondral ossification.
- Nutrition is carried through pedicle or via synovial fluid.
- Malignant change to chondrosarcoma may be there but is exceedingly rare.
- Knee followed by hip is the most common site of affection and this disease is the commonest cause of multiple loose bodies in the knee.

- Transient locking and grating sensations are the usual symptoms.
- On X-ray, only calcified/ossified bodies are visible, thus the actual number of loose bodies are always greater than that seen on X-ray (Fig. 18.15).
- The term "snowstorm appearance" is used to describe the appearance of this condition on arthroscopic evaluation of the knee.
- Symptomatic cases may need removal of loose bodies and synovectomy.
- The commonest cause of loose body in knee joint in young people is osteochondritis dissecans of knee. However, commonest cause overall and in elderly is OA knee and the commonest cause of multiple loose bodies in the knee joint is synovial chondromatosis.

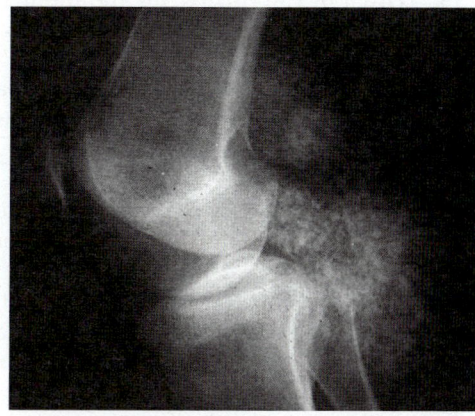

Fig.18.15: Synovial chondromatosis of knee

MULTIPLE CHOICE QUESTIONS

1. **Which type of cells predominantly seen in rheumatoid arthritis?**
   A. T cells   B. B cells
   C. Dendritic cells D. Giant cells
2. **Dactylitis is most commonly associated with:**
   A. Sickle cell anemia   B. Thalessemia
   C. Multiple myeloma D. Hemophilia
3. **Colchicine in acute gout helps by:**
   A. Mobilisation of uric acid
   B. Inhibits chemotaxis of neutrophils
   C. Increase of lymphocytes
   D. Affects purine metabolic pathway
4. **Daclizumab acts by binding to:**
   A. IL 2   B. IL 10
   C. TNF   D. INF alpha
5. **True about articular cartilage:**
   A. Is a type of elastic cartilage
   B. Is hyaline cartilage on the articular surface of bones
   C. Is type 1 cartilage providing compressive strength
   D. Is hyaline cartilage found in growth plate of bones
6. **Choose the correct statement about articular cartilage:**
   A. Zone 2 contains articular cartilage progenitor cell
   B. Zone 4 contains calcified cartilage
   C. Zone 3 has highest proteoglycans content
   D. Zone 1 has high water content
   E. All of the above
7. **Nutrient and oxygen reach the chondrocytes across perichondrium by:**
   A. Capillaries   B. Diffusion
   C. Along neurons   D. Active transport

8. **All of the following cause erosive arthritis** *except*:
   A. Rheumatoid arthritis
   B. Lupus arthritis/Jaccoud arthritis
   C. Tuberculous arthritis
   D. Septic arthritis
9. **In a patient with arthritis, examination of synovium aspirate, numerous lymphocytes, plasma cells and histocytes are found. What type of arthritis?**
   A. Acute pyogenic arthritis
   B. Chronic arthritis
   C. Granulomatous arthritis
   D. Rheumatoid arthritis
10. **Joint erosion is not a feature in:**
    A. SLE   B. Gout
    C. Psoriasis   D. Rheumatoid arthritis
11. **The father of joint replacement surgery is:**
    A. Manning   B. Girdlestone
    C. Charnley   D. Ponsetti
12. **In articular cartilage, most active chodrocytes are seen in:**
    A. Zone 1   B. Zone 2
    C. Zone 3   D. Zone 4
13. **Articular cartilage true is:**
    A. Very vascular structure
    B. Surrounded by thick perichondrium
    C. Has no nerve supply
    D. Fibrocartilage
14. **All of the following statements about synovial fluid are true,** *except*:
    A. Secreted primarily by type A synovial cells
    B. Follows non-Newtonian fluid kinetics
    C. Contains hyaluronic acid
    D. Viscosity is variable

15. **Which of the following statements about changes in articular cartilage with ageing is not true?**
   A. Total proteoglycan content is decreased
   B. Synthesis of proteogycans is decreased
   C. Enzymatic degradation of proteoglycans is increased
   D. Total water content of cartilage is decrease

16. **Synovial fluid of low viscosity is seen in all except:**
   A. Gout   B. Septic arthritis
   C. Osteoarthritis   D. Rheumatoid arthritis

17. **Deforming polyarthritis is associated with all of the following except:**
   A. Rheumatoid arthritis
   B. Psoriatic arthritis
   C. Behçet's syndrome
   D. Ankylosing spondylitis

18. **Erosion of bone is seen with all of the following except:**
   A. Gout
   B. SLE
   C. Psoriasis
   D. Rheumatoid arthritis

19. **Following X-ray changes are seen in:**

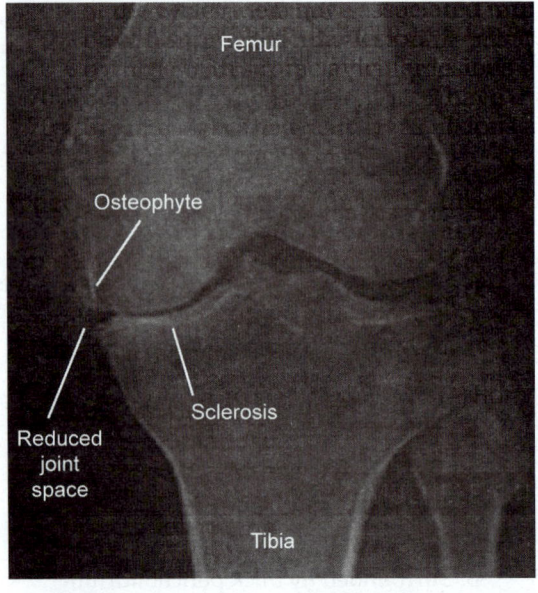

   A. OA   B. RA
   C. Psoriasis   D. Pseudogout

20. **Pain and arthritis of distal interphalangeal joints seen in:**
   A. Osteoarthritis
   B. Rheumatoid arthritis
   C. Ankylosing spondylitis
   D. de Quervain's disease

21. **Heberden's nodes are seen in:**
   A. Osteoarthritis of the distal interphalangeal joints
   B. Osteoarthritis of the proximal interphalangeal joint
   C. Rheumatoid arthritis of the 1st carpometacarpal joint
   D. Rheumatoid arthritis of the distal interphalangeal joints

22. **Bouchard's nodes are seen in:**
   A. Osteoarthritis of the distal interphalangeal joints
   B. Osteoarthritis of the proximal interphalangeal joint
   C. Rheumatoid arthritis of the 1st carpometacarpal joint
   D. Rheumatoid arthritis of the distal interphalangeal joints

23. **Osteoarthritis is not seen in:**
   A. Ankle joint
   B. Knee joint
   C. Hip joint
   D. 1st carpometacarpal

24. **Arthritis involving DIP, PIP, 1st carpometacarpal with sparing of MCP and wrist joint is typical of:**
   A. Osteoarthritis
   B. Rheumatoid arthritis
   C. Ankylosing spondylitis
   D. Psoriatic arthritis

25. **Which one of the following bursae always communicates with knee joint cavity?**
   A. Prepatellar
   B. Suprapatellar
   C. Superficial infrapatellar
   D. Deep infrapatellar

26. **A 58-year-old female patient presents with one-year history of anterior knee pain on climbing stairs. On examination crepitus was present. There was severe restriction of movements beyond 110 degrees. Examination of hip and back was normal. Diagnosis is:**
   A. Osteoarthritis   B. Psoriatic arthritis
   C. Osteonecrosis   D. Gout

27. **Joints not involved on osteoarthritis:**
   A. PIP   B. DIP
   C. MCP   D. Knee

28. **Which can cause loose body in the joint?**
   A. RA
   B. Ankylosing spondylitis
   C. OA
   D. SLE

29. **OA one of this is beneficial:**
   A. Glucosamine   B. Ketones
   C. Glucose   D. Citric acid

30. In patient with osteoarthritis of knee joint, atrophy occurs most commonly in which muscle?
  A. Quadriceps only
  B. Hamstrings only
  C. Both A and B
  D. Gastrocnemius

31. Heberden's arthropathy affects:
  A. Lumbar spine
  B. Symmetricaly large joints
  C. Sacroiliac joints
  D. Distal interphalangeal joints

32. True about osteoarthritis *except*:
  A. Commonly found in adult after 50 yrs
  B. Can involved single joints
  C. Lower limb deformity seen
  D. Ankylosis is seen

33. Severe disability in primary osteoarthritis of hip is best managed by:
  A. Arthrodesis
  B. Arthroplasty
  C. McMurray's hydrocortisone and physiotherapy
  D. Intra-articular hydrocortisone and physiotherapy

34. Proximal interphalangeal, distal interphalangeal and 1st carpometacarpal joint involvement and sparing of wrist is a feature of:
  A. Rheumatoid arthritis
  B. Pseudogout
  C. Psoriatic athropathy
  D. Osteoarthritis

35. A 62-year-old male complaints of pain bilateral knees R>L, he has difficulty in climbing stairs, squatting, sitting cross legged. His quadriceps muscle is wasted. On right knee X-ray there is subchondral sclerosis, tibial spine spiking obliterated medial joint space and reduced lateral joint space. AHLBACK grade 2 stage next step is:
  A. Conservative
  B. Arthroscopy
  C. Total knee replacement
  D. High tibial osteotomy

36. Boutonnière deformity has:
  A. Hyperextension of PIP joints and flexion of DIP joints
  B. Hyperextension of DIP joints and flexion of PIP joints
  C. Flexion of DIP joints and extension at metacarphalangeal joint
  D. Flexion of DIP joints

37. True about boutonnière deformity is/are:
  A. Rupture of extensor tendon
  B. Initially joints are mobile followed by rigidity

  C. Flexion at PIP joint and extension at DIP
  D. All of the above

38. In which of the deformities is the distal interphalangeal joint flexed and proximal interphalangeal joint extended?
  A. Boutonnière deformity
  B. Swan and neck deformity
  C. Z deformity
  D. Clawhand

39. Which of the following is difference between Rheumatoid arthritis and osteoarthritis?
  A. Osteophytes are seen in osteoarthritis
  B. Systemic symptoms are seen in osteoarthritis
  C. Rheumatoid arthritis is uncommon in hands and feet
  D. Osteoarthritis is an autoimmiune disease

40. In which of the following deformities is the distal interphalangeal joint extended?
  A. Boutonnière deformity
  B. Swan neck deformity
  C. Z deformity
  D. Claw hand

41. Rheumatoid arthritis affects which region of the spinal column?
  A. Cervical spine
  B. Thoracic spine
  C. Lumbosacral spine
  D. Equally affects all regions

42. All of the following are radiological features of rheumatoid arthritis *except*:
  A. Decreased joint space
  B. Aticular erosions
  C. Periarticular osteopenia
  D. Fibrous ankylosis

43. Hammertoe deformity is seen in:

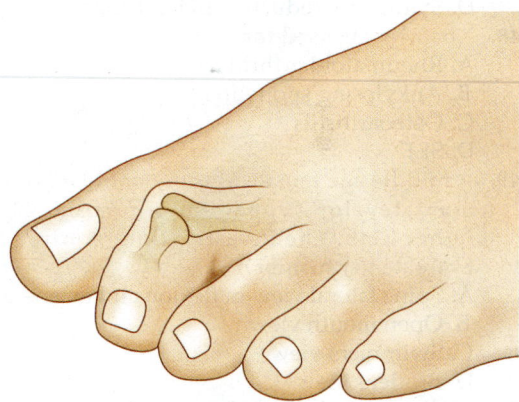

  A. Rheumatoid arthritis
  B. Fracture distal phalanx of great toe
  C. Bunion
  D. Osteochondritis

44. Windswept deformity of the knee is seen in:

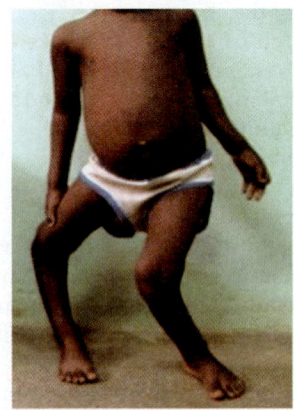

A. Osteoarthritis
B. Rheumatoid arthritis
C. Ankylosing sponylitis
D. Psoriatic arthritis

45. Swan neck deformity is seen in:
A. Osteoarthritis
B. Rheumatoid arthritis
C. Psoriatic arthritis
D. Gout

46. Distal interphalangeal joint involvement occur in:
A. Boutonnière deformity
B. Swan neck deformity
C. Dupuytren's contracture
D. All of the above

47. Which of the following is not a feature of rheumatoid arthritis?
A. Heberden's nodes
B. Swan neck deformity
C. Ulnar deviation of fingers at metacarpophalangeal joint
D. Symmetric reduction of joint space

48. Abatacept is used for:
A. Rheumatoid arthritis
B. Ankylosing sponylitis
C. Osteoarthritis
D. SLE

49. A middle age female of rheumatoid on treatment develops upper motor neuron signs in her limb. The investigation required to evaluate her further is:
A. Spine lateral view in flexion and extension.
B. Open mouth view
C. Swimmers view
D. Brodens view

50. Earliest radiological change in RA:
A. Decreased joint space
B. Articular erosion
C. Periarticular osteopenia
D. Subchondral cyst

51. Which arthritis causes no periosteal reaction?
A. Psoriatic arthritis
B. Reactive arthritis
C. Neruropathic arthritis
D. Rheumatoid arthritis

52. All are feature of seronegative spondylo-arthropathies except:
A. Uveitis   B. RA factor positive
C. HLA-B27 positive   D. Occur in young age

53. All are X-ray findings of RA except:
A. Reduced joint space
B. Soft tissue shadow
C. Periaticular new bone formation
D. Subchondral cyst

54. Joint spared in RA is:
A. Wrist   B. PIP
C. MCP   D. DIP

55. Pannus is seen in:
A. OA   B. RA
C. Psoriasis   D. Neurofibromatosis

56. A burn patient develops clawhand. Joint affected will be:
A. Flexion at proximal interphalangeal joint
B. Flexion at distal interphalangeal joint
C. Flexion at metacarpohalangeal joint
D. All of the above

57. Boutonnière deformity occur due to:
A. Flexion of proximal interphalangeal joint
B. Flexion at distal interphalangeal joint
C. Extension at metacarpophalangeal joint
D. Flexion at metacarpophalangeal joint

58. Joint not involved in rheumatoid arthritis according to 1987 modified ARA criterion:
A. Knee   B. Ankle
C. Tarsometatarsal   D. Metatarsophalangeal

59. What is pathognomic feature of rheumatoid arthritis?
A. Rheumatoid factor B. Rheumatoid nodule
C. Morning stiffness D. Ulnar drift of fingers

60. Which of the following is true regarding rheumatoid arthritis?
A. Typically involves small and large joints symmetrically but spares the cervical spine
B. Causes pleural effusion with low sugar
C. Pulmonary nodules are absent
D. Enthesopathy prominent

61. Swan neck deformity is:
A. Flexion of metacarpophalangeal joint and extension at interphalangeal joint
B. Extension at proximal interphalangeal joint and flexion at distal interphalangeal joint
C. Flexion at proximal interphalangeal joint and extension at distal interphalangeal joint
D. Extension at metacarpophalangeal joint and flexion a interphalangeal joint

62. **Distal interpahalangeal joint is not involved in:**
    A. Rheumatoid arthritis
    B. Psoriatic arthritis
    C. Multicentric hisiocytosis
    D. Neuropathic arthropathy

63. **"Windswept deformity" is seen in:**
    A. Ankylosing spondylitis
    B. Scurvy
    C. Rickets
    D. All of the above

64. **Windswept deformity in foot is seen in:**
    A. Rickets
    B. RA
    C. Hyperparathyroidism
    D. Scurvy

65. **HLA B27 is not seen in:**
    A. SLE
    B. Ankylosis spondylitis
    C. Reiter's syndrome
    D. Psoriatic arthritis

66. **Young male having pain with daily morning stiffness of spine for 30 minutes and reduced chest movements. Most probable diagnosis is:**
    A. Ankylosis spondylitis
    B. Rheumatoid arthritis
    C. Gouty arthritis
    D. Osteoarthritis

67. **Oligoarthritis with ascending joint involvement seen in:**
    A. Juvenile osteoarthritis
    B. Seronegative arthritis
    C. SLE
    D. Septic arthritis

68. **Spondyloarthropathy which is seronegative are all *except*:**
    A. AS   B. Psoriasis
    C. JRA   D. Reiter syndrome

69. **Arthritis with eye involvement is seen in:**
    A. Ankylosing spondylitis
    B. Psoriasis
    C. Gout
    D. Pseudogout

70. **Most common cause of reactive arthritis:**
    A. *Staph aureus*   B. *N. gonorrhoeae*
    C. *S. flexneri*   D. *E. coli*

71. **All are seronegative (spondyloepiphyseal) arthritis with ocular manifestation, *except*:**
    A. Ankylospondylitis
    B. Reiter's disease
    C. Rheumatoid arthritis
    D. Psoriatic arthritis

72. **Ankylosing spondylitis in associated with:**
    A. HLA-B27   B. HLA-B-8
    C. HLA-DW4/DR4   D. HLA-DR3

73. **Correct statement regarding AS:**
    A. Sacroiliitis is the earliest manifestation seen
    B. Gaenslen test done
    C. Peripheral joint involvement in 30% patients
    D. All of the above

74. **True regarding ankylosing spondylitis is:**
    A. Osteophytes grow in vertical directions
    B. Most common extra-articular manifestation is acute anterior uveitis
    C. HLA B27 is positive in more than 90% of cases
    D. All of the above

75. **A young man complaints of pain lower back his X-rays are shown below. Most likely diagnosis is:**

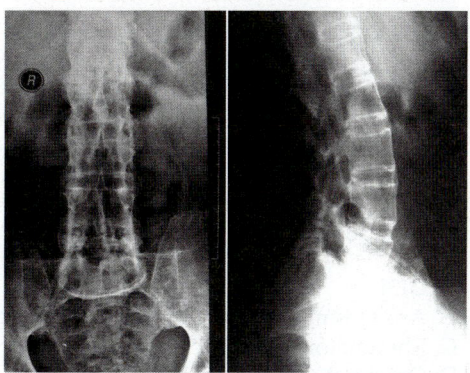

    A. AS   B. Spondylolisthesis
    C. Paget's disease   D. Osteoporosis

76. **Which of the following is not the extra-articular manifestations of ankylosing spondylitis?**
    A. Acute anterior uveitis
    B. Aortic valve disease
    C. Pulmonary fibrosis
    D. Dilated cardiomyopathy

77. **Identify the test performed:**

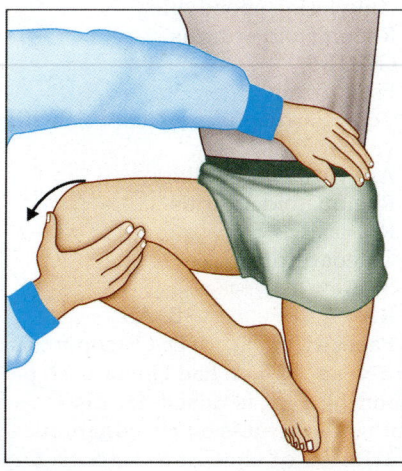

    A. FABER test   B. Thomas test
    C. SLR test   D. Gaenslen test

78. **Ankylosing spondylitis all is true *except*:**
   A. HLA B27 is found 90% of sufferers
   B. Uveitis is found in 40% of sufferers
   C. Condition is commoner in females
   D. Radiological changes do not can occur in spine before symptoms

79. **A 25-year-old man complaints of low backache decreased lumbar movements, morning stiffness which clinical examination will further help:**
   A. Head circumference
   B. Chest expansion
   C. Hyperextension of joints
   D. Plantar arch

80. **A young patient with complaints of severe low backache, with stiffness of back with reduced chest expansion is most probably suffering from:**
   A. Tuberculosis
   B. Ankylosing spondylitis
   C. Rheumatoid arthritis
   D. Metastasis

81. **In a middle aged male having back pain, syndesmophytes involving 4 continuous vertebrae are seen on X-ray. The patient has:**
   A. DISH
   B. Ankylosing spondylitis
   C. Rheumatoid arthritis
   D. Osteoarthritis

82. **True about ankylosing spondylitis are all *except*:**
   A. Affects males   B. 30–40 years
   C. 90% HLA-B5   D. Bamboo spine

83. **Bamboo spine with sacroiliitis:**
   A. Ankylosing spondylitis
   B. RA
   C. OA
   D. Psoriatic arthritis

84. **Scleritis with autommune disease involving joints:**
   A. Ankylosing spondylitis
   B. Rheumatoid arthritis
   C. GOUT
   D. Pseudogout

85. **Differential diagnosis of hand arthritis are all *excepts*:**
   A. Ankylosis spondylitis
   B. Rheumatoid arthritis
   C. Psoriasis
   D. Osteoarthritis

86. **Bechterew's disease:**
   A. RA   B. AS
   C. Paget's   D. Osteoporosis

87. **A 65-year-old man had H/o of back pain sine 3 months. ESR is raised. He also has dorso-lumbar tenderness on examination and mild restriction of chest movements. On X-ray syndesmophytes are present in vertebrae. Diagnosis is:**
   A. Ankylosing spondylitis
   B. Degenerative osteoarthritis of spine
   C. Ankylosing hyperostosis
   D. Lumbar canal stenosis

88. **A young male presents with joints and backache. X-ray of spine shows evidence of sacroiliitis. The most likely diagnosis is:**
   A. Rheumatoid arthritis
   B. Ankylosing spondylitis
   C. Polyarticular juvenile arthritis
   D. Psoriatic arthropathy

89. **Bamboo spine is seen in:**
   A. Tuberculosis
   B. Rheumatoid arthritis
   C. Ochronosis
   D. Ankylosis spondylitis

90. **CASPAR criteria is used in diagnosis of:**
   A. Psoriatic arthritis
   B. Rheumatoid arthritis
   C. Ankyosing spondylitis
   D. Reactive synovitis

91. **Pencil in cup deformity is seen in:**
   A. Rheumatoid arthritis
   B. Ankylosing spondylitis
   C. AVN
   D. Psoriatic arthritis

92. **Sausage digits is seen in:**
   A. Lyme arthritis   B. Osteoarthritis
   C. Psoriatic arthritis   D. None

93. **Resorption of distal phalanx is seen in:**
   A. Scleroderma
   B. Hyperparathyroidism
   C. Reiter's syndrome
   D. All

94. **True about psoriatic arthritis are all *except*:**
   A. HLA-Cw6 association
   B. Involvement of DIP joint
   C. More common in males
   D. Doc is methotrexate

95. **Psoriatic arthritis most commonly involves:**
   A. PIP   B. DIP
   C. MCP   D. Wrist

96. **All are true regarding psoriatic arthritis *except*:**
   A. Arthritis mutilans
   B. DIP involvement
   C. Ankylosis of small joints
   D. Lengthening of digits called telescoping

97. **A 35-year-old male develops involvements of PIP, DIP and metacarpophalangeal joints with sparing of wrist and metacarpophalangeal joints. The probable diagnosis is:**
   A. Psoriatic arthritis
   B. Osteoarthritis
   C. Rheumatoid arthritis
   D. Pseudogout

98. **Disease where distal interphalangeal joint is characteristically involved:**
   A. Psoriatic arthritis
   B. Rheumatoid
   C. SLE
   D. Gout

99. **In psoriatic arthropathy, treatment of choice is:**
   A. Methotrexate
   B. PUVA therapy
   C. Corticosteroids
   D. Indomethacin

100. **A 50-year-old alcoholic male with complaints of recurrent pain and swelling in foot joints. On examination red, shiny swollen joints seen which is the most appropriate investigation to be first done considering the X-ray showing:**

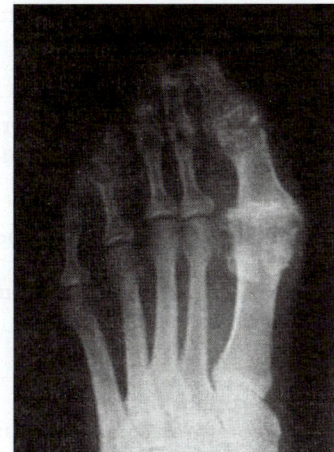

   A. HLA-B27
   B. PTH levels
   C. Uric acid levels
   D. Calcium levels

101. **Most common joint involved in gout is:**
   A. Knee
   B. Hip
   C. MP joint of great toe
   D. MP joint of thumb

102. **Drug of choice for the treatment of acute gout in patients in whom NSAIDs are contra-indicated is:**
   A. Colchicine
   B. Allopurinol
   C. Xyloric acid
   D. Paracetamol

103. **Needle-shaped crystals negatively birefringent on polarized microscopy is characteristic of which crystal associated arthropathy?**
   A. Gout
   B. CPPD
   C. Neuropathic arthropathy
   D. Hemophilic arthropathy

104. **This elderly male came with a history of recurrent attack of pain and swelling in the great toe in the past. This is the present X-ray of the hand. The diagnosis can be confirmed by:**

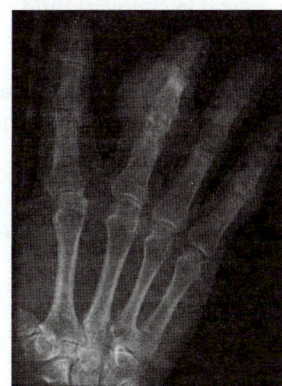

   A. X-ray of lumbosacral spine
   B. Polarized microscopy of tissue fluid aspirated
   C. Anti-CCP antibodies
   D. HLA B27

105. **A 40-year-old man presents with acute onset pain left great toe. On investigating punched out lesion is seen on phalanx and adjacent soft tissue. Most likely diagnosis is:**
   A. Reiter's arthritis   B. Psoriasis
   C. Rheumatoid   D. Gout

106. **A middle age male, known case of chronic renal failure develops MTP swelling. The test to be performed is:**
   A. Uric acid   B. HLAB 27
   C. RA factor   D. Calcium

107. **Drug used in acute gout:**
   A. Allopurinol   B. Probencid
   C. Colchicine   D. Sulfinpyrazone

108. **Acute gouty arthritis drug used is:**
   A. Probencid   B. Allopurinol
   C. Colchicine   D. Sulfinpyrazone

109. **A 35-year-old businessmen presents suddenly with severe pain, swelling and redness in left big toe in early morning. Most likely diagnosis is:**
   A. Rheumatoid arthritis
   B. Gouty arthritis
   C. Pseudogout
   D. Septic arthritis

110. **In a gouty arthritis, the characteristic X-ray findings includes:**
   A. Osteoporosis
   B. Erosion of joint
   C. Soft tissue calcification
   D. Narrowing of joint space

111. **Which of the following is not affected in gout?**
   A. Muscle   B. Skin
   C. Cartilage   D. Tendon

112. **In a patient of gouty arthritis best investigation is:**
    A. Serum uric acid
    B. Uric acid in urine
    C. Urate crystal in synovial fluid
    D. Serum calcium level

113. **What is not true about gout?**
    A. Abrupt increase in serum urate levels is more common a cause for acute gout than an abrupt fall in urate levels.
    B. Patient may be asymptomatic with high serum uric acid for years
    C. Development of arthritis correlates with level of serum uric acid
    D. Uric acid crystals are best seen by polarizing light microscope

114. **Which joint is most commonly affected in pseudogout:**
    A. Knee   B. Hip
    C. MP joint great toe   D. MP joint thumb

115. **Craniovertebral joint contains all *except*:**
    A. Wings of sphenoid B. Basiocciput
    C. Atlas   D. Axis

116. **The pathognomonic finding in pseudogout is:**
    A. CPPD crystals under microscope
    B. Polyarthritis with urinary sediment
    C. Juxta-articular osteopenia
    D. Bone spurs

117. **Periarticular calcification is seen in:**
    A. RA   B. Pseudogout
    C. OA   D. None of the above

118. **What change will be seen in vertebral column in ochronosis:**
    A. Calcification of disc
    B. Bamboo spine
    C. Increased disc space
    D. None

119. **In alkaptonuria heterotopic ossification occurs around:**
    A. Bone   B. Joint
    C. Soft tissue   D. None

120. **Calcification of menisci is seen in:**
    A. Hyperparathyroidism
    B. Pseudogout
    C. Renal osteodystrophy
    D. Acromegaly

121. **A lady presents with right knee swelling, aspiration was done in which CPPD crystals were obtained. Next best investigation is:**
    A. ANA   B. RF
    C. CPK   D. TSH

122. **X-ray of a young man shows heterotopic calcification around bilateral knee joints. Next investigation would be:**
    A. Serum phosphate
    B. Serum calcium
    C. Serum PTH
    D. Serum alkaline phosphatase

123. **Heterotrophic ossification—most important investigation you would do for management:**
    A. Alkaline phosphatase
    B. Serum potassium
    C. Acid phosphatase
    D. Calcium

124. **All of the following are associated with CV junction anomalies *except*:**
    A. Rheumatoid arthritis
    B. Ankylosing spondylosis
    C. Odontoid dysgenesis
    D. Basal degeneration

125. **Chondrocalcinosis is seen in:**
    A. Ochronosis
    B. Hypoparathyroidism
    C. Rickets
    D. Basal degeneration

126. **The earliest manifestation of alkaptonuria is:**
    A. Ankylosis of lumbodorsal spine
    B. Ochronosis
    C. Prostatic arthritis
    D. Pigmentation of tympanic membrane

127. **How to differentiate gout with pseudogout?**
    A. Large joint involvement
    B. Birefringent (particles) crystals
    C. Associated with hyperparathyroidism
    D. All of the above

128. **Characteristic crystals in pseudogout are:**
    A. Calcium pyrophosphate
    B. Sodium monourate
    C. Potassium urate
    D. Sodium pyrophosphate

129. **The most commonly involved joint in pseudogout:**
    A. Knee   B. Great toe
    C. Hip   D. Elbow

130. **Subluxation of atlanto-occipital joint is seen in all *except*:**
    A. Gout
    B. Odontoid dysgenesis
    C. Rheumatoid arthritis
    D. Ankylosis spondylitis

131. **Soft tissue calcification around the knee is seen in:**
    A. Scurvy
    B. Scleroderma
    C. Hyperparathyroidism
    D. Pseudogout

132. **Calcification of menisci is seen in:**
    A. Hyperparathyroidism
    B. Pseudogout
    C. Renal osteodystrophy
    D. Acromegaly

133. **Hemophilic arthropathy, which is not seen?**
    A. Subchondral bone cyst formation
    B. Increase in intercondylar distance
    C. Juxta-articular osteosclerosis
    D. Subchondral thining

134. Epiphyseal enlargement is seen in:
A. Rickets   B. Hemophilia
C. Septic arthritis   D. All of the above

135. Fracture are more common of hemophiliac because:
A. Joint stiffness   B. Osteopenia
C. Both A and B   D. Vascular pulsations

136. True about treatment of hemarthosis:
A. POP
B. Traction
C. Compression bandage
D. All of the above

137. Most common muscle for pseudotumar like growth in hemophilic arthopathy is:
A. Quadriceps femoris   B. Hamstring muscle
C. Gastrocnemius   D. Lliopsoas

138. All are feature of hemophilic knee joint, *except*:
A. Juxtra-articular osteosclerosis
B. Subcondral cyst formation
C. Widening of intercondylar notch
D. Squaring of patella

139. Arthroscopy is contraindicated in:
A. Chronic joint disease
B. Loose bodies
C. Hemophilia
D. Meniscal tear

140. Charcot's joint is another name for joint affected by:
A. Neuropathy
B. Osteoarthritis
C. Rheumatoid arthritis
D. Ankylosing spondylitis

141. Most common cause of neuropathy joint:
A. Leprosy   B. Tabes dorsalis
C. Diabetes   D. Nerve injury

142. Clutton's joint is seen in:
A. Primary syphilis   B. Secondary syphilis
C. Tertiary syphilis   D. Congenital syphilis

143. Neuropathic joint is seen in all *except*:
A. DM   B. Tabes dorsalis
C. Syringomyelia   D. Hypertension

144. Neuropathic joints are seen in all *except*:
A. Leprosy   B. Syringomyelia
C. Tuberculosis   D. Diabetes Mellitus

145. Not associated with neuropathic joint:
A. DM   B. Syringomyelia
C. Friedreich's ataxia   D. Tabes dorsalis

146. False about Charcot's joint in diabetes mellitus is:
A. Limitation of movements with bracing
B. Athrodesis
C. Total ankle replacement
D. Arthrocentesis

147. A 60-year-old man with diabetes mellitus presents with painless, swollen right ankle joint. Radiographs of the ankle show destroyed joint with large no. of loose bodies. The most probable diagnosis is:
A. Charcot's joint   B. Clutton's joint
C. Osteoarthritis   D. Rheumatoid arthritis

148. Neuropathic joint may arise in:
A. Syringomyelia   B. Tabes dorsalis
C. Leprosy   D. All of the above

149. In a patient suffering from tabes dorsalis Charcot's joint occurs most commonly at:
A. Elbow   B. Tarsometatarsal
C. Wrist   D. Knee

150. Most common Charcot's joints involved in diabetes mellitus are those of:
A. Shoulder   B. Ankle
C. Knee   D. Foot

151. Clutton's joints are:
A. Syphilitic joints
B. End stage tuberculosis joints
C. Associated with trauma
D. Usually painful

152. Joint least affected by neuropathy:
A. Shoulder   B. Hip
C. Wrist   D. Elbow

153. A 42 years male with frequent attacks of joint pain, underwent an X-ray showing soft tissue swelling, the likely diagnosis is:

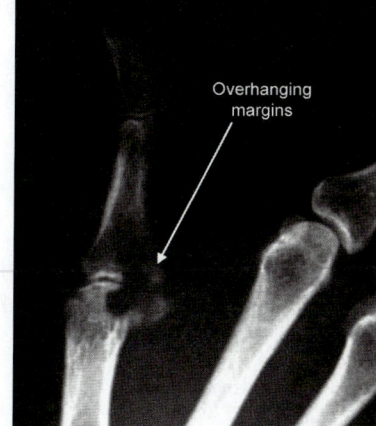

Overhanging margins

A. Gout   B. Parathyroid adenoma
C. Psoriasis   D. RA

154. Loose body in joint most common site is:
A. Knee   B. Hip
C. Elbow   D. Ankle

155. Multiple loose bodies are seen maximum in:
A. Osteochondritis dissecans
B. Synovial chondromatosis
C. Osteoarthritis
D. Rheumatoid arthritis

ANSWERS

1. A. T cells
   Rheumatoid arthritis (RA) is one of the most common chronic inflammatory syndromes. ... Evidence also supports a role for T-helper (Th) *cells*, Th17 *cells*, and impaired CD4+ CD25(hi) regulatory T cell (Treg) function in the pathogenesis of *RA*.

2. A. Sickle cell anemia
   One of the earliest clinical manifestations is dactylitis, presenting as early as six months of age, and may occur in children with sickle-cell trait.

3. B. Inhibits chemotaxis of neutrophils
   Colchicine is not used nowadays due to its increased side effects but can be used when NSAIDs are not useful in acute setting. It acts by inhibiting the chemotaxis of neutrophils, thus inhibiting the inflammatory pathway.

4. A. IL2
   Daclizumab is a therapeutic humanized monoclonal antibody used for the treatment of adults with relapsing forms of multiple sclerosis (MS). *Daclizumab* works by binding to CD25, the alpha subunit of the IL-2 receptor of T-cells.

5. B. Is hyaline cartilage on the articular surface of bones

6. B. Zone 4 contains calcified cartilage, C. Zone 3 has highest proteoglycans content and D. Zone 1 has high water content

7. B. Diffusion

8. B. Lupus arthritis/Jaccoud arthritis

9. C. Granulomatous arthritis

10. A. SLE

11. C. Charnely

12. C. Zone 3

13. C. Has no nerve supply

14. A. Secreted primarily by type A synovial cells

15. C. Enzymatic degradation of proteoglycans is increased

16. C. Osteoarthritis

17. C. Behçet's syndrome

18. B. SLE

19. A. OA

20. A. Osteoarthritis

21. A. Osteoarthritis of the distal interphalangeal joint

22. B. Osteoarthritis of the proximal interphalangeal joint

23. A. Ankle joint

24. A. Osteoarthritis

25. B. Suprapatellar

26. A. Osteoarthritis

27. C. MCP

28. C. OA

29. A. Glucosamine

30. A. Quadriceps only

31. D. Distal interphalangeal joints

32. D. Ankylosis is seen

33. B. Athroplasty

34. D. Osteoarthritis

35. A. Conservative
    • Next step is conservative but best would be TKR.

36. B. Hyperextension of DIP joints and flexion of PIP joints

37. D. All of the above

38. A. Boutonnière deformity

39. A. Osteophytes are seen in osteoarthritis

40. A. Boutonnière deformity

41. A. Cervical spine

42. D. Fibrous ankylosis

43. A. Rheumatoid arthritis

44. B. Rheumatoid arthritis

45. B. Rheumatoid arthritis

46. D. All of the above

47. A. Heberden's nodes

48. A. Rheumatoid arthritis

49. A. Spine lateral view in flexion and extension

50. C. Periarticular osteopenia

51. D. Rheumatoid arthritis

52. B. RA factor positive

53. C. Periaticular new bone formation

54. D. DIP

55. B. RA

56. D. All of the above

57. A. Flexion of proximal interphalangeal joint

58. C. Tarsometatarsal

59. B. Rheumatoid nodule

60. B. Causes pleural effusion with low sugar

61. B. Extension at proximal interphalangeal joint and flexion at distal interphalangeal joint

62. A. Rheumatoid arthritis

63. C. Rickets

64. B. RA

65. A. SLE

66. A. Ankylosis spondylitis

67. B. Seronegative arthritis

68. C. JRA

69. A. Ankylosis spondylitis

70. C. *S. flexneri*

71. C. Rheumatoid arthritis

72. A. HLA-B27

73. D. All of the above

74. D. All of the above

75. A. AS

76. D. Dilated cardiomyopathy
77. A. FABER test
78. C. Condition is commoner in females
79. B. Chest expansion
80. B. Ankylosing spondylitis
81. B. Ankylosing spondylitis
82. C. 90% HLA-B5
83. A. Ankylosing spondylitis
84. B. Rheumatoid arthritis
85. A. Ankylosis spondylitis
86. B. AS
87. A. Ankylosing spondylitis
88. B. Ankylosing spondylitis
89. D. Ankylosing spondylitis
90. A. Psoriatic arthritis
91. D. Psoriatic arthritis
92. C. Psoriatic arthritis
93. B. Hyperparathyroidism
94. C. More common in males
95. B. DIP
96. D. Lengthening of digits called telescoping
97. A. Psoriatic arthritis
98. A. Psoriatic arthritis
99. A. Methotrexate
100. C. Uric acid levels
101. C. MP joint of great toe
102. A. Colchicine
103. A. Gout
104. B. Polarized microscopy of tissue fluid aspirated
105. D. Gout
106. A. Uric acid
107. C. Colchicine
108. C. Colchicine
109. B. Gouty arthritis
110. C. Soft tissue calcification
111. A. Muscle
112. C. Urate crystal in synovial fluid
113. A. Abrupt increase in serum urate levels is more common a cause for acute gout than an abrupt fall in urate levels
114. A. Knee

115. A. Wings of sphenoid
116. A. CPPD crystals under microscope
117. B. Pseudogout
118. A. Calcification of disc
119. B. Joint
120. B. Pseudogout
121. D. TSH
122. A. Serum phosphate
123. A. Alkaline phosphatase
124. B. Ankylosing spondylosis
125. A. Ochronosis
126. B. Ochronosis
127. D. All of the above
128. A. Calcium pyrophosphate
129. A. Knee
130. A. Gout
131. D. Pseudogout
132. B. Pseudogout
133. C. Juxta-articular osteosclerosis
134. D. All of the above
135. C. Both A and C
136. D. All of the above
137. A. Quadriceps femoris
138. A. Juxtra-articular osteosclerosis
139. C. Hemophilia
140. A. Neuropathy
141. C. Diabetes
142. D. Congenital syphilis
143. D. Hypertension
144. C. Tuberculosis
145. C. Friendeich's ataxia
146. C. Total ankle replacement
147. A. Charcot's joint
148. D. All of the above
149. D. Knee
150. D. Foot
151. A. Syphilitic joints
152. D. Elbow
153. A. Gout
154. A. Knee
155. B. Synovial chondromatosis

Osteochondritis and AVN

AVASCULAR NECROSIS

Avascular necrosis (AVN), also called osteonecrosis or aseptic necrosis is a disease of impaired blood supply.

Common sites of AVN are:

Site of AVN	Eponym	Cause
1. Femoral head	Chandler disease	Discussed later
2. Proximal pole of scaphoid	Preiser disease (idiopathic AVN)	Fracture through waist of scaphoid
3. Distal femoral condyle	SPONK (spontaneous osteonecrosis of knee)	Idiopathic
4. Body of talus		Fracture through neck of talus
5. Proximal pole of lunate		Dislocation
6. Head of humerus		Neer's type IV fracture

Scaphoid

Scaphoid has a peculiar retrograde blood flow from distal to proximal through intra-osseous channels. Dorsal carpal branch supplies proximal pole distal to proximal as shown in Fig. 19.1 A and B. So, fracture through the waist of scaphoid leads to AVN of proximal pole.

Most of the blood supply of scaphoid enters through the dorsal ridge.

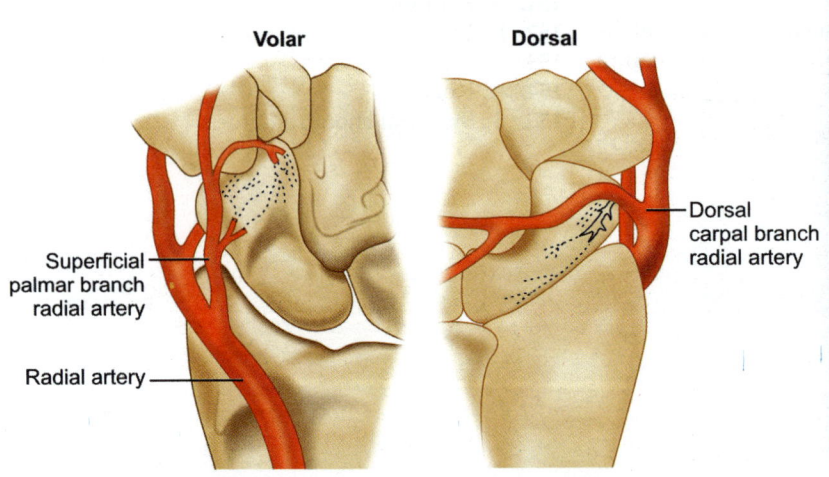

Fig. 19.1A: Blood supply of scaphoid

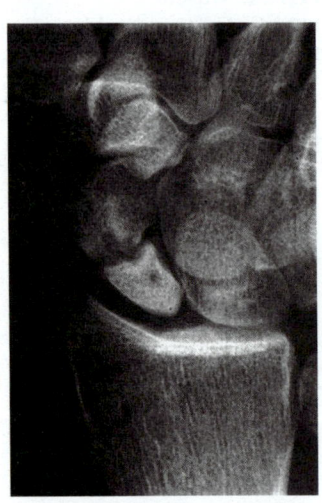

Fig. 19.1B: X-ray showing AVN of scaphoid

Talus

Fracture through neck of talus leads to AVN of body (Fig. 19.2) and is most commonly seen after Hawkins type IV fractures. More is the fracture displacement more is the soft tissue disruption near talus, more the chances of AVN after fracture.

On X-ray between 6 and 8 weeks, necrosed bone shows increased density (the earliest sign on X-ray) compared to the surrounding bone.

Hawkins sign (Fig. 19.3) describes subchondral lucency of the talar dome that occurs secondary to subchondral atrophy 6–8 weeks after a talar neck fracture. This indicates that there is sufficient vascularity in the talus, and is therefore unlikely to develop avascular necrosis later.

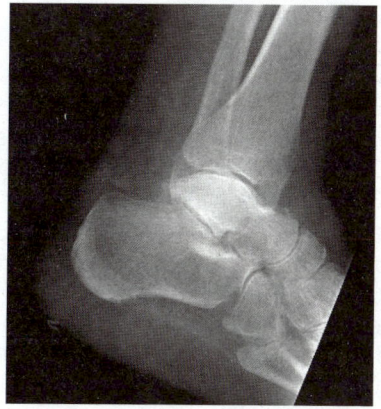

Fig. 19.2: X-ray showing AVN of talar body

Snow cap sign: *Snow cap sign* (Fig.19.4) or snow capping is defined as the appearance of dense sclerosis over the head of humerus or femur in cases of avascular necrosis as seen on plain radiographs, which resembles a snow capped mountain.

Head of Femur

Traumatic AVN occurs in head of femur commonly after a fracture neck of femur or posterior dislocation of hip joint (>12 hours duration). Femoral head is also the most common site of atraumatic AVN and the condition is called Chandler's disease. Anterolateral aspect is weight bearing area and is most commonly involved in AVN. The changes first begin in the subchondral bone beneath the articular cartilage of the head.

The causes of atraumatic AVN of the femoral head include:
1. Most common cause is idiopathic
2. Long term steroid intake, e.g. renal transplant, pemphigus, nephrotic syndrome, etc. (2nd commonest cause)
3. Coagulation disorder
4. Malignancy—leukemia, etc.
5. Substance abuse—alcohol
6. Storage disorder—Gaucher's disease
7. Infection—septic arthritis, osteomyelitis
8. Caisson disease—dysbaric osteonecrosis
9. Hyperlipidemia, nephrotic syndrome

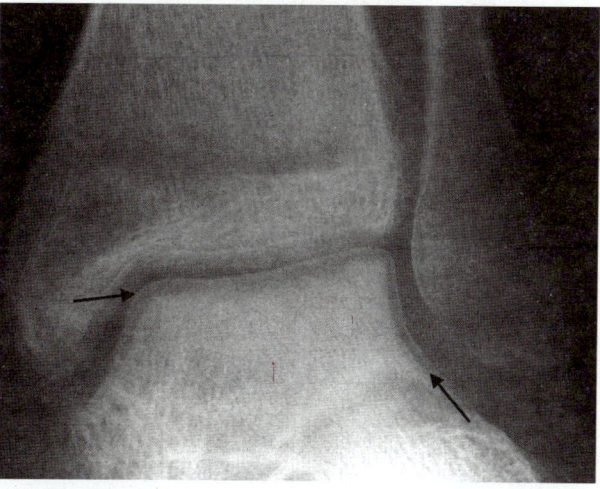

Fig. 19.3: X-ray showing Hawkins sign

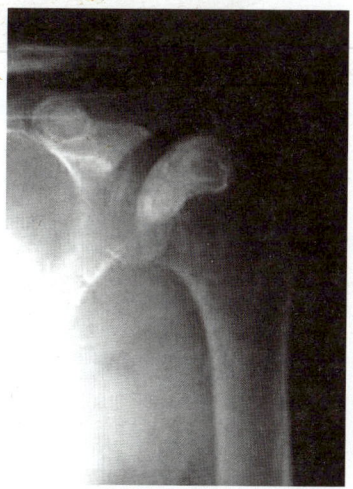

Fig. 19.4: Snow cap sign

10. Vasculitis—SLE, irradiation
11. Congenital disorder—SCFE, Perthes' disease
12. Chronic dialysis

Blood supply of femoral head (Fig. 19.5)
1. Branches of profunda femoris artery—MCFA (main) and LCFA.
2. Branch of obturator artery (foveal artery via ligamentum teres).
3. Metaphyseal artery.

Trueta's hypothesis: Trueta divided blood supply of femoral head according to age and gave an explanation of Perthes' disease being common in 4–8 years age group.

Cartilaginous growth plate starts appearing by 4 years of age and foveal artery appears at 8 years of age. Thus, in children <4 years of age metaphyseal artery can supply the head and in 4–8 years age group it cannot, as vessels cannot cross the growth plate. In adolescents/adults when growth plate disappears they can supply the head again.

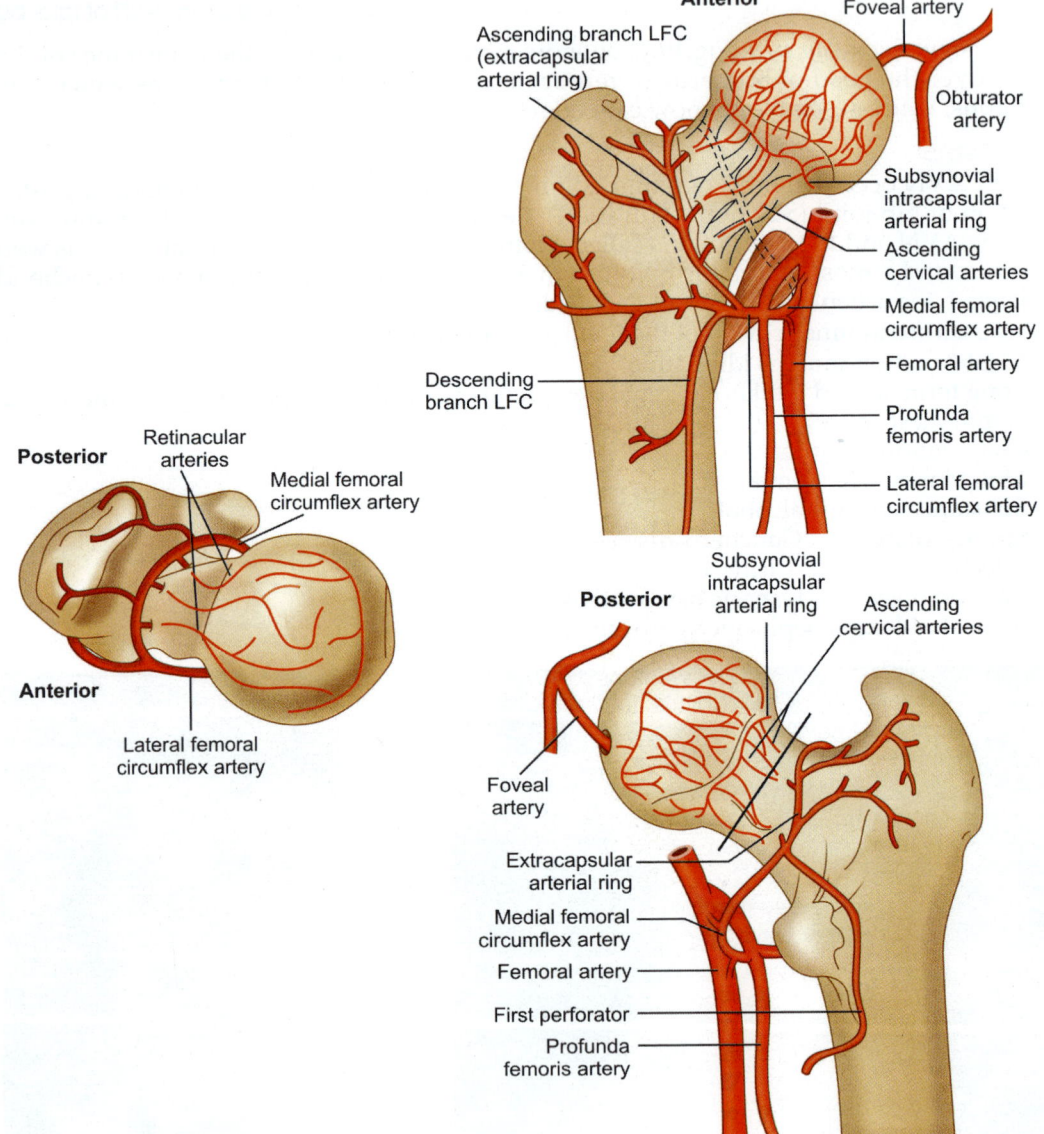

Fig. 19.5: Blood supply of femoral head

Age	Supply
<4 years	Metaphyseal artery
	Retinacular artery
4–8 years	Retinacular artery
>8 years	Retinacular artery
	Foveal artery
Adult	Metaphyseal
	Retinacular
	Foveal

Profunda femoris artery gives MCFA and LCFA which makes an extra-capsular arterial ring, anteriorly by LCFA and posteriorly by MCFA (main). From the extra-capsular arterial ring, arises ascending/retinacular arteries on the surface of the neck of femur, on its anterior/posterior/medial/lateral sides, lateral being the most important (branch of MCFA). At the junction of articular part of head/neck, a 2nd less distinct arterial ring called subsynovial intra-articular arterial ring arises. It is from this ring that vessels penetrate the head and are referred to as the epiphyseal arteries, the most important being the lateral epiphyseal group supplying the lateral weight bearing part of the head. These epiphyseal arteries anastomose with metaphyseal and foveal branches inside the head.

These vessels because of their proximity to neck are prone to injury in fracture NOF and more proximal is the lesion (fracture), more are the chances of AVN [subcapital (worst prognosis) >transcervical > basicervical is the order of development of AVN].

Clinical features
- Age: 20–50 years (male > female)
- Bilateral in 50% idiopathic cases and 80% of steroid induced cases (so, in management of AVN, contralateral hip should also be followed up for development of AVN).
- Deep pain in groin, antalgic gait.
- Decreased range of movement, especially internal rotation followed by abduction.
  This is a characteristic feature of altered femoral head shape and is seen in: AVN, SCFE, Perthes' disease.
- Sectoral sign.

X-ray (AP and frog lateral view)
X-ray changes take 3–6 months to appear.
Sclerosis, crescent sign (subchondral collapse of the necrotic segment, Fig 19.6).

MRI helps in earlier diagnosis and is the IOC when X-ray is normal, i.e. early in the course of the disease. Thus to screen contralateral hip in a diagnosed case of AVN, MRI becomes the IOC.

T1—single density line (demarcates normal ischemic bone interface).

T2—double density line.

Classification
1. Ficat and Arlet—crescent sign is stage IIB
2. Unversity of Pennsylvania—crescent sign is stage III
   <15% head involvement—mild AVN
   15–30% head involvement—moderate AVN
   >30% head involvement—severe AVN.

Differential diagnosis: Transient osteoporosis of hip.

Treatment
- Early stage—protected weight bearing
- Pre-collapse stage before appearance of crescent sign
  - Core decompression (FORAGE), name of surgery—Hungerford.
  - Drill holes are made which decrease the intraosseous pressure and increase vascularity.

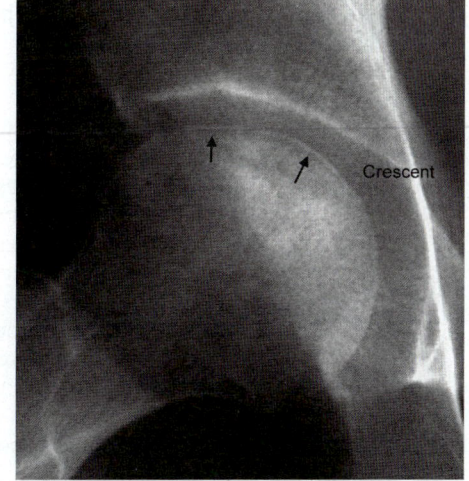

Fig. 19.6: Crescent sign in AVN of femoral head

- – Can be supplemented with vascularised/nonvascularised fibula graft. The peroneal blood vessels are anastomosed with branches of LCFA.
- – Muscle pedicle graft—can be fixed to increase vascularity.
- – Quadratus femoris—Meyer's graft.
- – Tensor fascia lata—Joshi's graft.
- Postcollapse:
  - – Osteotomy to bring the intact surface of femoral head in the weight bearing zone.
    - ▪ Transtrochanteric rotational osteotomy (Sugioka).
    - ▪ Intertrochanteric varus/valgus osteotomy.
- Arthritis (acetabular involvement)—total hip replacement is the most commonly performed procedure in AVN of femoral head, as most patients present in late stages.

OSTEOCHONDRITIS

These are a group of disorders characterized by interruption of the blood supply of a bone, in particular the epiphysis, followed by ischemic necrosis of osteoarticular fragment of bone leading to compression, fragmentation and separation. This disorder is defined as a focal disturbance of endochondral ossification and is regarded as having a multifactorial cause, so no one thing accounts for all aspects of this disease. It occurs mainly in the adolescent/growing age group, an often initiated by increased physical activity/trauma/repetitive stress.

Types

1. Splitting—due to increased wear during movement followed by ischemic changes. For example: Osteochondritis dissecans of knee (lower lateral part of medial femoral condyle).
2. Pulling/traction—pull of tendon/ligament causes separation of fragment. *For example*: Osgood-Schlatter's disease/Sever's/Johansson Larsen.
3. Crushing—due to increased pressure. *For example*: Kohler, Kienböck, Perthes, Scheuermann's, Calve's, Frieberg's, Islene.

Kienböck's Disease

- AVN of lunate, associated with ulna minus variant of hand.
- Patients are mostly manual laborers.

Type of osteochondritis	Bones involved
1. **Perthes**	Head of femur
2. **Panner**	Capitellum of humerus
3. **Preiser**	Scaphoid
4. **Pierson**	Symphysis pubis
5. **Schmier's**	Pisiform
6. **Kohler**	Navicular
7. **Kienböck**	Lunate
8. **Calve's**	Central bony nucleus of vertebrae
9. **Scheuermann**	Ring epiphysis of vertebrae
10. **Sever's**	Calcaneal epiphysis
11. **Dias**	Trochlea of talus
12. **Friedrich**	Medial clavicle
13. **Freiberg**	2nd metatarsal head
14. **Islene**	5th metatarsal head
15. **Dietrich**	Head of metacarpals
16. **Osgood-Schlatter**	Tibial tuberosity
17. **Johansson-Larsen**	Lower pole of patella
18. **Blount's**	Tibia
19. **Ahlback**	Medial femoral condyle (SPONK)
20. **Haglund**	Calcaneus
21. **Fleischner-Thiemann**	Phalanges
22. **Hass**	Head of humerus
23. **Burns**	Distal ulna

> Mnemonic: "Please C → **FOLKKS** → **MTP N**ot **L**egal in **C**ountry"
> Please (Panner's): 'C' (Capitellum)
> **F** (Freiberg's Ds): M
> **O** (Osgood Sy): T
> **L** (Larsen Sy): P
> **K** (Kohler Ds): N
> **K** (Keinbock Ds): L
> **S** (Sever Ds): C
> *Courtsey*: Dr Sanjiv (Mumbai)

- *Finsterer's sign*: Diagnostic for Kienböck's disease. The patient is asked to make a fist. There is tenderness at the base of the third metacarpal on tapping and its normal prominence is absent in patients with the disease.
- Negative ulnar variance is associated with Kienböck's disease, whereas positive ulnar variance is associated with ulnar impaction syndrome and injury to TFCC (triangular fibrocartilage complex).

Osgood-Schlatter's Disease

It is a traction apophysitis of the proximal tibial apophysis that mostly affects boys who are 12–15 years old. Although exact etiology is not known, repeated forceful contractions of the quadriceps causing small avulsion fractures of the secondary ossification center of the tibial tuberosity have been postulated as a cause. It is particularly common in adolescents playing sports like football, basketball, jumpers, runners, gymnastics, etc. which involve repeated forceful knee extension. Approximately 30% cases are bilateral. X-ray (Fig. 19.7) may show

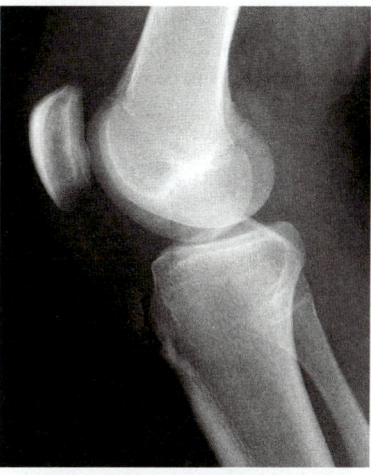

Fig. 19.7: X-ray of knee joint of a case of Osgood-Schlatter's disease

enlarged, fragmented or sclerosed tibial tubercle or calcification at the insertion of the patellar tendon.

Osteochondritis Dissecans

- An osteochondral fragment separates from the rest of the bone and forms a loose body in the joint.
- Knee (lateral surface of medial femoral condyle) is the commonest site affected followed by capitellum (2nd most common).
- The disease is two times more common in males and occurs generally during adolescence (10–20 years).
- Patients generally tend to come with a vague aching discomfort in the knee present for months.
- When these patients are made to sit on a couch with legs hanging, there is pain on internal rotation of the leg, which disappears as the leg is externally rotated (Wilson's test).
- X-ray: Intercondylar/tunnel view is more informative. Bone scan can provide early diagnosis, but MRI is the investigation of choice, provides earliest diagnosis and also aids in management.
- *Treatment*: Management depends upon the size of the defect created by separation of the fragment.
  - In smaller lesions, microfracture, i.e. multiple drilling of the crater is performed. Drilling leads to fresh pool of bleeding from marrow and the inflow of growth factors that cause the lesion to heal by fibrocartilage (not hyaline cartilage which is seen in normal joint).
  - In larger defects, a mosaicplasty or osteochondral autologous transplantation surgery is performed wherein an osteochondral graft is harvested from non-weight bearing area of the knee and transplanted into the crater.

Xtra edge

The commonest cause of loose body in knee joint is osteochondritis dissecans of knee. However, most common cause in elderly is OA knee. And the commonest cause of multiple loose bodies in the knee joint is synovial chondromatosis.

MULTIPLE CHOICE QUESTIONS

1. **Most common site of osteochondritis dissecans:**
   A. Lateral part of the medial femoral condyle
   B. Medial part of the medial femoral condyle
   C. Lateral part of the lateral femoral condyle
   D. Medial part of the lateral femoral condyle

2. **A 30-year-old HIV positive male who is on anti-retroviral therapy (protease inhibitors) has pain in the right hip joint for 2 months. He has difficulty in abduction and internal rotation. Which of the following is most likely diagnosis?**

A. Septic arthritis   B. Osteochondritis
C. Avascular necrosis D. Tubercular arthritis

3. **Potential causes of AVN include:**
   A. Prolonged intake of steroids
   B. Caisson's disease
   C. Sickle cell anemia
   D. Posterior dislocation hip
   E. Intracapsular fracture femur neck

4. **AVN of the hip may occur following which fractures?**
   A. Intertrochanteric fracture of the hip
   B. Subtrochanteric fracture
   C. Transcervical fracture of the neck of femur
   D. Fracture of posterior lip of the acetabulum

5. **AVN following transcervical neck femur fracture occurs due to damage to which of the following vessels?**
   A. Lateral retinacular branch of lateral circumflex femoral artery
   B. Lateral retinacular branch of medial circumflex femoral artery
   C. Medial retinacular branch of lateral circumflex femoral artery
   D. Obturator artery

6. **A patient with the history of trauma, a year back, comes with complain of wrist pain and the following X-ray, diagnosis is:**

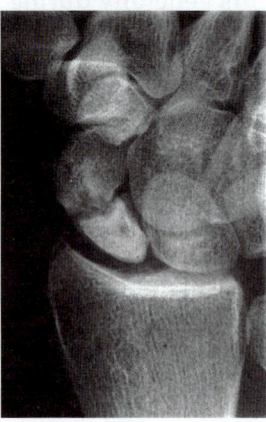

   A. Kohler's disease   B. Kienböck's disease
   C. AVN of scaphoid   D. Colles' fracture

7. **Most common cause of AVN of the hip is:**
   A. Idiopathic
   B. Alcoholism
   C. Caisson's disease
   D. Fracture neck of femur (post-traumatic)

8. **Which of the following part of the bone is not prone for AVN?**
   A. Proximal scaphoid B. Body of talus
   C. Femoral neck   D. Femoral head

9. **Kienböck's disease is osteochondritis of:**
   A. Scaphoid   B. Lunate
   C. Calcaneum   D. Tibial tuberosity

10. **Avascular necrosis investigation of choice:**
    A. X-ray   B. CT scan
    C. Bone scan   D. MRI

11. **Osteochondritis is seen in all *except*:**
    A. Fracture neck femur
    B. Sickle cell anemia
    C. Perthes' disease
    D. Paget's disease

12. **AVN affects all *except*:**
    A. Femur   B. Scaphoid
    C. Talus   D. Iliac crest

13. **Avascular necrosis of bone investigation of choice:**
    A. CT scan   B. MRI
    C. Bone scan   D. USG

14. **Avascular necrosis affects which part of femoral head?**
    A. Anteromedial   B. Anterolateral
    C. Posteromedial   D. Posterolateral

15. **Femur head avascular necrosis is due to damage to:**
    A. Medial circumflex arteries
    B. Lateral circumflex arteries
    C. Artery to ligament teres
    D. Obturator artery

16. **Avascular necrosis is seen at proximal pole of scaphoid because:**
    A. Blood supply enters proximal pole
    B. Blood supply enters through the waist
    C. Blood supply enters through the distal pole
    D. Proximal pole is intra-articular

17. **Post-traumatic avascular necrosis commonly occurs in which fracture?**
    A. Neck femur
    B. Surgical neck humerus
    C. Neck of talus
    D. Waist of scaphoid
    E. Neck radius

18. **AVN can occur at all *except*:**
    A. Femur neck   B. Body of talus
    C. Proximal scaphoid D. None

19. **Infraction of the distal epiphysis of the second metatarsal bone is:**
    A. Kienböck's   B. Kohler's disease
    C. Freiberg's disease D. Perthes' disease

20. **An elderly woman was admitted with a fracture of the neck of right femur which failed to unite. On examination an avascular necrosis of the head of femur was noted. The condition would have resulted most probably from the damage to:**
    A. Superior gluteal artery
    B. Inferior gluteal artery
    C. Acetabular branch of obturator
    D. Retinacular branches of circumflex femoral arteries

21. Avascular necrosis of head of the femur is most common:
    A. Subcapital fracture
    B. Basal fracture
    C. Fracture intertrochanteric
    D. Transcervical fracture

22. Caisson's disease the pain in joints and muscle is because of:
    A. N_2 B. O_2
    C. N_2O D. NO_2

23. Avascular necrosis of head of femur can occur in:
    A. Sickle cell anemia
    B. Caisson's disease
    C. Intracapsular fracture neck
    D. Trochanteric fracture

24. Osteochondritis in Osgood-Schlatter disease affect which bone:
    A. Capitulum's bone   B. Metacarpal
    C. Navicular   D. Tibial tuberosity

25. A 50-year-old man sustained posterior dislocation of left hip in an accident. Dislocation was reduced after 3 days. He started complaining of pain left after 6 months. X-ray of the pelvis was normal. The most relevant investigation at the stage will be:
    A. CRP levels in blood
    B. Ultrasonography of hip
    C. Arthrography of hip
    D. MRI of hip

26. A vascular necrosis can be a possible sequelae of fracture of all the following bones, *except*:
    A. Femur neck   B. Scaphoid
    C. Talus   D. Calcaneum

27. A woman of 45, a known cause of pemphigus vulgaris on a regular treatment with controlled primary disease presented with pain in the right hip and knee. Examination revealed no limb length discrepancy but the patient has tenderness in the Scarpa's triangle and limitation of abduction and internal rotation of the right hip joint as compared to the other side. The most probable diagnosis is:
    A. Stress fracture of neck of femur
    B. Avascular necrosis of femoral head
    C. Perthes' disease
    D. Transient synovitis of hip

28. Pathological changes in caisson's disease is due to:
    A. N_2 B. O_2
    C. CO_2 D. CO

29. Scheuermann's disease occurs in:
    A. Adults   B. Elderly
    C. Infants   D. Adolescents

30. Sever disease involves:
    A. Lunate   B. Tibial tubercle
    C. Calcaneum   D. Navicular

31. An adolescent male with complain of pain in knee for last few months after playing, with no history of trauma comes with this X-ray, diagnosis is:

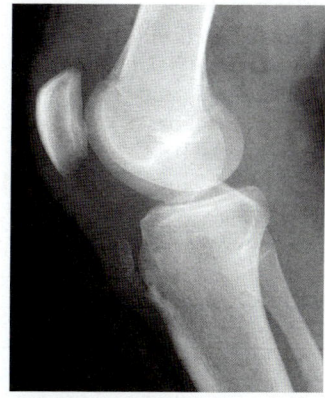

    A. Osteochondritis dessicans of femur
    B. Osteochondritis dessicans of patella
    C. Osgood-Schlatter disease
    D. Tibial tuberosity fracture

32. Osteonecrosis is not seen in:
    A. Ollier's disease   B. Kienboch
    C. Kohler's disease   D. Perthes' disease

33. Perthes' disease is:
    A. Fracture of femoral shaft
    B. Osteochondritis of femoral
    C. Infraction of femoral head
    D. Fracture dislocation of femoral neck

34. Which of the following is not a variety of osteochondritis?
    A. Pellegrini Stieda   B. Panner's
    C. Calves   D. Kohler's

35. Islene's disease is osteochondritis of:
    A. 2nd metacarpal   B. 5th metacarpal
    C. 2nd metatarsal   D. 5th metatarsal

36. In elbow, osteonecrosis usually involves:
    A. Olecranon   B. Trochlea
    C. Radius head   D. Capitulum

37. Sectoral sign is positive in:
    A. Avascular necrosis of femur head
    B. Osteochondritis of hip
    C. Protrusio acetabuli
    D. Slipped capital femoral epiphyses

38. Osgood-Schlatter disease:
    A. Involve the knee joint
    B. Kohler's disease
    C. Freiberg's disease
    D. Cervical spine

39. Osteochondritis is not seen in disease:
    A. Slipped capital femoral epiphysis
    B. Panner's disease
    C. Calve's disease
    D. Kohler's disease

40. Osteochondritis is not seen in disease:
A. Slipped capital femoral epiphysis
B. Panner's disease
C. Calve's disease
D. Kohler's disease

41. Freiberg's osteochondritis is:
A. 2nd metatarsal head
B. 5th metatarsal head
C. 2nd metatarsal base
D. 5th metatarsal base

42. Microfracture technique is carried out for:
A. Nonunion
B. Osteochondral defects
C. Tumors
D. Osteonecrosis

43. Which joint is commonly involved in osteochondritis dissecans?
A. Ankle joint
B. Knee joint
C. Wrist joint
D. Elbow joint

44. A patient is using oral steroids for a period of 5+ years and patient complaints of pain in the hip regions. Which one of the following is a diagnostic modality for confirmation of diagnosis?
A. Plain X-ray
B. CT scan
C. MRI
D. Isotope bone scan

45. After chronic use of steroids severe pain in right hip with immobility is due to:
A. Avascular necrosis
B. Perthes disease
C. Hip dislocation
D. Osteochondritis

ANSWERS

1. D. Medial part of the lateral femoral condyle
2. C. Avascular necrosis
3. ALL
4. C. Transcervical fracture of the neck of femur
5. B. Lateral retinacular branch of medial circumflex femoral artery
6. C. AVN of scaphoid
7. A. Idiopathic
8. C. Femoral neck
9. B. Lunate
10. D. MRI
11. D. Paget's disease
12. D. Iliac crest
13. B. MRI
14. B. Anterolateral
15. A. Medial circumflex arteries
16. C. Blood supply enters through the distal pole
17. A. Neck femur, C. Neck of talus, D. Waist of scaphoid
18. A. Femur neck
19. C. Freiberg's disease
20. D. Retinacular branches of circumflex femoral arteries—the major blood supply of femoral head is by lateral (superior) retinacular branch of medial circumflex artery
21. A. Subcapital fracture
22. A. N$_2$
23. A. Sickle cell anemia; B. Caisson's disease, C. Intracapsular fracture neck
24. D. Tibial tuberosity
25. D. MRI of hip
    • Diagnosis here is of AVN and it is best/ earliest picked by MRI

26. D. Calcaneum
27. B. Avascular necrosis of femoral head
    • Limitation of abduction and internal rotation in a patient with a disease where he might be taking steroids, makes the diagnosis of AVN of femoral head. Always look in the question, if any disease is mentioned, examiner is indirectly giving a clue of long term steroid intake.
28. A. N$_2$
29. D. Adolescents
30. C. Calcaneum
31. C. Osgood-Schlatter disease
32. A. Ollier's disease
33. B. Osteochondritis of femoral
34. A. Pellegrini Stieda
35. D. 5th metatarsal
36. D. Capitulum
37. A. Avascular necrosis of femur head
38. A. Involve the knee joint
39. D. Kohler's disease
40. A. Slipped capital femoral epiphysis
41. A. 2nd metatarsal head
42. B. Osteochondral defects
43. B. Knee joint
44. C. MRI
    • Whenever steroid/any disease where long term steroid intake may be a possibility, is mentioned in question, think of AVN
45. A. Avascular necrosis

Orthopedic Surgery and Evaluation

BONE CEMENT

Composition: One liquid (methyl methacrylate monomer) and one powder component (polymer, polymethyl methacrylate—PMMA). It is prepared by mixing the liquid monomer to the powder polymer (not vice versa). Barium sulfate is added for radiopacity.

Whole process divided into four phases:
1. *Mixing time*: Time taken by the powder and liquid to fully integrate.
2. *Dough time*: From the beginning of mixing to the point when the cement no longer sticks to surgical gloves.
3. *Working time*: Time during which the cement can be manipulated and the prosthesis can be inserted. The implant must be implanted before the end of working time.
4. *Setting time*: Time from the beginning of mixing until the time at which the exothermic reaction heats the cement (usually 10–12 minutes).

Xtra edge
- *Antibiotic impregnated bone cement*: Gentamicin, tobramycin, cefuroxime, vancomycin are commonly added antibiotics.
- Factors increasing bone cement dough and setting time.
  - *Decreased temperature of OT*
  - *Decreased humidity*
  - *Slow mixing*
- **Bone cement implantation syndrome** is characterised by sudden hypotension, hypoxia and may be loss of consciousness. It occurs during cementing/reaming of canal. Release of cement particles or emboli may be the cause. Most commonly the condition has been reported in hip replacement.
- **Tribology** is the branch of science and technology that deals with the study of friction, wear and lubrication characteristics of materials. It has its implications in long-term survival and function of the orthopedic implants and prostheses.
- **Biodegradable implants:** These implants (made up of polyglycolic acid, polydioxanone and polylevolactic acid) provide sufficient strength to the bone until fracture heals and then degrade spontaneously, thus eliminating need for second surgery for their removal.

ARTHROSCOPY

It is a minimally invasive procedure for joints done for diagnostic-cum-therapeutic purpose. Professor Kenji Takagi (Japanese surgeon) performed the first arthroscopic examination of the knee joint (tubercular knee), and is credited with the discovery of the arthroscope.
- Knee is the most common joint to undergo arthroscopic procedures, followed by shoulders, though virtually every major joint in the body can be scoped. Position of patient—supine. Common portals and their use is given in Table 20.1.
- *Shoulder*: Position of the patient—beach chair position or lateral decubitus position.
- *Complications*: Hemarthrosis and an iatrogenic damage to the articular cartilage. Extravasation of fluid leading to compartment syndrome. Improper portal placement may lead to neurovascular injuries.

Table 20.1: Common portals used in knee arthroscopy
• *Anterolateral*: Main viewing portal (established first) for diagnostic arthroscopy. Position: 1 cm above the lateral joint line and 1 cm lateral to the patellar tendon. It can view all structures except anterior horn of the lateral meniscus, periphery of posterior horn of the medial meniscus and posterior cruciate ligament (PCL).
• *Anteromedial*: This is a main working portal. It is made 1 cm above the medial joint line and 1 cm medial to the patellar tendon. It is used for viewing lateral compartment and also for inserting arthroscopic instruments inside the knee.
• *Posteromedial*: It is used for repair of posterior horn meniscal tears, PCL tears and loose body removal from posterior compartment.
• *Superolateral portal*: It is used for viewing the patellofemoral articulation.
• *Central transpatellar portal (Gillquist)*: It is located in midline 1 cm inferior to lower pole of patella. It is used in anterior cruciate ligament (ACL) reconstruction after the graft has been harvested.

(Taken from Fundamentals of Orthopedics by Mohindra and Jain, 2nd Ed., Jaypee Publishers)

- *Commercial arthroscope*: 4 mm portal and 30° oblique view is possible.
- *Triangulation*: It is an arthroscopic skill by which surgeon performs all arthroscopic maneuver. Triangle is made by tip of the instrument inside the joint (in one hand) and arthroscope in the other hand.

ARTHROPLASTY

It refers to a surgery where natural articulating surface is removed or replaced by natural or synthetic material.

Types

- Excision arthroplasty—a pseudojoint is created by removing one part of the joint.
    - Girdlestone arthroplasty—femoral head is removed from hip joint.
    - Radial head excision
    - Keller's operation—done in hallux valgus (phalanx of great toe removed).
- Interposition arthroplasty—interposition of synthetic/natural material b/w joint surfaces creating painless and stable joint.
    - *For example*: Interposition arthroplasty in rheumatoid elbow
- Replacement arthroplasty
    - Hemi—only one side of the joint is replaced (e.g. bipolar hemi hip arthroplasty)
    - Total—both articulating surface is replaced (THR, TKR).
  The most common indication for arthroplasty is pain.
  Goals—relieve pain > stability of joint > movement > correct deformity.

Hip Replacement

1. **Hemiarthroplasty**—only femoral head and neck is replaced, while acetabulum is retained. Most common indication is fracture NOF in elderly patient, in whom life expectancy is not much to consider a bigger surgery, i.e. THR.
   Hemiprosthesis can be:

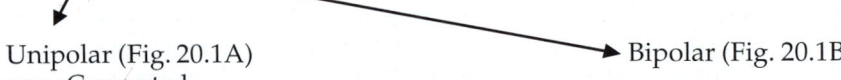

Unipolar (Fig. 20.1A)
(Thompson: Cemented;
 Austin Moore: Uncemented fixation)
The head is fixed to stem as a single piece.
Movement occurs only at one surface,
i.e. head and acetabular surface.

Bipolar (Fig. 20.1B)
An outer acetabular shell contains inside it a liner (polyethylene), inside which head revolves. Movement occurs at two surfaces—femoral head and liner, acetabular shell and acetabulum

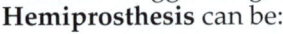

Disadvantage: Acetabulum erosion and protusio

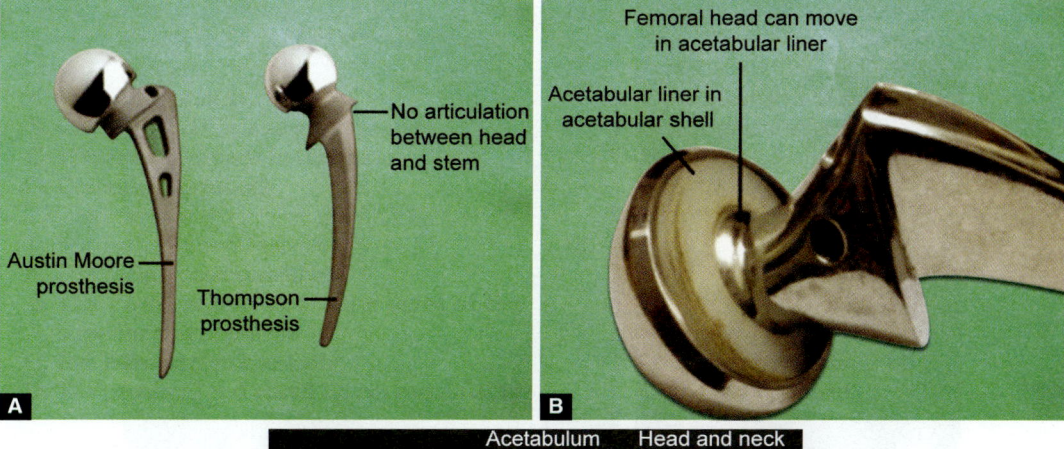

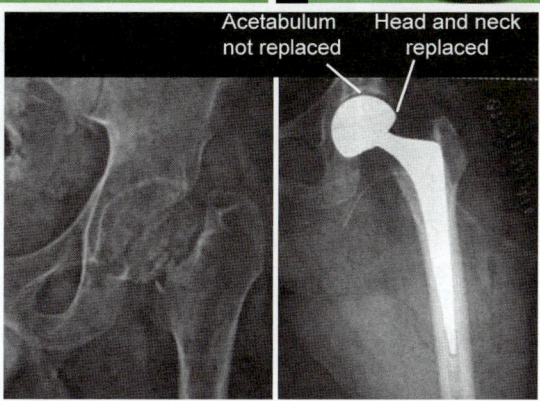

Fig. 20.1: (A) Unipolar prosthesis, (B) Bipolar prosthesis, (C) Bipolar arthroplasty X-ray

2. *Total hip replacement*: First performed by Dr John Charnley who is called the Father of Arthroplasty. His principle was low friction arthroplasty so he suggested a design where friction would be minimal.

Articulating surfaces: In THR, both head and acetabulum are replaced. Based on articulating surface of the prosthesis, THR may be:

– *Metal on polyethylene*—femoral head is of metal and acetabular liner is made of polyethylene.
– *Metal on metal*—both head and liner are made up of metal. It is contraindicated in patients with renal failure and women of childbearing age group.
– *Ceramic on polyethylene*—ceramic head and polyethylene liner.
– *Ceramic on ceramic*—both head and liner are made up of ceramic. Since ceramic is the hardest substance of all bearing materials, this combination offers the least wear rates. However, ceramic is brittle (i.e. not ductile) and chip fractures occur if neck and acetabular liner make contact in extreme range of joint motions. A complication unique to ceramic on ceramic bearing is squeaking sound (clicking sounds coming from joint).

Implant fixation: THR may be fixed with cement or may be uncemented where fixation initially is by press fit between prosthesis and bone and later it remains fixed by bone ingrowth over porous surface of the prosthesis. Cemented is done for elderly patients who need immediate stability and uncemented for younger patients (good bone stock) as it has longer life of the fixation and is a stronger fixation.

Complications
• Thromboembolism
• Subluxation or dislocation—risk factor—posterior approach to hip and malposition.
• Limb length discrepancy—lengthening is less tolerated than shortening.
• Nerve injury—sciatic nerve is the commonest.

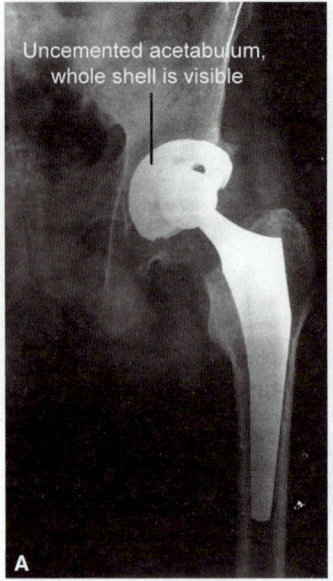
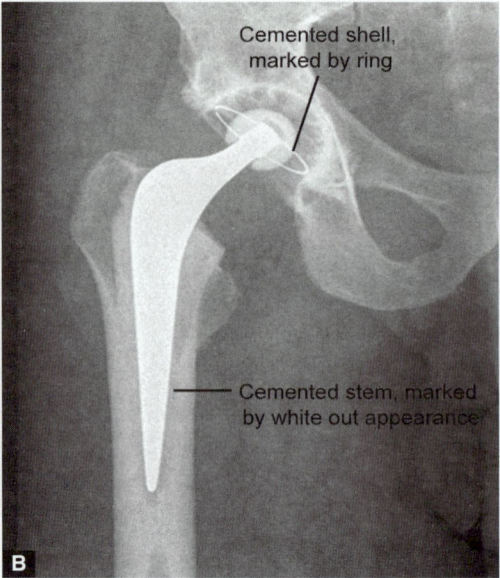

Fig. 20.2: Compare the two X-rays to differentiate between (A) Uncemented and (B) Cemented THR

- Heterotropic ossification—risk factor—anterolateral approach to hip.
- Periprosthetic fracture—femoral fracture > acetabulum. Classification—**Vancouver** system.
- Infection—classification—**Tsukayama**.
- Loosening—if it occurs without infection, called aseptic loosening. Particles of metal, cement or polyethylene can cause loosening, but polyethylene particles are the major contributor.

Knee Replacement

Most commonly performed arthroplasty in India is TKR. Commonest indication for the procedure is pain due to osteoarthritis.

Types

Total knee replacement (TKR): A type of resurfacing arthroplasty where complete joint articulating surface, i.e. femoral condyles, tibial surface and patella (+/–) are resected and replaced by prosthesis (Fig. 20.3B). Insall is credited with development of modern TKR prosthesis. In cruciate retaining TKR, PCL is retained.

Unicondylar knee replacement: When only one compartment of the three compartments (medial tibiofemoral, lateral tibiofemoral and patellofemoral) of the knee is affected, unicondylar knee replacement (UKR) is indicated. In this procedure, articulating bones of only one compartment (either medial or lateral tibiofemoral compartment) are resurfaced and polyethylene insert is placed (Fig. 20.3A). Rheumatoid arthritis is a contraindication because, it is an inflammatory disease and symmetrically involves both the compartments of the joint.

Complications

Patellar clunk syndrome: In this condition a fibrous nodule at the superior pole of the patella catches in the implant, leading to repeated catching/popping with movement of the joint.

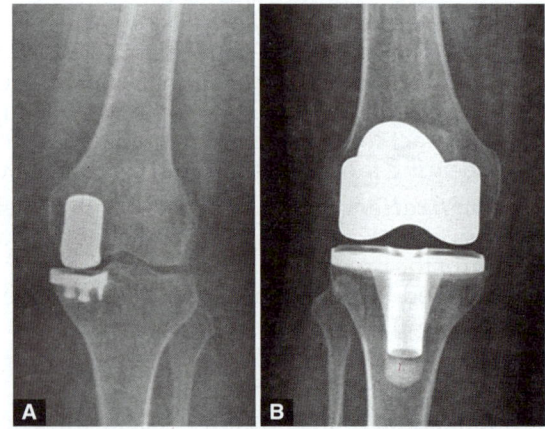

Fig. 20.3: (A) Unicondylar knee replacement, (B) Total knee replacement

High Tibial Osteotomy

Knee joint anatomy is such that, most of the load passes through the medial joint space. In OA most common deformity is varus, that leads to stress concentration on the medial side; while in RA, valgus is the commonest deformity that leads to stress on lateral side.

High tibial osteotomy is done in unicompartmental OA of knee, where knee joint is unloaded of the stress by correcting the malalignment and redistributing the stress on the joint.

Indications: Pain is the most common indication, that is caused by degenerative arthritis which is confined to one compartment with a corresponding varus or valgus deformity.

Contraindications
- Both compartments involved (lateral joint space decreased)
- Inflammatory arthritis, e.g. RA (it involves both compartments)
- More than 20° correction needed
- Knee flexion <90°
- Flexion contracture at knee >15°
- Medial compartment bone loss >3 mm
- Lateral tibial subluxation >1 cm.

Procedure: Osteotomy is performed near the joint line through cancellous bone, for better joint inclination and healing.

Complications: Compartment syndrome, knee stiffness, nonunion of osteotomy.

IMPORTANT SURGICAL APPROACHES
- Forearm:
    - Anterior approach—**Henry's** approach
    - Posterior approach—**Thompson's** approach
- Pelvis and acetabulum:
    - *Kocher-Langenbeck approach*: It is the posterior approach to the acetabulum which provides visualization of posterior wall and lateral aspect of the posterior column of the acetabulum. It allows complete exposure of posterior acetabular surface caudally, as far as the ischial tuberosity. The greater and lesser sciatic notch are also well visualized. However, the anterior and superior exposure are limited. Osteotomy of the greater trochanter can increase anterior iliac exposure but superior (proximal) exposure is still limited by the superior gluteal neuro-vascular bundle. If more superior/cranial exposure is necessary, an anterior approach would be a better option. Sciatic nerve is the commonest nerve to get injured in this approach. Indication—posterior wall fracture, posterior column fracture, transverse fracture, T-shaped fracture of acetabulum, approach to sciatic nerve, recurrent posterior dislocation of hip, etc.
    - *Ilioinguinal approach* and *iliofemoral approach*: These are anterior approaches used for anterior wall/anterior column fracture of acetabulum. The m/c nerve injured in this approach is lateral femoral cutaneous nerve.
- Hip:
    - Anterior approach—**Smith Peterson** approach.
    - Posterior approach—**Moore's** approach uses the same incision and tissue planes as Kocher-Langenbeck approach.
    - Anterolateral approach—**Watson-Jones** approach.
    - Direct lateral/transgluteal approach—**Harding's** approach.
    - Medial—**Ludloff's** approach.

MULTIPLE CHOICE QUESTIONS

1. **In uncemented arthroplasty of the hip, the stem remains attached to the bone by:**
   A. Bone ingrowth/overgrowth over the surface of the stem
   B. Mechanical bonding between the stem and bone
   C. Press fitting of the stem in the tight canal
   D. Adhesion between the stem and bone due to cohesive properties of the stem

2. **During performing a total hip replacement, the surgeon found destruction of the articular cartilage and multiple wedge-shaped subchondral depressions. What is this called?**

A. Osteolysis   B. Osteomyelitis
C. Osteonecrosis   D. Osteogenesis

3. **Patellar clunk syndrome is a known complication of which surgery?**
   A. Corrective osteotomy for genu valgum
   B. Total knee replacement
   C. Medial patella femoral ligament reconstruction
   D. Bicondylar plating of proximal tibia fracture

4. **Which of the following muscle seen on splitting tensor fascia lata during anterolateral approach before hip joint is exposed?**
   A. Gluteus maximus   B. Gluteus medius
   C. Gluteus minimus   D. Superior gemelli

5. **A patient after total hip replacement develops breathlessness. What is the definitive management?**
   A. Thrombolysis   B. Bronchodilators
   C. Steroids   D. Oxygen

6. **After knee replacement surgery, proprioceptors of joints are altered. Effect is:**
   A. Normal movement
   B. Complete loss of sensation at joint position at resting stage
   C. Loss of sensation of joint position at dynamic stage
   D. All type of sensation lost

7. **Metal on metal articulation should be avoided in:**
   A. Osteonecrosis
   B. Young female
   C. Inflammatory arthritis
   D. Revision surgery

8. **A patient developed breathlessness and chest pain, on second postoperative after a total hip replacement. Echocardiography showed right ventricular dilatation and tricuspid regurgitation. What is the most likely diagnosis?**
   A. Acute MI
   B. Pulmonary embolism
   C. Hypotensive shock
   D. Cardiac tamponade

9. **What is the most common cause of death after total hip replacement?**
   A. Infection
   B. Deep vein thrombosis
   C. Pulmonary embolism
   D. Pneumonia

10. **Indication of arthroplasty:**
    A. Osteoarthritis
    B. Rheumatoid arthritis
    C. Ankylosing spondylosis
    D. All of the above

11. **Aseptic loosening in cemented total hip replacement occurs as a result of hypersensitivity response to:**

A. Titanium debris
B. High density polyethylene debris
C. N, N-dimethyltryptamine
D. Free radicals

12. **Major indication (s) for arthroplasty:**
    A. Osteoarthritis of hip
    B. Ankylosis of elbow
    C. Ununited femoral neck fracture
    D. All of the above

13. **All of the following statements about high tibial osteotomy are true, *except*:**
    A. Magnitude of correction achieved is greater than 30 degree
    B. Indicated in unicompartmental osteoarthritis
    C. Performed through cancellous bone
    D. Recurrence is a long-term complication

14. **Which of the following is an absolute contraindication for total joint replacement?**
    A. Very young patients
    B. Recent or current joint sepsis
    C. Osteoporotic bone
    D. Limb length inequality

15. **Most common cause of death after total hip replacement is:**
    A. Infection
    B. Pulmonary embolism
    C. Deep vein thrombosis
    D. Pneumonia

16. **Tourniquet paralysis is an unfortunate complication that often leads to:**
    A. Neuropraxia   B. Axonotmesis
    C. Neurotmesis   D. None of the above

17. **Bone cement setting time is:**
    A. 30 sec   B. 1–2 min
    C. 8–10 min   D. >30 min

18. **Anterolateral arthroscopy of knee is done:**
    A. To see posterior cruciate ligament
    B. To see anterior portion of lateral meniscus
    C. To look for patella-femoral articulation
    D. To see the periphery of posterior horn of medial meniscus

19. **Watson-Jones procedure is done for:**
    A. Polio
    B. Neglected clubfoot
    C. Chronic ankle instability
    D. Muscle paralysis

20. **Watson-Jones approach is used for:**
    A. Neglected club foot
    B. Muscle paralysis
    C. Valgus deformity
    D. Hip replacement

21. **All of the following are used for giving traction *except*:**
    A. Bohler's stirrup   B. Steinmann
    C. K wire   D. Rush pin

22. **Which of the following approaches is best suited for performing triple arthodesis at the ankle?**
    A. Ollier's approach
    B. Gatellier and Chastang's approach
    C. Posterior approach to the ankle
    D. Colonna's approach

23. **All indicate that the intramedullary Kuntscher nail is properly seated** *except*:
    A. Slot facing posteromedially
    B. The distal end at about the level of the superior end of patella
    C. Eye faces posteromedially
    D. The proximal end about 2.5 cm proximal to the trochanter

24. **Kocher-Langenbeck approach is useful in acetabular fracture in all mentioned situations** *except*:
    A. Open fractures of acetabulum
    B. Sciatic nerve injury
    C. Recurrent dislocation despite of closed reduction
    D. Morel-Lavallée lesion

25. **Which of the following structures are not normally visualized during the arthroscopy of the knee?**
    A. Meniscus
    B. Cruciate ligaments
    C. Collateral ligament
    D. Patella articular surface

ANSWERS

1. A. Bone ingrowth/overgrowth over the surface of the stem
2. C. Osteonecrosis
3. B. Total knee replacement
4. B. Gluteus medius
5. A. Thrombolysis
6. A. Normal movement
   - The movement improves after replacement or at least is the same as preoperative range compared to an osteoarthritic knee.
7. B. Young female
8. B. Pulmonary embolism
9. C. Pulmonary embolism
10. D. All of the above
    - Any arthritis leading to pain is an indication of arthroplasty. But should be avoided in any active infections like tubercular/septic arthritis.
11. B. High density polyethylene debris
12. D. All of the above
13. A. Magnitude of correction achieved is greater than 30 degree

14. B. Recent or current joint sepsis
15. B. Pulmonary embolism
    - MI > pulmonary embolism is the leading cause of death in THR
16. A. Neuropraxia
17. C. 8–10 min
18. C. To look for patella-femoral articulation
    - Although best portal to see the patello-femoral articulation and patellar tracking during knee flexion is superolateral portal, the joint can also be viewed through anterolateral portal. All other structures are difficult to visualize via the anterolateral portal
19. C. Chronic ankle instability
20. D. Hip replacement
21. D. Rush pin
22. A. Ollier's approach
23. A. Slot facing posteromedially
24. D. Morel-Lavallée lesion
25. C. Collateral ligament